Dahlem Workshop Reports
Life Sciences Research Report 38
The Neural and Molecular Bases of Learning

The goal of this Dahlem Workshop is:
to generate a new synthesis
of neural and molecular
mechanisms of learning

Life Sciences Research Reports
Editor: Silke Bernhard

Held and published on behalf of the
Stifterverband für die Deutsche Wissenschaft

Sponsored by:
Senat der Stadt Berlin
Stifterverband für die Deutsche Wissenschaft

The Neural and Molecular Bases of Learning

J.-P. Changeux and M. Konishi,
Editors

Report of the Dahlem Workshop on
The Neural and Molecular Bases of Learning
Berlin 1985, December 8–13

Rapporteurs:
M. Baudry · M.F. Bear · Y. Dudai · W.J. Thompson

Program Advisory Committee:
J.-P. Changeux and M. Konishi, Chairpersons
R. Menzel · W. Singer · N. Tsukahara

A Wiley-Interscience Publication

John Wiley & Sons
Chichester New York Brisbane Toronto Singapore

Copy Editors: J. Lupp, K. Geue
Text Preparation: R. Rosing, J. Lambertz, L. Westacott, G. Custance
Photographs: E.P. Thonke

With 5 photographs, 54 figures, and 5 tables

British Library Cataloguing in Publication Data:

Dahlem workshop on the Neural and Molecular Bases of Learning. *(1985): Berlin)*
The neural and molecular bases of learning: report of the Dahlem Workshop on the Neural and Molecular Bases of Learning, Berlin 1985, December 8–13.—(Dahlem Workshop reports. Life sciences research report; 38).
1. Memory 2. Learning, Psychology of
3. Neuropsychology 4. Learning—Physiological aspects 5. Neurophysiology
I. Title II. Changeux, J.-P. III. Konishi, M.
IV. Stieterverband für die Deutsche Wissenschaft,
V. Series
599.01'88 QP408

ISBN 0 471 91569 6

Printed and Bound in Great Britain

Table of Contents

The Dahlem Konferenzen

Founders

Recognizing the need for more effective communication between scientists, the Stifterverband für die Deutsche Wissenschaft*, in cooperation with the Deutsche Forschungsgemeinschaft**, founded Dahlem Konferenzen in 1974. The project is financed by the founders and the Senate of the City of Berlin.

Name

Dahlem Konferenzen was named after the district of Berlin called *Dahlem*, which has a long-standing tradition and reputation in the sciences and arts.

Aim

The task of Dahlem Konferenzen is to promote international, interdisciplinary exchange of scientific information and ideas, to stimulate international cooperation in research, and to develop and test new models conducive to more effective communication between scientists.

The Concept

The increasing orientation towards interdisciplinary approaches in scientific research demands that specialists in one field understand the

---

* *The Donors Association for the Promotion of Sciences and Humanities, a foundation created in 1921 in Berlin and supported by German trade and industry to fund basic research in the sciences*

** *German Science Foundation*

needs and problems of related fields. Therefore, Dahlem Konferenzen has organized workshops, mainly in the Life Sciences and the fields of Physical, Chemical, and Earth Sciences, of an interdisciplinary nature.

Dahlem Workshops provide a unique opportunity for posing the right questions to colleagues from different disciplines who are encouraged to state what they do not know rather than what they do know. The aim is not to solve problems nor to reach a consensus of opinion, the aim is to define and discuss priorities and to indicate directions for further research.

Topics

The topics are of contemporary international interest, timely, interdisciplinary in nature, and problem oriented. Dahlem Konferenzen approaches internationally recognized scientists to suggest topics fulfilling these criteria. Once a year, the topic suggestions are submitted to a scientific board for approval.

Program Advisory Committee

A special Program Advisory Committee is formed for each workshop. It is composed of 6-7 scientists representing the various scientific disciplines involved. They meet approximately one year before the workshop to decide on the scientific program and define the workshop goal, select topics for the discussion groups, formulate titles for background papers, select participants, and assign them their specific tasks.Participants are invited according to international scientific reputation alone.Exception is made for younger German scientists. Invitations are not transferable.

Dahlem Workshop Model

Since no type of scientific meeting proved effective enough, Dahlem Konferenzen had to create its own concept. This concept has been tested and varied over the years. It is internationaaly recognized as the *Dahlem Workshop Model*. Four workshops per year are organized according to this model. It provides the framework for the utmost possible interdisciplinary communication and cooperation between scientists in a period of 4 1/2 days.

At Dahlem Workshops 48 participants work in four interdisciplinary discussion groups. Lectures are not given. Instead, selected participants write background papers providing a review of the field rather than a report on individual work. These papers, reviewed by selected participants, serve as the basis for discussion and are circulated to all participants before the meeting with the request to formulate written questions and comments to them. During the workshop, each of the four groups prepares reports reflecting their insights gained through the discussion. They also provide suggestions for future research needs.

Publication
The group reports written during the workshop together with the revised background papers are published in book form as the Dahlem Workshop Reports. They are edited by the editor(s) and the Dahlem Konferenzen staff. The reports are multidisciplinary surveys by the most internationally distinguished scientists and are based on discussions of advanced new concepts, techniques, and models. Each report also reviews areas of priority interest and indicates directions for future research on a given topic.

The Dahlem Workshop Reports are published in two series:

1) Life Sciences Research Reports (LS), and
2) Physical, Chemical, and Earth Sciences Research Reports (PC).

Director
Silke Bernhard, M.D.

Address
Dahlem Konferenzen
Wallotstrasse 19
D-1000 Berlin (West) 33

Tel.: (030) 891 5067

THE DAHLEM WORKSHOP MODEL

MONDAY	TUESDAY	WEDNESDAY	THURSDAY	FRIDAY
A. Opening (P) B. Introduction (P) C. Selection of Problems for the Group Agendas (S) 1 2 3 4	1 2 3 4	1 3	F. Report Session 1 2 3 4	G. Distribution of the Reports H. Reading Time I. Discussion of the Group Reports (P)
D. Presentation of Group Agendas (P) E. Group Discussions (S) 1 2		2 4		J. Groups Meet to Revise their Reports (S) 1 2 3 4

Key: (P) = Plenary Session;
(S) = Simultaneous Sessions;
○ = one discussion group

Explanation of the Dahlem Workshop Model

A. Opening
Background information is given about Dahlem Konferenzen and the Dahlem Workshop Model.

B. Introduction
The goal and the scientific aspects of the workshop are explained.

C. Selection of Problems for the Group Agenda
Each participant is requested to define priority problems of his choice to be discussed within the framework of the workshop goal and his discussion group topic. Each group discusses these suggestions and compiles an agenda of these problems for their discussions.

D. Presentation of the Group Agenda
The agenda for each group is presented by the moderator. A plenary discussion follows to finalize these agendas.

E. Group Discussions
Two groups start their discussions simultaneously. Participants not assigned to either of these two groups attend discussions on topics of their choice.
The groups then change roles as indicated on the chart.

F. Report Session
The rapporteurs discuss the contents of their reports with their group members and write their reports, which are then typed and duplicated.

G. Distribution of Group Reports
The four group reports are distributed to all participants.

H. Reading Time
Participants read these group reports and formulate written questions/comments.

I. Discussion of Group Reports
Each rapporteur summarizes the highlights, controversies, and open problems of his group. A plenary discussion follows.

J. Groups Meet to Revise their Reports
The groups meet to decide which of the comments and issues raised during the plenary discussion should be included in the final report.

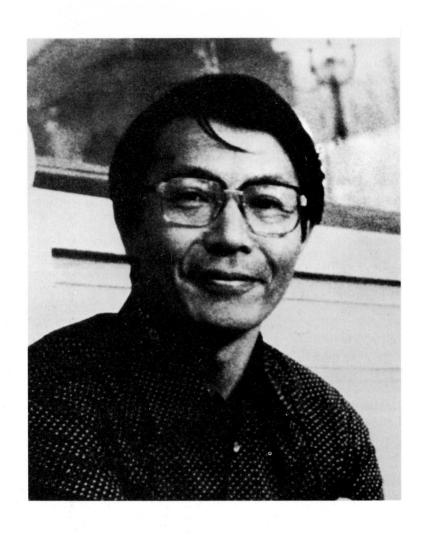

Nakaakira Tsukahara

Nakaakira Tsukahara

(1933-1985)

On August 12, 1985, a Boeing 747 crashed near Tokyo, taking the lives of more than 500 passengers on board. One of the people killed in this tragic accident was Professor Nakaakira Tsukahara, a man of genius in the field of neuroscience. At only 51 years of age, Nakaakira should have had many more productive years to complete his work on neural plasticity and synaptic sprouting and to continue to play a leading role in the ever expanding fields of neuroscience. He was one of the planners of the Dahlem Workshop on The Neural and Molecular Bases of Learning and this record of the workshop is dedicated to his memory.

Nakaakira was born in Kyoto in 1933. He graduated from the University of Tokyo Medical School in 1958 and took his Ph.D. at the Brain Research Institute where he studied under the late Professor T. Tokizane. After receiving his Ph.D. in 1963, he was appointed Assistant Professor in the Department of Physiology Faculty of Medicine at the University of Tokyo which was chaired by Professor K. Uchizone at that time. In 1965 he worked with Professor Vernon Brooks at New York Medical College and then with Sir John Eccles in Chicago and at Woods Hole. In 1970, a few years after his return to Japan, he was appointed to the chair of Stimulation Physiology at the newly established Institute of Biophysical Engineering at Osaka University.

I met Nakaakira at the University of Tokyo in 1962 upon my return from Sir John's Laboratory in Canberra. I was immediately struck by his brilliant ideas for research in brain and neuron assembly and by his commitment to achieve these goals. I still vividly recall our discussion on future prospects for neuroscience, a field in its infancy in the early 1960s. During the following three years Nakaakira worked on cat's red nucleus in conjunction with Dr. Toyama and Dr. Kosaka, discovering differential localization of cerebral cortical inputs in peripheral dendrites and cerebellar nuclear inputs in somata of red nucleus neurons. He continued to study cat's red nucleus in New York, but in Chicago and at Woods Hole he collaborated in research on dogfish shark cerebellum. Upon returning to Tokyo he took up his studies on cat's red nucleus again and discovered the remarkable reverberation phenomenon in the interposito-pontine nuclear circuit. Reverberation occurred in this circuit when interpositus nuclear neurons were deprived of Purkinje cell inhibition thereby causing a sustained depolarization in red nucleus neurons.

The main focus of Nakaakira's work, synaptic sprouting, was done in Osaka where he moved into new laboratories together with Dr. M. Udo and Dr. T. Bando who accompanied him from Tokyo. His initial finding that cerebral corticorubular fibers, originally impinging on peripheral dendrites, sprouted so as to make new synaptic contacts with somata of red nucleus neurons after lesion of cerebellar nuclei might not have been so striking because lesion-induced sprouting had already been demonstrated in the spinal cord. However, his subsequent discovery that similar sprouting occurred following cross-union of peripheral nerves remote from the red nucleus, reversing flexor-extensor relationships, was indeed amazing as it was commonly thought at that time that synaptic sprouting was an abnormal event following damage of brain tissues. This strongly suggested the involvement of synaptic sprouting in more normal mechanisms of motor compensation. He proceeded to demonstrate further that combined stimulation of limb skin and cerebral peduncle in Pavlovian conditioning paradigm also induced sprouting in the red nucleus as judged by electrophysiological indices. He eventually suggested that synaptic sprouting plays an essential role in learning and memory in the normal brain; this theory deserves serious attention and should be an important theme in future investigations of molecular and cellular bases of learning.

With this remarkable data in hand, Nakaakira delivered a special lecture at the 12th Annual Meeting of the Society for Neuroscience in Minneapolis in 1982 entitled, "Sprouting and the Neuronal Basis of Learning," followed by talks at numerous other congresses and symposia. His lectures intrigued audiences and his name became widely known in association with synaptic sprouting.

Although he was trained as a neurophysiologist, his interdisciplinary approach was best expressed in association with the field of neuroscience. In his last couple of years he seemed to be concentrating on a new approach to synaptic sprouting through molecular neuroscience. If he had lived, I am sure he would have become a leading scholar in this new and growing field of neuroscience.

In addition to his work on sprouting, he also participated in work on cerebellar control of pupillary light reflex and lens accommodation. His contribution to cable models of dendrites and spines was quite remarkable. In 1982 he joined Professor H. Asanuma as a Visiting Professor at

Rockefeller University to work on problems of sprouting in the cerebral cortex.

Although he was busy with laboratory work, Nakaakira never forgot the importance of organizations for researchers. In Tokyo he was an active leader of the Young Physiologists' Group. In Osaka he founded and led an excellent research group of graduate and postgraduate students in bioengineering. He was actively involved in the establishment of the National Institute of Physiology at Okazaki where he devoted himself to the operation of the center as a guest professor. In addition, he was always a promoting force of the Japan Neuroscience Society and chaired the 8th Annual Meeting in Osaka in 1984.

It is still hard to accept that we will never see him again. To his family he was always a kind, thoughtful, and dedicated husband and father. To his friends, colleagues, and students he was an inspiration who will always be remembered for his ambitious endeavors and impressive successes.

Masao Ito

The Neural and Molecular Bases of Learning,
eds. J.-P. Changeux and M. Konishi, pp. 5–12.
John Wiley & Sons Limited.

Introduction

J.-P. Changeux* and M. Konishi**

* Institut Pasteur
75724 Paris 15, France
** California Institute of Technology
Pasadena, CA 91125, USA

The word learning is commonly used to designate the rather widespread property of living organisms which exhibit lasting changes of behavior as a consequence of a defined interaction with their environment. Accordingly, learning is expected to cover a wide diversity of processes, from adaptative changes in the chemotactic response of bacteria to language and concept acquisition in humans. Faced with such a diversity, the search for common rules and mechanisms of learning, *a priori*, looks difficult if not impossible. However, persistent efforts have been made toward this aim over the past decades. To have some chance of success efforts must overcome severe methodological constraints: one such constraint deals with the careful utilization of the concept of "model," the other with a "level of organization."

Theoretical models are commonly used in the field of learning. They constitute formal and coherent representations of a given learning phenomenon or process and thus are necessarily limited in their applicability. They become useful, however, when they point to critical experimental tests and lead to specific and original predictions. Model building becomes essential in the investigation of systems as complex as the human brain. Models are used to delineate problems and raise pertinent questions, but in no instance should they be taken as accurate or exhaustive descriptions of reality. They are, instead, theoretical tools designed to approach such a description. Many pitfalls and useless debates in the discussion about learning might be avoided once such a distinction is made.

Experimental tests of theoretical models require adequate biological systems and often one has to rely on simple, or simplified, preparations such as invertebrate ganglia or slices of definite regions of the brain. The data obtained through such "model systems" may become essential to the understanding of higher order brain processes such as elementary building blocks, but in no instance can they integrally account for such processes. This leads us to the second methodological constraint: the *level of organization.*

Learning in unicellular organisms cannot usefully be compared with learning in the human brain unless one specifies the level of organization where the comparison may eventually become legitimate. Each level may possess its own rules which in turn depend on those of its elementary components. Accordingly, learning is studied at four levels: 1) the organism as a whole, 2) ensembles or populations of neurons, 3) individual nerve cells, and 4) that of their constitutive macromolecules.

The first level concerns the rules governing relationships among such units as stimuli, responses, and reinforcements. It deals primarily with behavior but also includes internal mental states referred to as representations, expectations, or cognitions. Two traditions of thought and experimental approaches have dominated this field: animal learning studied mainly in laboratory species and ethological studies in the field. The aim of a recent Dahlem workshop, organized by P. Marler and H.S. Terrace, was to attempt a synthesis of these two points of view and to "reconcile learning theory and natural behavior." The resulting book, entitled "The Biology of Learning" (5) dealt with biological and psychological aspects of learning and with questions of the relationship between learning at the behavioral and/or mental level and the underlying neural bases. As a result of that meeting and due to the recent, rapid development of cell physiology and molecular biology of the neuron, it was felt that the generation of a new synthesis of the neural and molecular *mechanisms* of learning would be timely. Hence, the planning of this workshop. Such a program, however, appeared too ambitious to several of us since in many instances only model systems are available. We decided, therefore, to utilize the term *bases* instead of *mechanisms.*

To generate a new synthesis often involves difficulties; however, the resulting synthesis was found at the crossroads of the rather distinct disciplines represented at the workshop, each having their own different experimental traditions and theoretical paradigms. Thus the workshop was successful in creating a dialog about the general significance of reported data and theories and their actual relevance to learning phenomena.

As expected, lively discussions took place about questions bridging distinct levels of organization such as the physiology of the nerve cell and its molecular biology or between the properties of single neurons and that of their assemblies coding for mental objects or symbols. Interestingly, no particular method was privileged and the "reductionist" approach (from the mental to the molecular) was equally balanced by the "synthetic" one (from cell and molecules to higher brain functions).

Discussions were focussed around four main topics which constitute the four main sections of this book. Each coincides with a distinct level of observation and analysis.

1. **Activity-dependent regulation of gene expression.** Storage of learning traces for lengths of time which exceed the metabolic half-life of the constitutive proteins of the neuron and its synapses is expected to involve protein synthesis, at least for the maintenance of these steady state concentrations. In addition, examples of differential regulation by electrical activity of particular sets of genes are known (see Changeux *et al.*, Thoenen and Acheson, and Henderson, all this volume), but evidence for the synthesis of novel protein species as a consequence (e.g., some splicing events as they occur in the immune system) has not yet been reported in the nervous system. Potential candidates exist for the second messengers which link electrical activity and gene expression, but regulatory proteins acting at the gene level have not yet been identified. Only one nucleus exists per nerve cell and this raises the question of the distribution of the gene products and of their channelling or targeting to particular synapses. Model systems and a rich panel of methods from molecular genetics and cell biology are available (see Yaniv, this volume) to approach and possibly answer these questions in the near future.

2. **Activity-dependent regulation of synaptic transmission and neuronal excitability.** Several well documented examples of activity-dependent changes of neuronal and/or synaptic properties have been reported in vertebrates (hippocampus (Anderson, this volume), cerebellum (Ito and Thompson, both this volume) and invertebrates

(*Aplysia* (Carew, this volume), *Hermissenda* (Alkon, this volume)). Target sites are either pre- or postsynaptic or both, but topological convergence and time coincidence of several signals are required to create "associative" links. Receptors for neurotransmitters may play the role of integrative units at the molecular level but other allosteric proteins, ion channels, or enzymes are possible candidates as well (see Changeux *et al.*, this volume). Covalent modifications are expected to make the change last longer. A key issue that remains is the identification of the molecular target(s) actually engaged in a physiologically unambiguous learning event with overt behavioral manifestations.

3. Activity-dependent modification of functional circuits. Neural circuits in development are subject to activity-dependent changes in synaptic connections. In several systems the outgrowth process and general topography of the projections appear independent of experience, whereas the subsequent events of synapse stabilization and elimination, which result in the final shaping of the neuronal circuits or maps, are regulated by the state of activity of the system (see Singer and Merzenich, both this volume). Rules of convergence and time coincidence also command this evolution which to a limited extent may persist in the adult where synapse turnover is considered to occur (see Cotman *et al.*, this volume). The elementary mechanisms of the activity-dependent regulation of synapse evolution (see Lømo and Changeux *et al.*, both this volume) remain a major area for future research as well as the precise relationship between learning-related changes in different areas of the cortex in the course of cognitive development.

4. Neuronal assemblies and memories. The search for the neural bases of higher brain functions is one of the most fascinating fields for future investigation with a pressing need for pertinent theory and novel methods of observation. A joint theoretical and experimental approach may lead to the identification of the still hypothetical, though widely mentioned, neuronal assemblies as coding units for internal representations and to the mechanisms of their selective storage in defined areas of the brain. In the near future theoretical models (von der Malsburg, this volume) may plausibly be developed to account for simplified experimental situations which actually exist in the invertebrate (Menzel and Bicker, this volume) and vertebrate (Thompson and Rolls, both this volume) nervous system and to decipher the spatio-temporal code of mental representations.

Cross-fertilization between the four groups was sufficient to reach a consensus about the usefulness and general application of cellular and molecular "model systems" from both invertebrates and vertebrates to higher level learning with, however, an expected diversity of elementary signalling mechanisms. The Hebb laws, in their general definition of a change of synapse efficacy and/or stability determined by the conjunction of activity (not exclusively firing) of converging pre- and postsynaptic elements, may serve as a general learning algorithm at the cellular and molecular level (1). Another line of consensus was the view that differentiation and learning takes place by selection (2) of preexisting neurons, synapses, molecules, and even molecular conformations. This contrasts the popular view that learning may "induce" the formation of new synapses and even new protein species. Nevertheless, specialized mechanisms, circuits, and even centers may exist in highly evolved brains (such as the human brain) to account for the successive steps of acquisition, storage, and retrieval and for short- and long-term memory storage that investigations on simple model systems are not expected to yield.

The knowledge of synaptic storage mechanisms alone is insufficient for an understanding of learning that is based on complex processes of coding. Neural coding involves both connections and signals between neurons. In simple systems, such as those mentioned above, the neuronal connections specify the relationships between stimulus and response. In complex systems, the neuronal connections may provide many possible input-output functions, each of which depends on various contingencies. If encoding of information involves many neurons, learning may likewise engage many neurons and synapses. To determine the spatial and temporal distribution of these neurons and synapses may be an essential step for understanding the neural mechanisms of learning. Thus, technical innovations such as recording many neurons simultaneously may become a prerequisite for the study of learning. On the other hand, it may also serve to identify single neurons that can represent the operation of a network. Such neurons may represent the role of the network in learning: for example, early experience shapes the stimulus selectivity of orientation-sensitive neurons in the visual cortex (Singer, this volume) and that of song-specific neurons in the bird's song control system (4). Thus even when learning involves many neurons, single-neuron recording techniques can help elucidate the neural mechanisms of learning (3).

Finally, one particularly vivid enigma remains to be answered: how do memories persist in the brain for years in a state that resists synapse and molecular turnover? Theoretical models are available (Changeux *et al.* and Kennedy, both this volume), yet data is scarce!

Acknowledgements. We would like to express our special thanks to Siemens AG for their generous help in providing Dahlem Konferenzen, free of charge, with their *Bürosystem 5800* for the production of this book. The timely appearance of this volume was only possible through the dedicated work and cooperation between Wolfgang Kahoun and Peter J. Schwieger of Siemens AG, Berlin and the Dahlem Konferenzen staff.

REFERENCES

(1) Changeux, J.-P., and Heidmann, T. 1986. Allosteric receptors and molecular models of learning. In *New Insights into Synaptic Function*, eds. G. Edelman, W.E. Gall, and W.M. Cowan. London: John Wiley Publishers, in press.

(2) Changeux, J.-P.; Heidmann, T.; and Patte, P. 1984. Learning by selection. In *The Biology of Learning*, eds. P. Marler and H.S. Terrace, pp. 115-133. Dahlem Konferenzen. Berlin, Heidelberg, New York, Tokyo: Springer-Verlag.

(3) Konishi, M. 1984. A logical basis for single-neuron study of learning in complex neural systems. In *The Biology of Learning*, eds. P. Marler and H.S. Terrace, pp. 311-324. Dahlem Konferenzen. Berlin, Heidelberg, New York, Tokyo: Springer-Verlag.

(4) Margoliash, D., and Konishi, M. 1985. Auditory representation of autogenous song in the song system of white-crowned sparrows. *Proc. Natl. Acad. Sci.* 82: 5997-6000.

(5) Marler, P., and Terrace, H.S., eds. 1984. The Biology of Learning. Dahlem Konferenzen. Berlin, Heidelberg, New York, Tokyo: Springer-Verlag.

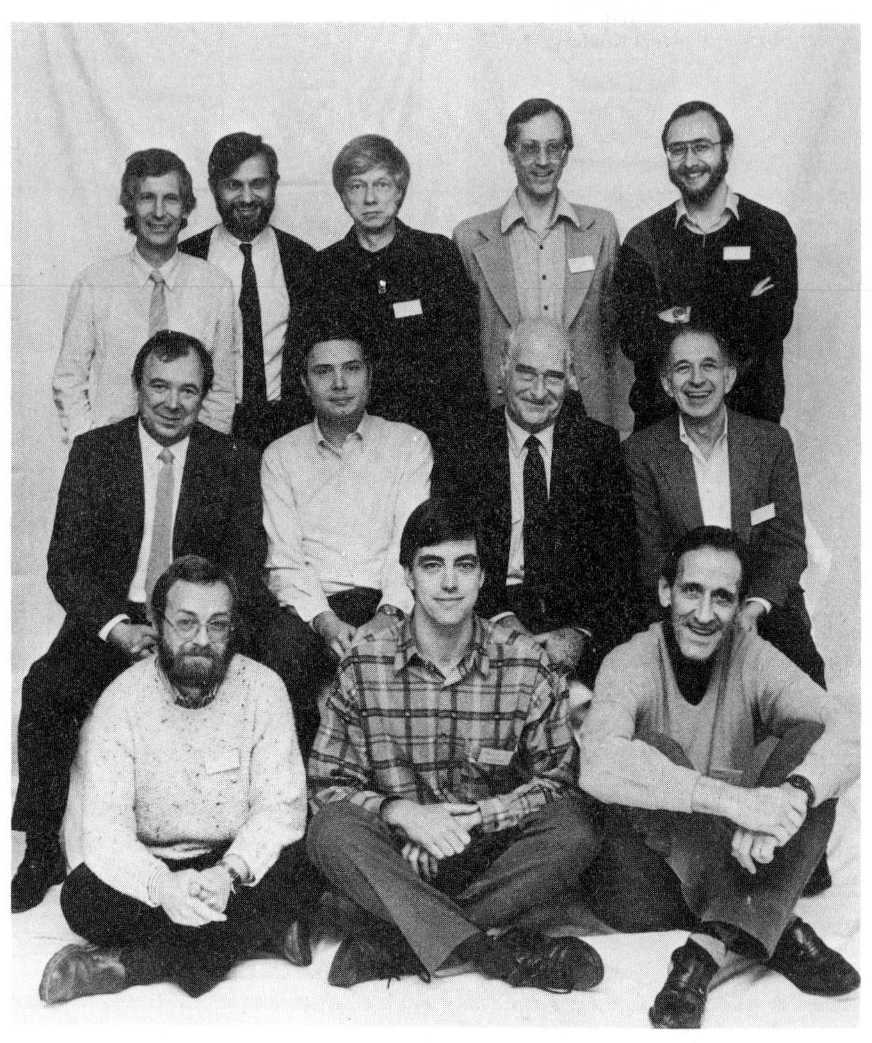

Back row, left to right:
Moshe Yaniv, Jacques Mallet, Martin Heisenberg, Ted Ebendal, Wieland Huttner

Middle row, left to right:
Jean-Pierre Changeux, Wes Thompson, Gunther Stent, Eric Kandel

Front row, left to right:
Gerd Bicker, Chris Henderson, Hans Thoenen

The Neural and Molecular Bases of Learning,
eds. J.-P. Changeux and M. Konishi, pp. 13–30.
John Wiley & Sons Limited.

Activity-dependent Regulation of Gene Expression

Group Report

W.J. Thompson, Rapporteur

G. Bicker
J.-P. Changeux
T.L. Ebendal
M. Heisenberg
C.E. Henderson
W. Huttner
E.R. Kandel
J.B. Mallet
G.S. Stent
H. Thoenen
M. Yaniv

INTRODUCTION

There are probably several mechanisms by which memory can be stored in nervous tissue without changes in gene expression, and some of these are discussed in the other group reports in this volume. In our deliberations, however, we adopted the position that formation of some long-term memories probably does involve qualitative changes or quantitative changes, or both, in gene expression within nerve cells. A qualitative change in gene expression (i.e., an expression of a novel protein) might arise from transcription from a previously untranscribed gene; a change in the processing (splicing) of a previously transcribed primary mRNA, creating a new mRNA by combination of different exons; or genomic rearrangements, such as those occurring in the immune system. A quantitative change in gene expression might arise from a change in the rate of transcription of a gene previously transcribed at a lower (or higher) rate, a change in stability of a previously transcribed mRNA, or a change in efficiency with which an existing mRNA is translated into protein. Although there are known examples of regulation of the expression of eukaryotic proteins by each of these processes, the most common mode of regulation is believed to be at the level of gene trans-cription. Accordingly, we considered some of the evidence for changes in gene expression in the formation of long-term memory, discussed how neural activity might affect gene expression, delineated some examples of neural activity-related changes in neural protein and gene expression, and finally, considered some approaches that one might take in identifying changes in the expression of specific genes underlying long-term memory.

EVIDENCE FOR THE INVOLVEMENT OF GENE REGULATION IN LEARNING AND MEMORY

One of our first topics was the evidence for the involvement of gene expression in learning. The evidence we considered was obtained from conditioning studies carried out with mammals and fish more than a decade ago and more recently with molluscs.

About ten years ago Agranoff, Barondes, Squire, and others, following up an earlier finding of Flexner, found that administration of protein synthesis inhibitors and actinomycin D (a nonspecific inhibitor of RNA polymerase) to experimental animals interferes with their acquisition of long-term memory (26). These inhibitors did not affect the acquisition of short-term memory and were effective only if given during or within a few hours of the training session. While these experiments suggested that protein synthesis and RNA synthesis are necessary for the formation of long-term memory, they nonetheless had both methodological and conceptual weaknesses. From the methodological point of view, these inhibitors had some nonspecific effects, such as making the animal ill or producing seizures. From the conceptual point of view, it proved difficult to relate RNA synthesis or protein synthesis, or both, to formation of long-term memory without knowing the identity of the molecular species in the brain whose synthesis is actually required in the learning process. Hence, these kinds of experiments came to be largely abandoned by the late 1970s.

Recently Goelet, Castellucci, Schwartz, Schacher, Montarolo, and Kandel (Carew, this volume, and Kandel, personal communication) have reopened this line of investigation using the mollusc *Aplysia* as experimental material. As described by Carew (this volume), the learning associated with the gill withdrawal reflex of *Aplysia* comprises both a short-term and a long-term form of sensitization of the reflex, depending on the training paradigm. Work carried out by Kandel, Schwartz, and their colleagues (16) has indicated that the short-term form of sensitization is mediated by a chemical modification of a preexisting channel in the membrane of one of the cells in the reflex arc. Frost *et al.* (11) have recently shown that the same monosynaptic pathway from sensory neuron to motor neuron, which is modified under the short-term training paradigm leading to sensitization of the reflex, is also modified under the long-term sensitization paradigm as well: training increases the amplitude of the excitatory postsynaptic potentials (EPSPs) elicited by the sensory neurons in the motor neurons twofold. Blumenthal and Castellucci have shown that the acquisition of long-term, but not of short-term, sensitization can be blocked by administration of a protein synthesis inhibitor to the preparation (Kandel, personal communication). Rayport and Schacher (27) and Montarolo *et al.* (21) have reconstituted the monosynaptic sensory neuron to the motor neuron pathway of the reflex in dissociated cell culture. They have shown that the single synapse in the pathway undergoes a short-term enhancement of EPSP amplitude in response to a single 5 minute exposure to serotonin and a long-term enhancement in response to five such exposures to serotonin. They have also shown that the long-term enhancement induced by serotonin is blocked by exposure of the preparation to protein synthesis inhibitors (anisomycin or emetine) or RNA synthesis inhibitors (actinomycin or alpha-amanitin) while the short-term enhancement is unaffected by such treatments ((21) and Kandel, personal communication). Furthermore, as in mammals and fish, in the molluscan preparation the protein or RNA synthesis inhibitors need to be present only during or briefly after the training session in order to block the acquisition of the long-term sensitization. Inhibitors applied some time after the training session do not affect the acquisition of long-term sensitization. In work in progress Goelet, Castellucci, Schwartz, and Kandel have surveyed the proteins extracted from the neurons of the reflex on two-dimensional gels and have found in preliminary experiments that several new proteins are expressed during acquisition of long-term sensitization (Kandel, personal communication). Taken together these results suggest that acquisition of long-term sensitization involves genes and proteins not involved in short-term sensitization. Some of the new proteins identified might be involved in the initial events of induction of gene expression and the subsequent modifications of the sensory neuron leading to an enchancement of its synaptic efficacy (e.g., by increasing the number and size of active zones of its axon terminals presynaptic to the motor neuron). Alternatively, these proteins could reflect the stabilization of constitutively expressed proteins.

HOW COULD NEURONAL ACTIVITY CHANGE THE RATE OF TRANSCRIPTION OF GENES?

As pointed out in the *INTRODUCTION* and in the background paper by Yaniv, regulation of protein synthesis can occur at several levels but the most common level of regulation is a modulation of the rate of gene transcription. The rate of transcription of eukaryotic genes appears to be modulated by several regulatory proteins ("transcription factors") which bind to specific gene regions usually located upstream from the initiation site for RNA polymerase. The binding of these proteins can exert either a positive or negative effect on the rate of initiation of transcription by the polymerase.

Therefore, in order for neural activity to change the rate of gene transcription it would have to cause an alteration of some transcription factors within the neuron. It was suggested that events occurring at the cell membrane as a result of neural activity might alter transcription factors through two means (see Changeux, this volume). First, an allosteric modification of the affinity of the transcription factor protein for its DNA binding site could occur, due to induction by neural activity of a change in the intracellular concentration of an ion species or of a second messenger molecule. Second, activity might induce a cascade of enzymatic reactions leading to a covalent modification of a transcription factor, e.g., by protein phosphorylation (22) or proteolysis. There are indications that both types of modification of transcription factors occur in other eukaryotic cells (see Yaniv, this volume).

Given a means by which neural activity can modulate the rate of gene transcription, we still had to deal with some special problems in the case of long-term memory. The first problem concerns the generally short duration of an activity signal responsible for induction of a long-term memory. Any protein newly synthesized as a consequence of such an activity signal would be expected to be subject to turnover. How then could the memory be made long-lasting? Two possibilities were proposed. First, the transcription factor modified by the activity signal during training might in fact be stable. Yaniv reported (this volume) that transcription factors usually remain tightly bound to their DNA binding sites, unless the cell undergoes DNA replication in preparation for mitosis. Since neural cells are generally postmitotic, it is possible that a modified transcription factor remains stably bound to the DNA in the long term. Second, the change in the rate of expression of a particular gene induced by a transient activity signal might be stabilized in the long term by permanently switching the metabolic pathway of the nerve cell from one steady state to another. For instance, we may consider the flip-flop metabolic circuit proposed by Delbrück in 1948 (6):

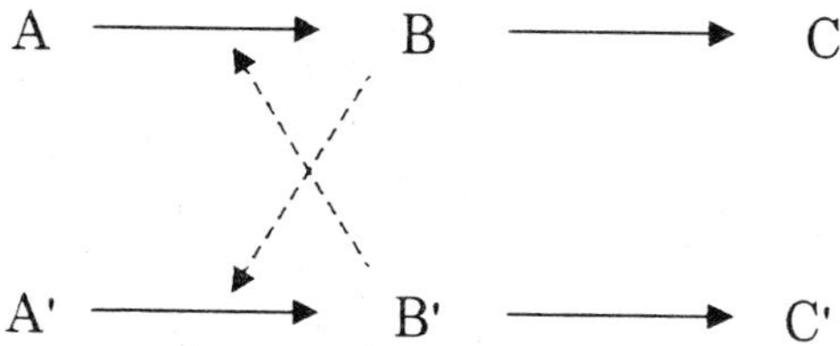

where the metabolites B and B' reciprocally inhibit the enzymes catalyzing their own production. According to this circuit a nerve cell can be in two alternative steady states: in one state only substance C and in the other only substance C' is produced. Suppose C' is an effector molecule which activates a particular protein species P (a transcription factor) which is constitutively synthesized in the neuron. When activated by C', P can bind to a particular region of DNA, activating the expression of a particular gene, G. Prior to delivery of the stimulus to the nerve cell, the cell produces only C but not C', and hence G is inactive. Now suppose that the transient training stimulus inhibits the production of B. This will permit the production of B' and reinforce the inhibition of the production of B, thus throwing the cell into the other steady state under which C' instead of C is produced. The presence of C' will activate the expression of G. This activation will be permanent despite any turnover of P since there will always be enough P molecules to be activated by C'. A number of different mechanisms of this general type are possible.

The second problem concerns the diversity of activity-dependent changes in neuronal gene expression. While it is presently unclear what protein changes underlie the acquisition of long-term memory and whether these changes are qualitative or quantitative, we asked whether it would be possible for activity to regulate a large number of different genes in different neurons? On first thought it might appear that a large ensemble of activity-regulated genes would require the specific activation of a large number of different transcription factors by neuronal activity. However, this need not necessarily be the case. During embryonic development of the nervous system, as neurons become committed to their differentiated fates, an ensemble of genes is presumably brought into a potentially active state by structural changes of the chromatin in which it is embedded (Yaniv, this volume; (4)). As different neurons develop, they may obtain a commitment of different gene ensembles. Thus one and the same transcription factor may activate a different ensemble of genes in different neurons depending on which ensemble had been made potentially activatable at an earlier stage of development in any given cell.

The third problem concerns the complex geometry of neurons. Generally, the synapses which produce neuronal activity and which are presumably the substrate for modifications underlying the acquisition of memory are located at remote sites on the neuron's dendritic tree, far from the cell nucleus. Therefore, any second messenger or modified transcription factor generated at a synaptic site in the dendritic tree would have to be transported to the nucleus to cause activation of its cognate gene ensemble. Moreover, how are products, resulting from such gene activation and responsible for modification of synapses "targeted" only to the particular synapses, to be modified in the memory acquisition? Maybe in some instances no such targeting occurs and the modifications are generalized over entire neurons. However, evidence from long-term potentiation (LTP) in the pyramidal cells of the mammalian hippocampus indicates that the potentiation is not generalized to all synapses in the neuron but pertains only to those activated by the stimulus (Andersen, this volume). Of course it has not been shown as yet that LTP requires protein synthesis for its acquisition, but the question of targeting the products of gene activation should nonetheless be addressed. As possible mechanisms of such targeting, we considered the following ideas:

a) A local, transient synaptic change underlying short-term memory may mark the changed synapses as candidates for subsequent long-term modification. In this case the gene product responsible for the long-term modification might not need to be especially targeted to a specific site for its action. Rather, the product might be transported through all the dendrites of a neuron but act only at the synaptic or perisynaptic sites already marked as candidates for change.

b) Polysomes are known to be located in the dendrites of neurons and even concentrated at synaptic sites (32). These polysomes, even if they are identical throughout the dendrites, might encode proteins of general relevance to long-term synaptic or dendritic modifications. Therefore, local activation of protein synthesis and utilization of its products might be possible.

c) Finally, proteins to be utilized in converting a short-term into a long-term memory might be targeted for transport only to the very dendrites, and possibly even the very synapses, where they are to act. It is certainly the case that neurons appear to be capable of targeting transport of some macromolecular components (e.g., ribosomes and vesicle types) to different major portions of the cell, e.g., axon versus dendrites. Examples of targeting of viral proteins to the apical and basolateral membrane surfaces of polarized epithelial cells have been described (31). It will be interesting to see in the future whether neurons are capable of targeting macromolecules to specific dendrites and/or synapses.

EXAMPLES OF ACTIVITY-DEPENDENT REGULATION OF GENE EXPRESSION

There exist some well-analyzed examples of the regulation by activity of mRNA levels in excitable tissues. Four examples have been discussed in this volume (see Changeux, Thoenen and Acheson, and Henderson, all this volume): the acetylcholine receptor, myosin, catecholamine-synthesizing enzymes, and growth factors which will be considered briefly below.

Acetylcholine Receptor

It has been shown that the supersensitivity to acetylcholine of denervated muscle fibers results from an increase in the rate of synthesis of the acetylcholine receptor (Changeux, this volume). This denervation-induced increase in synthesis is, at least in large measure, due to the paralysis of the muscle: stimulating a denervated muscle directly prevents the increase in the content of acetylcholine receptor in the fiber membrane without changing the rate of turnover of the receptor. Moreover, it is possible to induce an increase in the receptor content of the cell membrane of spontaneously contracting chick muscle cells in primary culture by exposure of the cells to tetrodotoxin (TTX) which abolishes impulse activity and hence muscle contraction. Addition of actinomycin D to such muscle cultures prevents the tetrodotoxin-induced increase in receptor content, indicating that RNA synthesis is required for the TTX induction. Recently, by use of a cDNA probe for the α-subunit of the chick receptor, Klarsfeld and Changeux (17) have shown that exposure of such muscle cultures to TTX results in an approximately 14-fold increase in the cellular content of α-subunit mRNA. While most of the evidence suggests that this TTX induction occurs at the level of transcription of the receptor gene, an activity effect on mRNA stability cannot as yet be excluded.

Muscle Myosin

Vertebrates carry several different myosin heavy and light chain genes in their genomes. Different contractile types of muscle fibers are created by the differential expression of these genes. Three primary classes of fibers are usually recognized: slow-oxidative (SO), fast fatigue-resistant (FR), and the fast fatigable (FF).

It is known from the experiments of Buller *et al.* (3) and work that has since followed (24) that the expression of myosin genes in a given muscle fiber is plastic: for example, when a muscle comprised predominantly of SO fibers is innervated by a motor nerve which normally innervates a muscle composed of fast (FR and FF) fibers, these "cross-reinnervated" fibers are transformed from slow to fast over the course of weeks. How does the innervating nerve exert this influence on the muscle? The best experimental evidence suggests that the influence is activity-mediated. Motor neurons innervating fast or slow muscles differ in activity; they are active for different amounts of time and at different frequencies. A recent, convincing demonstration of this difference has been produced by Hennig and Lømo (14). They have shown that motor neurons innervating a muscle in the hind limb of the rat are of three types corresponding to one of the three types of muscle fibers: SO, FR, and FF. The SO motor neurons in this muscle are active about 30% of the day, and during their active periods they produce action potentials at a frequency of about 20 Hz. The FR and FF motor neurons, in contrast, are active at 50-90 Hz for only 2-5% and 0.1% of the day, respectively. Thus the SO motor neurons give a large number of action potentials at low frequency continuously over a given time period, whereas the FR and FF motor neurons give fewer total action potentials per unit time although when they are active they generate action potentials in high frequency bursts. Pette and collaborators (23) have shown that if a low frequency (10 Hz) stimulus pattern (analogous to the slower activity of SO motor neurons) is extrinsically imposed on the nerve supplying a fast muscle in the rabbit, this fast muscle is almost completely transformed into a slow muscle. The nerve is not even necessary for this transformation: Lømo and his collaborators have shown that a denervated muscle stimulated directly via implanted electrodes can be induced to transform its fiber types (19). A fast-like activity pattern (intermittent stimulation at high frequency) makes slow fibers more fast-like; fast fibers can be made more slow-like if they are given a slow-type activity pattern. Lømo has thus shown that each fiber is plastic and can change its contractile apparatus so that a range of contractile properties are possible; each type of fiber is said to have an "adaptive range," and the particular properties it assumes depend on the total amount and pattern of activation it receives (Lømo, personal communication). This adaptive range in contractile properties is apparantly determined by proteins in addition to the myosin heavy and light chains: other proteins regulate the calcium fluxes across the sarcoplasmic reticulum and the interactions between actin and myosin. Nonetheless, there is good evidence from analysis of the myosin heavy and light chains expressed in muscle fibers following these manipulations, from use of antibodies directed against different myosin isoforms, and from emerging studies using cDNA probes of muscle myosin genes that the particular genes being expressed are changed by activity (2).

This is a particularly intriguing and unexploited example of the influence of activity on an excitable cell. Not only does activity apparently change gene expression but what change is made depends upon the amount and pattern of this activity.

Catecholamine-synthesizing Enzymes

A non-muscle example, for which it is reasonably clear that nerve activity causes a change in mRNA levels, is the selective increase in levels of catecholamine-synthesizing enzymes (tyrosine hydroxylase and dopamine ß-hydroxylase) occurring in sympathetic ganglion cells or adrenal medullary cells in response to stimulation of their cholinergic innervation. As Thoenen and Acheson have outlined (this volume), this phenomenon, designated "transsynaptic induction," consists of a 50-200% increase in enzyme levels in a sympathetic ganglion beginning about 20 hours after stimulation of its preganglionic axons at 10 Hz for 10 min. The enzyme levels reach a peak about 48 hours after stimulation and then return to basal values in about a week. Mallet and colleagues (10) have recently studied changes in the levels of tyrosine hydroxylase mRNA in the adrenals, locus coeruleus, and substantia nigra as a consequence of increased activity. Reserpine was used to induce this activity: this drug depletes the catecholamine stores of the cells in the sympathetic nervous system, deprives their targets of normal activation, and reflexively increases the activity of the preganglionic cholinergic inputs to these ganglion cells. He found up to a fivefold increase in the levels of tyrosine hydroxylase mRNA following administration of reserpine, which preceded the rise in tyrosine hydroxylase activity. In contrast to the case of muscle myosin described above, some information is available regarding the potential signalling mechanisms for this transsynaptic induction. As described by Thoenen and Acheson (this volume), nerve stimulation brings about a substantial increase in the Na^+ concentration of the postsynaptic neuron. This change in Na^+ results from the activation of the cholinergic nicotinic receptor, rather than simply from depolarization.

Growth Factors

Activity-induced changes in growth factor levels were also considered because of their potential for explaining a) the sprouting of neurons to form new connections and/or b) the regression of synaptic connections as inputs compete for factor(s) (discussed by Henderson, this volume). The best evidence for an activity-dependent regulation of a growth factor is provided by experiments in which a reduction in neuromuscular activity of chicken embryos has been found to result in an increased level of trophic support for motor neurons (see review by Henderson, this volume). Unfortunately, the trophic factor has yet to be characterized in this case. The case for activity-regulation of the well-known neurotrophic factor NGF is less convincing. While denervation of the adult rat iris leads to an increase in the synthesis and release of NGF (1, 8, 9), there is no direct evidence that the changes are due to the inactivity of the postsynaptic target cells. Moreover, the situation is made more complex by the ambiguity of the cellular origin of the NGF produced in the iris or in other sympathetic targets. It cannot be taken for granted that the postsynaptic cells are synthesizing NGF: other candidates are glial cells and fibroblasts.

Another common assumption about trophic factors is that their uptake by the innervating axons is activity-dependent. In no case has this assumption yet been proven. Indeed, evidence in the case of NGF indicates that its uptake by innervating axons is activity-independent. Specifically, the uptake by sympathetic axons of ^{125}I-NGF injected into the anterior chamber of the eye is not altered upon reducing activity by decentralization of the superior cervical ganglion or by administration of ganglionic blocking agents (33). Neither is NGF uptake enhanced by increasing the activity of the sympathetic axons during cold stress (33). This manipulation of activity does, however, clearly affect vesicle recycling: augmentation of sympathetic activity increases the retrograde transport of dopamine-ß-hydroxylase antibodies injected into the eye chamber (18).

Recent experiments with the neuromuscular junction indicate that in addition to soluble growth factors, such as those being investigated by Henderson *et al.* (13), molecules associated with cell membranes and extracellular matrices are also important in regulating axonal growth and synapse formation. Sanes and his colleagues (5, 29, 30) have followed up on the observation, by Jansen *et al.* (15), that the refractoriness of a normally innervated muscle to innervation by an implanted nerve is due to the activity evoked in the muscle fibers by their intact innervation: if an innervated muscle is paralyzed then synapse formation occurs; conversely, if a denervated muscle is stimulated to activity then the formation of new synapses which would otherwise occur is prevented. Sanes and his collaborators have recently been able to show that several molecules on the surface of skeletal muscle fibers change their expression in an activity-dependent fashion. N-CAM (a neural cell adhesion molecule) and J1 (a new adhesion molecule, so far shown to mediate neuron-astrocyte adhesion *in vitro*) are both present at low levels in normal adult muscle, but accumulate following denervation; in each case, the effects of denervation can be largely mimicked by pharmacological (TTX) paralysis of innervated muscles (5, 30). *In vitro*, accumulation of JS-1, a synapse specific basal lamina antigen, is reversibly stimulated when myotubes are chronically paralyzed by addition of TTX or lidocaine to their medium. This elevation in JS-1 expression occurs despite the fact that paralyzed myotubes accumulate less basal lamina overall than do spontaneously active myotubes (29). A coordinate, activity-dependent (or, more properly, inactivity-dependent) response involving soluble, membrane bound, and extracellular matrix-associated neuroactive molecules may thus account for the greatly enhanced susceptibility of denervated muscle fibers to synapse formation.

PROBLEMS IN DETERMINING THE LINK BETWEEN A CHANGE IN GENE EXPRESSION AND NEURAL ACTIVITY

Even given the identification of a gene whose expression is changed by neural activity, it may not be entirely straightforward to determine how the link between the two is established. One would expect at least one of the stages is represented by a quantitatively small biochemical change (for example, by formation of a second messenger molecule or by activation of a transcription factor). This presents special, additional problems in the nervous system because these changes are probably occurring in a small number of cells. Therefore, the small amounts of material available for biochemical analysis probably present considerable obstacles for the identification of the link. For example, Yaniv (personal communication) estimated that 10^7 cells would be needed to search for a DNA binding protein once the particular gene, including its regulatory sequence, is cloned.

Thoenen and Acheson (this volume) emphasized that one must be cautious in attempting to overcome this limitation on the amount of available material by the use of stable cell lines. Such cell lines may not exhibit responses which are those typical of the nontransformed cells for which they are used as models (Thoenen and Acheson, this volume). Moreover, additional considerations when using *in vitro* model systems are the potential regulatory effects of a) the culture conditions themselves, specifically cell-substrate and cell-cell interactions, and b) the developmental stage of the source of cells for primary culture, as effects of a given stimulus can be influenced by both of these factors (Thoenen and Acheson, this volume).

Group members, therefore, urged caution in the interpretation of data from cell cultures: one must make sure that *in vitro* observations mimic the *in vivo* situation. Nonetheless, any *in vitro* cell response may represent an interesting example of trophic factor or activity control of neuronal properties.

SCREENING FOR MACROMOLECULES INVOLVED IN LEARNING

If acquisition of long-term memory does involve a change in gene expression then one might hope to detect differences in the macromolecules expressed in nervous tissue as the result of a training session. Many members of the group were of the opinion that the modern molecular, biochemical, immunological, and genetic approaches which are now available have made the identification of the macromolecular changes attending the acquisition of memory feasible and timely. A rather straightforward biochemical approach is provided by the modern, sensitive techniques for two-dimensional electrophoresis of proteins. In fact, Kandel discussed preliminary results from his laboratory indicating the successful application of this procedure to the case of a nonassociative learning in *Aplysia* (Carew, this volume, and above).

It was felt that the most promising approach is provided by the new methods in molecular cloning, which offer the possibility of comparing the differences in mRNA sequences present in the nervous system of trained and untrained animals. The basic procedure is to prepare a cDNA library in bacteria from mRNA extracted from neural tissue of trained animals, preferably from a portion of the brain suspected to be involved in the particular learning task. Next, identical copies of this library would be probed with radioactive cDNA: one copy with probe prepared from mRNA from the untrained animal and the second copy with probe prepared from mRNA from the trained animal. With this technique one would hope to detect differences in the hybridization of the probes from the trained vs. the untrained animal. If new mRNAs were present as a result of training, one would expect some cDNA clones to be recognized only by the probes prepared from the trained animal.

Similarly, if certain mRNAs were present in greater abundance in the trained animal then some cDNA clones should show a greater degree of hybridization with the probes prepared from the trained animal. In practice this technique can apparently detect a messenger as rare as only one copy in 10,000 and quantitative differences in messenger levels as low as fivefold (Mallet, personal communication). The sensitivity of the method can be further increased to detect an mRNA of abundance as low as one copy per 100,000 molecules by enriching the cDNAs for sequences likely to be of interest by "subtractive hybridization." This subtractive procedure (28) takes advantage of specific cDNA-mRNA hybridization: single-stranded cDNAs prepared from mRNA from nervous tissue of trained animals would be combined with mRNA extracted from a piece of nervous tissue suspected not to be involved in the learning. The cDNAs unique to the experienced tissue would then be unhybridized and could be purified by chromatographic procedures. These unique cDNAs could be used to prepare an initial library enriched for sequences that are not involved in general housekeeping fuctions in neurons. If clones containing sequences whose expression is induced or enhanced as a result of learning can be identified, then it will be possible to translate these sequences into proteins (or peptide segments) and then to use antibodies prepared against these proteins or peptides to identify their cellular location and hopefully their function. In some limited cases it might even be possible to prove the involvement of a particular mRNA in a learning task through the use of an anti-sense mRNA (12). A number of laboratories, including those of some of the group members, are now employing these cloning techniques to investigate experience-related changes in gene transcription in the nervous system.

Novel macromolecules present in nerve tissue as a result of learning might also be detectable by use of immunological screening. It was suggested that this could be accomplished by a two-step immunization procedure with nervous tissue. In the first step, immunization would be with nervous tissue from untrained subjects. During the immune response to this material, cytotoxic drugs which destroy the responding immune cells are given (20). The second immunization would be with nervous tissue from the trained animal. The immune response to this second challenge would supposedly be to antigenic determinants novel to the nervous tissue of the trained animal. These antibodies could then be used to identify the macromolecules whose expression was changed by the training procedure. While this method, unlike the cloning techniques, has the advantage of possibly detecting macromolecular differences other than those present in the amino acid sequence of proteins (e.g., polysaccharide components), we felt this method to be much more cumbersome and less sensitive for primary changes in proteins than the cloning methods.

It is our belief that classical genetics should also be helpful in identifying macromolecules involved in long-term memory. A feasible approach here would be to search for *Drosophila* mutants defective in long-term memory. For example, one promising mutant is amnesiac. This mutant has a memory whose lifetime is distinctly shorter than that of typical long-term memories, but which is longer than most short-term memories in the wild-type fly (7, 25). An indication of the promise of this approach is that analysis of *Drosophila* mutants has already allowed the identification of some proteins involved in acquisition and retention of short-term memory (25).

CONCLUSION

The regulation of gene expression in the nervous system has recently become an object of investigation in many laboratories. Insofar as long-term memory involves any change in gene expression, one should be able to apply the methodologies of modern molecular biology to the study of learning and memory. Further, as a number of examples of activity-related changes in neuronal gene expression are now becoming known, we hope that it will soon be possible to discover how neural activity really manages to regulate gene expression.

REFERENCES

(1) Barth, E.-M.; Korsching, S; and Thoenen, H. 1984. Regulation of nerve growth factor synthesis and release in organ cultures of rat iris. *J. Cell Biol.* 99: 839-843.

(2) Barton, P.J.R., and Buckingham, M.E. 1985. The myosin alkali light chain proteins and their genes. *Biochem. J.* 231: 249-261.

(3) Buller, A.J.; Eccles, J.C.; and Eccles, R.M. 1960. Interactions between motoneurones and muscles in respect of characteristic speeds of their responses. *J. Physl.* 150: 417-439.

(4) Changeux, J.-P. 1986. Coexistence of neuronal messengers and molecular selection. *Progr. Brain Res.*, in press.

(5) Covault, J., and Sanes, J.R. 1985. Neural cell adhesion molecule (N-CAM) accumulates in denervated and paralyzed skeletal muscles. *Proc. Natl. Acad. Sci.* 82: 4544-4548.

(6) Delbrück, M. 1949. Discussion remarks. In *Unités Biologiques Douées de Continuité Génétique*, ed. A. Lwoff, pp. 33-35. Paris: Editions du Centre National de la Recherche Scientifique.

(7) Dudai, Y. 1985. Genes, enzymes and learning in *Drosophila*. *Trends in Neurosciences* 8: 18-22.

(8) Ebendal, T.; Olson, L.; and Seiger, A. 1983. The level of nerve growth factor (NGF) as a function of innervation. A correlative radioimmunoassay and bioassay study of the rat iris. *Exp. Cell Res.* 148: 311-317.

(9) Ebendal, T.; Olson, L.; Seiger, A.; and Hedlung, K.-O. 1980. Nerve growth factors in the rat iris. *Nature* 286: 25-28.

(10) Faucon Biguet, N.; Buda, M.; Lamouroux, A.; Samolyk, D.; and Mallet, J. 1986. Time course of the changes of TH mRNA in rat brain and adrenal medulla after a single injection of reserpine. *EMBO J.* 5: 287-291.

(11) Frost, W.N.; Castellucci, V.F.; Hawkins, R.D.; and Kandel, E.R. 1985. Monosynaptic connections made by the sensory neurons of the gill- and siphon-withdrawal reflex in *Aplysia* participate in the storage of long-term memory for sensitization. *Proc. Natl. Acad. Sci.* 82: 8266-8269.

(12) Harland, R., and Weintraub, H. 1985. Translation of mRNA injected into *Xenopus* oocytes is specifically inhibited by antisense RNA. *J. Cell Biol.* 101: 1094-1099.

(13) Henderson, C.E.; Huchet, M.; and Changeux, J.-P. 1984. Neurite-promoting factors for embryonic spinal neurons and their developmental changes in the chick. *Develop. Biol.* 104: 336-347.

(14) Henning, R., and Lømo, T. 1985. Firing patterns of motor units in normal rats. *Nature* 314: 164-166.

(15) Jansen, J.K.S.; Lømo, T.; Nicolaysen, K.; and Westgaard, R.H. 1973. Hyperinnervation of skeletal muscle fibers: dependence on muscle activity. *Science* 181: 559-561.

(16) Kandel, E.R., and Schwartz, J.H. 1982. Molecular biology of learning: modulation of transmitter release. *Science* 218: 433-443.

(17) Klarsfeld, A., and Changeux, J.-P. 1985. Activity regulates the levels of acetylcholine receptor α-subunit mRNA in cultured chicken myotubes. *Proc. Natl. Acad. Sci.* 82: 4558-4562.

(18) Lees, G.J.; Geffen, L.B.; and Rush, R.A. 1981. Phentolamine increases neuronal binding and retrograde transport of dopamine-ß-hydroxylase antibodies. *Neurosci. L.* 22: 115-118.

(19) Lømo, T.; Westgaard, R.W.; and Dahl, H.A. 1974. Contractile properties of muscle: control by pattern of muscle activity in the rat. *P. Roy. Soc. Lon. B* 187: 99-103.

(20) Matthew, W.D., and Patterson, P.H. 1983. The production of a monoclonal antibody that blocks the action of a neurite outgrowth-promoting factor. *Cold S. H. Quant. Biol.* 48: 625-631.

(21) Montarolo, G.P.: Castellucci, V.F.; Goelet, P.; Kandel, E.R.; and Schacher, S. 1985. Long-term faciliation of the monosynaptic connection between sensory neurons and motor neurons of the gill-withdrawal reflex in *Aplysia* in dissociated cell culture. *Soc. Neurosci. Abstr.* 11: 795.

(22) Nestler, E.J., and Greengard, P. 1983. Protein Phosphorylation in the Nervous System. New York: Wiley

(23) Pette, D.; Muller, W.; Leisner, E.; and Vrbova, G. 1976. Time dependent effects on contractile properties, fibre population, myosin light chains and enzymes of energy metabolism in intermittently and continuously stimulated fast twitch muscles of the rabbit. *Pflugers Arch.* 364: 103-112.

(24) Pette, D., and Vrbova, G. 1985. Invited review: neural control of phenotypic expression in mammalian muscle fibers. *Muscle and Nerve* 8: 676-689.

(25) Quinn, W.G. 1984. Work in invertebrates on the mechanisms underlying learning. In *The Biology of Learning*, eds. P. Marler and H.S. Terrace, pp. 197-246. Dahlem Konferenzen. Berlin, Heidelberg, New York, Tokyo: Springer-Verlag

(26) Rainbow, T.C. 1979. Role of RNA and protein synthesis in memory formation. *Neurochem. Res.* 4: 297-312.

(27) Rayport, S.G., and Schacher, S. 1986. Synaptic plasticity *in vitro*: cell culture of identified *Aplysia* neurons mediating short-term habituation and sensitization. *J. Neurosci.* 6: 759-763.

(28) Rhyner, T.A.; Faucon Biguet, N.; Berrard, S.; Borbely, A.A.; and Mallet, J. 1986. An efficient approach for the selective isolation of specific transcripts from complex brain mRNA populations. *J. Neurosci. Res.* 16: 167-181.

(29) Sanes, J.R., and Lawrence, J.C. 1983. Activity-dependent accumulation of basal lamina by cultured myotubes. *Develop. Biol.* 97: 123-136.

(30) Sanes, J.R.; Schachner, M.; and Covault, J. 1986. Expression of several adhesive macromolecules (N-CAM, L1, J1, NILE, uvomorulin, laminin, fibronectin, and a heparan sulfate proteoglycan) in embryonic, adult, and denervated adult skeletal muscles. J. *Cell Biol.* 102: 420-431.

(31) Simons, K., and Fuller, S.D. 1985. Cell surface polarity in epithelia. *Ann. R. Cell. Biol.* 1: 243-288.

(32) Steward, O., and Falk, P.M. 1985. Polyribosomes under developing spine synapses: growth specializations of dendrites at sites of synaptogenesis. *J. Neurosci. Res.* 13: 75-88

(33) Stockel,K.; Dumas, M.; and Thoenen, H. 1978. Uptake and subsequent retrograde axonal transport of nerve factor (NGF) are not influenced by neuronal activity. *Neurosci. L.* 10: 61-64.

The Neural and Molecular Bases of Learning,
eds. J.-P. Changeux and M. Konishi, pp. 31–84.
John Wiley & Sons Limited.

The Acetylcholine Receptor and Molecular Models for Short- and Long-term Learning

J.-P. Changeux, A. Klarsfeld, and T. Heidmann
Neurobiologie Moléculaire
Institut Pasteur
75724 Paris 15, France

INTRODUCTION

The involvement of cholinergic mechanisms in central learning processes has been repeatedly mentioned in the past ((251); see also Singer, this volume), yet this review will not address this question. Its aim is to report briefly on the recent progress on the structure, biophysics, and molecular genetics of a peripheral receptor, the acetylcholine nicotinic receptor from fish electric organ and vertebrate neuromuscular junction (8, 52), and to utilize this information to build theoretical models for short- and long-term learning mechanisms at the cellular and molecular level.

Such an attempt hinges upon several difficulties. The nicotinic receptor is postsynaptic and presynaptic mechanisms have often been invoked in cellular mechanisms of learning (review (106); see also Carew, this volume). It is linked to a cation selective ion channel (130) and thus is distinct from other groups of receptors known to regulate cytoplasmic enzymes (see (236)). It is synthesized by nonneuronal, electrocyte, or muscle cells which are multinucleated. However, those neuronal receptors known to have similar characteristics, such as the glycine receptor (206) or the γ-amino butyric acid receptor (13, 195), show strikingly analogous structural and functional properties, and this legitimates the present approach.

This paper will cover three main aspects of acetylcholine receptor research:

1) the regulatory or "allosteric" properties of the acetylcholine receptor

as a model for short-term regulation of synapse efficacy at the postsynaptic level;
2) the activity-dependent regulation of acetylcholine receptor biosynthesis as a model for regulation of receptor number in the time scale of hours and days; and
3) diverse biochemical properties of the membrane-bound or purified receptor which may potentially account for long-term changes of synaptic properties.

ALLOSTERIC TRANSITIONS OF THE ACETYLCHOLINE RECEPTOR AND MODELS OF SHORT-TERM REGULATION OF SYNAPSE EFFICACY AT THE POSTSYNAPTIC LEVEL

Allosteric proteins (47, 176, 178) constitute a group of specialized proteins which act as biological transducers. They recognize, or are sensitive to, regulatory signals (in general, small molecules), possess a biological activity, and mediate the interaction between the site for the regulatory signals and the biologically active site. Examples of such regulatory proteins are hemoglobin (11), regulatory enzymes (82, 141, 142, 182), and DNA-binding proteins (7, 68). In all these systems, as initially stated (45, 176, 178), the regulatory interaction takes place between topograpically distinct sites (sometimes carried by distinct subunits) and is mediated by conformational transitions - or allosteric transitions - of the protein molecule between a small number of discrete states. In general, these proteins exhibit threshold responses due to positive cooperative interactions for ligand binding which are assigned to the cooperative assembly of their constitutive subunits into symmetrical oligomers (178).

These concepts have been extended to the proteins involved in intercellular communication, typified in the nervous system by the receptors for neurotransmitters (46, 47, 49, 55, 127). The neurotransmitter would serve as a regulatory signal acting on the external face of the receptor molecule. The biologically active site would either be a transmembrane ion channel or an enzyme catalytic site oriented toward the inside of the cell (review (49, 52, 53)).

Allosteric Properties of the Acetylcholine Receptor

The smallest molecular weight unit of the acetylcholine receptor from the fish electric organ and vertebrate neuromuscular junction is a heterologous pentamer made up of four different subunits (review (8, 52, 62, 128)) of exact protein molecular weight α = 50,116; β = 53,681; γ = 56,279; δ = 57,565 (189, 191-193), with the stoichiometry $\alpha_2\beta\gamma\delta$ (211, 214). The cDNAs coding for the four subunits have been cloned and sequenced in *Torpedo* (12, 58, 71, 94, 191-193, 255) and in high vertebrates (see ref. in (194)), and the inferred amino acid sequence of the four chains show striking homologies (10-60% identity, average 40%) (192, 211). Accordingly, the five subunits are viewed as making a transmembrane bundle with a rotational axis of quasi-symmetry perpendicular to the plane of the membrane (26, 32) (Fig. 1). In *Torpedo*, the molecule may also exist as a dimer of two $\alpha_2\beta\gamma\delta$ oligomers cross-linked by a disulfide bridge between the δ-chains (review (62)).

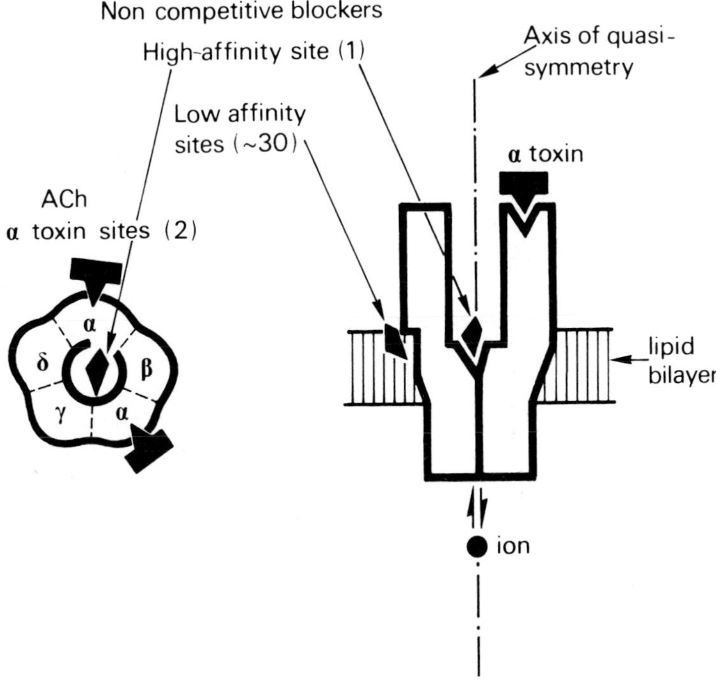

FIG. 1 – Diagrammatic representation of the acetylcholine receptor protein. Left: "en face" view from the synaptic cleft (the arrangement of the subunits is that proposed in (103), but is still under debate). Right: side view of the transmembrane organization of the molecule. Two main categories of sites are shown: the two high-affinity sites for acetylcholine or snake venom α-toxins and the "allosteric" sites for noncompetitive blockers. The unique high-affinity site for noncompetitive blockers is, according to the model proposed (113), located in the quasi-symmetry axis of the molecule.

The two α-chains carry the two primary acetylcholine and α-toxin binding sites which exhibit positive cooperative interactions, even though they differ in several of their pharmacological properties. Reconstitution experiments (review (8, 9, 47, 62, 207, 234)) further show that the $\alpha_2\beta\gamma\delta$ oligomer contains the ionic channel and that all subunits are required for the regulation of its opening (175). In addition, the membrane-bound receptor carries binding sites for other categories of ligands which affect the properties of the acetylcholine binding sites and/or the opening of the ion channel. The most typical ones are the "noncompetitive blockers," local anesthetics, chlorpromazine, phencyclidine, and the frog toxin histrionicotoxin, which are viewed as interfering directly and/or indirectly with the ion channel (review (1, 47)). They bind to two main categories of sites (114): "high-affinity" sites, sensitive to histrionicotoxin and present as a unique copy per receptor pentamer, and "low-affinity" sites, insensitive to histrionicotoxin, much more numerous (10-20 times the number of α-bungarotoxin sites) and lipid-dependent (114) (Fig. 1). Binding of noncompetitive blockers to their site at equilibrium enhances the binding of cholinergic ligands to the acetylcholine binding site ((60), review (114, 200)). Conversely, cholinergic ligands potentiate their binding (98, 114, 143). Reciprocal allosteric interactions take place under equilibrium conditions between these two classes of sites.

All four subunits of the receptor contribute to the unique high affinity site for noncompetitive blockers (104, 125, 179, 198, 199, 201), and its simplest location is the central hydrophilic funnel (visualized by electron microscopy in the axis of quasi-symmetry of the molecule) where the distances to all five chains are minimal (109) (Fig. 1). Since binding of ligands to this site blocks the ion channel when it opens, it appears likely (though still hypothetical) that it is related, and even possibly belongs, to this channel. The amino acid labeled by chlorpromazine at the level of its high-affinity site on the δ-subunit has been identified by photolabeling as serine 262 (93). This amino acid belongs to the putative transmembrane hydrophobic segment referred to as helix II (58, 71, 192). This segment is clearly nonhomologous of the peptides of the α-subunit labeled by affinity labeling reagents of the agonist binding site which are located in the NH2-terminal large hydrophilic domain (70, 126). Accordingly, the interaction between the acetylcholine binding site and the high-affinity site for noncompetitive blockers would be indirect or allosteric and mediated by conformational transition of the receptor molecule.

In parallel, rapid kinetic analysis of fluorescent (110, 209) or radioactive agonist binding (30, 183) and channel opening (114, 119, 184) leads to the distinction of two main categories of conformational transitions: 1) the still unresolved primary reaction of *activation*, which results in the opening of the ion channel in the micro-to-millisecond time scale; and 2) slower secondary transitions referred to as *desensitization*, which regulate the ability of the receptor molecule to be activated and are resolved in a minimum of two processes (80, 114, 183, 230, 273, 274) – a fast one, at the rate of 2-75 s^{-1}, and a slow one, at the rate of 0.01-0.1 s^{-1}. The rapid phase leads to a 1,000-fold decrease in initial flux, the slow one to undetectable ion transport (review (119)). Very slow transitions on the time scale of several hours have been recently demonstrated (43), yet their relationship to the state of opening of the ion channel remains unclear.

The simplest minimal model (111, 184), which fits the rapid binding and flux data, is an adapted version of the concerted model for allosteric transitions (178), and that proposed in a different context by Katz and Thesleff (133) for pharmacological desensitization:

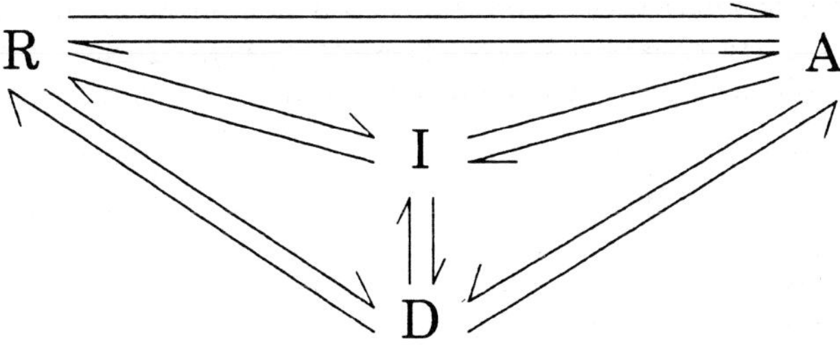

where A corresponds to the active state, with the channel open, and I and D correspond respectively to the rapidly and slowly desensitized states. All these states are discrete, interconvertible, and for some of them A (124) and D (110) are present *before* ligand binding. Their respective dissociation constants are 50-100 μM (R), less than 1 μM (I), and up to 5 nM (D) for the fluorescent agonist dansyl 6 choline (110) and acetylcholine (30). Under resting conditions, in the absence of agonist, the R state would be dominant.

During physiological transmission the cleft concentration of acetylcholine rapidly jumps up to 0.1-1 mM, yielding near saturation of the R state. On the other hand, exposure to low concentrations of acetylcholine yields the high-affinity, D, state with a dissociation constant which interestingly falls in the range of the non-quantal leak concentration of acetylcholine in the synaptic cleft (132).

In agreement with the model, the noncompetitive blockers shift the receptor towards the D state to greater or lesser extents, depending on the structure of the compound and its relative affinity for the R and D states and via their high-affinity site and/or their multiple, low affinity, lipid-dependent ones (109). In both cases the noncompetitive blockers behave as regulatory ligands of the response to acetylcholine. Ca^{2+} ions also play this role. At equilibrium they preferentially stabilize the D state (59, 110) but also accelerate the slow transition towards the same state (197). Substance P enhances desensitization in cells derived from the neural crest (57, 252). Electric fields also affect these transitions: hyperpolarization accelerates rapid desensitization while depolarization has the opposite effect (see ref. in (258)).

A Model of Short-term Regulation of Synapse Efficacy

The basic postulate directly inspired from the mentioned allosteric properties of the acetylcholine receptor (48, 53, 112) is that the response efficacy of neuronal receptors is governed by the ratio of a minimum of two conformations of the receptor: an activatable A and an inactivatable (desensitized) I which are discrete, present before ligand binding, and interconvertible within a time scale several orders of magnitude longer than that of the activation reaction, and differ by their relative affinities for the various classes of ligands binding to the receptor, by the oriented electrical dipolar moment of the protein, and, of course, by the biological activity which characterizes the A state (channel opening, enzyme activation, etc.). Binding of the different categories of ligands shifts the $A \rightleftharpoons I$ equilibrium to an extent determined by their relative affinities to the A and I states, and electric fields affect the transition as a function of the difference in dipole moment between the states (Fig. 2a).

The model can be applied to multi-protein receptor systems (see (89, 90, 236)) and to ion channels in general which may also be viewed as transmembrane allosteric proteins (see (42, 190, 259)). The short-term transitions may be extended to longer time scales by covalent modifications such as phosphorylation (see section on *Phosphorylation*, (67, 182, 247, 267), and Carew, this volume).

Since receptors for neurotransmitters and ion channels in the adult have a defined and stable distribution, such membrane-bound allosteric proteins may spatially integrate multiple converging signals. The signals could be either the principal neurotransmitter released by the overlying nerve ending or coexisting neuronal messengers such as peptides (see (89, 90, 121)) which may originate from the same or neighboring nerve terminal or varicosity. To these "external" primary signals might be added "internal" second messengers (see (182)) produced by closely located synapses on their cytoplasmic face or by "ambient" signals such as hormones (see (89, 256)). Finally, the electrical potential of the postsynaptic cell, and in particular (though not necessarily) the action potential, may serve as "global" signals regulating the allosteric transitions of a given receptor or ion channel as a function of the whole state of activity of the cell.

Timing relationships between multiple ligands are known to exist at the level of the catalytic site of enzymes with several substrates. They are evident in the case of regulatory proteins, the functions of which are governed by cooperative transitions simultaneously affecting the binding properties of *several* categories of sites (53, 110) (Fig. 2b).

In short, membrane-bound allosteric receptors and ion channels may mediate the integrations in space *and* time of multiple signals from both the outside *and* inside of nerve cells, thus making possible their association.

Application of the Model to Experimental Systems

The basic kinetic equations of the model have been derived (53, 112) and computer simulations obtained for specific cases. In Fig. 2 "efficacy" has been expressed in terms of n_a, the fraction of receptors (or ion channels) in the activatable conformation (A), compared to a critical value, n_{ac}, above which the local change of membrane potential will be sufficient to either trigger or prevent action potential generation at the hillock of the neuron.

Homosynaptic regulation. The state of activity of the considered synapse regulates the fraction of its own postsynaptic receptors in the activatable conformation. The neurotransmitter and/or a co-released messenger may exhibit a preferential affinity either for the desensitized state, thereby leading to depression, or, alternatively, for the activatable state resulting in facilitation or potentiation (Fig. 2c1 and Fig. 3).

The data of Magleby and Pallota (157) on the neuromuscular junction can simply be accounted for by such a model (53). In this particular case, repetitive release of acetylcholine (at a rather high but still physiological frequency) leads to the acceleration of rapid desensitization and to a reversible short-term decrease of response amplitude.

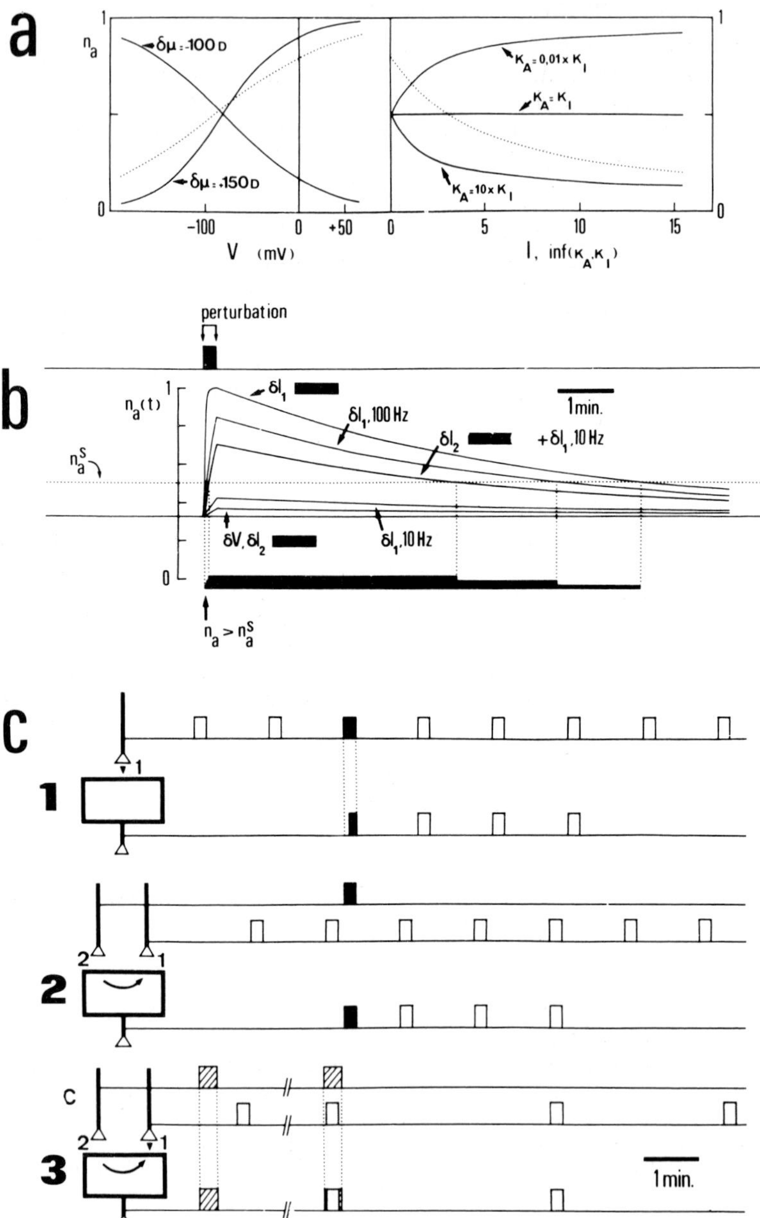
a
n_a
$\delta\mu = -100$ D
$\delta\mu = +150$ D
$K_A = 0,01 \times K_I$
$K_A = K_I$
$K_A = 10 \times K_I$
-100
0
+50
V (mV)
0
5
10
15
I, inf(K_A,K_I)
b
perturbation
$n_a(t)$
n_a^s
δI_1
δI_1, 100 Hz
δI_2
$+\delta I_1$, 10 Hz
1 min.
δV, δI_2
δI_1, 10 Hz
$n_a > n_a^s$
c
1
2
3
C
1 min.

FIG. 2 – A model of regulation of synapse efficacy based on the allosteric transitions of a postsynaptic receptor (from (50, 111)).

a) Variation of the fractional concentration n_a of receptors in the activatable conformation as a function of the transmembrane electrical potential, V, and of the concentration, l, of endogenous effector. Left: variation of n_a (V,0) as a function of V for two values of the change $\delta\mu$, of the electrical dipolar moment normal to the plane of the membrane associated with the I $\rightleftharpoons$ A interconversion; arbitrarily $n_a = 0.5$ when V = 80 mV. The dotted line represents the variation of n_a (V,0) for the acetylcholine receptor calculated from the rates of desensitization measured *in vivo* at the neuromuscular junction and from n_a at zero membrane electrical potential measured *in vitro* on acetylcholine receptor-rich membrane fragments from *Torpedo*. Right: variation of n_a (0,1) as a function of l calculated from $K_A = K_I$, $K_A = 10xK_I$, and $K_A = 0.01xK_I$ with inf (K_A, K_I) as the units for the abscissa; arbitrarily $n_a = 0.5$ in the absence of effector. The dotted line represents the variation of n_a (0,1) for the cholinergic receptor and acetylcholine measured *in vitro* ($K_I = 2$ nM, $K_A = 70$ µM, n_a (0,0) = 0,8).

b) Variation of the fractional concentration n_a of receptors in the activatable conformation as a function of time for square-pulse perturbations or perturbations "in burst" of variable frequency. Variation of n_a calculated from equations (2) and (4) in (111) for square-pulse perturbations of 15 s duration and from equations (4) and (5) in (111) for perturbations "in burst" of identical duration and composed of square pulses of 2 ms duration. The rate constants k_+ and k_- were chosen respectively equal to 0.002 and 0.001 s^{-1} in the absence of effector, to 0.002 and 0.5 s^{-1} in the presence of l_1 and to 0.002 and 0.005 s^{-1} in the presence of l_2 at the same membrane potential. A change of 100 D in the electrical dipolar moment associated with the I $\rightleftharpoons$ A interconversion was selected, and a variation of 100 mV of the transmembrane electrical potential for the δV perturbation. The threshold value,

$$n_a^s$$

is arbitrarily equal to 0.5 and the time interval is represented on the figure for the various perturbations when

$$n_a^s > n_{ac}.$$

c) 1) Homosynaptic regulation, 2) heterosynaptic regulation, and 3) classical conditioning. The efficacy of synapse 2 is assumed to be invariant; the receptor of synapse 1 and the effectors l_1 and l_2 have identifical properties to those in Fig. 2b. The presynaptic stimuli are square-pulses (▨), or "bursts" of 1 Hz (□), 10 Hz (⊡), or 50 Hz (■). The receptors of synapse 1 are regulated by the effector l_1 released by the presynaptic terminal of synapse 1 (case 1) by the effector l_2 released by synapse 2 (case 2), or by both (case 3).

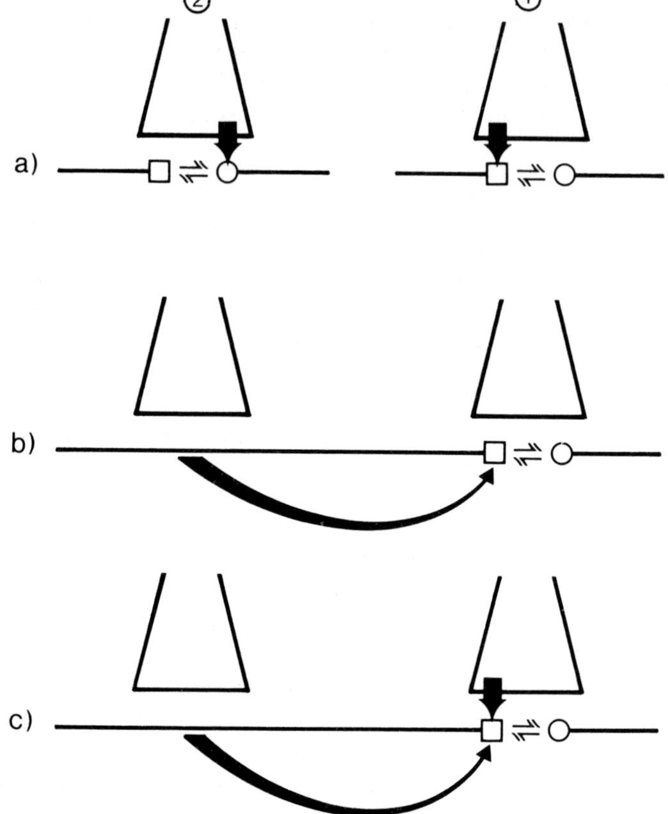

FIG. 3 – Schematic representation of the differential effect of external and internal signals on two allosteric states of the postsynaptic receptor under the conditions described in Fig. 1. a) Homosynaptic depression and facilitation, b) heterosynaptic facilitation, and c) classical conditioning and Hebb synapse.

Heterosynaptic regulations. The efficacy n_a of one synapse (1) is regulated by the activity of another synapse (2) via an external (or internal) messenger and in the direction of a facilitation (or of a depression). In the case of Fig. 2c (2 and 3) and Fig. 3 (b and c), two situations have been considered. In one case (Fig. 2c, $2c_2$), the postsynaptic receptor from synapse 1 is regulated exclusively by signals originating from synapse 2 (Fig. 3b). In the other (Fig. 2c, $2c_3$) two signals, one released by the terminal of synapse 1 and the other emitted by synapse 2, converge on the receptor of synapse 1 (Fig. 3c). Interestingly, in the first case, no stringent timing relationships are required between the firings of synapse 1 and 2 to change the efficacy of synapse 1. On the other hand, in the second case (Fig. 2c, $2c_3$), the coincidence of the firings of synapses 1 and 2 is required for a change of efficacy to occur at synapse 1. This last scheme is analogous to classical conditioning and can equally lead to a potentiation or a depression.

This second scheme may plausibly account for the heterosynaptic depression of the parallel fiber-Purkinje cell synapse which occurs in the cerebellum as a consequence of its concomitant firing with the climbing fiber synapse ((123) and Ito, this volume). Also, the joint activation of the serotonin-linked adenylate cyclase by both serotonin (released by an interneuron) and intracellullar Ca^{2+}, raised by the firing of the postsynaptic (sensory) cell and postulated as the central mechanism of cellular conditioning in *Aplysia* (see (106, 107) and Carew, this volume), might be tentatively interpreted in similar terms. In both cases the neurotransmitter released presynaptically and an internal postsynaptic signal (e.g., Ca^{2+}) might be viewed as stabilizing in a cooperative (or synergistic) manner, a privileged conformation of the receptor-channel or -enzyme complex: a desensitized state in the case of the Purkinje cell, an activatable one in the case of *Aplysia*. The postsynaptic receptor thus serves as a "molecular integrator" in time and space of multiple converging signals. It yields a simple molecular device which accounts for Hebb's general rules of topological convergence and time-coincidence as a prerequisite for the establishment of an associative link.

Finally, the model may also account for eventual effects of the electrical activity of the postsynaptic neuron on the receptors present on its own surface, since the allosteric transitions of the postsynaptic receptor might be sensitive to electric fields. It fits with the recent observation and interpretation of Wigström and Gustafsson (279) (see Andersen, this volume) about long-term potentiation in the hippocampus. They assign to the transition of the voltage-sensitive, transmitter-dependent N-methyl-D-aspartate (glutamate) receptor an "active" conformation as a consequence of the simultaneous presynaptic transmitter release and postsynaptic depolarization. The model also takes into account the actual firing of the postsynaptic cell.

ACTIVITY-DEPENDENT REGULATION OF THE BIOSYNTHESIS OF THE ACETYLCHOLINE RECEPTOR AND OTHER POSTSYNAPTIC PROTEINS

The second part of this paper no longer deals with reversible structural properties of the acetylcholine receptor in the time range of milliseconds to hours. We are concerned here with longer-term, activity-dependent changes in receptor number which are known to occur in the course of the development of the motor endplate. Even though a large part of this development takes place *in ovo* or *in utero*, several of its steps may be regulated by the neurally elicited activity of the muscle and of its innervation. In chick embryo, for example, spontaneous movements appear around day 3.5 of incubation, reach a peak by around 13-16 days, and are of neurogenic origin (102, 216). Even growth cones release acetylcholine (56, 60, 134).

In vertebrate embryonic muscle fibers, before the arrival of the exploratory motor axons, the acetylcholine receptor is diffusely distributed along the whole fiber, exhibits significant lateral motion (10), possesses rapid turnover time (half-life 17-22 hours) (16, 44, 72), and the mean open time of its ionic channel is 3-10 ms (131, 181). In contrast, in the adult muscle the acetylcholine receptor is highly localized at the endplate with a density about 1,000 times higher than in nonsynaptic areas (28, 163, 231), is immobile (27, 28, 85, 219, 220), turns over slowly (half-life ~ 10 days or more), and possesses (except in birds) a mean open time 3-5 times shorter than the embryonic receptor and an intrinsic conductance significantly larger (see section on *Clustering, Stabilization, and Chemical Maturation of the Acetylcholine Receptor and Other Postsynaptic Proteins*).

The development of the endplate thus involves two main parallel processes: 1) the local aggregation, stabilization, and maturation of the acetylcholine receptor (and other proteins) under the motor nerve ending; and 2) elimination of the extrajunctional receptor. Only the latter process, which involves an activity-dependent regulation of receptor number, will be discussed in this chapter.

Regulation by Electrical Activity of Extrajunctional Receptor Biosynthesis

In the developing muscle the evolution of the acetylcholine receptor content consists of three main phases (review (47, 79, 172)). First, the receptor content increases in a dramatic manner (19, 20, 27, 36, 37, 91) and this accumulation, which can be reproduced with primary cultures of myoblasts ((202), review (168)), coincides with their fusion into myotubes. It involves a *de novo* synthesis of receptor molecules as demonstrated by the incorporation of radioactive (169, 173) or heavy isotope (72, 73) labeled amino acids into the receptor protein. Chronic injection of neuromuscular blocking agents *in ovo* does not significantly affect this initial onset.

The second phase of the evolution corresponds to a significant decrease of receptor content which starts around day 15 in chick embryo (breast muscle) (19, 20, 36, 37) and parallels the elimination of extrajunctional receptor (19). Such a decrease might possibly result either from an enhanced degradation of the receptor, for instance, as a consequence of the inversion of electrical potential (253), or from a repression of its biosynthesis. Measurements of the metabolic degradation rate of the receptor throughout this evolution show that this rate does not change. Thus a *repression of receptor biosynthesis* takes place (19, 20, 36, 37). Interestingly, this regulation becomes effective soon after the newly formed endplates start to transmit nerve impulses.

To test for a contribution of the spontaneous neurogenic activity of the muscle fibers in this repression, chick embryos were chronically paralyzed by botulinum toxin (92), d-tubocurarine (36, 37), or flaxedil (20, 27). Unambiguously, chronic paralysis maintains a high receptor content without changing its degradation rate. The neurally evoked spontaneous activity of the embryonic muscles is thus responsible for the disappearance of the acetylcholine receptor in nonjunctional areas. A similar activity-dependent regulation can be reproduced in the adult as a consequence of denervation (review (79, 101, 105, 156) and Lømo, this volume) and in chick embryonic myotubes in culture by blocking their spontaneous electrical activity with tetrodoxin (21, 244).

The observed changes of receptor content are accompanied by changes in specific mRNA assayed with α-subunit cDNA probes. In adult mouse or rat muscle after denervation (95, 170) the content in α-subunit mRNA increases between 7-fold in rat diaphragm (95) to 50- to 100-fold in mouse leg muscle (170). In the case of chick mytotubes in culture, blocking of spontaneous electrical activity by tetrodotoxin causes an approximate 13-fold increase in α-subunit mRNA (135) whereas surface receptor augments only 2- to 3-fold. The activity-dependent regulation of receptor biosynthesis thus primarily affects mRNA production, most likely at the level of transcription (an additional effect on mRNA stability yet cannot be excluded).

Southern blot hybridization indicates the existence of a single locus for the α-subunit in chick (135), mouse (172), and *Torpedo* (136). Thus the activity-dependent regulation of acetylcholine receptor biosynthesis affects, at least for the α-subunit, the expression of a single copy gene coding for a polypeptide chain common to *both* junctional and extrajunctional receptor (see, in addition, the section on *Intrinsic and*

Extrinsic Modifications of the Acetylcholine Receptor As Potential Elements for Long-term Changes of Endplate Properties).

At the third and latest stage of endplate formation in the adult, new molecules of receptor are steadily inserted into the postsynaptic membrane but not into extrajunctional areas, and the total number of receptor molecules may increase up to 30-fold (165). Muscle fibers contain multiple nuclei, some of which (about 1%) appear closely associated with the endplate (63). This raises the possibility that the receptor genes are differentially expressed in junctional and non-junctional nuclei. Indeed, synapse-rich and synapse-free samples of mouse diaphragm contain different amounts of acetylcholine receptor α- and δ-subunit mRNA (2- to 14-fold) (171). A differential transcription of acetylcholine receptor genes may thus take place in subsynaptic vs. extrasynaptic nuclei, although differential mRNA stability could also play a role.

Neural Regulation of Other Muscle Proteins Biosynthesis

Denervation and/or paralysis of skeletal muscle in the adult (or in the embryo) may (or may not) affect the production of distinct groups of proteins in addition to the acetylcholine receptor (Table I).

First, the muscle content in a vast majority of proteins grouped under the name Family I does not significantly change after denervation (at least before the onset of muscle atrophy). It includes, in addition to the housekeeping proteins, most of the contractile proteins (some of which are nevertheless neurally regulated) (see (162), and Lømo, this volume).

A second group of proteins referred to as Family II evolves in a manner similar, if not identical, to the acetylcholine receptor. Among the best studied are the several species of voltage-sensitive Na^+ channels (42, 86, 246). In cultured rat muscle, chronic blockade of the spontaneous electrical activity leads to a nearly twofold increase in the sarcolemmal density of the tetrodotoxin-sensitive species (245) without change of its metabolic half-life (246). Also, their density immediately adjacent to the endplate is 5- to 10-fold higher (expressed as Na currents) than in nonjunctional areas (15).

In addition, denervation (and/or blocking of synaptic transmission) increases the production by the muscle of several proteins involved in endplate formation and stabilization, in particular a neurite outgrowth promoting factor active on chick spinal neurons ((116-118), see also Henderson, this volume) and the cell adhesion molecule N-CAM (64, 215). A similar regulation may also affect some basal lamina

TABLE 1 - Patterns of genes expressed in embryonic and adult junctional and extrajunctional nuclei.

Proteins	Nucleus Type			DNA regulatory sequence
	embryonic	extra-junctional	junctional	
Family I "housekeeping" contractile	+	+	+ (?)	M
Family II Acetylcholine receptor, Na^+ channel, muscle growth factor, N-CAM	+	-	+	MAN
Family III Acetylcholinesterase forms	+	+ (or -)	+	MAN

components (see (232)). Finally, the cytoskeletal 43KD protein v_1, which selectively interacts with the acetylcholine receptor on its cytoplasmic face (41, 87, 140, 186, 248), is also a potential candidate for such a regulation. Yet for most of them the actual demonstration that electrical activity regulates their biosynthesis is still lacking (see Henderson, this volume, for discussion).

A third group of proteins, referred to as Family III, is composed of the different molecular forms of the acetylcholine degradative enzyme acetylcholinesterase (review (153, 161)). In the chick, paralysis of the embryo by injection of snake venom α-toxin in the egg yolk from day 3 to 12 causes a disappearance of endplate acetylcholinesterase detected by the Koelle method ((91), see also (20, 27, 196)). After chronic paralysis *in vivo*, or motor neuron-muscle co-cultures *in vitro* (224, 225, 269-271), the heavy 16-19.5 S form disappears (but cf. (250)). Conversely, electrical stimulation of the muscle (154, 155, 224, 225) reverses this effect. Activity of the muscle thus regulates the production and localization of endplate heavy form of acetylcholinesterase in a direction opposite to that of the extrajunctional receptor and of the proteins from Family II. Since chronic blocking of the endplate interferes with the localization of the esterase to a larger extent than with that of the receptor (20, 27, 22), it yields functional junctions but with a "modified" endplate potential ((225), see also (146)), thus offering a postsynaptic model for long-term change of synapse efficacy without any necessary change in receptor property (see Lømo, this volume).

Intracellular Second Messengers Linking Membrane Electrical Activity and Acetylcholine Receptor (and Other Muscle Proteins) Gene Expression

The intracellular second messenger(s) which link(s) the electrical activity of the muscle cell with gene expression has (have) not yet been identified with certainty. Studies with the mouse mutant muscular dysgenesis, where electrical activity still regulates acetylcholine receptor biosynthesis despite uncoupling of the excitation-contraction process, makes a major contribution of muscle mechanical activity to this particular regulation unlikely.

A role of Ca^{2+} (and/or Na^{+}) ions which enter the voltage-sensitive Na^{+} channel during activity has been suggested in the case of the acetylcholine receptor (21, 22, 83, 166, 167, 205, 210, 222, 276), the tetrodotoxin-sensitive Na^{+} channel (245, 246), and acetylcholinesterase (222). In cultured muscle cells the calcium ionophore A23187 may cause a marked reduction of the density of both acetylcholine receptor (167) (after prior elevation by TTX treatment) and Na^{+} channels (245) and an increase in the production of acetylcholinesterase (222). Similar results are obtained with Ryanodin, an alkaloid which at low concentrations elicits the release of Ca^{2+} from the sarcoplasmic reticulum without a generalized ionophoric action (205, 246). Cytosolic Ca^{2+} thus appears to be involved in this regulation. Also, anti-calmodulin agents such as trifluoroperazine exert an effect in a direction opposite to that of Ca^{2+} (235, 246), supporting a mediation of the Ca^{2+} effect via calmodulin.

Ascorbic acid has been shown to cause a three- to fivefold increase in acetylcholine receptor content of cultured myogenic L_5 line (139) accompanied by a dramatic increase in α-subunit mRNA without change of myosin light chain two (LC_2) mRNA (138). In frog and mammalian skeletal muscles, ascorbic acid levels are low (~50 μ/gm of tissue) but increase up to two-fold five days after denervation (in rat) (see (139)).

A contribution of cyclic nucleotides as second messengers has also been suggested (21, 226). The addition of dibutyryl cAMP to chick muscle cells in culture increases the number of surface acetylcholine receptor (21, 25) whereas dibutyryl cGMP has the opposite effect ((21) but cf. (25, 167)). A similar increase by 8 bromo cAMP occurs in the case of the Na^+ channel in cultured rat muscle cells, although in this system dibutyryl cGMP has no effect (246). On the other hand, dibutyryl cGMP and/or electrical stimulation promotes the production of acetylcholinesterase heavy form ((153-155, 224, 225), see Lømo, this volume). An eventual link between the Ca^{2+}-dependent and cyclic nucleotide-dependent regulatory systems has been suggested (18, 21, 246). However, an increase of intracellular cAMP brings about a general stimulation of cellular protein synthesis in addition to that of the channel proteins ((21) but cf. (25, 167)) which is not observed upon blocking electrical activity or ascorbic acid treatment. cAMP action thus appears more "pleiotropic" than that of intracellular Ca^{2+} suggesting a parallel rather than sequential effect of these two putative second messengers.

Finally, depolarization is known to induce inositol phosphate turnover in several tissues including smooth muscle (see ref. in (17, 187)), yet the contribution of inositol phospholipids in the activity-dependent regulation of skeletal muscle proteins appears plausible but remains to be investigated.

Models for the Activity-dependent Regulation of Muscle Protein Biosynthesis

In the course of embryonic development, two main classes of regulatory mechanisms at the gene level have been distinguished: 1) the determination (or commitment) of sets of genes characteristic of a given cell category (e.g., skeletal muscle vs. mesenchymal cell) which involves a transition of the local conformation of the chromatin switching a specific gene from a buried "closed" conformation to an "open" or "ready-to-be-transcribed" state and, conversely (see Yaniv, this volume), 2) the actual transcription of the open genes into RNA and the processing export and stabilization (vs. destabilization) of the mature mRNA, which are the initial steps in the expression of the determined genes into proteins, globally referred to as differentiation.

We will be concerned here exclusively with the second of these processes, i.e., the regulation of the expression of already determined genes. As discussed in the case of the nerve cells (see (48)), the number of determined genes may be larger than the number of those actually transcribed by a given differentiated cell nucleus. One may hypothesize that this is indeed the case in skeletal muscle for the extrajunctional nuclei compared to the junctional ones and possibly of the adult junctional nuclei compared to the embryonic ones (see (171)). Accordingly, the pattern of genes actively transcribed would correspond to a selection among the population of determined genes (48). A minimum of three differentiated states of these nuclei may thus be distinguished on the basis of the genes expressed and of the regulatory elements involved (Fig. 2).

In the embryonic state (which may include several substates to account for the various patterns of contractile proteins observed), a large majority of the determined genes are transcribed including those coding for the contractile proteins, the channel proteins, the esterases, and the synapse formation proteins (i.e., Families I, II, and III). These genes are turned on at the early stages of myoblasts/myotubes differentiation. A set of *cis*-acting DNA sequences (marked M in Fig. 4) would then be involved, and one may envision that some of the relevant *trans*-acting proteins are directly or indirectly regulated by cyclic AMP or other pleiotropic second messengers.

In the adult extrajunctional nuclei the genes of Family I and III are switched on and those of Family II switched off. As a consequence the muscle fiber becomes refractory to innervation. Specific DNA sequences, marked **A** in Fig. 4, may be postulated and the second messengers directly or indirectly acting on the concerned regulatory proteins might include Ca^{2+} and/or ascorbic acid.

In the adult junctional nuclei the genes of Family II are switched on as those of Family III, yet little can be said about their ability to express contractile proteins. On the other hand, the steady-state production of the "synapse formation" proteins, in particular of MNGF, might be essential for the maintenance of the synapse, in particular of the motor axon terminal. The second messengers involved at the subneural level are able to counteract the effect of electrical activity on the expression of the Family II genes. Distinct signals are thus involved in these two regulations. The nature of the anterograde signals released by the nerve is not known: neuronal coexisting messengers such as calcitonin-gene-related-peptide (CGRP) (121), ascorbic acid, and of course acetylcholine are possible candidates. A pending question is whether the internal "second messengers" involved affect the same regulatory protein as that acting on the sequences **A** (but in opposite direction as

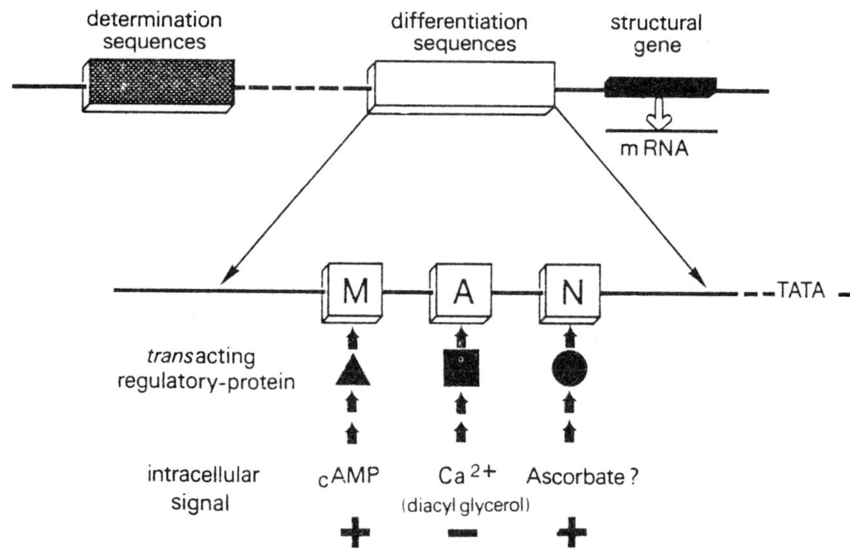

FIG. 4 – Schematic representation of *hypothetical* regulatory DNA sequences regulating the expression of muscle-specific genes. **M** stands for the DNA sequences responsible for the turning-on, at some stage of myoblast/myotube differentiation, of muscle-specific genes of all three Families (see text). cAMP may play a role in this process. **A** represents the activity-sensitive element(s) involved in the control of Family II and Family III genes (a subdivision may, however, exist between the two families) by muscle electrical activity. Ca^{2+} ions most likely play a role in the signalling pathway leading to this control element and are responsible for turning off class II genes in the extrasynaptic nuclei as a consequence of electrical activity. **N** is perhaps the most speculative feature of this model and is introduced to account for persisting class II gene expression in the junctional nuclei of electrically active muscle. It is equally plausible that neural control is achieved by interfering with the activity-dependent regulation at any one of its steps (up to and including the binding of the relevant *trans*-activating factor(s) to the **A** element) or even that junctional nuclei are not accessible to this regulatory pathway, e.g., because of their special assocation with the endplate subneural apparatus.

Ca^{2+}) or whether an additional regulatory protein and thus DNA sequence (marked **N** in Fig. 4) are involved.

The extension of these models to nerve cells remains speculative (48). Activity-dependent regulation of protein biosynthesis has been described for enzymes of neurotransmitter biosynthesis such as tyrosine hydroxylase (see Thoenen, this volume; (158)), for neuropeptides (see (23, 24)), and for the acetylcholine receptor (18). Denervation hypersensitivity has been reported in the case of peripheral (145) and central (see (242)) neurons but may result from changes in the production of neurotransmitter degradative enzymes (74) rather than, or in addition to, neurotransmitter receptors. Moreover, the regulation will concern a unique postmitotic nucleus. Nevertheless, such activity-dependent regulation of gene expression might be critical for the selection of the adult phenotype of the nerve cell, i.e., the pattern of transmitters it synthesizes and releases, of receptors it produces, and of growth factors it liberates. It may as well play a role in the long-term regulation of this phenotype in the adult brain. To account for the polarity of the nerve cell and the highly anisotropic distribution of its components, in particular of its receptors for neurotransmitters, additional "epigenetic" posttranscriptional mechanisms have to be postulated for their "targeting" and for their eventual local modulation by activity (see below and (48, 51) for discussion). Finally, the time range of such activity-dependent effects on number of molecules will be limited by the metabolic half-life of the relevant molecules, i.e., in the order of a day for extrajunctional receptor. Additional mechanisms have to be postulated to account for their long-term resistance to turnover (see below).

LONG-TERM POSTSYNAPTIC CHANGES IN THE DEVELOPING MOTOR ENDPLATE

Concomitant with the elimination of the extrajunctional receptor, the postsynaptic membrane differentiates under the motor nerve ending. Before the arrival of the exploratory motor axons, the components of the postsynaptic membrane (acetylcholine receptor, acetylcholinesterase, N-CAM, 43,000 protein, and other cytoskeletal proteins) are present in a dispersed form in the muscle cell. The contact of the growth cone with the surface of the sarcolemma rapidly causes their clustering, followed (at least for some of them) by a metabolic stabilization and eventually a change of functional properties. This "assemblage" and "maturation" of the postsynaptic membrane may to some extent be regulated by the activity of the neuromuscular junction, at least by two distinct mechanisms: 1) the direct regulation of their assemblage into a defined supramolecular organization, and 2) the availability of these components and, in particular, the size of their "stock" in the muscle cell when the synapses form. Still, only limited information is available on the molecular mechanisms involved, yet several biochemical reactions known to affect the properties of the acetylcholine receptor might plausibly take part in these processes.

Clustering, Stabilization, and Chemical Maturation of the Acetylcholine Receptor and Other Postsynaptic Proteins: Effects of Activity

A few hours after the growth cone from a cholinergic neuron contacts a skeletal muscle fiber *in vitro*, the surface density of acetylcholine receptors increases in the postsynaptic membrane up to more than tenfold (4, 84, 217) as a consequence of the migration and local aggregation of receptor molecules diffusely distributed in the muscle membrane (4, 5, 148, 283) and, in some systems, the preferential insertion of newly formed receptor molecules at the junctional site (39, 217).

The anterograde signal(s) responsible for the patching of acetylcholine receptors (investigated with neuron-muscle co-cultures) is most likely not acetylcholine but a coexisting molecule whose biosynthesis is co-regulated with that of the proteins engaged in acetylcholine metabolism (237). A component of the basal lamina from *Torpedo californica* electric organ, which causes acetylcholine receptor to aggregate in chick myotubes (188) and is antigenically similar to molecules concentrated at neuromuscular junctions (78), is a plausible candidate for such a factor, among many others (6, 233). However, postively charged latex beads elicit, in the absence of nerve, postsynaptic differentiations resembling the folded subneural apparatus of a rather mature motor endplate (203, 204).

The accumulation of acetylcholinesterase in the basal lamina (165) of the developing endplates closely follows that of the acetylcholine receptor in the subneural sarcolemma (19, 155, 223, 225) and is elicited by the same aggregating factor from the basal lamina (275).

The metabolic stabilization of the acetylcholine receptor does not coincide but rather follows its aggregation with a significant delay (36, 37, 81, 224, 225, 240): about 2.5 weeks after hatching in the chick (20, 36, 37) or just before birth in rat or mouse diaphragm (16, 149, 174, 213, 254). Similarly, in non-innervated muscle, the esterases turn over with a half life of about ~ 50 h (218), while in the adult the junctional esterases have a metabolic half-life of about 20 days (129).

During the development of the endplates the physiological and pharmacological properties of the acetylcholine receptor undergo significant changes. The most significant one is the threefold decrease of mean open time of the ionic channel (from about 4.5-1.5 ms) (81, 229) which follows the metabolic stabilization of the receptor protein in frog and rat (between postnatal days 8-18 in rat soleus) (229), but not in birds (238), and affects both junctional and nonjunctional receptors (145, 239).

In rat (but not in *Xenopus* (147)) denervation at birth arrests, or at least delays, the developmental decrease in channel mean open time (239) and electrical stimulation of the muscle restores its normal evolution ((31), Lømo, this volume). A control of ion channel kinetics by the type of innervating axon has been recently demonstrated in parasympathetic ganglion cells (160). Channel conversion thus appears as a candidate mechanism for neurally evoked long-term changes of synaptic properties.

The topology of the endplates in skeletal muscle fibers does not show diversity or variability comparable to that of the synapses on a nerve cell. A rather original situation is nevertheless offered with the chick wing muscles, *latissimus dorsi*, which receive two distinct types of innervation (29). The slow anterior muscle (ALD) shows several endplates distributed at approximately equal distances along the muscle fiber, whereas the fast posterior muscle (PLD) receives a single focal endplate in the middle of the fiber. Cross-innervation experiments in the embryo have shown that the nerve, not the muscle, determines the pattern of endplates (120, 282), and during development the programs of neurally evoked spontaneous activity differ in the two muscles. In 15-day-old embryos the ALD shows a sustained low activity of around 0.2-1 Hz, whereas the PLD shows high-frequency bursts of activity around 8 Hz interrupted by periods of silence (97).

Electric pulses delivered to the spinal cord by chronically implanted electrodes at 0.5 Hz frequency from day 10-15 of incubation cause a significant increase (by a factor of 1.8-2.0) in the number of clusters of acetylcholine receptor (265) and of patches of acetylcholinesterase activity (266) per individual PLD muscle fiber and per total PLD muscle. However, the distribution of the multiple clusters of acetylcholine receptor which appear in the normally focal-innervated PLD is not as regular as in ALD.

A theoretical mechanism (50) has been proposed to account for the epigenetic dependence of the ALD and PLD synaptic topologies upon the afferent input on the basis of the management of a finite and limited stock of receptor via a) the interconversion of the receptor protein into a form which aggregates under a nerve terminal but still diffuses laterally in the nerve membrane and b) the release by the nerve endings of an "anterograde factor" which triggers this interconversion in amounts directly linked to the afferent message. The computer simulation of the model confirms that the biochemical hypotheses made are sufficient to obtain a distibuted pattern of acetylcholine receptor clusters when the afferent message is continuous and a focal pattern when it occurs in bursts.

Intrinsic and Extrinsic Modifications of the Acetylcholine Receptor as Potential Elements for Long-term Changes of Endplate Properties

The correlation of the elementary steps of the postsynaptic membrane genesis and long-term maturation with defined molecular processes remains fragmentary. However, recent progress on the biochemistry and physical chemistry of the membrane-bound and purified receptor offers possible candidate mechanisms for such changes, which might tentatively be used as "building blocks" to elaborate models for long-term changes of synaptic properties. They might be classified as either "intrinsic" covalent modifications of the receptor molecule or "extrinsic" differences in membrane environment (228).

Immunoreactivity toward myasthenic sera. Early work on the purified junctional and extrajunctional (or embryonic) receptor from muscle revealed few intrinsic differences between the two categories of receptor (3, 33, 34, 61, 88, 180) except their reactivity with antireceptor antibodies from patients with *Myasthenia gravis* (2, 150, 277). Hall and collaborators (100) have recently found, among 35 sera from myasthenic patients, one which interferes with the binding of ^{125}I α-bungarotoxin to extrajunctional receptor from denervated muscle or C2 mouse muscle cell line (99) but has no effect on the binding of the toxin to the adult junctional receptor and which silences selectively the channels with long opening times (241, 272). Moreover, in the chick where this type of channel persists in the adult, this serum stains the adult endplate. Thus the postnatal loss of immunoreactivity noticed at the endplate appears directly related to the "conversion" of the ionic channel. However, the antigenic determinants associated with this transition have not yet been identified.

The ε-subunit. The molecular processes occurring during endplate genesis and maturation are complex enough to allow a regulation of gene expression to play a role in addition to that already mentioned in the course of the elimination of the nonjunctional receptor (see section on *ACTIVITY-DEPENDENT REGULATION OF THE BIOSYNTHESIS OF THE ACETYLCHOLINE RECEPTOR AND OTHER POSTSYNAPTIC PROTEINS*). A suggestion in favor of such a possibility is the recent cloning and sequencing of a DNA complementary to a messenger mRNA present in fetal calf which codes for a novel polypeptide called an ε-subunit (257) and shows an amino acid sequence homology with the γ-subunit (according to recent work γ would be "embryonic" at ε "adult").

Disulfide bonding of the receptor light form into heavy form dimer. Reconstitution of the pure acetylcholine receptor heavy and light forms into planar lipid bilayer and statistical analysis of single channels on rat myotubes (279) have shown that two light forms may cooperate within the dimer and undergo simultaneous opening and closing with an overall conductance approximately twice that of a single $\alpha_2\beta\gamma\delta$ oligomer (234). Also, during embryonic and postnatal development of the electric organ the ratio of light/heavy form, initially strongly in favor of the light form, subsequently shifts towards the heavy form dimer which is almost exclusively present in the adult electric organ (122).

Phosphorylation. Early experiments with *E. electricus* crude receptor extracts revealed NaF-sensitive interconversion between two isoelectric forms of the receptor protein suggesting a contribution of phosphorylation-dephosphorylation reactions in this interconversion (260, 261). Phosphorylation of the receptor was subsequently demonstrated by direct *in vitro* incorporation of ^{32}P into the receptor polypeptides (96, 262). Phosphoserines have also been identified by chemical analysis of the purified chains of *T. californica* receptor (268). Finally, several protein kinases have been isolated from extracts of electric organ and shown to phosphorylate respectively the γ and δ chains of the acetylcholine receptor (review (182)) at the level of a peptide located in the COOH-terminal region of the chain. Pharmacological activation of protein kinase C reversibly enhances desensitization of the acetylcholine response of cultured mouse myotubes (77) and *in vitro* phosphorylation accelerates desensitization of *T. californica* purified receptor (Huganir and Greengard).

Phosphorylation also affects structural parameters of the receptor protein. Treatments at acid pH or by *E. coli* alkaline phosphatase under conditions known to dephosphorylate phosphoproteins enhance the susceptibility to heat inactivation of the receptor protein in its membrane-bound and detergent-extracted forms (227, 228), and the state of phosphorylation of the membrane-bound receptor changes during the maturation of the electric organ.

Basal lamina. The role of components of the basal lamina as aggregating factors for the acetylcholine receptor and esterase has already been mentioned. Regeneration experiments in adult frog muscle suggest that the basal lamina plays the role of a long-term organizing matrix under which the receptor molecules are continuously replaced (see above).

43,000 dalton protein and cytoskeleton. In the electric organ a protein with an apparent molecular weight of 43KD on SDS gels (248, 249) is strongly bound to the postsynaptic membrane on its cytoplasmic side (278) and distributes along with the acetylcholine receptor (87, 186, 243). Brief exposure of the receptor-rich membrane to pH 11 (184) or lithium diiodosalicylate (76) releases the 43K protein without significant changes of receptor functional properties (76, 115, 185) but it destabilizes the receptor to heat treatment (228) or proteolytic attack (137) and enhances its motion as monitored with spin-labeled (219-221) or phosphorescent (152) derivatives of α-bungarotoxin via electron microscopy (14, 41). The close relation between intermediate filaments and the 43K protein suggests that this highly insoluble, cystein-rich molecule (249) may serve as an intermediate piece between the cytoskeleton and the postsynaptic membrane (40, 140). It is detected with anti-43K monoclonal antibodies in newly formed acetylcholine receptor clusters at the early steps of synapse formation (38) and as early as 12 hours after application of polypeptide-coated latex beads to cultured *Xenopus laevis* muscle cells, where it accompanies the patches of receptor (204).

The 43K protein can be phosphorylated *in vitro* (226). This opens the possibility of a regulation of the 43K protein attachment to the receptor and/or the cytoskeleton by phosphorylation-dephosphorylation reactions (226, 280).

Models for Long-term Changes of Postsynaptic Properties Resistant to Molecular Turnover

The diverse intrinsic and extrinsic modifications of the acetylcholine receptor mentioned above might be tentatively used in a purely speculative manner as elements to build models for long-term changes of synapse properties at the postsynaptic level. Two categories of models may be *a priori* distinguished. In a first group, the short-term changes are made long lasting within the metabolic lifetime of the constitutive macromolecules of the synapses (see section on *ALLOSTERIC TRANSITIONS OF THE ACETYLCHOLINE RECEPTOR AND MODELS OF SHORT-TERM REGULATION OF SYNAPSE EFFICACY AT THE POSTSYNAPTIC LEVEL*). In a second group, the trace persists beyond the half-life of the components of the postsynaptic membrane (and of the synapse) and thus may be termed "self-sustained" (review (53)). Three of them will be mentioned:

1) **Self-sustained metabolic steady states.** The postsynaptic side of the synapse (or dendritic spine) can be viewed as an open thermodynamic system which may exist under multiple steady states (208). The logical structures which enable such a system to generate multiple steady states have been analyzed in detail (263). The simplest case is pure autocatalysis: a loop with only one, postive element. For instance (53), in addition to the allosteric receptor, nearby in the cytoplasm an enzyme E may exist such that one has the following sequence of reactions:

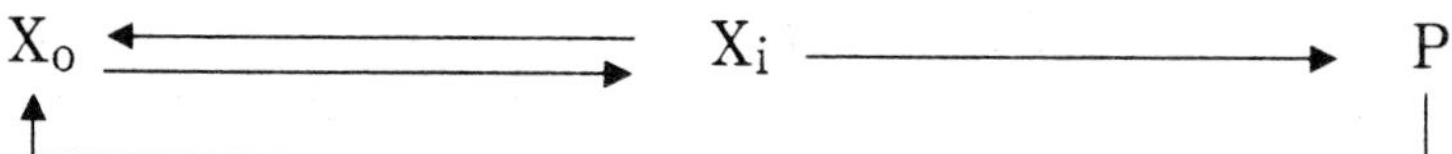

where X is a permeant ion which enters the cytoplasm by the open receptor ion channel ($X_o \rightleftharpoons X_i$) and serves as a substrate (or activator) of the enzyme yielding the compound P. If P now stabilizes the receptor in the A state, a positive feedback loop is established which after a conditioning train of impulses may shift synapse efficacy to a stable state robust to molecular turnover (as long as the steady-state input and the concentrations of enzyme and receptor remain constant). A related mechanism based on a kinase that is activated by phosphorylation and capable of intermolecular autophosphorylation has been recently proposed ((151), see also Kennedy this volume). Other mechanisms might be invented (53). These might include negative feedback loops, but in *even* numbers ((263) but also positive ones (69)), and might affect the state of activity of an enzyme or ion channel, also that of gene repressors and/or activators thus leading to stable switches of gene patterns (177).

2) **Conservation of symmetry in oligomeric protein molecules.** Molecular mechanisms have been identified (212) or postulated (35) for the maintenance (or propagation) of a determined (or differentiated) state of DNA through molecular turnover and/or DNA replication. For instance, propagation of the methylated state of DNA occurs via an enzyme which methylates the "new" strand of the DNA molecule exclusively when the complementary "old" one is methylated (212). A similar mechanism (66) has been proposed for a protein molecule (such as the acetylcholine receptor or an enzyme) that is an essential part of a synapse and can exist in two states (active and inactive), forming a dimer, probably with a twofold rotation axis that can be modified chemically by, for example, the attachment of a phosphate group. For instance, a protein kinase would exist which phosphorylates a freshly replaced monomer in a dimer exclusively when the complementary monomer from the same dimer is in a phosphorylated state, e.g., as a consequence of a former activity-dependent step.

Experimental demonstration of the relative enrichment in dimers of the population of receptor molecules during maturation of the electric organ (122) (see above) does not yet suffice to bring support to this still hypothetical mechanism.

3) **Protein template.** The basal lamina plays the role of an "organizing matrix" in the development of the postsynaptic membrane and thus acts as a "template" for self-sustained changes in receptor properties (review in (53)). A quantitative model for such changes has been developed on the cytoplasmic side in the case of the cytoskeletal 43,000 protein v_1 assumed to interact directly with the receptor. v may exist under two states and only one of them, v_A, cross-links two receptor molecules (280). When it does, the openings of the two channels are no longer independent and the postsynaptic ionic response is potentiated. If the conversion to v_A (for instance, by a phosphorylation) is catalyzed by an enzyme (for instance, a kinase) which is itself activated by an ion which enters the channel of the receptor (for instance, Ca^{2+}), then the postsynaptic potentiation may become self-perpetuating without any covalent modification of the receptor as long as a minimum activity steadily traverses the synapse. Such a mechanism (among many others) illustrates how a long-term "local" modification of synaptic properties may become established at the posttranslational level.

CONCLUSION

In addition to the traditional behavioral approaches, learning may be investigated at several different levels of organization: 1) at the molar level of large cooperative assemblies ((54, 108, 113, 264) and von der Malsburg, this volume) or groups (75) of neurons; 2) at the cellular level of the individual nerve cells, the connections they establish, and of their ability to generate nerve impulses; and 3) at the molecular level of the regulatory or allosteric proteins able to integrate multiple communication signals in time and space.

The acetylcholine nicotinic receptor has been selected as a model for such a membrane-bound allosteric molecule despite the fact that evidence for its involvement in physiologically relevant learning mechanisms is still largely missing. It is thus in a strictly speculative manner, and at our own risk, that the knowledge available for this protein of muscular origin has been extended to higher neuronal processes. Our justification, however, is that this protein plausibly shares with central receptors, ion channels, and even cytoplasmic enzymes several structural and functional features which might be critical in central learning. We are not of the opinion that complex learning processes will ever be reduced to the properties of a unique molecular species. On the other hand, such processes might plausibly involve networks of molecules within a given nerve cell, with already parallel and hierarchical properties and with multiple external and internal messengers within a wide range of time scales, and allosteric proteins are expected to play the role of critical elementary knots in such networks.

A possible approach may thus be the attempt to reconstitute (rather than reduce) learning phenomena occurring at high levels of organization from ensembles of such simple mechanisms, with the distinction of those involved in the associative links between pathways (which may satisfy the general rule of topological convergence and time correlation of Hebb (108)) and those engaged in their storage or readout, which might not be nessarily the same.

Allosteric transitions of regulatory proteins, analogous to those displayed at the membrane level by the acetylcholine receptor, may account for the first group of mechanisms. An extension of the time scale of these transitions might be achieved by covalent modifications within, however, the limits of the metabolic lifetime of the protein. In a longer term time range, changes in the number of molecules will result from a regulation of their biosynthesis at any step from the gene to the synaptically localized protein. The examples presented in the case of the acetylcholine receptor deal primarily with regulatory mechanisms which take place during the development of the muscle but persist in the adult, for instance, after denervation. They thus may account for the turnover of the components of the synapse and eventually for that of the synapse itself. They primarily concern the quantitative expression of a set of preexisting genes without any known gene recombination or splicing event.

The self-perpetuation of a learning trace through molecular turnover might be achieved by a variety of mechanisms which are not necessarily unique to nerve cells. Indeed, the self-perpetuation of a given differentiated state occurs in many cellular systems and two main groups of processes have been discussed: the self-replication of a molecular structure and/or the switch from a nonequilibrium steady-state regime to another one within a "dissipative" system (208) composed of feedback-regulated chains of reactions.

Selectionist versus instructionist models of learning have already been extensively discussed (see (54, 75, 159, 264)) and are beyond the scope of this review. Nevertheless, one may emphasize that several processes of selection at the molecular level have been encountered in this presentation: among preexisting conformations of allosteric proteins such as receptors, kinases, or gene repressors and among molecules with distinct topological distribution on the surface of the cell during the formation of the subsynaptic membrane. Selection may also occur, in addition, among nerve endings (see (51, 65), and Henderson, this volume) and at the level of large ensemble of cells (see (113, 264)). The spontaneous activity occurring in neuronal networks during development and in the adult is expected to play a crucial part in this selection. Future work should lead to an evaluation of the extent to which the data gathered with the neuromuscular as a model system may be extended to nerve cells and neuronal networks.

REFERENCES

(1) Adams, P.R. 1981. Acetylcholine receptor kinetics. *J. Membr. Biol.* 58: 161-174.

(2) Almon, R.R., and Appel, S.H. 1975. Interactions of myasthenic serum globulin with the acetylcholine receptor. *Biochim. Biophys. Acta* 393: 66-77.

(3) Alper, R.; Lowry, J.; and Smith, J. 1974. Binding properties of acetylcholine receptors extracted from normal and from denervated rat diaphragm. *FEBS Lett.* 48: 130-132.

(4) Anderson, M.J., and Cohen, M.W. 1977. Nerve induced and spontaneous redistribution acetylcholine receptors on cultured muscle cells. *J. Physl. Lon.* 268: 757-773.

(5) Anderson, M.J.; Cohen, M.W.; and Zorychta, E. 1977. Effects of innervation on the distribution of acetylcholine receptors on cultured cells. *J. Physl. Lon.* 268: 731-756.

(6) Anderson, M.J., and Fambrough, D.M. 1983. Aggregates of acetylcholine receptors are associated with plaques of a basal lamina heparan sulfate proteoglycan on the surface of skeletal muscle fibers. *J. Cell Biol.* 97: 1396-1411.

(7) Anderson, J.; Ptashne, M.; and Harrison, S.C. 1984. Cocrystals of the DNA binding domain of phage 434 repressor and a synthetic phage 434 operator. *Proc. Natl. Acad. Sci.* 81: 1307-1311.

(8) Anholt, R.; Fredkin, D.R.; Deerinck, T.; Ellisman, M.; Montal, M.; and Lindstrom, J. 1982. Incorporation of acetylcholine receptors into liposomes. *J. Biol. Chem.* 257: 7122-7134.

(9) Anholt, R.; Lindstrom, J.; and Montal, M. 1985. The molecular basis of neurotransmission: structure and function of the nicotinic acetylcholine receptor. In *The Enyzmes of Biological Membranes*, ed. A.N. Martonosi, vol. 3, pp. 335-401. New York: Plenum.

(10) Axelrod, D.; Ravdin, P.M.; Koppel, D.E.; Schlessinger, J.; Webb, W.W.; Elson, E.L.; and Podleski, T.R. 1976. Lateral motion of fluorescently labeled acetylcholine receptors in membranes of developing muscle fibers. *Proc. Natl. Acad. Sci.* 73: 4594-4595.

(11) Baldwin, J., and Chothia, C. 1979. Haemoglobin: the structural changes related to ligand binding and its allosteric mechanism. *J. Mol. Biol.* 129: 175-220.

(12) Ballivet, M.; Patrick, J.; Lee, J.; and Heinemann, S. 1982. Molecular cloning of cDNA coding for the delta-subunit of *Torpedo* acetylcholine receptor. *Proc. Natl. Acad. Sci.* 79: 4466-4470.

(13) Barnard, E.A.; Beeson, D.; Bilbe, G.; Brown, D.A.; Constanti, A.; Conti-Tronconi, B.M.; Dolly, J.O.; Dunn, S.M.J.; Mehraban, F.; Richards, B.M.; and Smart, T.G. 1983. Acetylcholine and GABA receptors: subunits of central and peripheral receptors and their encoding nucleic acids. *Cold S.H. Quant. Biol.* 48: 109-124.

(14) Barrantes, F.J.; Meugebauer, D.-Ch.; and Zingheim, H.P. 1980. Peptide extraction by alkaline treatment is accompanied by rearrangement of the membrane-bound acetylcholine receptor from *Torpedo marmorata*. *FEBS Lett.* 112: 73-78.

(15) Beam, K.G.; Caldwell, J.H.; and Campbell, D.T. 1985. Na channels in skeletal muscle concentrated near the neuromuscular junction. *Nature* 313: 588-590.

(16) Berg, D.K., and Hall, Z.M. 1975. Loss of alpha-bungarotoxin from junctional and extrajunctional acetylcholine receptors in rat diaphragm muscle *in vivo* and in organ culture. *J. Physl. Lon.* 252: 771-789.

(17) Berridge, M., and Irvine, R.F. 1984. Inositol triphosphate, a novel second messenger in cellular signal transuctions. *Nature* 312: 315-321.

(18) Betz, H. 1983. Regulation of alpha-bungarotoxin receptor accumulation in chick retina cultures: effects of membrane depolarization, cyclic nucleotide derivatives, and Ca^{2+}. *J. Neurosci.* 3: 1333-1341.

(19) Betz, H.; Bourgeois, J.P.; and Changeux, J.-P. 1977. Evidence for degradation of the acetylcholine (nicotinic) receptor in skeletal muscle during the development of the chick embryo. *FEBS Lett.* 77: 219-224.

(20) Betz, H.; Bourgeois, J.P.; and Changeux, J.-P. 1980. Evolution of cholinergic proteins in developing slow and fast skeletal muscles from chick embryo. *J. Physl.* 302: 197-218.

(21) Betz, H., and Changeux, J.-P. 1979. Regulation of muscle acetylcholine receptor synthesis *in vitro* by derivatives of cyclic nucleotides. *Nature* 278: 749-752.

(22) Birnbaum, M.; Reiss, M.; and Shainberg, A. 1980. Role of calcium in the regulation of acetylcholine receptor synthesis in cultured muscle cell. *Pflug. Arch.* 385: 37-43.

(23) Black, I.B.; Adler, J.E.; Dreyfus, C.F.; Jonakait, G.M.; Katz, D.M.; Lagamma, E.G.; and Markey, K.M. 1984. Neurotransmitter plasticity at the molecular level. *Science* 225: 1266-1270.

(24) Black; I.B.; Adler, J.E.; and Lagamma, E.F. 1986. Impulse activity differentially regulates co-localized transmitters by altering messenger RNA levels. *Prog. Brain Res.*, in press.

(25) Blosser, J.C., and Appel, S.H. 1980. Regulation of acetylcholine receptor by cyclic AMP. *J. Biol. Chem.* 253: 3088-2093.

(26) Bon, F.; Lebrun, E.; Gomel, J.; Van Rappenbusch, R.; Cartaud, J.; Popot, J.L.; and Changeux, J.-P. 1984. Image analysis of the heavy form of the acetylcholine receptor from *Torpedo marmorata*. *J. Mol. Biol.* 176: 205-237.

(27) Bourgeois, J.P.; Betz, H.; and Changeux, J.-P. 1978. Effets de lat paralysie chronique de l'embryon de poulet par le flaxédil sur le

développement de la jonction neuro-musculaire. *C.R. Acad. Sci. Paris* 286D: 773-776.

(28) Bourgeois, J.P.; Popot, J.L.; Ryter, A.; and Changeux, J.-P. 1973. Consequentces of denervation on the distribution of the cholinergic (nicotinic) receptor sites from *Electrophorus electricus* revealed by high resolution autoradiography. *Brain Res.* 62: 557-563.

(29) Bourgeois, J.P., and Toutant, M. 1982. Innervation of avian *Latissimus dorsi* muscle and axonal outgrowth pattern in the *Posterior latissimus dorsi* motor nerve during embryonic development. *J. Comp. Neur.* 208: 1-15.

(30) Boyd, N.D., and Cohen, J.B. 1980. Kinetics of binding of [^{3}H] acetylcholine and [^{3}H] carbamoylcholine to *Torpedo* postsynaptic membranes: slow conformational transitions of the cholinergic receptor. *Biochemiostry* 19: 5344-5358.

(31) Brenner, H.R.; Meier, T.; and Widmer, B. 1983. Early action of nerve determines motor endplate differentiation in rat muscle. *Nature* 395: 536-537.

(32) Brisson, A., and Unwin, P.N.T. 1985. Quaternary structure of the acetylcholine receptor. *Nature* 315: 474-477.

(33) Brockes, J.P.; Berg, D.; and Hall, Z.W. 1976. The biochemical properties and regulation of acetylcholine receptors in normal and denervated muscle. *Cold S.H. Quant. Biol.* 40: 253-262.

(34) Brockes, J.P., and Hall, Z.W. 1975. Acetylcholine receptors in normal and denervated rat diaphragm muscle. I. Purification and interaction with [^{125}I]-alpha-bungarotoxin. *Biochemistry* 14: 2092-2106.

(35) Brown, D. 1984. The role of stable complexes that repress and activate eucaryotic genes. *Cell* 37: 359-365.

(36) Burden, S. 1977. Acetylcholine receptors at the neuromuscular junction: developmental change in receptor turnover. *Dev. Biol.* 61: 79-85.

(37) Burden, S. 1977. Development of the neuromuscular junction in the chick embryo. The number, distribution and stability of the acetylcholine receptor. *Dev. Biol.* 57: 317-329.

(38) Burden, S.J. 1985. The subsynaptic 43 KD protein is concentrated at developing nerve-muscle synapses *in vitro*. *Proc. Natl. Acad. Sci.* 82: 7805-7809.

(39) Bursztajn, S., and Fischbach, G.D. 1984. Evidence that coated vesicles transport acetylcholine receptors to the surface membrane of chick myotubes. *J. Cell. Biol.* 98: 498-506.

(40) Cartaud, J.; Kordeli, C.; Nghiêm, H.O.; and Changeux, J.-P. 1983. La proteine 43000 daltons nu 1: pièce intermédiaire assurant l'ancrage du recepteur cholinergique au cytosquelette sous-neural? *C.R. Acad. Sci. Paris* 297: 285-289.

(41) Cartaud, J.; Sobel, A.; Rousseleet, A.; Devaux, P. F.; and Changeux, J.-P. 1981. Consequences of alkaline treatment for the ultrastructure of the acetylcholine-receptor-rich membranes from *Torpedo marmorata* electric organ. *J. Cell. Biol.* 90: 418-426.

(42) Catterall, W.A. 1980. Neurotoxins that act on voltage-sensitive sodium channels. *Ann. R. Pharm. Tox.* 20: 15-43.

(43) Chang, H.W.; Bock, E.; and Neumann, E. 1984. Long-lived metastable states and hysteresis in the binding of acetylcholine to *Torpedo califonica* acetylcholine receptor. *Biochemistry* 23: 4546-4556.

(44) Chang, C.C., and Huang, M.C. 1975. Turnover of junctional and extrajunctional acetylcholine receptors of the rat diaphragm. *Nature* 253: 643-644.

(45) Changeux, J.-P. 1961. The feedback control mechanism of biosynthetic L-threonine deaminase by L-isoleucine. *Cold S.H. Quant. Biol.* 26: 313-318.

(46) Changeux, J.-P. 1966. Responses of acetylcholinesterase from *Torpedo marmorata* to salts and curarizing drugs. *Molec. Pharm.* 2: 369-392.

(47) Changeux, J.-P. 1981. The acetylcholine receptor: an "allosteric" membrane protein. *Harvey Lect.* 75: 85-254.

(48) Changeux, J.-P. 1986. Coexistence of neuronal messengers and molecular selection. *Prog. Brain Res.*, in press.

(49) Changeux, J.-P.; Bon, F.; Cartaud, J.; Devillers-Thiéry, A.; Giraudat, J.; Heidmann, T.; Holton, B.; Nghiêm, H.O.; Popot, J.L.; Van Rapenbush, R.; and Tzartos, S. 1983. Allosteric properties of the acetylcholine receptor protein from *Torpedo marmorata*. *Cold S.H. Quant. Biol.* 48: 35-52.

(50) Changeux, J.-P.; Courrège, Ph.; Danchin, A.; and Lasry, J.M. 1981. Un mécanisme biochimique pour l'épigénèse de la jonction neuromusculaire. *C.R. Acad. Sci. Paris* 292: 449-453.

(51) Changeux, J.-P., and Danchin, A. 1976. Selective stabilization of developing synapses as a mechanism for the specification of neuronal networks. *Nature* 264: 705-712.

(52) Changeux, J.-P.; Devillers-Thiéry, A.; and Chemouilli, P. 1984. Acetylcholine receptor: an allosteric protein. *Science* 225: 1335-1345.

(53) Changeux, J.-P., and Heidmann, T. 1986. Allosteric receptors and molecular models of learning. In *New Insights into Synaptic Function*, eds. G. Edelman, W.E. Gall, and W.M. Cowan. New York: Wiley, in press.

(54) Changeux, J.-P.; Heidmann, T.; and Patte, P. 1984. Learning by selection. In *The Biology of Learning*, eds. P. Marler and H.S. Terrace, pp. 115-133. Dahlem Konferenzen. Berlin, Heidelberg, New York, Tokyo: Springer-Verlag.

(55) Changeux, J.-P.; Thiéry, J.P.; Tung, Y.; and Kittel, C. 1967. On the cooperativity of biological membranes. *Proc. Natl. Acad. Sci.* 57: 335-341.

(56) Chow, I., and Poo, M.M. 1985. Release of acetylcholine from embryonic neurons upon contact with muscle cell. *J. Neurosci.* 5: 1076-1082.

(57) Clapham, D.E., and Neher, E. 1984. Substance P reduces acetylcholine-induced current in isolated bovine chromaffin cells. *J. Phys. Lon.* 347: 255-277.

(58) Claudio, T.; Ballivet, M.; Patrick, J.; and Heinemann, S. 1983. Nucleotide and deduced amino acid sequences of *Torpedo califonica* acetylcholine receptor subunit. *Proc. Natl. Acad. Sci.* 80: 1111-1115.

(59) Cohen, J.B.; Weber, M.; and Changeux, J.-P. 1974. Effects of local anesthetics and calcium on the interaction of cholinergic ligands with the nicotinic receptor protein from *Torpedo marmorata*. *Molec. Pharm.* 10: 904-932.

(60) Cohen, S.A. 1980. Early nerve msucle synapses *in vitro* release transmitter over post synaptic membrane having low acetylcholine sensitivity. *Proc. Natl. Acad. Sci.* 77: 644-648.

(61) Colquhoun, D., and Rang, H.P. 1976. Effects of inhibitors on the binding of iodinated alpha-bungarotoxin to acetylcholine receptors in rat muscle. *Molec. Pharm.* 12: 519-535.

(62) Conti-Tonconi, B.M., and Raftery, M.A. 1982. The nicotinic cholinergic receptor: correlation of molecular structure with functional properties. *Ann. R. Biochem.* 51: 491-530.

(63) Couteaux, R. 1973. Structure and Function of Muscle, ed. G.H. Bourne, vol. 2, pp. 483-530. New York: Academic Press.

(64) Covault, J., and Sanes, J. 1985. Neural cell adhesion molecule (N-CAM) accumulates in denervated and paralyzed skeletal muscles. *Proc. Natl. Acad. Sci.* 82: 4544-4548.

(65) Cowan, M.W.; Fawcett, J.W.; O'Leary, D.; and Stanfield, B.B. 1984. Regressive phenomena in the development of the vertebrate nervous system. *Science* 225: 1258-1265.

(66) Crick, F. 1984. Memory and molecular turnover. *Nature* 312: 101.

(67) Curtis, B.M., and Catterall, W.A. 1985. Phosphorylation of the calcium antagonist receptor of the voltage-sensitive calcium channel by cAMP-dependent protein kinase. *Proc. Natl. Acad. Sci.* 82: 2528-2532.

(68) De Combrugghe, B.; Busby, S.; and Buc, H. 1984. Activation of transcription by the cyclic AMP receptor protein. In *Biological Regulation and Development*, eds. R. Golberger and C. Yamamoto, pp. 129-167. New York: Plenum.

(69) Delbrück, M. 1949. In *Unités Biologiques Douées de Continuité Génétique CNRS* 8: 33-35.

(70) Dennis, M.; Giraudat, J.; Hibert, F.; Hirth, C; Goeldner, M.; Chang, J.Y.; and Changeux, J.-P. 1985. Structural analysis of the cholinergic binding sites of the acetylcholine receptor from *Torpedo mamorata.* International Symposium on "Molecular Aspects of Neurobiology" Florence, Italy. Abstract Nr. 22.

(71) Devillers-Thiéry, A.; Giraudat, J.; Bentaboulet, M.; and Changeux, J.-P. 1983. Complete mRNA coding sequence of the acetylcholine binding alpha-subunit of *Torpedo marmorata* acetylcholine receptor: a model for the transmembrane organization of the polypeptide chain. *Proc. Natl. Acad. Sci.* 80: 2067-2071.

(72) Devreotes, P.N., and Fambrough, D.M. 1975. Turnover of acetylcholine receptors in skeletal muscle. *Cold S.H. Quant. Biol.* 40: 237-251.

(73) Devreotes, P.N.; Garnder, J.M.; and Fambrough, D.M. 1977. Kinetics of biosynthesis of acetylcholine receptor and subsequent incorporation into plasma membrane of cultured chick skeletal muscle. *Cell* 10: 365-373.

(74) Dunn, P.M., and Marshall, L.M. 1985. Lack of nicotinic supersensitivity in frogs sympathetic neurons following denervation. *J. Physl. Lon.*363: 211-225.

(75) Edelman, G.M., and Finkel, L. 1984. Neuronal group selection in the cerebral cortex. In *Dynamic Aspects of Neocortical Function*, eds. G. Edelman, W.E. Gall, and W.M. Cowan, pp. 653-695. New York: Wiley.

(76) Elliott, J.; Blanchard, S.G.; Wu, W.; Miller, J.; Strader, C.D.; Hartig, P.; Moore, H.P.; Racs, J.; and Raftery, M.A. 1980. Purificaton of *Torpedo californica* post-synaptic membranes and fractionation of their constituent proteins. *Biochem. J.* 185: 667-677.

(77) Eusebi, F.; Molinaro, M.; and Zani, B. 1985. Agents that activate protein kinase C reduce acetylcholine sensitivity in cultured myotubes. *J. Cell Biol.* 100: 1339-1342.

(78) Fallon, J.; Nitkrin, R.M.; Reist, N.E.; Wallace, B.G.; and McMahan, U.J. 1985. Acetylcholine receptor aggregating factor is similar to molecules concentrated at neuromuscular junction. *Nature* 315: 571-574.

(79) Fambrough, D. 1979. Control of acetylcholine receptors in skeletal muscle. *Physiol. Rev.* 59: 165-227.

(80) Feltz, A., and Trautmann, A. 1980. Interaction between nerve-released acetylcholine and bath applied agonists at the frog end plate. *J. Physl. Lon.* 299: 533-552.

(81) Fischbach, G.D., and Schuetze, S.M. 1980. A postnatal decrease in acetylcholine channel open time at rat end-plates. *J. Physl. Lon.* 303: 125-137.

(82) Fletterick, R.J., and Madsen, N.B. 1980. The structures and related functions of phosphorylase a. *Ann. R. Biochem.* l49: 31-61.

(83) Forrest, J.W.; Mills, R.G.; Bray, J.J.; and Hubbard, J.I. 1981. Calcium-dependent regulation of the membrane potential and extrajunctional acetylcholine receptors of rat skeletal muscle. *Neuroscience* 6: 741-749.

(84) Frank, E., and Fischbach, G.D. 1979. Early events in neuromuscular junction formation *in vitro*. *J. Cell Biol.* 83: 143-158.

(85) Frank, E.; Gautvik, K.; and Sommer-Schild, H. 1975. Cholinergic receptors at denervated mammalian endplates. *Acta Physl. Scand.* 95: 66-76.

(86) Frelin, C.; Lombet, A.; Vigne, P.; Romey, G.; and Lazdunski, M. 1981. The appearance of voltage sensitive Na+ channels during the *in vitro* differentiation of embryonic chick skeletal muscle cells. *J. Biol. Chem.* 254: 3600-3607.

(87) Froehner, S.C.; Gulbrandsen, V.; Hyman, C.; Jeng, A.Y.; Neubig, R.R.; and Cohen, J.B. 1981. Immunofluorescence localization at the mammalian neuromuscular junction of the M_r 43,000 protein of *Torpedo* postsynaptic membranes. *Proc. Natl. Acad. Sci.* 78: 5230-5234.

(88) Froehner, S.C.; Reiness, C.G.; and Hall, Z.W. 1977. Subunit structure of the acetycholine receptor from denervated rat skeletal muscle. *J. Biol. Chem.* 252: 8589-8696.

(89) Fuxe, K.; Agnati, L.; Andersson, K.; Martire, M.; Ogren, S.O.; Giardino, L.; Battistini, N.; Grimaldi, R.; Farabeloli, C.; Härfstrand, A.; and Toffano, G. 1984. Receptor-receptor

interactions in the central nervous system, evidence for the existence of heterostatic synaptic mechanisms. In *Regulation of Transmitter Function*, eds. E.S. Vizi and K. Magyars. Proc. 5th Meeting Eur. Soc. Neurochem.

(90) Fuxe, K.; Agnati, L.; Härfstrand, A.; Janson, A.; Anderson, K.; Ruggeri, M.; Zoli, M.; and Goldstein, M. 1986. Morphofunctional studies on the neuropeptide Y/adrenaline costoring nerve terminal systems in the dorsal cardiovascular region of the medulla obloryata. Focus on receptor-receptor interactions in co-transmission. *Prog. Brain Res.*, in press.

(91) Giacobini, G.; Filogamo, G.; Weber, M.; Boquet, P.; and Changeux, J.-P. 1973. Effect of a snake-neurotoxin on the development of innervated motor muscles in chick embryo. *Proc. Natl. Acad. Sci.* 70: 1708-1712.

(92) Giacobini-Robecchi, M.G.; Giacobini, G.; Filogamo, G.; and Changeux, J.-P. 1975. Effect of the type A toxin from *C. botulinum* on the development of skeletal muscles of their innervation in chick embryo. *Brain Res.* 83: 107-121.

(93) Giraudat, J.; Dennis, M.; Heidmann, T.; Chang, J.Y.; and Changeux, J.-P. 1986. Structure of the high affinity binding site for noncompetitive blockers of the acetylcholine receptor: amino acid of the delta-subunit labeled by ^{3}H chlorpromazine. *Proc. Natl. Acad. Sci.* 83: 2719-2723

(94) Giraudat, J.; Devillers-Thiéry, A.; Auffray, C.; Rougeon, F.; and Changeux, J.-P. 1982. Identification of a cDNA clone coding for the acetylcholine binding subunit of *Torpedo marmorata* acetylcholine receptor. *EMBO J.* 1: 713-717.

(95) Goldman, D.; Boulier, J.; Heinemann, S.; and Patrick, J. 1985. Muscle denervation increases the levels of two mRNAs coding for the acetylcholine receptor alpha-subunit. *J. Neurosci.* 5: 2553-2558.

(96) Gordon, A.; Davis, G.; and Diamond, I. 1977. Phosphorylation of membrane proteins at a cholinergic synapse. *Proc. Natl. Acad. Sci.* 74: 263-267.

(97) Gordon, T.; Purves, R.; and Vrbova, G. 1977. Differentiation of electrical and contractile properties of slow and fast muscle fibers. *J. Physl. Lon.* 269: 535-547.

(98) Grünhagen, H.H., and Changeux, J.-P. 1976. Studies on the electrogenic action of acetylcholine with *Torpedo marmorata* electric organ. Quinacrine: a fluorescent probe for the conformational transitions of the cholinergic receptor protein in its membrane bound state. *J. Mol. Biol.* 106: 497-516.

(99) Gu, Y.; Silberstein, L.; and Hall, Z. 1985. The effects of a myasthenic serum on the acetylcholine receptors of C2 myotubes. I. Immunological distinction between the two toxin-binding sites of the receptor. *J. Neurosci.* 5: 1909-1916.

(100) Hall, Z.; Gorin, P.; Silberstein, L.; and Bennett, C. 1985. A postnatal change in the immunological properties of the acetylcholine receptor at muscle endplates. *J. Neurosci.* 5: 730-734.

(101) Hall, Z., and Reiness, C.G. 1977. Electrical stimulation of denervated muscles reduces incorporation of methionine into the ACh receptor. *Nature* 268: 655-657.

(102) Hamburger, V. 1970. Embryonic mobility in vertebrates. In *The Neurosciences: Second Study Program*, ed. F.O. Schmitt, pp. 141-151. New York: Rockefeller University Press.

(103) Hamilton, S.L.; Pratt, D.R.; and Eaton, D.C. 1985. Arrangement of the subunits of the nicotinic acetylcholine receptor of *Torpedo californica* as determined by alpha-neurotoxin cross-linking. *Biochemistry* 24: 2210-2219.

(104) Haring, R.; Kloog, Y.; and Sokolovsky, M. 1984. Localization of phencyclidine binding sites on alpha- and beta-subunits of the nicotinic acetylcholine receptor from *Torpedo ocellata* electric organ using azido phencyclidine. *J. Neurosci.* 4: 627-637.

(105) Harris, W.A. 1981. Neural activity and development. *Ann. R. Physl.* 43: 689-710.

(106) Hawkins, R.D.; Abrahms, S.W.; Carew, T.J.; and Kandel, E.R. 1983. A cellular mechanism of classical conditioning in *Aplysia*: activity dependent enhancement of presynaptic facilitation. *Science* 219: 400-405.

(107) Hawkins, R., and Kandel, E. 1984. Is there a cell-biological alphabet for simple forms of learning? *Psychol. Rev.* 91: 375-391.

(108) Hebb, D.O. 1949. The Organization of Behavior: A Neuropsychological Theory. New York: Wiley.

(109) Heidmann, T.; Bernhardt, J.; Neumann, E.; and Changeux, J.-P. 1983. Rapid kinetics of agonist binding and permeability response analysed in parallel on acetylcholine receptor rich membranes from *Torpedo marmorata*. *Biochemistry* 22: 5452-5459.

(110) Heidmann, T., and Changeux, J.-P. 1979. Fast kinetic studies on the interaction of a fluorescent agonist with the membrane-bound acetylcholine receptor from *Torpedo marmorata*. *Eur. J. Bioch.* 94: 281-296.

(111) Heidmann, T., and Changeux, J.-P. 1980. Interaction of a fluorescent agonist with the membrane-bound acetylcholine

receptor from *Torpedo marmorata* in the millisecond time range: resolution of an "intermediate" conformational transition and evidence for positive cooperative effects. *Biochem. Biophys. Res. Comm.* 97: 889-896.

(112) Heidmann, T., and Changeux, J.-P. 1982. Un modèle moléculaire de régulation d'efficacité d'une synapse chimique au niveau postsynaptique. *C.R. Acad. Sci.*295: 665-670.

(113) Heidmann, A.; Heidmann, T.; and Changeux, J.-P. 1984. Stabilisation selective de représentations neuronales par résonance entre "pré-représentations" spontanées du réseau cérébral et "percepts" évoqués par interaction avec le monde extérieur. C.*R. Acad. Sci. III* 299: 839-844.

(114) Heidmann, T.; Oswald, R.E.; and Changeux, J.-P. 1983. Multiple sites of action for noncompetitive blockers on acetylcholine receptor rich membrane fragments from *Torpedo marmorata*. *Biochemistry* 22: 3112-3127.

(115) Heidmann, T.; Sobel, A.; Popot, J.L.; Changeux, J.-P. 1980. Reconstitution of an acetylcholine receptor. Conservation of the conformational and allosteric transition and recovery of the permeability response; role of lipids. *Eur. J. Bioch.* 110: 35-55.

(116) Henderson, C.E.; Huchet, M.; and Changeux, J.-P. 1981. Neurite outgrowth from embryonic chicken spinal neurons is promoted by media conditioned muscle cells. *Proc. Natl. Acad. Sci.* 78: 2625-2629.

(117) Henderson, C.E.; Huchet, M.; and Changeux, J.-P. 1984. Neurite-promoting activities for embryonic spinal neurons and their developmental changes in chick. *Develop. Biol.* 104: 336-347.

(118) Henderson, C.E.; Benoit, P.; Guénet, J.L.; Huchet, M.; and Changeux, J.-P. 1986. Increase of neurite-promoting activity for spinal neurons in muscles of "paralysé" mice and tenotomised rats. *Dev. Brain Res.* 25: 65-70.

(119) Hess, G.P.; Cash, D.J.; and Aoshima, H. 1983. Acetylcholine receptor-controlled ion translocation: chemical kinetic investigations of the mechanisms. *Ann. Rev. Bioph. Bioeng.* 12: 443-473.

(120) Hnik, P.; Jirmanova, I.; Vyklicky, L.; and Zeena, J. 1967. Fast and slow muscle of the chick after nerve cross-union. *J. Physl. Lon.* 193: 309-325.

(121) Hökfelt, T.; Holets, V.R.; Staines, W.; Meister, B.; Melander, T.; Schalling, M.; Schultzberg, M.; Freedman, J.; Björklund, H.; Olson, L.; Lindk, B.; Elfvin, L.G.; Lundberg, J.; Lindgren, J.A.; Samuelsson, B.; Terenius, L.; Post, C.; Everitt, B.; and Goldstein, M. 1986. Coexistence of peptides neuronal messengers – an overview. *Prog. Brain Res.*, in press.

(122) Holton, B.; Tzartos, S.J.; and Changeux, J.-P. 1984. Comparison of embryonic and adult *Torpedo* acetylcholine receptor by sedimentation characteristics and antigenicity. *Int. J. Dev. Neurosci.* 2: 549-555.

(123) Ito, M.; Sakurai, M.; and Tongroach, P. 1982. Climbing fibre induced depression of both mossy fibre responsiveness and glutamate sensitivity of cerebellar Purkinje cells. *J. Physl. Lon.* 324: 113-134.

(124) Jackson, M. 1984. Spontaneous openings of the acetylcholine receptor channel. *Proc. Natl. Acad. Sci.* 81: 3901-3904.

(125) Kaldany, R.R.J., and Karlin, A. 1983. Reaction of quinacrine mustard with acetylcholine receptor from *Torpedo californica:* functional consequences and sites of labeling. *J. Biol. Chem.* 258: 6232-6242.

(126) Kao, P.; Dwork, A.; Kaldany, R.; Silver, M.; Wideman, J.; Stein, S.; and Karlin, A. 1984. Identification of the alpha-subunit half-cystine specifically labeled by an affinity reagent for the acetylcholine receptor binding site. *J. Biol. Chem.* 259: 11662-11665.

(127) Karlin, A. 1967. On the application of "a plausible model" of allosteric proteins to the receptor for acetylcholine. *J. Theor. Biol.* 16: 306-320.

(128) Karlin, A. 1983. Anatomy of a receptor. *Neuroscience Comm.* 1: 111-123.

(129) Kasprzak, H., and Salpeter, M.M. 1985. Recovery of acetylcholinesterase at intact neuromuscular junctions after *in vivo* inactivation with Di-isopropylfluorophosphate. *J. Neurosci.* 5: 951-955.

(130) Katz, B. 1966. Nerve Muscle and Synapse. New York: McGraw Hill.

(131) Katz, B., and Miledi, R. 1972. The statistical nature of the acetylcholine potential and its molecular components. *J. Physl. Lon.* 224: 665-699.

(132) Katz, B., and Miledi, R. 1977. Transmitter leakage from motor nerve endings. *Proc. Roy. Soc. Lon. B* 196: 59-72.

(133) Katz, B., and Thesleff, S. 1957. A study of the "desensitization" produced by acetylcholine at the motor end-plate. *J. Physl. Lon.* 138: 63-80.

(134) Kidokoro, Y., and Yeh, E. 1982. Initial synaptic transmission at the growth cone in *Xenopus* nerve-muscle cultures. *Proc. Natl. Acad. Sci.* 79: 6727-6731.

(135) Klarsfeld, A., and Changeux, J.-P. 1985. Activity regulates the level of acetylcholine receptor alpha-subunit mRNA in cultured chick myotubes. *Proc. Natl. Acad. Sci.* 82: 4558-4562.

(136) Klarsfeld, A.; Devillers-Thiéry, A.; Giraudat, J.; and Changeux, J.-P. 1984. A single gene codes for the nicotinic acetylcholine receptor alpha-subunit in *Torpedo marmorata*: structural and developmental implications. *EMBO J.* 3: 35-41.

(137) Klymkowsky, M.W.; Heuser, J.E.; and Stroud, R.M. 1980. Protease effects on the structure of acetylcholine receptor membranes from *Torpedo californica*. *J. Cell. Biol.* 85: 823-838.

(138) Knaack, D.; Admon, S.; Podleski, T.; Oswald, R.; and Salpeter, M. 1985. Ascorbic acid treatment increases acetylcholine receptor mRNA levels in cultured myogenic cells. *Soc. Neurosci. Abstr.* 223.1.

(139) Knaack, D., and Podleski, T. 1985. Ascorbic acid mediates acetylcholine receptor increase induced by brain extract on myogenic cells. *Proc. Natl. Acad. Sci.* 82: 575-579.

(140) Kordeli, C.; Cartaud, J.; Nghiêm, O.H.; Pradel, L.A.; Dubreuil, C.; Paulin, D.; and Changeux, J.-P. 1985. Evidence for a polarity in the distribution of proteins from the cytoskeleton in *T. marmorata* electrocytes. *J. Cell. Biol.* 102: 748-761.

(141) Krause, K.; Volz, K.; and Lipscomb, W. 1985. Structure at 2.9.A resolution of aspartate carbamoyl transferase complexed with the bisubstrate analogue N-(phophon-acetyl)-L-aspartate. *Proc. Natl. Acad. Sci.* 82: 1643-1647.

(142) Krebs, E.G. 1981. Phosphorylation and dephosphorylation of glycogen phosphorylase: a prototype of reversible covalent modification. *Curr. T. Cell. Reg.* 18: 401-419.

(143) Krodel, E.K.; Beckman, R.A.; and Cohen, J.B. 1979. Identification of a local anesthetic binding site in nicotinic post-synaptic membranes isolated from *Torpedo marmorata* electric tissue. *Molec. Pharm.* 15: 294-312.

(144) Kuffler, S.W.; Dennis, M.J.; and Harris, A.J. 1971. The development of chemosensitivity in extrasynaptic areas of the neuronal surface after denervation of para sympathetic ganglion cells in the heart of the frog. *P. Roy. Soc. B* 177: 555.

(145) Kullberg, R., and Kasprzak, H. 1985. Gating kinetics of nonjunctional acetylcholine receptor channels in developing *Xenopus* muscle. *J. Neurosci.* 5: 970-976.

(146) Kullberg, R.W.; Mikelberg, F.S.; and Cohen, M.W. 1980. Contribution of cholinesterase to developmental decrease in the

time course of synaptic potentials at an amphibian neuromuscular junction. *Develop. Biol.* 75: 255-267.

(147) Kullberg, R.; Owens, J.L.; and Vickers, J. 1985. Development of synaptic currents in immobilized muscle of *Xenopus laevis*. *J. Physl.* 364: 57-68.

(148) Kuromi, H.; Brass, B.; and Kidokoro, Y. 1985. Formation of acetylcholine receptor clusters at neuromuscular junction in *Xenopus* cultures. *Develop. Biol.* 109: 165-176.

(149) Levitt, T.A., and Salpeter, M.M. 1981. Denervated endplates have a dual population of junctional acetylcholine receptors. *Nature* 91: 239-241.

(150) Lindstrom, J. 1985. Immunobiology of myasthenia gravis, experimental autoimmune myasthenia gravis, and Lamber-Eaton syndrome. *Ann. R. Immun.* 3: 109-131.

(151) Lisman, J. 1985. A mechanism of memory storage insensitive to molecular turnover: a bistable autophosphorylating kinase. *Proc. Natl. Acad. Sci.* 82: 3055-3057.

(152) Lo, M.M.S.; Garland, P.B.; Lamprecht, J.; and Barnard, E.A. 1980. Rotational mobility of the membrane-bound acetylcholine receptor of *Torpedo* electric organ measured by phosphorescence depolarisation. *FEBS Lett.* 111: 407-412.

(153) Lømo, T.; Massoulié, J.; and Vigny, M. 1985. Stimulation of denervated rat soleus muscle with fast and slow activity patterns induces different expression of acetylcholinesterase molecular forms. *J. Neurosci.* 5: 1180-1187.

(154) Lømo, T., and Slater, C.R. 1976. Control of neuromuscular synapse formation. In *Synaptogenesis*, ed. L. Tauc, pp. 9-31. Naturalia and Biologia.

(155) Lømo, T., and Slater, C.R. 1980. Control of junctional acetylcholinesterase by neural and muscular influences in the rat. *J. Physl. Lon.* 303: 191-202.

(156) Lømo, T., and Westgaard, R.H. 1975. Further studies on the control of Ach sensitivity by activity in the rat. *J. Physl. Lon.* 252: 603-626.

(157) Magleby, K.L., and Pallota, B.S. 1981. A study of desensitization of acetylcholine receptors using nerve-released transmitter in the frog. *J. Physl. Lon.* 316: 225-250.

(158) Mallet, J.; Faucon, N.; Buda, M.; Lamouroux, A.; and Samolyk, D. 1983. Detection and regulation of the tyrosine hydroxylase mRNA levels in rat adrenal medulla and brain tissues. *Cold S.H. Quant. Biol.* 48: 305-308.

(159) Marler, P. 1984. Song learning: innate species differences in the learning process. In *The Biology of Learning*, eds. P. Marler and H. Terrace, pp. 289-311. Dahlem Konferenzen. Berlin, Heidelberg, New York, Tokyo: Springer Verlag.

(160) Marshall, L. 1985. Presynaptic control of synaptic channel kinetics in sympathetic neurons. *Nature* 317: 621-623.

(161) Massoulié, J., and Bon, S. 1982. The molecular forms of cholinesterase and acetylcholinesterase in vertebrates. *Ann. R. Neur.* 5: 57-106.

(162) Matsuda, R.; Spector, D.; and Strokman, R.C. 1984. Denervated skeletal muscle displays discoordinate regulation for the synthesis of several myofibrillar proteins. *Proc. Natl. Acad. Sci.* 81: 1122-1125.

(163) Matthews-Bellinger, J., and Salpeter, N. 1978. Distribution of AchR receptors at frog neuromuscular junctions with a discussion of some physiological implications. *J. Physl.* 279: 197-213.

(164) Matthews-Bellinger, J., and Salpeter, M. 1983. Fine structural distribution of acetylcholine receptors at developing mouse neuromuscular junctions. *J. Neurosci.* 3: 644-657.

(165) McMahan, U.J.; Sanes, J.R.; and Marshall, L.M. 1978. Cholinesterase is associated with the basal lamina at the neuromuscular junction. *Nature* 271: 172-174.

(166) McManaman, J.L.; Blosser, J.C.; and Appel, S.H. 1981. The effect of calcium on acetylcholine receptor synthesis. *J. Neurosci.* 1: 771-776.

(167) McManaman, J.L.; Blosser, J.C.; and Appel, S.H. 1982. Inhibitors of membrane depolarization regulate acetylcholine receptor synthesis by a calcium-dependent, cyclic nucleotide independent mechanism. *Biochem. Biophys. Acta* 720: 28-35.

(168) Merlie, J. 1984. Biogenesis of the acetylcholine receptor, a multisubunit integral membrane protein. *Cell* 36: 573-575.

(169) Merlie, J.P.; Changeux, J.-P.; and Gros, F. 1978. Skeletal muscle acetylcholine receptor. Purification, characterization, and turnover in muscle cell cultures. *J. Biol. Chem.* 253: 2882-2891.

(170) Merlie, J.P.; Isenberg, K.E.; Russell, S.D.; and Sanes, J.R. 1984. Denervation supersensitivity in skeletal muscle: analysis with a cloned cDNA probe. *J. Cell. Biol.* 99: 332-335.

(171) Merlie, J., and Sanes, J. 1985. Concentration of acetylcholine receptor mRNA in synaptic regions of adult muscle fibers. *Nature* 317: 66-68.

(172) Merlie, J.P.; Sebbane, R.; Gardner, S.; Olson, E.; and Lindstrom, J. 1983. The regulation of acetylcholine receptor expression in mammalian muscle. *Cold S.H. Quant. Biol.* 48: 135-146.

(173) Merlie, J.P.; Sobel, A.; Changeux, J.-P.; and Gros, F. 1975. Synthesis of acetylcholine receptor during differentiation of cultured embryonic muscle cells. *Proc. Natl. Acad. Sci.* 72: 4028-4032.

(174) Michler, A., and Sakmann, B. 1980. Receptor stability and channel conversion in the subsynaptic membrane of the developing mammalian neuromuscular junction. *Develop. Biol.* 80: 1-17.

(175) Mishina, M.; Kurosaki, T.; Tobimatsu, T.; Morimoto, Y.; Noda, M.; Yamamoto, T.; Terao, M.; Lindstrom, J.; Takahashi, T.; Kuno, M.; and Numa, S. 1984. Expression of functional acetylcholine receptor from cloned cDNAs. *Nature* 307: 604-608.

(176) Monod, J.; Changeux, J.-P.; and Jacob, F. 1963. Allosteric proteins and cellular control systems. *J. Mol. Biol.* 6: 306-328.

(177) Monod, J., and Jacob, F. 1961. General conclusions: teleonomic mechanisms in cellular metabolism, growth and differentiation. *Cold S.H. Quant. Biol.* 26: 389-401.

(178) Monod, J.; Wyman, J.; and Changeux, J.-P. 1965. On the nature of allosteric transitions: a plausible model. *J. Mol. Biol.* 12: 88-118.

(179) Muhn, P., and Hucho, F. 1983. Covalent labeling of the acetylcholine receptor from *Torpedo* electric tissue with the channel blocker [^{3}H] triphenylmethylphophonium by ultraviolet irradiation. *Biochemistry* 22: 421-425.

(180) Nathanson, N.M., and Hall, Z.W. 1979. Subunit structure and peptide mapping of junctional and extrajunctional acetylcholine receptors from rat muscle. *Biochemistry* 18: 3392-3401.

(181) Neher, E., and Sakmann, B. 1976. Single channel currents recorded from membrane of denervated frog muscle fibers. *Nature* 260: 799-802.

(182) Nestler, E., and Greengard, P. 1984. Protein Phosphorylation in the Nervous System. New York: Wiley.

(183) Neubig, R.R.; Boyd, N.D.; and Cohen, J.B. 1982. Conformations of *Torpedo* acetylcholine receptor associated with ion transport and desensitization. *Biochemistry* 21: 3460-3467.

(184) Neubig, R.R., and Cohen, J.B. 1980. Permeability control by cholinergic receptors in *Torpedo* post synaptic membranes: agonist dose response relations measured at second and millisecond times. *Biochemistry* 19: 2770-2779.

(185) Neubig, R.R.; Krodel, E.K.; Boyd, N.D.; and Cohen, J.B. 1979. Acetylcholine and local anesthetic binding to *Torpedo* nicotinic postsynaptic membranes after removal of nonreceptor peptides. *Proc. Natl. Acad. Sci.* 76: 690-694.

(186) Nghiêm, H.O.; Cartaud, J.; Dubreuil, C.; Kordeli, C.; Buttin, G.; and Changeux, J.-P. 1983. Production and characterization of a monoclonal antibody directed against the 43,000 M.W. nu 1 polypeptide from *Torpedo marmorata* electric organ. *Proc. Natl. Acad. Sci.* 80: 6403-6407.

(187) Nishizuka, Y. 1984. Turnover of inositol phopholipids and signal transduction. *Science* 225: 1365-1370.

(188) Nitkin, R.M.; Wallace, B.G.; Spira, M.E.; Godfrey, E.W.; and McMahan, U.J. 1983. Molecular components of the synaptic basal lamina that direct differentiation of regenerating neuromuscular junctions. *Cold S.H. Quant. Biol.* 48: 653-665.

(189) Noda, M.; Furutani, Y.; Takahashi, H.; Toyosato, M.; Tanabe, T.; Shimizu, S.; Kikyotani, S.; Kayano, T.; Hirose, T.; Inayama, S.; and Numa, S. 1983. Cloning and sequence analysis of calf cDNA and human genomic DNA encoding alpha-subunit precursor of muscle acetylcholine receptor. *Nature* 305: 818-823.

(190) Noda, M.; Shimizu, S.; Tanabe, T.; Takai, T.; Kayano, T.; Ikeda, T.; Takahashi, H.; Nakayama, H.; Kanaoka, Y.; Minamino, N.; Kangawa, K.; Matsuo, H.; Raftery, M.A.; Hirose, T.; Inayama, S.; Hayashida, H.; Miyata, T.; and Numa, S. 1984. Primary structure of *Electrophorus electricus* sodium channel deduced from cDNA sequence. *Nature* 312: 121-127.

(191) Noda, M.; Takahashi, H.; Tanabe, T.; Toyosato, M.; Furutani, Y.; Hirose, T.; Asai, M.; Inayama, S.; Miyata, T.; and Numa, S. 1982. Primary structure of alpha-subunit precursor of *Torpedo californica* acetylcholine receptor deduced from cDNA sequence. *Nature* 299: 793-797.

(192) Noda, M.; Takahashi, H.; Tanabe, T.; Toyosato, M.; Kikyotani, S.; Furutani, Y.; Hirose, T.; Takashima, H.; Inayama, S.; Miyata, T.; and Numa, S. 1983. Structural homology of *Torpedo californica* acetylcholine receptor subunits. *Nature* 302: 528-532.

(193) Noda, M.; Takahashi, H.; Tanabe, T.; Toyosato, M.; Kokyotani, S.; Hirose, T.; Asai, M.; Takashima, H.; Inayama, S.; Miyata, T.; and Numa, S. 1983. Primary structures of alpha- and beta-subunit precursors of *Torpedo californica* acetylcholine receptor deduced from cDNA sequences. *Nature* 301: 251-255.

(194) Numa, S.; Noda, M.; Takahashi, H.; Tanabe, T.; Toyosato, M.; Furutani, Y.; and Kikyotani, S. 1983. Molecular structure of the nicotinic acetylcholine receptor. *Cold S.H. Quant. Biol.* 48: 57-69.

(195) Olsen, R.W. 1981. GABA-benzodiazepine-barbiturate receptor interactions. *J. Neurochem.* 37: 1-13.

(196) Oppenheim, R.W.; Pittman, R.; Gray, M.; and Madredrut, J.L. 1978. Embryonic behavior, hatching and neuromuscular development in the chick following a transient reduction of spontaneous mobility and sensory input by neuromuscular blocking agents. *J. Comp. Neur.* 179: 619-640.

(197) Oswald, R.E. 1983. Effects of calcium on the binding of phencyclidine to acetylcholine receptor-rich membrane fragments from *Torpedo californica* electroplaque. *J. Neurochem.* 41: 1077.

(198) Oswald, R., and Changeux, J.-P. 1981. Selective labeling of the delta subunit of the acetylcholine receptor by a covalent local anesthetic. *Biochemistry* 20: 7166-7174.

(199) Oswald, R., and Changeux, J.-P. 1981. Ultraviolet light-induced labeling by noncompetitive blockers of the acetylcholine receptor from *Torpedo* electroplaque. *Molec. Pharm.* 25: 360-368.

(200) Oswald, R.E.; Heidmann, T.; and Changeux, J.-P. 1983. Multiple affinity states for noncompetitive blockers revealed by ^{3}H-phencyclidine binding to acetylcholine receptor rich membranes fragments from *Torpedo marmorata. Biochemistry* 22: 3128-3136.

(201) Oswald, R.; Sobel, A.; Waksman, G.; Roques, B.; and Changeux, J.-P. 1980. Selective labeling by [^{3}H-]trimethisoquin azide of polypeptide chains present in acetylcholine receptor rich membranes from *Torpedo marmorata. FEBS Lett.* 111: 29-34.

(202) Patrick, J.; Heinemann, S.; Lindstrom, J.; Schubert, D.; and Steinbach, J. 1972. Appearance of acetylcholine receptors during differentiation of a myogenic cell line. *Proc. Natl. Acad. Sci.* 69: 2762-2768.

(203) Peng, H.B., and Cheng, P.C. 1982. Formation of postsynaptic specializations induced by latex beads in cultured muscle cells. *J. Neurosci.* 2: 1760-1774.

(204) Peng, H.B., and Froehner, S.C. 1985. Association of the postsynaptic 43K protein with newly formed acetylcholine receptor clusters in cultured muscle cells. *J. Cell Biol.* 100: 1698-1705.

(205) Pezzementi, L., and Schmidt, J. 1981. Ryanodine alters the rate of acetylcholine receptor synthesis in chick skeletal muscle cell cultures. *J. Biol. Chem.* 256: 12651-12654.

(206) Pfeiffer, K.; Simler, R.; Grenningloh, G.; and Betz, H., 1984. Monoclonal antibodies and peptide mapping reveal structural similarities between the subunits of the glycine receptor of rat spinal cord. *Proc. Natl. Acad. Sci.* 81: 7224-7227.

(207) Popot, J.L. 1983. Structural and functional properties of the acetylcholine receptor: studies using reconstituted vesciles. In *Basic Mechanisms of Neuronal Hyperexcitability*, ed. H.H. Jasper and N.M. Van Gelder, pp. 137-170. New York: Alan Riss.

(208) Prigogine, I. 1961. Introduction to the Thermodynamics of Irreversible Processes. New York: Interscience.

(209) Prinz, H., and Maelicke, A. 1983. Interaction of cholinergic ligands with the purified acetylcholine receptor protein: equilibrium binding studies. *J. Biol. Chem.* 258: 10263-10271.

(210) Prives, J.D. 1976. Appearance of specialized cell membrane components during differentiation of embryonic skeletal muscle cells in culture. In *Surface Membrane Receptors*, eds. R.A. Bradshaw, W.A. Frazier, R.C. Merrell, D.I. Gottlieb, and R.A. Hogue-Angeletti, pp. 363-375.

(211) Raftery, M.A.; Hunkapiller, M.; Strader, C.D.; and Hood, L.E. 1980. Acetylcholine receptor: complex of homologous subunits. *Science* 208: 1454, 1457.

(212) Razin, A., and Friedman, J. 1981. Methylation and its possible biological role. In *Progress in Nucleic Acid Research and Molecular Biology*, ed. W.E. Cohn, vol. 25, pp. 33-52. New York: Academic Press.

(213) Reiness, C., and Weinberg, C. 1981. Metabolic stabilization of acetylcholine receptors at newly formed neuromuscular junction in rat. *Develop. Biol.* 84: 247-254.

(214) Reynolds, J.A., and Karlin, A. 1978. Molecular weight in detergent solution of acetylcholine receptor from *Torpedo californica*. *Biochemistry* 17: 2035-2038.

(215) Rieger, F.; Grumet, M.; and Edelman, G. 1985. N-CAM at the vertebrate neuromuscular junction. *J. Cell. Biol.* 101: 285-293.

(216) Ripley, K.L., and Province, R.R. 1972. Neural correlates of embryonic mobility in the chick. *Brain Res.* 45: 127-134.

(217) Role, L.; Matossian, V.R.; O'Brien, R.; and Fischbach, G.D. 1985. On the mechanism of acetylcholine receptor accumulation at newly formed synapses on chick myotubes. *J. Neurosci.* 5: 2197-2204.

(218) Rotundo, R.L., and Fambrough, D.M. 1980. Secretion of acetylcholinesterase: relation to acetylcholine receptor metabolism. *Cell* 22: 595-602.

(219) Rousselet, A.; Cartaud, J.; and Devaux, P.F. 1979. Importance des interactions protéine dans le maintien de la structure des fragments excitable de l'organe électrique de *Torpedo marmorata*. *Comp. Rendus Acad. Sci. Paris D* 289: 461-463.

(220) Rousselet, A.; Cartaud, J.; Devaux, P.F.; and Changeux, J.-P. 1982. The rotational diffusion of the acetylcholine Receptor in *Torpedo marmorata* membrane fragments studies with a spin-labelled alpha-toxin: importance of the 43.000 protein(s). *EMBO J.* 1: 439-445.

(221) Rousselet, A.; Cartaud, J.; Saitoh, T.; Changeux, J.-P.; and Devaux, P. 1980. Factors influencing the rotational diffusion of the acetylcholine receptor-rich membranes from *Torpedo marmorata* investigated by saturation transfer electron spin resonance spectroscopy. *J. Cell. Biol.* 90: 418-426.

(222) Rubin, L.L. 1985. Increase in muscle Ca^{++} mediate changes in acetylcholinesterase and acetylcholine receptors caused by muscle contraction. *Proc. Natl. Acad. Sci.* 82: 7121-7125.

(223) Rubin, L.L.; Schuetze, S.M.; and Fischbach, G.D. 1979. Accumulation of acetylcholinesterase at newly formed nerve-muscle synapses. *Develop. Biol.* 69: 46-58.

(224) Rubin, L.L.; Schuetze, S.M.; Weill, C.; and Fischbach, G.D. 1978. The appearance of acetylcholinesterase at newly formed neuromuscular junctions is regulated by nerve-muscle activity. *Neuroscience Abstr.* 4: 1193.

(225) Rubin, L.L.; Schuetze, S.M.; Weill, C.L.; and Fischbach, G.D. 1980. Regulation of acetylcholinesterase appearance at neuromuscular junctions *in vitro*. *Nature* 283: 264-267.

(226) Saitoh, T., and Changeux, J.-P. 1980. Phosphorylation *in vitro* of membrane fragments from *Torpedo marmorata* electric organ. *Eur. J. Biochem.* 105: 51-62.

(227) Saitoh, T., and Changeux, J.-P. 1981. Change in state of phosphorylation of acetylcholine receptor during maturation of the electromotor synapse in *Torpedo marmorata* electric organ. *Proc. Natl. Acad. Sci.* 78: 4430-4434.

(228) Saitoh, T.; Wennogle, L.P.; and Changeux, J.-P. 1979. Factors regulating the suspectibility of the acetylcholine receptor protein to heat inactivation. *FEBS Lett.* 108: 489-494.

(229) Sakmann, B., and Brenner, H.R. 1978. Changes in synaptic channel gating during neuromuscular development. *Nature* 274: 68-70.

(230) Sakmann, B.; Patlak, J.; and Neher, E. 1980. Single acetylcholine activated channels show burst-kinetics in presence of desensitizing concentrations of agonist. *Nature* 286: 71-73.

(231) Salpeter, M.; Smith, C.; and Matthews-Bellinger, J.A. 1984. Acetylcholine receptor at neuro-muscular junctions by E.M.

autoradiography using mask a analysis and linear source. *J. Electr. Microsc. Tech.* 1: 63-81.

(232) Sanes, J.R., and Chiu, A.Y. 1983. The basal lamina of the neuromuscular junction. *Cold S.H. Quant. Biol.* 48: 667-678.

(233) Sanes, J.R., and Hall, Z.W. 1979. Antibodies that bind specifically to synaptic sites on muscle fiber basal lamina. *J. Cell Biol.* 83: 357-370.

(234) Schindler, H.; Spillecke, F.; and Neumann, E. 1984. Different channel properties of *Torpedo* acetylcholine receptors monomers and dimers reconstituted in planar membranes. *Proc. Natl. Acad. Sci.* 81: 6222-6226.

(235) Schneider, M.; Shieh, B.H.; Pezzementi, L.; and Schmidt, J. 1984. Trifluoperazine stimulates acetylcholine receptor synthesis in cultured chick myotubes. *J. Neurochem.* 42: 1350-1401.

(236) Schramm, M., and Selinger, Z. 1984. Message transmission: receptor controlled adenylate cyclase system. *Science* 225: 1350-1356.

(237) Schubert, D.; Heinemann, S.; and Kidokoro, Y. 1977. Cholinergic metabolism and synapse formation by a rat nerve cell line. *Proc. Natl. Acad. Sci.* 74: 2579-2583.

(238) Schuetze, E. 1980. The acetylcholine channel open time in chick muscle is not decreased following innervation. *J. Physl. Lon.* 303: 111-124.

(239) Schuetze, S.M., and Vicini, S. 1984. Neonatal denervation inhibits the normal postnatal decrease in endplate channel open time. *J. Neurosci.* 4: 2297-2302.

(240) Schuetze, S.M.; Frank, E.F.; and Fischbach, G.D. 1978. Channel open time and metabolic stability of synaptic and extrasynaptic acetylcholine receptors on cultured chick myotubes. *Proc. Natl. Acad. Sci.* 75: 520-523.

(241) Schuetze, S.M.; Vicini, S.; and Hall, Z.W. 1985. Myasthenic serum selectively blocks acetylcholine receptors with long channel open times at developing rat endplates. *Proc. Natl. Acad. Sci.* 82: 2533-2537.

(242) Schwartz, J.C.; Llorens Cortes, C.; Rose, C.; Quach, T.T.; and Pollard, H. 1983. Adaptative changes of neurotransmitter receptor mechanisms in the central nervous system. *Prog. Brain Res.* 58: 117-130.

(243) Sealock, R.; Wray, B.E.; and Froehner, S.C. 1984. Ultrastructural localization of the M_r 43.000 protein and the acetylcholine receptor in *Torpedo* postsynaptic membranes using monoclonal antibodies. *J. Cell. Biol.* 98: 2239.

(244) Shainberg, A., and Burstein, M. 1976. Decrease of acetylcholine receptor synthesis in muscle cultures by electric stimulation. *Nature* 264: 348-349.

(245) Sherman, S.J., and Catteral, W.A. 1984. Electrical activity and cytosolic calcium regulate levels of tetrodotoxin sensitive sodium channels in cultured rat muscle cells. *Proc. Natl. Acad. Sci.* 81: 262-266.

(246) Sherman, S.J.; Chrivia, J.; and Catterall, W.A. 1985. Cyclic adrenosine 3' : 5' - monophosphate and cytosolic calcium exert opposing effects on biosynthesis of tetrodoxtoxin - sensitive sodium channels in rat muscle cells. *J. Neurosci.* 5: 1570-1576.

(247) Shuster, M.J.; Camardo, S.A.; Siegelbaum, S.A.; and Kandel, E. 1985. Cyclic AMP-dependent protein kinase clones the serotonin-sensitive K+ channels of *Aplysia* sensory neurons in cell free membrane patches. *Nature* 313: 392-395.

(248) Sobel, A.; Weber, M.; and Changeux, J.-P. 1977. Large scale purification of the acetylcholine receptor protein in its membrane-bound and detergent extracted forms *Torpedo marmorata* electric organ. *Eur. J. Biochem.* 80: 215-224.

(249) Sobel, A.; Heidmann, T.; Hofler, J.; and Changeux, J.-P. 1978. Distinct protein components from *Torpedo marmorata* membranes carry the acetylcholine receptor site and the binding site for local anesthetics and histrionicotoxin. *Proc. Natl. Acad. Sci.* 75: 510-514.

(250) Sohal, G.S., and Wrenn, R.W. 1984. Appearance of high-molecular-weight acetylcholinesterase in aneural muscle developing *in vivo*. *Develop. Biol.* 101: 229-234.

(251) Squire, L.R., and Davis, H.P. 1981. The pharmacology of memory: a neurobiological perspective. *Ann. R. Pharm. Tox.* 21: 323-356.

(252) Stallcup, W.B., and Patrick, J. 1980. Substance P enhances cholinergic receptor desensitization in a clonal nerve cell line. *Proc. Natl. Acad. Sci.* 77: 634-638.

(253) Stent, G. 1973. A physiological mechanism for Hebb's postulate of learning. *Proc. Natl. Acad. Sci.* 70: 997-1001.

(254) Steinbach, J.H.; Merlie, J.; Heinemann, S.; and Bloch, R. 1979. Degradation of junctional and extrajunctional acetylcholine receptors by developing rat skeletal muscle. *Proc. Natl. Acad. Sci.* 76: 3547-3551.

(255) Sumikawa, K.; Houghton, M.; Smith, J.C.; Bell, L.; Richards, B.M.; and Barnard, E.A. 1982. The molecular cloning and characterization of cDNA coding for the alpha subunit of the acetylcholine receptor. *Nucl. Acid R.* 10: 5809-5822.

(256) Swanson, L.W.; Sawchenko, P.E.; and Lind, R. 1986. Regulation of multiple peptides in C.R.S. parvocellular neurosecretory neurons: implications for the stress response. *Prog. Brain Res.*, in press.

(257) Takai, T.; Noda, M.; Mishina, M.; Shimizu, S.; Furutani, Y.; Kayano, T.T.; Ikeda, T.; Kubo, T.; Takahashi, H.; Takahashi, T.; Kuno, M.; and Numa, S. 1985. Cloning, sequenching and expression of cDNA for a novel subunit of acetylcholine receptor for calf muscle. *Nature* 315: 761-764.

(258) Takeyasu, K.; Udgaonkar, J.B.; and Hess, G.P. 1983. Acetylcholine receptor: evidence for a voltage-dependent regulatory site for acetylcholine. Chemical kinetic measurements in membrane vesicles using a voltage clamp. *Biochemistry* 22: 5973-5978.

(259) Talvenheimo, J.A.; Tamkun, M.M.; Hartshorne, R.P.; Messner, D.J.; Sharkey, R.G.; Costa, M.R.C.; and Catterall, W.A. 1983. Structure and functional reconstitution of the voltage-sensitive sodium channel from rat brain. *Cold S.H. Quant. Biol.* 48: 155-164.

(260) Teichberg, V.T., and Changeux, J.-P. 1976. Presence of two forms with different isoelectric points of the acetylcholine receptor in the electric organ of *Electrophorus electricus* and their catalytic interconversion *in vitro*. *FEBS Lett.* 67: 264-268.

(261) Teichberg, V.T., and Changeux, J.-P. 1977. Evidence for protein phosphorylation and dephosphorylation in membrane fragements isolated from the electric organ of *Electrophorus electricus*. *FEBS Lett.* 74: 71-76.

(262) Teichberg, V.T.; Sobel, A.; and Changeux, J.-P. 1977. *In vitro* phosphorylation of acetylcholine receptor. *Nature* 267: 540-542.

(263) Thomas, R. 1981. On the relation between the logical structure of systems and their ability to generate multiple steady-states or sustained oscillations. *Spr. Ser. Syn.* 9: 180-193.

(264) Toulouse, G.; Dehaene, S.; and Changeux, J.-P. 1986. Spin glass model of learning by selection. *Proc. Natl. Acad. Sci.* 83: 1695-1699.

(265) Toutant, M.; Bourgeois, J.P.; Toutant, J.P.; Renaud, D.; Le Douarin, G.H.; and Changeux, J.-P. 1980. Chronic stimulation of the spinal cord in developing chick embryo causes the differentiation of multiple clusters of acetylcholine receptor in the *posterior latissimus dorsi* muscle. *Develop. Biol.* 76: 384-395.

(266) Toutant, M.; Toutant, J.P.; Renaud, D.; Le Douarin, G.; and Changeux, J.-P. 1981. Effet de la stimulation médullaire, chronique sur le nombre total de sites d'activité acétyl-

cholinérastique du muscle *posterior latissimus dorsi* de l'embryon de poulet. *C.R. Acad. Sci.* 292: 771-775.

(267) Tsien, R.W. 1983. Calcium channels in excitable cell-membrane. *Ann. R. Physl.* 45: 341-358.

(268) Vandlen, R.L.; Wu, W.C.-S.; Eisenach, J.C.; and Raftery, M.A. 1979. Studies of the composition of purified *Torpedo californica* acetylcholine receptor and of its subunits. *Biochemistry* 10: 1845-1854.

(269) Vigny, M.; Bon, S., Massoulié, J.; and Leterrier, F. 1978. Active site efficiency of acetylcholinesterase molecular forms in *Electrophorus, Torpedo,* rat and chicken. *Eur. J. Biochem.* 85: 317-323.

(270) Vigny, M.; Digiamberardino, L.; Couraud, J.Y.; Reiger, F.; and Koenig, J. 1976. Molecular forms of chicken acetylcholinesterase: effect of denervation. *FEBS Lett.* 69: 277-280.

(271) Vigny, M.; Koenig, J.; and Rieger, F. 1976. The motor endplate specific form of acetylcholinesterase: appearance during embryogenesis and reinnervation of rat muscle. *J. Neurochem.* 27: 1347-1353.

(272) Villu, A.; Gu, Y.; Hestrin, S.; and Hall, Z. 1985. The effects of a myasthenic serum on the acetylcholine receptors of C2 myotubes II. Functional inactivation of the receptors. *J. Neurosci.* 5: 1917-1924.

(273) Walker, J.W.; McNamee, M.G.; Pasquale, E.; Cash, D.J.; and Hess, G.P. 1981. Acetylcholine receptor inactivation in *Torpedo californica* electroplax membrane vesicles. Detection of two processes in the millisecond and second time region. *Biochem. Biophys. Res. Comm.* 100: 86-90.

(274) Walker, J.W.; Takeyasu, K.; and McNamee, M.G. 1982. Activation and inactivation kinetics of *Torpedo californica* acetylcholine receptor in reconstituted membranes. *Biochemistry* 21: 5384-5389.

(275) Wallace, B.G.; Nitkin, R.M.; Reist, N.E.; Fallon, J.R.; Moayeri, N.; and McMahan, U.J. 1985. Aggregates of acetylcholinesterase induced by acetylcholine receptor-aggregating factor. *Nature* 315: 574-577.

(276) Weidoff, P.M.; McNamee, M.G.; and Wilson, B.W. 1979. Modulation of cholinergic proteins and RNA by ouabain in chick muscle cultures. *FEBS Lett.* 100: 389-393.

(277) Weinberg, G.C., and Hall, Z. 1979. Antibodies from patients with *myasthenia gravis* recognize determinants unique to extgra

junctional acetylcholine receptors. *Proc. Natl. Acad. Sci.* 76: 504-508.

(278) Wennogle, L.R., and Changeux, J.-P. 1980. Transmembrane orientation of proteins present in acetylcholine receptor-rich membranes from *Torpedo marmorata* studied by selective proteolysis. *Eur. J. Biochem.* 106: 381-393.

(279) Wigström, H., and Gustafsson, B. 1986. Postsynaptic control of hippocampal long-term potentiation. *J. Physl. Paris*, in press.

(280) Yéramian, E., and Changeux, J.-P. 1986. Un modèle de changement d'efficacité synaptique à long terme fondé sur l'interaction du récepteur de l'Ach avec la protéine sous synaptique de 43 000 daltons. *C.R. Acad. Sci. Série III, No. 17* 302: 609-616.

(281) Yéramian, E.; Trautman, A.; and Claverie, P. 1986. Acetylcholine receptors are not functionally independent. *Biophys. J.* 50: 253-263 .

(282) Zelena, J.; Vycklicky, L.; and Jirmanova, I. 1967. Motor end-plates in fast and slow muscles of the chick after cross-union of their nerves. *Nature* 214: 1010-1011.

(283) Ziskind-Conhaim, L.; Inestrosa, N.C.; and Hall, Z.W. 1984. Acetylcholine is functional in embryonic rat muscle before its accumulation at the sites of nerve muscle contact. *Develop. Biol.* 103: 369-377.

The Neural and Molecular Bases of Learning,
eds. J.-P. Changeux and M. Konishi, pp. 85–98.
John Wiley & Sons Limited.

Activity-dependent Regulation of Gene Expression

H. Thoenen* and A. Acheson**

* Abt. Neurochemie
Max-Planck-Institut für Psychiatrie
8033 Planegg-Martinsried, F.R. Germany
** School of Medicine
Case Western Reserve University
Cleveland, OH 44106, USA

Abstract. The activity-dependent modulation of gene expression is a characteristic feature of higher integrated nervous systems such as the human brain. This type of activity-dependent "hardware adaptation" greatly expands the functional capacity of the brain. We discuss the peripheral sympatho-adrenal nervous system as a model for function-dependent regulation of gene expression. It has been demonstrated *in vivo* and in organ culture that presynaptic nerve impulse flow regulates the gene expression of both catecholamine biosynthetic enzymes and peptides in postsynaptic sympatho-adrenal cells. This phenomenon, called "transsynaptic induction," has been extensively characterized on a descriptive level, but little is known about the biochemical signalling mechanism(s) by which the presynaptic cholinergic input alters gene expression, since an adequate *in vitro* model system has not yet become available. Such a system would be necessary for a detailed molecular analysis of the signalling mechanism(s) involved and requires sufficient quantities of homogeneous neurons or neuron-like cells. Activity-dependent regulation of gene expression in the sympatho-adrenal system is discussed in the context of regulatory mechanisms intrinsic to the structure of the tissue, such as cell-cell contact and the interaction of cells with components of the extracellular matrix. These structural regulatory factors have to be taken into account when evaluating the effects of regulators which act via chemical signalling, such as presynaptic nerve input, hormones or neurotrophic factors, on alterations in gene expression.

INTRODUCTION

With the rapidly increasing use of computers in science it has become customary to compare the functioning of the brain with that of a computer. Indeed, many brain functions can be mimicked by computers, and in many respects they are even more efficient and reliable than the human brain. However, there is a fundamental difference between the two: the higher vertebrate brain has the capability of modifying its macromolecular composition, including its morphology, according to functional changes or, teleologically speaking, according to functional requirements. This capability of function-dependent "hardware adaptation" expands the capacity of the brain to an almost unimaginable extent. Although the existence of function-dependent changes in the nervous system is well established, the underlying mechanisms are generally poorly understood. In order to study them at a biochemical or molecular level it is necessary to apply reductionist experimental principles and to use simple model systems. Together with the relatively primitive nervous systems of molluscs or insects, the neuromuscular junction and the peripheral sympathetic nervous system have been the favored models for studying function-dependent regulation of gene expression. The use of the neuromuscular junction as such a model system will be discussed in a separate chapter of this volume (see Changeux *et al.*, this volume) and we will concentrate here on the peripheral sympathetic nervous system, including the adrenal medulla. In this system, activity-dependent regulation of gene expression has been demonstrated, the consequences of which are changes in the levels of specific transmitter-synthesizing enzymes and neuronal peptides. We will summarize the activity-regulated changes in the sympathetic nervous system and will put this information in the context of more recent insights into the role of structural regulatory phenomena, such as cell-cell and cell-extracellular matrix (ECM) contact, in modulating the effects of regulation by chemical signalling, such as by neuronal activity and neurotrophic factors.

ACTIVITY-MEDIATED TRANSSYNAPTIC REGULATION OF THE SYNTHESIS OF CATECHOLAMINE BIOSYNTHETIC ENZYMES

It is well established that the consequences of nerve impulse activity are not confined to neurotransmitter-mediated changes in the ionic permeability of the postsynaptic membrane, resulting in depolarization or hyperpolarization. The response of the postsynaptic cell to input also involves alterations in posttranslational (covalent) modifications of proteins, for example in their state of phosphorylation (for a review see (32)), and changes in the rate of synthesis of a variety of macromolecules involved in many cellular functions. The peripheral sympatho-adrenal medullary system has proved to be a useful model for the analysis of activity-dependent changes in gene expression because it is easily accessible, is organized relatively simply, and much is known about its physiological functions and biochemical properties. Increased activity of the preganglionic cholinergic fibers, resulting from drug administration, stressful stimuli such as cold, forced swimming or restraint, or direct electrical stimulation of the preganglionic nerves themselves brings about an increase in the levels of tyrosine hydroxylase (TH). This increase does not become apparent before 12-24 hours and reaches a maximum 48 hours after the onset of the increase in activity (for a review of the early literature see (37); for a more recent review see (40); see also (46)). Direct stimulation of the preganglionic nerves for 30 minutes at 10 Hz is sufficient to obtain the full increase in TH levels 48 hours later (45).

That the increase in TH levels does not reflect a general increase in protein synthesis can be deduced from the fact that the overall incorporation of amino acids into protein is not significantly elevated and that the increase in specific enzyme activities is very selective (40). The specific activities of TH and dopamine-beta-hydroxylase (DBH) both increase, whereas that of the third enzyme involved in noradrenaline biosynthesis, aromatic amino acid decarboxylase (DDC), remains unchanged. No change is observed in the specific activity of lactate dehydrogenase (LHD), a cytoplasmic marker enzyme. The increase in TH and DBH specific activities results from enhanced synthesis of these proteins, as has been directly demonstrated by immunotitration experiments (evidence for increased number of enzyme molecules) and immunoprecipitation after pulse-labelling, which revealed increased incorporation of amino acids into the molecules (15, 19, 47).

More recently, it has been demonstrated that the increased synthesis of TH is preceded by a corresponding increase in levels of mRNA coding for TH (5, 13, 35, 36). These direct measurements are in agreement with earlier observations that the transsynaptic induction of TH could be blocked by inhibitors of RNA synthesis only in the first few hours after the initiation of the response by increased preganglionic activity. At later stages (after 12 hours), the increase in TH synthesis could no longer be blocked by such inhibitors. In contrast, inhibitors of protein synthesis interfered with the increase in TH activity when administered at any time during which the TH activity was still increasing (40).

Transsynaptic induction of TH and DBH can be completely blocked by ganglion blocking agents, and the effect of increased preganglionic activity can be mimicked by nicotinic agonists in sympathetic ganglia in organ culture (8, 40). These two pieces of evidence indicate that the effect is mediated by acetylcholine, the physiological transmitter of the preganglionic cholinergic nerves, rather than by peptides which may be co-released with acetylcholine. The enhanced enzyme synthesis is closely linked to the activation of the nicotinic cholinergic receptors and not to the resulting propagation of action potentials mediated by the tetrodotoxin-sensitive "fast sodium channels" (6). In contrast to nicotinic blocking agents, direct inhibitors of the sodium channel, like tetrodotoxin, do not interfere with transsynaptic induction (39). In addition, depolarization of sympathetic neurons by high potassium or veratridine does not result in increased enzyme levels (33). The lack of importance of action potential propagation and depolarization for the phenomenon is further supported by the work of Chalazonitis and Zigmond (9), who showed that the electrical stimulation of the preganglionic fibers of the superior cervical ganglion of the rat, and not of the postganglionic fibers, was necessary for the increase in TH levels. It must be mentioned that all the results referred to so far are derived from observations made *in vivo* in adult animals or in organ culture systems using sympathetic ganglia or adrenal glands obtained from adult animals. In contrast, in cultures of dissociated sympathetic neurons from newborn rat, potassium depolarization resulted in a calcium-dependent increase in TH levels, but carbachol, a long-acting acetylcholine agonist, had no effect (17). High potassium-mediated TH induction disappeared with increasing age of the cultures, whereas a small and variable increase in TH activity brought about by carbachol treatment appeared (Gnahn and Thoenen, unpublished observations), suggesting the existence of a developmentally regulated mechanism. In other words, TH could be induced by depolarization at earlier developmental stages but would be strictly controlled by a nicotinic receptor-mediated mechanism at later stages.

POSSIBLE SIGNALLING MECHANISMS FOR TRANSSYNAPTIC INDUCTION

Although it is clear that increased preganglionic activity brings about an increased synthesis of TH and DBH, which is preceded, at least in the case of TH, by an increase in mRNA levels, the biochemical events which link the activation of the nicotinic receptor to the subsequent increase in mRNA levels are not known. The possible involvement of cAMP as a second messenger was a matter of controversy (for example, cf. (16) with (38)). However, the following data are incompatible with such a role for cAMP: in sympathetic ganglia transsynaptic induction occurs without detectable increases in cAMP levels, and markedly increased cAMP levels produced by cholera toxin or isoproterenol (both of which lead to increases in cAMP in neurons rather than non-neuronal cells) do not mimic the effect of preganglionic stimulation. The increases in cAMP which occur in the adrenal gland after stressful stimuli have been shown to originate from the adrenal cortex, since they can be eliminated by hypophysectomy or administration of glucocorticoids, neither of which treatment alters the phenomenon of transsynaptic induction in rat adrenal medulla (38). In addition, it is possible to bring about enzyme induction in primary cultures of bovine adrenal chromaffin cells by 8-bromo-cAMP, a permeant cAMP analog (2, 25). However, the pattern of enzymes induced by cAMP is different from that resulting from increased preganglionic cholinergic input to the adrenal gland; not only are TH, DBH, and phenylethanolamine-N-methyltransferase (PNMT), the enzyme converting noradrenaline to adrenaline, induced but the activities of DDC and acetylcholinesterase are also increased (2).

Unfortunately, in contrast to what has been shown using sympathetic ganglia, it has so far been impossible to initiate enzyme induction in organ cultures of adrenal gland or in primary cultures of adrenal chromaffin cells with nicotinic agonists. It may be that this failure is due to the large amounts of catecholamines which are released by this treatment, which could interfere with the inducing effect. The quantities of catecholamines stored in chromaffin granules are much higher than those stored in cell bodies of sympathetic neurons, and thus the amounts released would be much greater in the adrenal system. The discrepancy between the *in vivo* and *in vitro* situations could be explained by the fact that *in vivo* the released catecholamines are rapidly removed by the efficient venous drainage of the adrenal medulla. This possibility is also supported by the finding that the enzyme induction in sympathetic ganglia brought about by nicotinic agonists can be inhibited by catecholamines. The blockade of the nicotinic receptor-mediated enzyme induction by catecholamines is correlated with a blockade of the bulk sodium influx which occurs via these receptors; the contribution of the tetrodotoxin-sensitive sodium channels is negligible (6). This bulk sodium influx results in an increase in the intracellular sodium concentration from 20 to 100 mM within 5-10 minutes of exposure to 200 μM carbamylcholine (7). The importance of bulk sodium influx is also supported by the observation that replacement of sodium by lithium or Tris in the culture medium abolishes carbachol-mediated TH induction in sympathetic ganglion organ cultures (39). Moreover, preliminary experiments in primary cultures of bovine adrenal chromaffin cells indicate that treatment with a sodium ionophore results in an increase in TH activity (Krauss *et al*., unpublished observations). In spite of all these correlations, no causal relationship has yet been established between sodium influx and the induction mechanism. Even if bulk sodium influx could be shown to be causally linked to the phenomenon, the major question would still remain unanswered, namely, in which manner is sodium linked to an increase in TH mRNA levels?

The involvement of calcium in the signalling process responsible for transsynaptic induction is not yet clear. TH induction by nicotinic agonists in sympathetic ganglia in organ culture was not affected by the absence of calcium in the medium, nor even by the presence of 10mM EGTA (39). Nonetheless, these data do not exclude the possibility that mobilization of endogenous calcium plays a role in the phenomenon.

The transsynaptic induction of TH can be enhanced by glucocorticoids (39). However, this effect may be an indirect one. In contrast to the unambiguous localization of glucocorticoid receptors in the nuclei of satellite cells in rat sympathetic ganglia, no glucocorticoid receptors could be demonstrated in the nuclei of neurons by autoradiography (42). Glucocorticoids could thus act on the non-neuronal cells to enhance somehow the effect of preganglionic stimulation indirectly. An additional way in which glucocorticoids could indirectly enhance the effect of presynaptic nerve stimulation would be to increase transmitter release from the preganglionic nerves (40).

STRUCTURAL FACTORS REGULATING THE LEVELS OF CATECHOLAMINE BIOSYNTHETIC ENZYMES

It is important to remember that preganglionic stimulation is not occurring in a vacuum. In addition to the effect of cholinergic nerve input on the levels of the catecholamine biosynthetic enzymes, there are at least two additional structural factors which can regulate the levels of these enzymes: contact with other cells and contact with some components of the ECM. In referring to these two types of interactions as "structural," we do not mean to imply that these factors are not also subject to regulation, only that they are inherent to the structure of the tissue at any given stage of development. Cell contact-mediated regulation of TH levels was first studied in PC12 pheochromocytoma cells (30) and has subsequently been studied in greater detail in primary cultures of bovine adrenal chromaffin cells. In this system, increased cell density (and thereby increased cell-cell contact) brings about increases in the specific activities of TH, DBH, and PNMT whereas those of DDC, LDH, and acetylcholinesterase remain unaffected (1, 3). For TH, the increased enzymatic activity has been shown to be due to an increase in the number of enzyme molecules, and, since the effect can be blocked by alpha-amanitin, an inhibitor of mRNA synthesis is likely to be due to an increase in TH synthesis (3). Conditioned medium from high-density cultures cannot mimic the effect of increased density (3), but adrenal medullary plasma membranes and plasma membrane extracts can completely mimic the effect of increased density in terms of time course, selectivity, and magnitude (Saadat and Thoenen, unpublished observations).

It has recently been observed that components of the ECM, particularly laminin, can promote neurite outgrowth (31) and can also potentiate the survival and neurite-promoting effects of the soluble neurotrophic molecules nerve growth factor (NGF) and brain-derived neurotrophic factor (10, 28). Thus, the "structural" influence of the ECM can alter the ability of a neuron to respond to the chemical signalling mediated by the neurotrophic factor. It has also been shown that laminin has a direct effect on the specific activities of the catecholamine biosynthetic enzymes TH, DBH, and PNMT in cultures of calf chromaffin cells (1). Exposure of calf chromaffin cells to a laminin substrate results in an approximately 100% rise in TH activity after 2 days, which can also be shown to be due to an increase in the number of TH molecules by immunotitration and is blocked by alpha-amanitin.

Furthermore, it has been shown on the light microscopic level that chromaffin cells *in vivo* appear to be in contact with both one another and with laminin. Localization of both TH and laminin on frozen sections of calf adrenal medulla using indirect immunofluorescence reveals clusters of TH-positive chromaffin cells which appear to be in close apposition to each other without a basement membrane in between. These clusters are then surrounded by a laminin-positive sheath (1). Preliminary electron microscopic evidence obtained from mouse adrenal medulla supports these observations (Kreutzberg, unpublished observations). Thus, cell-cell and cell-ECM contact, influences inherent to the structure of the tissue *in vivo* which can be mimicked to some extent *in vitro*, can be shown to regulate levels of the same enzymes as does preganglionic nerve input. In the chromaffin cell system, cell contact-mediated TH induction is not additive with that mediated by NGF or by laminin. Nonetheless, NGF-mediated and cell contact-mediated effects are pharmacologically separable, implying that their mechanisms of action differ at some level. It is not known to what extent all of these factors, ECM, contact with other cells, neurotrophic factors and other hormones (such as glucocorticoids) which may be present in the circulation, and preganglionic nerve activity, interact with each other *in vivo*. Nonetheless, at least *in vitro*, the chromaffin cell system offers a clear-cut example of the ability of structural influences to alter response of the cell to chemical signals. Another such example is cortisol-mediated induction of the enzyme glutamine synthetase in gliocytes. In this system it has been shown that direct contact between gliocytes and neurons is required for the cortisol-mediated effect (29). It has also been demonstrated that cell-cell contacts between embryonic retinal cells in culture play a role in maintaining the activity of cytoplasmic cortisol receptors (34). The implications of the interactions between structural influences and chemical signals for *in vitro* studies is clear: as many variables as possible have to be controlled in order to study one regulatory mechanism independently of the others.

REGULATION OF PEPTIDES

Presynaptic nerve impulse flow has also been shown to regulate levels of peptides in both the adrenal medulla and in sympathetic ganglia. However, in both systems the effects on peptides are not as well understood as are those on catecholamine biosynthetic enzymes. This is partly because the enzymes responsible for peptide processing and degradation have not yet been identified or characterized. Measurements of peptide levels alone are not sufficient to distinguish among changes in synthesis, processing, or degradation rates, any or all of which might be affected by various stimuli. In addition, peptide release can also be regulated, which adds another level of complexity to the interpretation of changes in peptide levels.

Keeping these reservations in mind, it has been demonstrated that levels of enkephalins in the adrenal medulla are increased *in vivo* by splanchnic nerve stimulation with about the same time course as is seen for elevation of TH levels (41). This increase is blocked by inhibitors of both protein and RNA synthesis (41). However, denervation of the rat adrenal gland and pharmacological blockade of synaptic transmission *in vivo* have also been shown to increase adrenal enkephalin content via an increase in the biosynthesis of enkephalin precursors (14, 26, 27). An increase in preproenkephalin mRNA levels has also been demonstrated in denervated adrenals *in vivo* (24). Rat adrenal medullae explanted to culture (and thus denervated) show a time-dependent increase in both enkephalin levels (26) and in preproenkephalin mRNA levels (27) as well. The rises in both peptide and mRNA levels can be prevented by treatment of the explants with depolarizing agents (26, 27).

Enkephalin levels and TH have been shown to be coordinately regulated by *in vitro* reserpine treatment of cultured bovine adrenal chromaffin cells (43). This may be unrelated to the effect of reserpine *in vivo*, reflecting rather a direct effect of the drug on the enzymes involved. Increased cAMP levels can also increase enkephalin levels in cultured chromaffin cells (11). However, reflecting the complexity of peptide measurements, Eiden and co-workers (11) have also shown that, while cAMP increases levels of preproenkephalin mRNA, reserpine treatment actually decreases mRNA levels, although both treatments increase levels of the mature peptides (11, 44). It has also been shown that nicotinic receptor stimulation (over a period of 2 days) stimulates enkephalin release from bovine chromaffin cells in culture, as well as producing increases in preproenkephalin mRNA levels and enkephalin precursor biosynthesis (12).

In the superior cervical ganglion the situation is even more complicated. Two peptide transmitters, substance P and somatostatin, are co-localized in sympathetic neurons with noradrenaline (18, 21). Nerve impulse activity and membrane depolarization decrease levels of both substance P (21, 23) and somatostatin (20). However, levels of these peptides are also regulated by other factors, both structural and chemical, which are influencing the neurons. For example, if the sympathetic ganglion is removed from the influence of its target tissue, by decentralization or by being put into explant culture, there is a massive increase in substance P levels (21, 23). However, if the neurons are dissociated and brought into culture, substance P levels remain constant (22), suggesting that not only the target tissue (perhaps via soluble factors) but also the other cells present in the ganglion regulate peptide levels. Additionally, it has recently been demonstrated that neuron-neuron contact regulates the levels of substance P in sympathetic neurons. In this case increased cell density brought about a 7-fold increase in the levels of substance P per neuron (4). That direct neuron-neuron contact is important for this effect was suggested by a) the almost total absence of non-neuronal cells in the cultures, b) the fact that the actual degree of neuronal aggregation increased with increasing cell density, and c) the absence of effect of high-density conditioned medium (4). Yet another complicating factor comes from the fact that all of the studies mentioned above deal only with neonatal rat sympathetic neurons. At least some of the regulatory phenomena described may be developmentally regulated as well. For instance, the target tissue-mediated effects on peptide levels are not seen in the adult animal (23).

As is the case for catecholamine biosynthetic enzymes, interactions of neurons or chromaffin cells with the ECM could also be involved in peptide homeostasis. It is not known how the regulatory influences on peptide levels interact with one another, nor is it clear whether increased presynaptic nerve input actually has any effect on peptide gene expression. It is clear, however, that other regulatory factors besides nerve input are important for the maintenance of peptide levels and that their roles must be better understood before that of nerve activity can be clarified.

CONCLUDING REMARKS

When one looks back over the history of the phenomenon originally described as "transsynaptic induction" in 1969, one realizes that in the ensuing 16 years the problems have not been solved by any means. There is no *in vitro* model system available to study the biochemical mechanism of the phenomenon, and no new information about the series of biochemical events linking the binding of acetylcholine to its receptor to the eventual alterations in gene expression, beyond the possible involvement of sodium, have been put forward. Nonetheless, it remains a fairly well characterized example of the activity-dependent regulation of gene expression, and since both TH and PNMT have recently been cloned (see (13, 35, 36) and B. Kaplan, unpublished results), it should be possible to study the regulation of both of these enzymes at the mRNA level. Perhaps these new tools will generate renewed interest in the phenomenon itself and lead to the development of an adequate model system for studying the biochemical events involved. Such a model system, whether consisting of primary cultures or cell lines, should provide sufficient quantities of homogeneous material to allow the analysis of biochemical processes using molecular genetics techniques.

REFERENCES

(1) Acheson, A.; Edgar, D.; Timpl, R.; and Thoenen, H. 1986. Laminin increases both levels and activity of tyrosine hydroxylase in calf adrenal chromaffin cells. *J. Cell Biol.* 102: 151-159.

(2) Acheson, A.L.; Naujoks, K.; and Thoenen, H. 1984. Nerve growth factor-mediated enzyme induction in primary cultures of bovine adrenal chromaffin cells: specificity and level of regulation. *J. Neurosci.* 4: 1771-1780.

(3) Acheson, A.L., and Thoenen, H. 1983. Cell contact-mediated regulation of tyrosine hydroxylase synthesis in cultured bovine adrenal chromaffin cells. *J. Cell Biol.* 97: 925-928.

(4) Adler, J.A., and Black, I.B. 1985. Sympathetic neuron density differentially regulates transmitter phenotypic expression. *Proc. Natl. Acad. Sci.* 82: 4296-4300.

(5) Black, I.B.; Chikaraishi, D.M.; and Lewis, E.J. 1985. Trans-synaptic increase in RNA coding for tyrosine hydroxylase in a rat sympathetic ganglion. *Brain Res.* 339: 151-153.

(6) Boenisch, H.; Otten, U.; and Thoenen, H. 1980. The role of sodium influx mediated by nicotinic receptors as an initital event in trans-synaptic induction of tyrosine hydroxylase in adrenergic neurons. *Naunyn-Schmiedeberg's Arch. Pharmacol.* 313: 199-203.

(7) Brown, D.A., and Scholfield, C.N. 1974. Movements of labelled sodium ions in isolated rat superior cervical ganglia. *J. Physl. Lon.* 242: 321-351.

(8) Chalazonitis, A.; Rice, P.J.; and Zigmond, R.E. 1980. Increased ganglionic tyrosine hydroxylase and dopamine-beta-hydroxylase activities following preganglionic nerve stimulation: role of nicotinic receptors. *J. Pharmacol. Exp. Ther.* 213: 139-143.

(9) Chalazonitis, A., and Zigmond, R.E. 1980. Effects of synaptic and antidromic stimulation on tyrosine hydroxylase activity in the rat superior cervical ganglion. *J. Physl. Lon.* 300: 525-538.

(10) Edgar, D.; Timpl, R.; and Thoenen, H. 1984. The heparin-binding domain of laminin is responsible for its effects on neurite outgrowth and neuronal survival. *EMBO J.* 3: 1463-1468.

(11) Eiden, L.E.; Giraud, P.; Affolter, H.-U.; Herbert, E.; and Hotchkiss, A.J. 1984. Alternative modes of enkephalin biosynthesis regulation by reserpine and cyclic AMP in cultured chromaffin cells. *Proc. Natl. Acad. Sci.* 81: 3949-3953.

(12) Eiden, L.E.; Giraud, P.; Dave, J.R.; Hotchkiss, A.J.; and Affolter, H.-U. 1984. Nicotinic receptor stimulation activates enkephalin release and biosynthesis in adrenal chromaffin cells. *Nature* 312: 661-663.

(13) Faucon Biguet, N.; Buda, M.; Lamouroux, A.; Samolyk, D.; and Mallet, J. 1986. Time course of changes of TH mRNA in rat brain and adrenal medulla after a single injection of reserpine. *EMBO J.*, in press.

(14) Fleminger, G.; Lahm, H.-W.; and Udenfriend, S. 1984. Changes in rat adrenal catecholamines and proenkephalin metabolism after denervation. *Proc. Natl. Acad. Sci.* 81: 3587-3590.

(15) Gagnon, C.; Otten, U.; and Thoenen, H. 1976. Increased synthesis of dopamine-beta-hydroxylase in cultured rat adrenal medullae after *in vivo* administration of reserpine. *J. Neurochem.* 27: 259-265.

(16) Guidotti, A., and Costa, E. 1977. Trans-synaptic regulation of tyrosine 3-mono-oxygenase biosynthesis in rat adrenal medulla. *Bioch. Pharm.* 26: 817-823.

(17) Hefti, F.; Gnahn, H.; Schwab, M.E.; and Thoenen, H. 1982. Induction of tyrosine hydroxylase by nerve growth factor and by elevated K^+ concentrations in cultures of dissociated sympathetic neurons. *J. Neurosci.* 2: 1554-1566.

(18) Hoekfelt, T.; Elfvin, L.G.; Elde, R.; Schultzberg, M.; Goldstein, M.; and Luft, R. 1977. Occurrence of somatostatin-like immunoreactivity in some peripheral sympathetic noradrenergic neurons. *Proc. Natl. Acad. Sci.* 74: 3587-3591.

(19) Joh, T.H.; Gegliman, C.; and Reis, D. 1973. Immunochemical demonstration of increased accumulation of tyrosine hydroxylase protein in sympathetic ganglia and adrenal medulla elicited by reserpine. *Proc. Natl. Acad. Sci.* 70: 2767-2771.

(20) Kessler, J.A.; Adler, J.E.; Bell, W.O.; and Black, I.B. 1983. Substance P and somatostatin metabolism in sympathetic and special sensory ganglia *in vitro*. *Neurosience* 9: 309-318.

(21) Kessler, J.A.; Adler, J.E.; Bohn, M.C.; and Black, I.B. 1981. Substance P in principal sympathetic neurons: regulation by impulse activity. *Science* 214: 335-336.

(22) Kessler, J.A.; Adler, J.E.; Jonakait, G.M.; and Black, I.B. 1984. Target organ regulation of substance P in sympathetic neurons in culture. *Develop. Biol.* 103: 71-79.

(23) Kessler, J.A., and Black, I.B. 1982. Regulation of substance P in adult rat sympathetic ganglia. *Brain Res.* 234: 182-187.

(24) Kilpatrick, D.L.; Howells, R.D.; Fleminger, G.; and Udenfriend, S. 1984. Denervation of rat adrenal glands markedly increases preproenkephalin mRNA. *Proc. Natl. Acad. Sci.* 81: 7221-7223.

(25) Kumakura, K.; Guidotti, A.; and Costa, E. 1979. Primary cultures of chromaffin cells: molecular mechanisms for the induction of tyrosine hydroxylase by 8-Br-cyclic AMP. *Molec. Pharm.* 16: 865-876.

(26) LaGamma, E.F.; Adler, J.E.; and Black, I.B. 1984. Impulse activity differentially regulates [leu]enkephalin and catecholamine characters in the adrenal medulla. *Science* 224: 1102-1104.

(27) LaGamma, E.F.; White, J.D.; Adler, J.E.; Krause, J.E.; McKelvy, J.F.; and Black, I.B. 1985. Depolarization regulates adrenal preproenkephalin mRNA. *Proc. Natl. Acad. Sci.* 82: 8252-8255.

(28) Lindsay, R.M.; Thoenen, H.; and Barde, Y.-A. 1985. Placode and neural crest-derived sensory neurons are responsive at early developmental stages to brain-derived neurotrophic factors (BDNF). *Develop. Biol.* 112: 319-328.

(29) Linser, P., and Moscona, A.A. 1983. Hormonal induction of glutamine synthetase in cultures of embryonic retina cells: requirement for neuron-glia contact interactions. *Develop. Biol.* 96: 529-534.

(30) Lucas, C.A.; Edgar, D.; and Thoenen, H. 1979. Regulation of tyrosine hydroxylase and choline acetyltransferase activities by cell density in the PC12 rat pheochromocytoma clonal cell line. *Exp. Cell Res.* 121: 79-86.

(31) Manthorpe, M.; Engvall, E.; Ruoslahti, E.; Longo, F.; Davis, G.E.; and Varon, S. 1983. Laminin promotes neuritic regeneration from cultured peripheral and central neurons. *J. Cell Biol.* 97: 1882-1890.

(32) Nestler, E.J., and Greengard, P. 1983. Protein phosphorylation in the brain. *Nature* 305: 583-588.

(33) Otten, U., and Thoenen, H. 1976. Mechanisms of tyrosine hydroxylase and dopamine-beta-hydroxylase induction in organ cultures of rat sympathetic ganglia by potassium depolarization and cholinomimetics. *Naunyn-Schmiedeberg's Arch. Pharmacol.* 292: 153-159.

(34) Saad, A.D.; Soh, B.M.; and Moscona, A.A. 1981. Modulation of cortisol receptors in embryonic retina cells by changes in cell-cell contacts: correlations with induction of glutamine synthetase. *Biochem. Biophys. Res. Comm.* 98: 701-708.

(35) Stachowiak,M.; Sebbane, R.; Stricker, E.M.; Zigmond, M.J.; and Kaplan, B.B. 1985. Effect of chronic cold exposure on tyrosine hydroxylase mRNA in rat adrenal gland. *Brain Res.* 359: 356-359.

(36) Tank, A.W.; Lewis, E.J.; Chikaraishi, D.M.; and Weiner, N. 1985. Elevation of RNA coding for tyrosine hydroxylase in rat adrenal gland by reserpine treatment and exposure to cold. *J. Neurochem.* 45: 1030-1033.

(37) Thoenen, H. 1972. Neuronally mediated enzyme induction in adrenergic neurons and adrenal chromaffin cells. *Biochem. Soc. Symp.* 36: 3-15.

(38) Thoenen, H. 1975. Transynaptic regulation of neuronal enzyme synthesis. In *Handbook of Psychopharmacology*, eds. L.L. Iversen,

S.D. Iversen, and S.H. Snyder, vol. 3, pp. 443-475. New York: Plenum Press.

(39) Thoenen, H., and Otten, U. 1978. Trans-synaptic enzyme induction: ionic requirements and modulatory role of glucocorticoids. In *Structure and Function of Monoamine Enzymes*, eds. E. Usdin, N. Weiner, and M.B.H. Youdim, pp. 439-464. New York: Marcel Dekker.

(40) Thoenen, H.; Otten, U.; and Schwab, M. 1979. Orthograde and retrograde signals for the regulation of neuronal gene expression: the peripheral sympathetic nervous system as a model. In *The Neurosciences Fourth Study Program*, eds. F.O. Schmidt and F.G. Worden, pp. 911-928. Cambridge, MA: MIT Press.

(41) Viveros, O.H.; Diliberto, E.J.; Hazum, E.; and Chang, K.-J. 1980. Enkephalins as possible adrenomedullary hormones: storage, secretion and regulation of synthesis. In *Neural Peptides and Neuronal Communication, Advance in Biochemistry and Psychopharmacology*, eds. E. Costa and M. Trabucchi, vol. 22, pp. 191-204. New York: Raven Press.

(42) Warenbourg, M.; Otten, U.; and Schwab, M.E. 1981. Labelling of Schwann and satellite cells by 3H-dexamethasone in a rat sympathetic ganglion and sciatic nerve. *Neuroscience* 6: 1139-1143.

(43) Wilson, S.P.; Abou-Donia, M.M.; Chang, K.-J.; and Viveros, O.H. 1981. Reserpine increases opiate-like peptide content and tyrosine hydroxylase activity in adrenal medullary chromaffin cells in culture. *Neuroscience* 6: 71-79.

(44) Wilson, S.P.; Chang, K.-J.; and Viveros, O.H. 1980. Synthesis of enkephalins by adrenal medullary chromaffin cells: reserpine increases incorporation of radiolabelled amino acids. *Proc. Natl. Acad. Sci.* 77: 4364-4368.

(45) Zigmond, R.E., and Ben-Ari, Y. 1977. Electrical stimulation of preganglionic nerve increases tyrosine hydroxylase activity in sympthetic ganglia. *Proc. Natl. Acad. Sci.* 74: 3078-3080.

(46) Zigmond, R.E., and Chalazonitis, A. 1979. Long-term effects of preganglionic stimulation on tyrosine hydroxylase activity in the rat superior cervical ganglion. *Brain Res.* 164: 137-152.

(47) Zigmond, R.E.; Chalazonitis, A.; Lau, H.; and Joh, T. 1978. Preganglionic nerve stimulation increases the number of tyrosine hydroxylase molecules in a sympathetic ganglion. *Fed. Proc.* 37: 825.

The Neural and Molecular Bases of Learning,
eds. J.-P. Changeux and M. Konishi, pp. 99–118.
John Wiley & Sons Limited.

Activity and the Regulation of Neuronal Growth Factor Metabolism

C.E. Henderson

Neurobiologie Moléculaire
Institut Pasteur
75724 Paris 15, France

Abstract. Evidence concerning the role of neuronal growth factors in the development and maintenance of the peripheral and central nervous systems continues to accumulate, although only three of the molecules involved have been purified and characterized. There is indirect evidence in several systems that inactive postsynaptic cells produce higher levels of neuronal growth factor than do their active counterparts, but in no case is there rigorous proof of this. Such activity-dependent regulation may underlie competition between neurons during the period of cell death and between nerve terminals during synaptic rearrangement. Models have been proposed in which active presynaptic terminals receive trophic award in the form of growth factors during synapse elimination. The data and models are critically discussed.

INTRODUCTION

Many types of postmitotic neurons are now known to respond, *in vivo* or *in vitro*, to the extracellular presence of certain molecules by increased growth as measured by one or more of the following parameters: cell survival, axonal or dendritic growth (13). Such molecules are collectively referred to as neuronal growth factors (GFs) although only in one case, that of the nerve growth factor (NGF), has a physiological role been demonstrated (32, 49). In the absence of concrete data about many of the other proposed candidates for neuronal GF status, it is hard to define the distinction between GFs and other "housekeeping" nutrients, but useful working criteria might be: a) a certain selectivity for neuronal cells, b) the presence of specific GF receptors on the neuronal surface, and c) action over relatively short distances.

The synthesis of many GFs is thought to occur in target tissues with which the growing neuron is, or is about to be, in contact during development, regeneration, or, perhaps to a lesser extent, adult life. This observation has given rise to two connected hypotheses, stated here in their most general form: a) GFs provide a mechanism whereby target tissues can specify, select, and/or modify neuronal connections; b) regulation of GF metabolism (synthesis, liberation, uptake) by the activity of the system could be a means of epigenetically influencing the structure of neuronal circuits.

The aim of this article is to discuss the evidence for an influence of activity on GF metabolism and to consider the roles that have been proposed for GFs in synapse selection and modulation. Such a discussion is by its very nature speculative, for two major reasons. First, many of the "GFs" alluded to are only tentatively identified by their activity *in vitro* or *in vivo*. Aside from NGF only two of the candidate GFs have been characterized at the molecular level, as discussed in the following section. Second, in no case has the effect of activity on the production or uptake of a known GF been unambiguously demonstrated.

THREE MOLECULES WITH NEUROTROPHIC ACTIVITY

Before coming to a more oriented discussion on the possible role of activity in the regulation of GF metabolism, I shall briefly review the molecular and functional data available on the only three neurotrophic molecules whose purification to homogeneity has been reported. This seems important as many of our ideas about the roles GFs could play *in vivo* are based on the existing models. I shall complete the section with a selective overview of "candidate GFs," *in vitro* activities of interest which have not yet been fully characterized at a molecular level.

Nerve Growth Factor (NGF)

β-NGF is the only purified GF whose importance *in vivo* has been demonstrated (32, 49). Appropriately timed treatment of animals with antibodies to NGF results in the almost complete destruction of populations of both sensory and sympathetic neurons. Several observations (30, 46, 49) support the proposal that NGF is synthesized in target organs where it functions to regulate survival and differentiation of responsive neurons. First, NGF applied to sympathetic or sensory nerve terminals binds to specific receptors and is internalized and retrogradely transported to the cell body. Second, axotomy results in neuronal death, while administration of NGF can prevent both experimentally induced and naturally occurring cell death. Finally, at least *in vitro* (9), NGF is effective under conditions in which it is only available to distal regions of axons and their terminals.

Recently, the presence of NGF protein and its specific mRNA has been unambiguously demonstrated for the first time in innervated sympathetic effector organs *in situ*, using sensitive two-site enzyme immunoassays (30) and radioactive single-stranded RNA or DNA probes (24, 46). The expression of β-NGF is strikingly correlated with the density of sympathetic innervation in effector organs, although the cellular site of synthesis has not been identified.

NGF has almost certainly other roles to play in the developing and adult nervous system. Its possible function in the hippocampus is discussed below (see section on *Adult Rat Hippocampus*). Another important property, demonstrated *in vitro* and *in vivo*, is the chemotactic (neurotropic) effect of a concentration gradient of NGF on the direction of axonal outgrowth (17, 33).

Brain-derived Neurotrophic Factor (BDNF)

Although sensory neurons constitute the classical NGF-dependent population, not all dorsal root ganglion (DRG) neurons have a requirement for NGF and those that do are apparently dependent on NGF only at a certain stage of their development. Barde *et al.* (1) have purified a protein from pig brain capable of supporting the surivival *in vitro* of some DRG neurons that do not respond to NGF. This brain-derived neurotrophic factor (BDNF), a basic protein of molecular weight 12,300, is clearly distinguishable from NGF.

In addition to its action on sensory neurons, BDNF has a marked effect on survival and neurite outgrowth from cultured neurons of the embryonic chick nodose ganglion, which are derived from the neural placode and do not respond to NGF (34). Furthermore, preparations enriched for BDNF enhance the growth of fetal rat retinal neurons. To date, no published data is available on the *in vivo* effects of injection of BDNF or its blocking antibodies.

Ciliary Neuronotrophic Factor (CNTF)

Neurons of the cholinergic, neural crest-derived ciliary ganglion will only survive in culture in the presence of extracts of tissues such as the target muscles of the eye (35). This CNTF activity can not be mimicked by NGF or BDNF and has been shown to reside in a slightly acidic protein of molecular weight 20,500. Purified CNTF will also support the survival *in vitro* of dorsal root and sympathetic ganglion neurons from day 11 chick embryos but not neurons from the nodose ganglion. Recently it has become apparent that although CNTF is concentrated in eye muscles during the period of target-dependent cell death, high levels of very similar molecules are found in sources as different as adult rat sciatic nerve. The biological role of the CNTF molecules thus appears to be less narrow than originally hypothesized and awaits further definition.

Other Growth-promoting Activities

Characterization of putative neuronal growth factors in other regions of the nervous system is less advanced although many studies *in vitro* have suggested their existence. The spinal motoneuron has been the subject of particular attention, both because its development and that of the neuromuscular junction are relatively well documented and because of possible pathological implications (for a review see (20)). Thus activities have been described which promote survival, neurite outgrowth or sprouting, and/or acetylcholine synthesis in cultured motoneurons. Some of these activities are described in more detail in the section on *SYSTEMS IN WHICH ACTIVITY MAY MODULATE GF EXPRESSION*. However, no molecular species has yet been identified as a motoneuron GF. Recently, a neurite extension factor for chicken embryo cerebral cortical neurons cultured in serum-free defined medium was purified to apparent homogeneity (28). In the presence of reducing agents it migrated in SDS polyacrylamide gels as a single band with an apparent molecular weight of 6500 and appeared to be, in fact, a disulfide-bonded form of S100β. Other growth-promoting activities probably associated with novel molecules are currently under study for hippocampal neurons, forebrain neurons, and peripheral ganglia (for a review see (13)).

SYSTEMS IN WHICH ACTIVITY MAY MODULATE GF EXPRESSION

Probably the best example of a molecule whose expression is regulated by activity is that of the nicotinic acetylcholine receptor (see Changeux *et al.*, this volume). Our present understanding of that system would suggest that there exists a basic developmental program for the expression of the receptor at different stages of muscle differentiation but that this program can be modulated by, amongst other factors, the spontaneous or evoked activity of the system. This type of regulation could be of importance both in synaptogenesis and in regeneration. The possible functional implications of activity-dependent regulation within the central nervous system, in which patterns of evoked activity are both precise and varied, need not be underlined.

The aim of this section is to present data addressing the question of whether there is activity-dependent regulation of GF expression. No published data exists for BDNF or CNTF in this context and so, apart from those on NGF, all results reported concern "candidate GFs" supposed to exist from their activities *in vivo* or *in vitro*. Some of the problems in interpreting such results will be discussed later in more detail.

NGF in the Rat Iris

With the exception of the male mouse submaxillary gland and certain other exceptional sources, the rat iris contains amongst the highest levels of NGF protein and mRNA of any tissue tested, as can be expected from its dense sympathetic innervation (30, 46). Levels of NGF in this tissue were increased by at least one order of magnitude ten days after sensory or sympathetic denervation and fell back to barely detectable levels concomitant with the reinnervation of iris grafts (15). This observation has been confirmed using sensitive immunoassays in both denervated and explanted irides (2, 14). The situation at the RNA level is less clear. Whereas explantation had a marked effect on *de novo* synthesis, as shown by measuring levels of specific NGF mRNA (46), no corresponding change was observed in irides whose sympathetic and sensory innervation had been surgically removed *in situ* (47).

Adult Rat Hippocampus

The adult rat hippocampus contains the highest levels of NGF protein and mRNA thus far detected in the central nervous system, whereas embryonic rat brain contains no detectable NGF mRNA but similar levels of an NGF-like protein suggested to be a fetal form of NGF (29, 51). Medial septal neurons will specifically transport NGF injected into the hippocampal formation, and exogenous NGF enhances cholinergic properties of septal neurons both *in vivo* (neonatal rat hippocampus, deafferented adult rat hippocampus) and *in vitro* (fetal septal neurons) (13). These results suggest that NGF may play a physiological role in the central nervous system, although clear effects of blocking antibodies remain to be demonstrated.

Several phenomena have been observed subsequent to hippocampal deafferentation (for a review see (13)). Septohippocampal denervation leads to sprouting of sympathetic axons from the cerebral vasculature; injection of NGF antiserum into the hippocampal formation under these conditions reduces the extent of sprouting. Removal of the entorhinal, but not the commissural, projection to the hippocampus results in sprouting of septohippocampal axons and a concomitant increase of NGF-like activity. Using intracerebral grafting techniques it was shown that neonatal rat superior cervical neurons, which have an absolute requirement for NGF or similar GFs for their survival, will survive in the hippocampal formation of adult rats only in the presence of a denervating fimbria-fornix lesion.

It should be noted, however, that no change in hippocampal NGF mRNA levels was detected 15 or 30 days after transection of the fimbria of adult rats (51), whereas an increase was found when the same operation was performed on one week-old rats (T. Ebendal, personal communication).

Motoneuron Cell Death

During the course of normal development in the chick embryo about 50% of the motoneurons initially generated in the anterior horn of the spinal cord undergo cell death, starting on embryonic day 5. In embryos in which the limb bud has been extirpated at early stages, 100% of the motoneurons destined to innervate the limb die during the same period. On the other hand, implantation of a supernumerary limb before the onset of cell death results in the rescue of some of the motoneurons that would normally have died. These classical experiments were among the first to suggest the existence of a GF (as yet uncharacterized) on which motoneurons depend for their survival (19).

Since cell death occurs in many systems soon after axons have reached their destination, the most common hypothesis is that neurons compete at the periphery for a limited supply of GF (and/or synaptic space), and only those which are successful in this competition will survive. There is evidence for this proposal both in the spinal cord and in the ciliary ganglion (CG). In the latter case, when the number of CG cells initially innervating the eye was experimentally reduced, a greater proportion of the remaining ganglionic neurons survived to maturity (39). However, several results obtained using the amphibian spinal cord are not easily explained by peripheral competition and alternative mechanisms such as selective cell death or central competition have been invoked (31).

More recently the effects of activity on motoneuron cell death have been studied. Embryos immobilized with pre- or postsynaptic neuromuscular blocking agents during the period of naturally occurring cell death exhibited increased numbers (hypothanasia) of motoneurons over controls at the end of this period (40). In contrast, electrical stimulation of hindlimbs increased motoneuron death while leaving cell numbers in dorsal root ganglia unaltered (38).

Interpreted in terms of peripheral competition for a muscle-derived motoneuron GF, these findings prompted the following hypothesis. Inactive (noninnervated) myotubes produce GF in sufficient quantity to maintain the whole of the initially generated motoneuron pool. Transmission at newly formed nerve-muscle contacts results in a diminution of GF production, and GF levels become limiting, leading to competition. Quantitative selection of the innervating population is thus initiated by activity. Blocking transmission keeps GF production at its original levels; direct stimulation hastens the shutdown of synthesis.

Polyneuronal Innervation at the Neuromuscular Junction
In vertebrate fast skeletal muscles at late embryonic stages, each muscle fiber receives at a single endplate up to 5 (or more) motor axon terminals from different motoneurons, all but one of which are eliminated in the course of the following weeks. In all probability the regression of polyneuronal innervation occurs mainly by the retraction of axon collaterals (the average motor unit size decreases at the same time), although some changes in neuron and muscle fiber number may occur during this period. It is likely that terminals at a given endplate compete for stabilization: when motor unit size is measured in rat lumbrical muscles deprived of all but a single axon, the remaining motor unit fails to decrease in size (6). However, the generality of this result is not clear.

Regression of polyneuronal innervation is retarded when neuromuscular activity is reduced by tenotomy (section of tendons) in neonatal rats (4) or by local anesthesia in adults undergoing regeneration (5), whereas direct stimulation accelerates the process of regression (37). One of many possible hypotheses (10) is that multiple terminals are maintained at the endplate by a supply of GF. GF supply becomes limiting in an activity-dependent manner leading to competition between neighboring terminals and retraction of the losers. Reduction of activity keeps GF levels high for longer, whereas direct stimulation has the opposite effect. If this hypothesis is correct then the type of activity is also important, since acceleration of synapse elimination by chronic neuromuscular stimulation is dependent on the temporal pattern in which the stimuli are presented (50).

Motor Nerve Sprouting
In adult skeletal muscles that have been partially denervated or inactivated by agents such as botulinum toxin, motor axons remaining

within the muscle sprout either at the terminal or first node of Ranvier so as to reinnervate the muscle fibers that have been denervated (Fig. 1a). Elegant *in vivo* evidence exists to suggest that this sprouting occurs in response to a "sprouting signal" released by the denervated fibers and capable of diffusing a limited distance within the muscle (8).

Antibodies to a muscle-derived protein of 56,000 molecular weight inhibit sprouting induced by treatment with botulinum toxin (18). Furthermore, the 56K protein itself is reported to enhance the survival of cultured embryonic spinal neurons. Confirmation of the GF status of this antigen, however, will require the study of the effects of monospecific antibodies on normal development *in vivo*.

Whatever its nature, production of the sprouting signal by denervated muscle fibers is regulated by activity: direct stimulation of partially denervated muscles strongly inhibits the formation of sprouts (7).

Spinal Neurons and Motoneurons *in Vitro*

Survival-promoting factors. Extracts of skeletal muscle contain as yet unidentified substances that enhance the *in vitro* survival of motoneurons labeled *in situ* by retrograde transport of HRP. Levels of these survival-promoting activities increase following denervation (48); this increase is reported to be prevented by direct stimulation of the denervated muscles (25).

Neurite-promoting factors. Media conditioned by embryonic myotubes and extracts of neonatal muscle contain protein factors distinct from laminin that enhance neurite outgrowth in cultures of embryonic spinal neurons taken at an age at which motoneurons should have a high relative abundance (23). Levels of activity were developmentally regulated in leg muscle of post-hatch chicks, increasing tenfold during the course of the first 3 days after hatching and subsequently falling back to basal levels. Denervation of neonatal chick leg muscle resulted in increases of up to 15-fold in the specific neurite-promoting activity of muscle extracts as compared to controls (22). The time course of appearance of this activity was similar to that for the detection of sprouts in partially denervated mammalian muscles (Fig. 1b). Two other experimental models were investigated in which muscle activity was lowered without sectioning the nerve. The mutant mouse "paralysé" exhibits a spontaneous regression of motor nerve endings with concomitant paralysis. Neurite-promoting activity in mutant muscle extracts was up to tenfold higher than in extracts from control littermates, and the difference between them tended to increase with

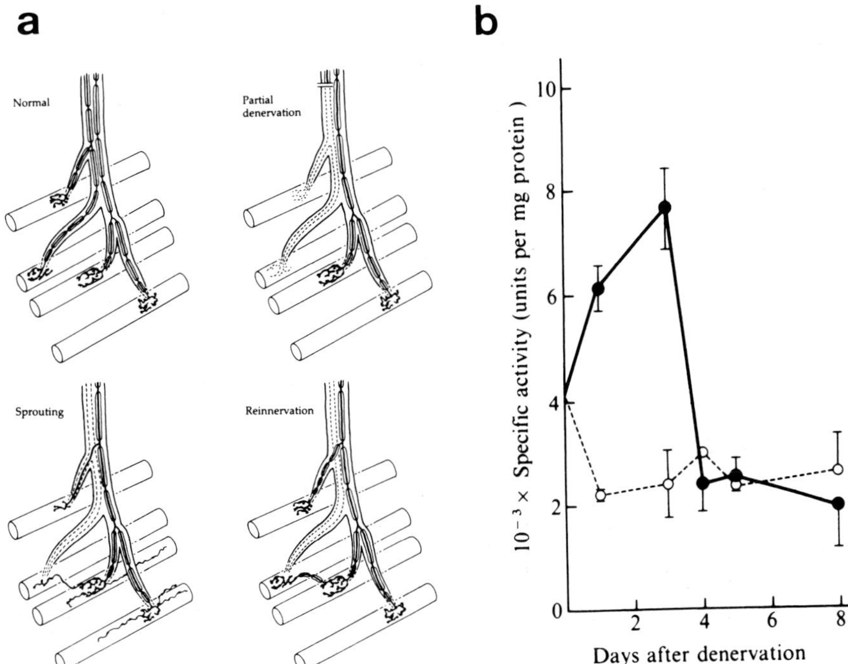

FIG. 1 – Sprouting of motor axons at the neuromuscular junction. a) Following inactivation or partial section of the motor nerve, sprouts appear both at terminals and at nodes of Ranvier. Some of these successfully reinnervate the denervated muscle fibers (reproduced with permission from the Annual Review of Neuroscience, see (8), by Annual Reviews Inc.).
b) Neurite-promoting activity for cultured spinal neurons in extracts of skeletal muscle in the days following denervation. In extracts of denervated chick leg muscle (●) there was a sharp rise in neurite-promoting activity, reaching a peak at 3 days after denervation. No corresponding change was observed in muscles of contralateral legs (o). From 4 days after denervation, denervated muscles were visibly atrophied (reprinted by permission from Nature, see (22)).

age until death. Tenotomy, too, caused a significant increase in neurite-promoting activity in muscles of neonatal rats (21).

Polyneuronal Innervation of Cerebellar Purkinje Cells

Adult Purkinje cells each receive innervation from one climbing fiber originating from the inferior olive. To attain this adult configuration the Purkinje cell undergoes a transient period of functional polyneuronal innervation early in postnatal life (12, 36). Regression of multiple innervation is greatly retarded in animals such as X-irradiated rats or "staggerer" or "weaver" mutant mice in which the Purkinje cells receive reduced synaptic input (36). Arguments similar to those discussed for the neuromuscular junction in the section on *Polyneuronal Innervation at the Neuromuscular Junction* may also be applied here.

Plasticity in the Central Nervous System

The formation of ocular dominance columns in the developing visual cortex is thought to involve synaptic rearrangement and elimination. In this system, when one eye of a monkey is occluded during the first weeks of life, the columns corresponding to the deprived eye shrink (26). In addition, chronic blockade of visual activity with tetrodotoxin impedes the segregation of ocular dominance columns whereas direct stimulation induces segregation. Comparable phenomena are observed at the level of the transcallosal connections between cortical areas (27).

PRESYNAPTIC RESPONSES TO NEURONAL GFs: MODELS OF SYNAPSE SELECTION

There is considerable variation in the degree of convergence of synaptic inputs onto postsynaptic cells in different regions of the nervous system; the number of innervating axons can vary from one to tens of thousands (41). The different functional modes associated with these configurations suggest that the quantitiative regulation of synapse numbers is in itself of fundamental importance. In most cases studied, the formation of the adult configuration occurs during development by the competitive rearrangement and/or elimination of contacts initially formed. This suggests the possibility that qualitative selection of synapses may also occur during the establishment or modification of specific neuronal circuits.

One of the best-studied examples of synapse elimination is the developing neuromuscular junction (see above). Changeux and his collaborators have constructed mathematical models (10, 16) for the selective stabilization of muscle innervation during development based on competition of the active nerve terminals for a postsynaptic retrograde factor, μ. At the peak of multiple innervation the synthesis of μ by the muscle fiber stops, possibly as a consequence of muscle electrical and/or mechanical activity, and the stock of μ becomes limited. Within each nerve ending μ undergoes an autocatalytical reaction, initiated by the nerve impulses reaching the terminal, which results in the production of a presynaptic stabilization factor, s. A nerve terminal is stabilized when its internal concentration of s reaches a threshold

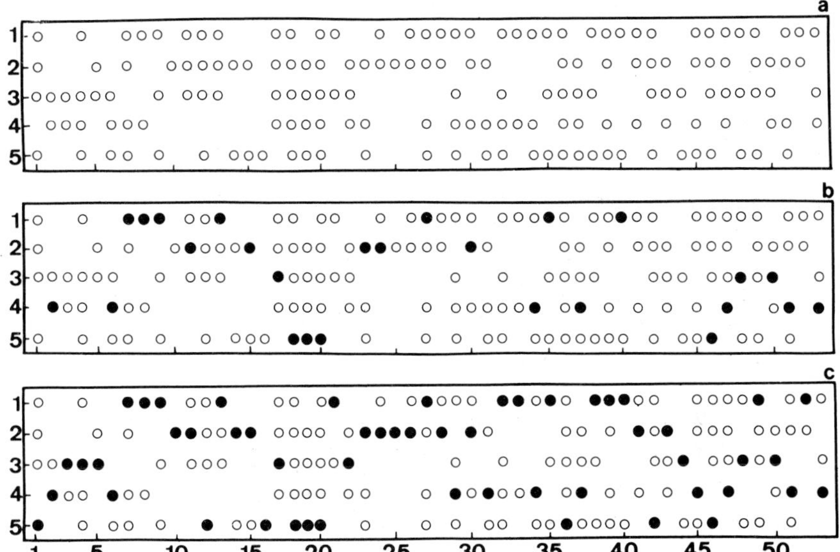

FIG. 2 – Computer simulation of the selective stabilization model for the development of muscle innervation. a) Starting configuration in which 5 neurons polyneuronally innervate 53 muscle fibers; the circles represent the initial nerve endings. b) Intermediate situation after 600 iterations; black dots represent stabilized nerve endings. c) Final situation after 1218 iterations; there is a single stabilized nerve ending per muscle fiber, and the dispersion in size of the motor units remains unchanged (reprinted by permission from (16)).

value. Starting from a polyneuronally innervated situation, computer simulation of this model predicts that only one nerve terminal will be stabilized per muscle fiber, that all fibers will remain innervated, and that the dispersion in size of motor units will remain constant (Fig. 2). The authors claim that this model accounts for the effects of lowered or increased activity on the development of polyneuronal innervation (see above) and suggest that μ might be one of the motoneuron GFs discussed above and that s might be involved in stabilizing the presynaptic cytoskeleton.

Another model for synaptic stabilization was inspired by the observation of the restriction of innervation by a given axon to a few distributed target cells in some autonomic ganglia (41). In the rat submandibular ganglion, for instance, there is marked polyneuronal innervation at birth while at maturity each neuron receives only one preganglionic

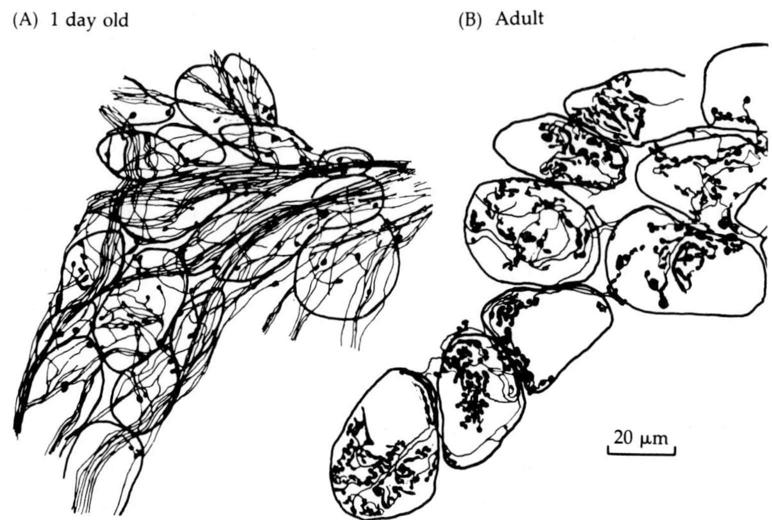

FIG. 3 – The number of synapses on ganglion cells increases during early life. Camera lucida drawings of neurons from the submandibular ganglion of neonatal (A) and adult (B) rats treated with zinc iodide-osmium. This reagent preferentially stains synaptic boutons. The number of boutons on neurons increases during the period of synapse elimination, a fact confirmed in this and other autonomic ganglia by electron microscopy (reprinted by permission from (41)).

axon input (Fig. 3). As in muscle, regression takes place at a period when populations of innervating and target cells are not greatly varying in number; there is thus a concomitant reduction in the "neural unit." However, in apparent contrast with the neuromuscular junction, the number of synapses actually increases during the period when some inputs are being eliminated. The distribution of these synapses comes to be concentrated on particular cells rather than territories. A comparable rearrangement of climbing fiber synapses on Purkinje cell dendrites occurs during cerebellar development (36).

Based on these observations, and the original suggestion by Hebb of the importance of coincident presynaptic and postsynaptic activity, Purves and Lichtman (41) have proposed that trophic factor is released by active postsynaptic cells in proportion to depolarization and can only be taken up by a simultaneously active terminal. The greater the postsynaptic activity generated, the greater the presynaptic trophic award. Because all of the synaptic terminals arising from a particular axon have synchronous activity, a strongly innervated target cell would progressively encourage the establishment of additional terminals by that axon. No simulation of this model is currently available.

These are clearly not the only models that have been put forward for the activity-dependent regulation of synapse elimination; others involving stabilization of postsynaptic components, for instance, are outside the scope of this article. Direct experimental testing of the models presented will not be simple until some of the molecular components have been better identified. However, one prediction of both models discussed (and others) is that active terminals will be favored in competition over their less active neighbors. Measurements of the size of motor units in adult rat muscles reinnervated by active and inactive motor axons do indeed suggest that active nerve terminals have a competitive advantage over inactive terminals during synapse elimination (42).

One apparent difference between the models, proposed by Gouze *et al.* (16), is that an active postsynaptic cell produced less GF than its inactive counterpart, whereas for Purves and Lichtman (41) the converse is true. At first sight, experimental results on the effects of activity on synapse elimination would seem to be consistent with the former view. It would be possible to reconcile the two postulates, however, by supposing the involvement of two GF-like activities (see section on *GFs versus Stabilization Factors*). One would support the presence of multiple nerve terminals at the synapse; its synthesis would be reduced in an activity-dependent fashion thus triggering competition between terminals. In certain experimental situations its synthesis could be maintained, thus retarding regression. The other would be involved in synapse stabilization *per se*, would be produced in greater quantities by active postsynaptic cells, and assimilated more efficiently by active terminals.

DISCUSSION OF THE DATA AND MODELS

The general conclusion from the results discussed earlier might be that production (synthesis or release) of GFs by target cells is at its highest when the cells are inactive, as is the case for the nicotinic acetylcholine receptor. In this section, however, I wish to outline some of the problems involved in interpreting the data and to mention some questions that must be answered before GF involvement in the specification of neuronal networks can be tested. Underlying the whole discussion, of course, is the problem that until more molecular data become available the true multiplicity of GF species and the range of their actions can not be realistically appreciated.

Site of Synthesis of Neuronal GFs

One underlying assumption of models in which GFs regulate interactions between neurons and their target cells (postsynaptic neuron, muscle fiber) is that GFs are produced by the target cell and act in a retrograde fashion upon the innervating neuron. Despite the demonstration of NGF synthesis in sympathetic effector organs there is remarkably little firm evidence for this supposition, and indeed immunofluorescence studies suggest that in the rat iris NGF is mainly localized in the Schwann cells associated with the axon fascicles (44). Until *in situ* hybridization techniques for the localization of mRNA have been further perfected, all the results reported above are subject to this proviso. In particular, it is not impossible that some of the apparent effects of activity or denervation on GF expression are in fact mediated via the incompletely understood effects of activity on glial metabolism and proliferation, both centrally and peripherally. This element is lacking from the theoretical models presented.

Effects of Denervation

Many of the experimental data presented earlier purport to show an increase of GF activity subsequent to denervation. However, the problems of interpreting the results in terms of GF production are twofold. First, denervation has effects on the target cell other than the reduction of activity and effects on other cell types in the vicinity. Although in principle these can be controlled for by direct stimulation of the denervated tissue, this has been done only in a few of the cases cited (3, 7, 25). Another approach has been to compare the effects on GF levels of quite different experimental treatments known to affect the activity of the system in a parallel fashion (21, 22). Second, apparent increases in GF production following denervation could in theory result not from an increased rate of synthesis in the target organ but only by the interruption of retrograde transport of GF by the lesioned neurons. This criticism has been excluded in the case of the explanted rat iris by measurement of mRNA levels but seems pertinent to studies on deafferented adult hippocampus and irides denervated *in situ* (see corresponding sections).

Quantitative and Qualitative Regulation of Presynaptic Elements

One of the major purposes of the commonly observed phenomena of overproduction of neurons followed by cell death and polyneuronal innervation followed by synaptic rearrangement must be to ensure *quantitative matching* between partners within presynaptic and postsynaptic populations: each innervating neuron can only sustain a certain neural or motor unit, each target cell requires a certain number of inputs in order to function normally (41). There now exists quite suggestive evidence in several of the systems discussed (NGF (49), motoneuron cell death (3), motor nerve sprouting (8)) that GFs might be involved in such quantitative matching and that essential competitive interactions might be triggered by activity.

A quite separate proposition is that within a group of pre- and postsynaptic cells there are mechanisms to determine which individual presynaptic cell remains in contact with which postsynaptic cell. This could be referred to as *qualitative matching* (41). Both theoretical models of synapse selection discussed earlier represent mechanisms for qualitative matching on the basis of impulse activity (see section on *PRESYNAPTIC RESPONSES TO NEURONAL GFs*). However, in the systems they treat (skeletal muscle and autonomic ganglia) – as opposed to, say, the visual cortex – the potential importance of qualitative rather than quantitative matching is not clear. Activity-linked regulation in these systems may be simply a mechanism for ensuring that the appropriate number of synapses remain, whereas the formation of specific neuronal circuits in other systems may involve completely different processes.

GFs versus Stabilization Factors

All the GFs discussed here were tentatively identified by their action on the survival or axonal outgrowth of certain neuronal populations. The relation between such GFs and molecules involved in the short- or long-term stabilization of certain synaptic contacts has not been demonstrated for any known GF although it is known that in the absence of NGF, applied peripherally *in vitro*, axonal branches of sympathetic neurons will wilt and retract (9). The relation between growth and stabilization is conceptually less clear in systems where the number of synapses actually increases during the regression of polyneuronal innervation, such as the submandibular ganglion.

It is important to consider the possible role in synapse stabilization of such molecules as N-CAM, or other synaptic antigens (45), and that of electrical fields created by ion translocation at the synapse. Interestingly, levels of N-CAM on skeletal muscle cells are increased following denervation (43) or paralysis (11). Studies are required on the effect of blocking antibodies to these and other molecules on the process of synapse elimination.

Essential Features of the Regulating Activity

It would be premature to attempt to define the necessary physicochemical features (transmission, action potential, contractile, etc.) of the spontaneous or evoked activity suggested to have effects on GF metabolism. One question seems worth asking, however: how could activity regulate GF metabolism in many different systems and at different developmental stages? One possibility comes from the observations that different patterns of imposed activity can differentially modulate phenomena including synthesis of myosin isoforms, synaptic efficacy, and synapse elimination. Synthesis, liberation, and uptake of a given GF could be regulated only by a given activity pattern. Thus differences in GF metabolism between "active" and "inactive" cells discussed above may in fact occur between active cells having qualitatively different activity patterns.

CONCLUSIONS

It now seems likely that neuronal GFs play an important role in the establishment and maintenance of neuronal connections, both in the peripheral and central nervous systems. Three molecules with neurotrophic activity have now been characterized including NGF, by far the most studied example. Even in the case of NGF, however, important questions remain to be answered concerning its cellular site of synthesis and the regulation of its production during development. Our knowledge of the candidate GFs identified by their *in vitro* or *in vivo* activities is even less complete.

Many experiments have been directed to the study of an intuitively attractive activity-dependent regulation of GF metabolism (synthesis, secretion, or uptake) and others can be interpreted in this light. However, it seems fair to conclude at present that in none of the systems discussed is there unambiguous evidence for such regulation. Problems in interpreting the results presented stem both from methodological considerations and from the lack, until relatively recently, of tools such as cDNA probes which should allow the problem to be addressed more directly. At the present state of our knowledge, arguably the most convincing evidence for activity-dependent regulation of GF metabolism comes from a system in which the molecules involved have not yet been characterized, that of motor nerve sprouting at the neuromuscular junction.

Models of synapse stabilization have been put forward that involve activity-dependent regulation (either up- or down-) of GF production. However, only when the molecules involved have been better characterized will it be possible for them to be tested.

REFERENCES

(1) Barde, Y.-A.; Edgar, D.; and Thoenen, H. 1982. Purification of a new neurotrophic factor from mammalian brain. *EMBO J.* 1: 549-553.

(2) Barth, E.M.; Korsching, S.; and Thoenen, H. 1984. Regulation of NGF synthesis and release in organ cultures of rat iris. *J. Cell Biol.* 99: 839-843.

(3) Bennett, M.R. 1983. Development of neuromuscular synapses. *Physiol. Rev.* 63: 915-1048.

(4) Benoit, P., and Changeux, J.-P. 1975. Consequences of tenotomy on the evolution of multi-innervation in developing rat soleus muscle. *Brain Res.* 99: 354-358.

(5) Benoit, P., and Changeux, J.-P. 1978. Consequences of blocking the nerve with a local anaesthetic on the evolution of multi-innervation at the regenerating neuromuscular junction of the rat. *Brain Res.* 149: 89-96.

(6) Betz, W.J.; Caldwell, J.H.; and Ribchester, R.R. 1980. The effects of partial denervation at birth on the development of muscle fibres and motor units in rat lumbrical muscle. *J. Physl.* 303: 265-279.

(7) Brown, M.C., and Holland, R.L. 1979. A central role for denervated tissues in causing nerve sprouting. *Nature* 282: 724-726.

(8) Brown, M.C.; Holland, R.L.; and Hopkins, W.G. 1981. Motor nerve sprouting. *Ann. R. Neurosci.* 4: 17-42.

(9) Campenot, R.B. 1982. Development of sympathetic neurons in compartmentalized cultures. II. Local control of neurite-survival by NGF. *Develop. Biol.* 93: 13-24.

(10) Changeux, J.-P., and Danchin, A. 1976. Selective stabilisation of developing synapses as a mechanism for the specification of neuronal networks. *Nature* 264: 705-712.

(11) Covault, J., and Sanes, J.R. 1985. Neural cell adhesion molecule (N-CAM) accumulates in denervated and paralysed skeletal muscles. *Proc. Natl. Acad. Sci.* 82: 4544-4548.

(12) Crépel, F.; Mariani, J.; and Delhaye-Bouchaud, N. 1976. Evidence for multiple innervation of Purkinje cells by climbing fibers in immature rat cerebellum. *J. Neurobiol.* 7: 567-578.

(13) Crutcher, K.A. 1986. The role of growth factors in neuronal development and plasticity. *Crit. Rev. Clin. Neurobiol.*, in press.

(14) Ebendal, T.; Olson, L.; and Seiger, A. 1983. The level of NGF as a function of innervation. *Exp. Cell Res.* 148: 311-317.

(15) Ebendal, T.; Olson, L.; Seiger, A.; and Hedlund, K.O. 1980. Nerve growth factors in the rat iris. *Nature* 286: 25-28.

(16) Gouzé, J.-L., Lasry, J.-M.; and Changeux, J.-P. 1983. Selective stabilization of muscle innervation during development: a mathematical model. *Biol. Cybern.* 46: 207-215.

(17) Gundersen, R.W., and Barrett, J.N. 1980. Characterization of the turning response of dorsal root neurites toward nerve growth factor. *J. Cell Biol.* 87: 546-554.

(18) Gurney, M.E. 1984. Suppression of terminal sprouting at the neuromuscular junction by immune sera. *Nature* 307: 546-548.

(19) Hamburger, V. 1977. The developmental history of the motor neuron. *Neurosci. Res. Progr. Bull.* 15S: 1-37.

(20) Henderson, C.E. 1986. Neurite-promoting factors for spinal neurons. In *Glial-Neuronal Communication in Development and Regeneration*, eds. H. Althaus and W. Seifert. NATO ASI Series, in press.

(21) Henderson, C.E.; Benoit, P.; Huchet, M.; Guénet, J.-L.; and Changeux, J.-P. 1986. Increase of neurite-promoting activity for spinal neurons in muscles of "paralysé" mice and tenotomised rats. *Develop. Brain Res.* 25: 65-70.

(22) Henderson, C.E.; Huchet, M.; and Changeux, J.-P. 1983. Denervation increases a neurite-promoting activity in extracts of skeletal muscle. *Nature* 302: 609-611.

(23) Henderson, C.E.; Huchet, M.; and Changeux, J.-P. 1984. Neurite-promoting factors for embryonic spinal neurons and their developmental changes in the chick. *Develop. Biol.* 104: 336-347.

(24) Heumann, R.; Korsching, S.; Scott, J.; and Thoenen, H. 1984. Relationship between levels of NGF and its messenger RNA in sympathetic ganglia and peripheral target tissues. *EMBO J.* 3: 3183-3189.

(25) Hill, M.A.; Dangain, J.; and Bennett, M.R. 1985. Motoneurone growth factor activity in muscle regulated by impulse traffic. *Neurosci. L.* 19S: 71.

(26) Hubel, D.H.; Wiesel, T.N.; and Le Vay, S. 1977. Plasticity of ocular dominance columns in monkey striate cortex. *Phil. Trans. R. Soc. B* 278: 377-409.

(27) Innocenti, G.M. 1981. Growth and reshaping of axons in the establishment of visual callosal connections. *Science* 218: 824-827.

(28) Kligman, D., and Marshak, D.R. 1985. Purification and characterization of a neurite extension factor from bovine brain. *Proc. Natl. Acad. Sci.* 82: 7136-7139.

(29) Korsching, S.; Auburger, G.; Heumann, R.; Scott, J.; and Thoenen, H. 1985. Levels of nerve growth factor and its mRNA in the central nervous system of the rat correlate with cholinergic innervation. *EMBO J.* 4: 1389-1393.

(30) Korsching, S., and Thoenen, H. 1983. Nerve growth factor in sympathetic ganglia and corresponding target organs of the rat: correlation with density of sympathetic innervation. *Proc. Natl. Acad. Sci.* 80: 3513-3516.

(31) Lamb, A.H. 1979. Evidence that some developing limb motoneurons die for reasons other than peripheral competition. *Develop. Biol.* 71: 8-21.

(32) Levi-Montalcini, R., and Angeletti, P. 1968. Nerve growth factor. *Physiol. Rev.* 48: 534-569.

(33) Levi-Montalcini, R.; Chen, M.G.M.; and Chen, J.S. 1978. Neurotropic effects of the nerve growth factor in chick embryo and in neonatal rodents. *Zoon* 6: 201-212.

(34) Lindsay, R.M.; Thoenen, H.; and Barde, Y.-A. 1986. Placode and neural crest-derived sensory neurons are responsive at early developmental stages to BDNF. *Develop. Biol.* 112: 319-328.

(35) Manthorpe, M., and Varon, S. 1985. Regulation of neuronal survival and neuritic growth in the avian ciliary ganglion by trophic factors. In *Growth and Maturation Factors*, ed. G. Guroff, vol. 3, pp. 77-117. New York: Wiley.

(36) Mariani, J. 1983. Elimination of synapses during the development of the central nervous system. *Prog. Brain Res.* 58: 383-392.

(37) O'Brien, R.A.D.; Ostberg, A.J.; and Vrbova, G. 1978. Observations on the elimination of polyneuronal innervation in developing mammalian skeletal muscle. *J. Physl.* 282: 571-582.

(38) Oppenheim, R.W., and Nùnez, R. 1982. Electrical stimulation of hindlimb increases neuronal cell death in chick embryos. *Nature* 295: 57-59.

(39) Pilar, G.; Landmesser, L.; and Burstein, L. 1980. Competition for survival among developing ciliary ganglion cells. *J. Neurophysl.* 43: 233-254.

(40) Pittman, R., and Oppenheim, R.W. 1979. Cell death of motoneurons in the chick embryo spinal cord. IV. Evidence that a functional neuromuscular interaction is involved in the regulation

of naturally occurring cell death and the stabilization of synapses. *J. Comp. Neur.* 187: 425-446.

(41) Purves, D., and Lichtman, J.W. 1985. Principles of Neural Development, 1 vol. Sunderland: Sinauer Assoc. Inc.

(42) Ribchester, R.R., and Taxt, T. 1983. Motor unit size and synaptic competition in rat lumbrical muscles reinnervated by active and inactive motor axons. *J. Physl.* 344: 89-111.

(43) Rieger, F.; Grumet, M.; and Edelman, G. 1985. N-CAM at the vertebrate neuromuscular junction. *J. Cell Biol.* 101: 285-293.

(44) Rush, R.A. 1984. Immunohistochemical localization of endogenous nerve growth factor. *Nature* 312: 364-366.

(45) Rutishauser, U. 1984. Developmental biology of neural cell adhesion molecule. *Nature* 310: 549-553.

(46) Shelton, D.L., and Reichardt, L.F. 1984. Expression of the beta-nerve growth factor gene correlates with the density of sympathetic innervation in effector organs. *Proc. Natl. Acad. Sci.* 81: 7951-7955.

(47) Shelton, D.L., and Reichardt, L.F. 1985. Denervation of the rat iris does not increase the level of mRNA encoding beta nerve growth factor. *Soc. Neurosci. Abstr.* 11: 939.

(48) Slack, J.R., and Pockett, S. 1982. Motor neurotrophic factor in denervated adult skeletal muscle. *Brain Res.* 247: 138-140.

(49) Thoenen, H., and Barde, Y.-A. 1980. Physiology of nerve growth factor. *Physiol. Rev.* 60: 1284-1335.

(50) Thompson, W. 1983. Synapse elimination in neonatal rat muscle is sensitive to pattern of muscle use. *Nature* 302: 614-616.

(51) Whittemore, S.R.; Ebendal, T.; Lärksfors, L.; Olson, L.; Seiger, A.; Strömberg, I.; and Persson, H. 1986. Developmental and regional expression of beta-nerve growth factor messenger RNA and protein in the rat central nervous system. *Proc. Natl. Acad. Sci.* 83: 817-821.

The Neural and Molecular Bases of Learning,
eds. J.-P. Changeux and M. Konishi, pp. 119–136..
John Wiley & Sons Limited.

Molecular Mechanisms of the Regulation of Eukaryotic Gene Transcription

M. Yaniv

Département de Biologie Moléculaire
Institut Pasteur
75724 Paris 15, France

INTRODUCTION

Living organisms regulate the expression of many of their genes in response to external stimulus. Similarly, during development and differentiation in multicellular organisms, many gene products are temporally and locally regulated. The pioneering work of Jacob and Monod (26) laid out the concepts of regulatory circuits in bacteria. In the past 25 years, through a combined effort of bacterial geneticists and molecular biologists, many of the mechanisms that control gene expression in bacteria were elucidated. A typical bacterial promoter includes two conserved elements: the Pribnow box (TATAAT) and the TTGACA box preceding the initiation site of transcription by roughly 10 base pairs (bp) and 35 bp. For regulated operons the transcription can be repressed in many cases by a repressor molecule binding to an operator sequence, usually overlapping the transcription initiation site. In other cases positive regulatory proteins, binding to sequences overlapping or located in close proximity to an imperfect -35 box, stimulate transcription from these promoters. Furthermore, in several systems, such as the classical lactose operon, both negative and positive regulators (*lac* repressor and cAMP-binding proteins) modulate the activity of this promoter (see reviews in (41, 43)).

The enzyme assuming this transcription is the bacterial RNA polymerase composed of four subunits (β'βα2), the core polymerase, and a fifth subunit, sigma (σ), required for the formation of the active holoenzyme to confer promoter specificity to the core enzyme. In several cases, such as sporulation of *Bacillus subtilis* or in certain phage infections, a new protein with a novel specificity replaces the bacterial σ subunit resulting in preferential activation of a new class of promoters. In still other bacteriophage infections (T7) a new RNA polymerase, coded by the phage genome, specifically transcribes the phage late genes. The activity of the bacterial RNA polymerase can be monitored *in vitro*, faithful initiations being obtained in the presence of the σ factor. Repression or activation can be obtained in many cases by the addition of the pure repressor or activating proteins.

Contrary to the normal bacterial cell with a single enzyme, three distinct RNA polymerases exist in all eukaryotic cells. The first, RNA polymerase I (or A), is responsible for the transcription of ribosomal RNA genes. The second, RNA polymerase III (or C), transcribes the genes coding for tRNA or 5S RNA. The third, RNA polymerase II (B), transcribes all the genes coding for proteins and several genes coding for low-molecular-weight RNA. The three eukaryotic enzymes are more complex than their bacterial homologues: they are composed of roughly 10 subunits each, some of these subunits may be common to all three enzymes. Furthermore, the specific initiation by these enzymes certainly requires more than one additional factor.

The steady-state level of a specific mRNA in the cytoplasm of eukaryotic cells can be regulated by the frequency of RNA chain initiation, by the rate of processing (splicing, export to cytoplasm, etc.), and by the stability of the mature RNA in the cytoplasm. The synthesis of the protein coded by mRNA can be further modulated by the efficiency of its translation by the protein-synthesizing machinery. In this paper I will discuss exclusively the transcription of protein coding genes by RNA polymerase II with emphasis on the elements that control the rate of initiation.

EUKARYOTIC PROMOTERS

Analysis of the protein content or enzymatic functions of different tissues or cells of an organism shows that a large fraction of proteins are common to all cells. These include metabolic enzymes and structural proteins common to all cells, frequently defined as housekeeping genes. However, some of the proteins are cell-specific. These include many of the excreted proteins that are synthesized by specific cells (e.g., insulin and chemotrypsin secreted by the endocrine and exocrine cells of the pancreas, albumin secreted by liver cells, ovalbumin secreted by oviduct cells, immunoglobulins excreted by B lymphocytes, etc.). Other cell-specific proteins are intracellular such as the muscle-specific isomers of actin and myosin, α- and β-globins, biosynthetic enzymes for specific neurotransmitters, etc. The study of the abundance of mRNA coding for specific proteins has shown that in most cases the regulation of protein synthesis occurs at the level of RNA. Liver cells, for example, contain large amounts of mRNA coding for albumin, a liver-specific protein, whereas no such mRNA is found in any other cell of the adult animal. Furthermore, nuclear run-on experiments have shown that this gene is actively transcribed only in liver cells. Similarly, only mature B lymphocytes contain mRNA coding for the light and heavy chains of the excreted immunoglobulins.

For other gene products it has been shown that the increase in the level of protein is correlated with the increase in the rate of synthesis of RNA. Induction of specific cell proteins by stress, such as heat shock, or by toxic agents, such as cadmium, is accompanied by the simultaneous increase in the level of heat shock-specific or metallothionein-specific mRNAs. Recent work by Klarsfeld and Changeux (28) shows that the increase in the rate of synthesis of acetylcholine receptor upon blocking the spontaneous activity of myotubes is coupled with the increase in specific mRNA level.

Advances in elucidating the control mechanisms of transcription in eukaryotes were hampered by the higher complexity of their genome and lack of powerful genetic tools in higher eukaryotes. Only the recent advent of techniques that permit gene cloning, rapid DNA sequencing, directed mutagenesis, gene transfer, and analysis of sequence-specific DNA-binding proteins has permitted progress in the understanding of eukaryotic systems. Three approaches were mainly used in an attempt to identify sequences that are important for the control of gene activity: a) DNA transfer into cells, b) sequence comparison, and c) transcription *in vitro*.

Foreign DNA can be introduced into eukaryotic cells by several techniques including microinjection, calcium phosphate coprecipitation, DEAE-dextran facilitated uptake, recombinant virus infection, etc. Microinjection is frequently used for the introduction of DNA into oocytes, fertilized eggs, or embryos. The transient expression of the exogenous DNA before its integration can be assayed between one to four days post-transfection or injection. Alternatively, its expression can be assayed at a later time after its stable integration in the recipient cells or in the transgenic animals obtained from microinjected fertilized eggs. The rate or level of expression can be tested by several experimental approaches: analysis of the rate of transcription of the specific gene in isolated nuclei (nuclear run-on), analysis of the level of stable mRNA (S1 or northern), measuring the level of the gene product by immunological assay, and, finally, measuring the activity of an enzyme coded by the transfected or injected DNA. In this conjuncture, many studies are carried out with plasmid constructions where an eukaryotic promoter is cloned upstream of a DNA fragment coding for a bacterial gene such as chloramphenicol acetyltransferase (CAT) or β-galactosidase. Transcription of such chimeric plasmids gives rise to a specific mRNA that is translated in the cytoplasm. The enzymatic activity, absent in nontransfected cells, is a good indication for the strength of the promoter used (20).

One of the most studied eukaryotic promoters is that of the herpes virus thymidine kinase gene (tk). By deletion analysis McKnight and Kingsbury (30) have shown that 105 bp of DNA preceding the RNA start site are sufficient to confer full activity to this promoter after injection into *Xenopus* oocytes. Furthermore, the same sequences allow for maximal activity of this promoter in short- or long-term expression assays in tissue culture cells. Linker scanning replacement mutagenesis and point mutations analysis have shown that four oligonucleotide blocks (an AT-rich sequence, two GC-rich elements, and a CCAAT sequence) are crucial for promoter activity within this region. Similar conclusions were obtained for the rabbit β-globin gene by Dierks *et al.* (8).

Such studies, and the parallel comparison of the sequence of a large number of eukaryotic genes with the location of the 5' ends of the mature mRNA (cap site), showed that certain consensus sequences are found upstream of RNA initiation sites. The 5' nucleotide (+1) of the RNA is usually a purine surrounded by pyrimidines. An AT-rich sequence with a consensus

$$TATA^{A}_{T}A^{A}_{T}$$

(TATA box or Goldberg-Hogness box) is located about 30 nucleotides before this 5' end (-30). Further upstream (about -80) another sequence

$$GG^{C}_{T}C^{T}_{A}AT$$

(CAAT box) is found in a certain number of genes (5). A third sequence element, frequently present upstream from the initiation site, is the hexanucleotide GGGCGG (10). The -30 and -80 elements are usually defined as the *proximal and distal upstream elements* of the promoter (see Fig. 1). The tk promoter contains a TATA box, a CAAT box in a reversed orientation, and two GGGCGG blocks. When compared with bacterial promoters the TATA box can be considered the homologue of the Pribnow box, the CAAT box, or similar distal upstream sequence

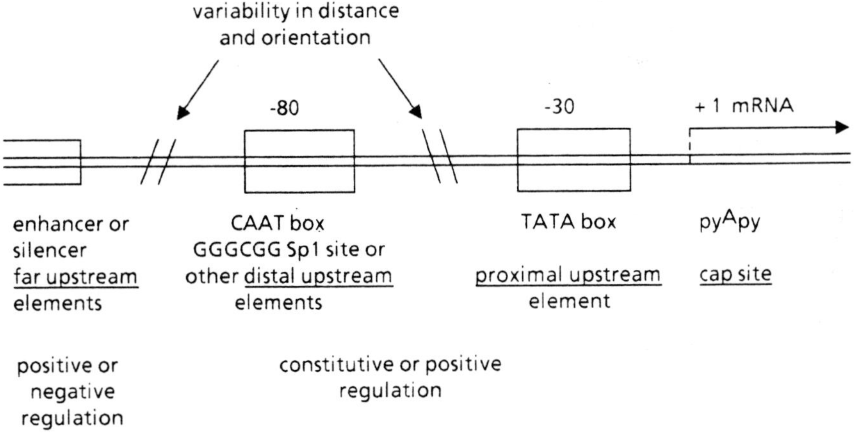

FIG. 1 – Eukaryotic transcription control sequences.

elements as the homologues of the -35 bacterial sequence. A substantial difference concerns the distance between the different elements. In bacteria, DNase I footprint experiments have shown that the RNA polymerase interacts with residues including the -10 and -35 boxes. Furthermore, the distance between these two elements is crucial and cannot be varied considerably. The extended distance between the eukaryotic elements and the transcription initiation sites, the great variability in distance, and the orientation independence of the distal element raise difficulties in adapting a similar scheme for eukaryotes in spite of the presence of extra subunits in the eukaryotic enzymes.

ENHANCERS

The situation became apparently more complex when the early promoter of SV40 virus was studied by similar techniques. The first 110 bp preceding the cap site confer certain basal activity to this promoter, roughly similiar to that of the tk promoter. However, the 170 bp upstream of this fragment (positions -110 to -280 relative to the cap site) increase the activity of this promoter by a factor of ten to one hundred (3,22). This element was defined as the *far upstream control element*. It contains a repetition of 72 bp, with a single 72 bp element bearing about half of the wild-type activity. The surprise arose when several groups realized that this viral element can activate or enhance the transcription *in vivo* from cellular promoters such as β-globin, con-albumin, or α-collagen when cloned 5' or 3' to a transcription unit in both possible orientations. This *cis*-acting element was named *enhancer*, similar elements have since been found in the far upstream sequences of many viral promoters (2, 16 24, 32). Furthermore, enhancer elements were found in an intron located in the middle of the rearranged gene coding for the heavy and light chains of immunoglobulins (1, 18, 33). Contrary to the viral enhancers that function in many cell types, these are cell specific: they function only in lymphocytes. The fact that enhancers can function in an orientation- and position-independent manner distinguishes them from the bacterial positive regulatory sequences where the positive activator protein is probably interacting directly with the RNA polymerase by protein-protein contacts (25).

UPSTREAM SEQUENCES THAT CONFER INDUCTION OF TISSUE SPECIFICITY

Analysis of the abundance of specific RNA discussed above strongly suggested that in many cases control of gene activity occurs at the level of transcription initiation. Only in rare cases is DNA rearrangement associated with the onset of specific transcriptions as in the case of immunoglobulins. It became important to test whether cell specificity or induction of transcription are operating at sequences found upstream of the mRNA cap site. Gene transfer studies have shown that in many cases such controls are indeed operating at the promoter level and not in the body or coding sequences. Insulin promoter, when coupled to a test gene such as CAT or SV40 large T antigen coding sequences, is active in the β-endocrine cells of the pancreas but not in any other cell of the organism (23, 46). Similarly, the albumin promoter is active only in adult liver cells and not in any other cell type tested (35). Chimeric plasmids, containing the *Drosophila* heat shock 70 kd promoter or the metallothionein promoter linked to a test gene, clearly show that induction occurs by the increase in the promoter strength. The basal level of these promoters can be increased ten- to one hundred-fold by the specific stimuli. Table 1 summarizes some of the known examples of *cell-specific* and *inducible* or *modulated promoters*. It includes also the third class of *constitutive promoters* that function in most or all cell types tested. Many strong viral promoters such as the SV40 early promoter or the long terminal repeat (LTR) of Rous sarcoma virus (RSV) are included in this class. The distinction between constitutive and modulated promoters is somewhat arbitrary. The activity of some constitutive promoters can be modulated by either the physiological state of the cell, by transformation, or viral infection. As an example, α-collagen

Table 1 – Diversity of eukaryotic promoters.

Constitutive	Inducible or modulated (a)	Cell-specific (b)
SV40 early	herpes virus tk (viral infection	Insulin (endocrine pancreas cells
LTR of RSV	hsp 70 (heat shock)	chemotrypsin
α-collagen	metallothionein (Zn, Cd)	α-amylase {exocrine
α-tubulin	β-interferon (poly IC)	elastase } pancreas cells
β-actin	histone H4 (cell cycle)	globin (erythroid cells)
	LTR of LAV (HTLV-III) (viral infection)	albumin (liver)
	E2, E3, E4 of adenovirus (viral Ela)	α-antitrypsin (liver)
	BPV1 promoter (viral E2)	α-crystallin (len cells)
	fos (serum, growth factors)	immunoglobulin (B lymphocytes)
	LTR of MMTV (glucocorticoids)	α-actin (muscle)
		ovalbumin (oviduct)

(a) The nature of the inducer is indicated in parentheses.
(b) The specific tissue is indicated in parentheses.

promoter activity decreases in slow-growing cells (G. Moore and M. Yaniv, submitted for publication).

What are the exact sequences that regulate either the cell specificity of certain promoters or their response to external stimuli? To try to answer this question several groups generated plasmid construction with a series of deletions, removing more and more of the promoter upstream sequences. These plasmids were tested after transfection into the corresponding cells. For different promoters, sequences upstream of the cap site, including roughly 70-80 bp (hsp 70 (38); metallothionein (9)), 120-140 bp (β-globin (8); albumin (P. Herbomel *et al.*, unpublished results), 200-280 bp (elastase (34); insulin (46)), or even 425 bp (ovalbumin (P. Chambon, personal communication)), were required for strong regulated expression. Thus, in many cases, sequences beyond the TATA (-30) and CAAT (-80) boxes are necessary for tissue-specific expression. In several cases a sequence element common to a class of co-regulated genes (globins, immunoglobins, pancreas exocrine functions) could be identified upstream of the CAAT box. Some of these promoter distal, tissue-specific elements can act as moderate (three- to tenfold) tissue-specific enhancers when placed 5' or 3' to a test promoter such as tk (19). Upstream sequences found in inducible promoters such as the LTR of MMTV, metallothionein, β-interferon, and *fos* protooncogene also act as inducible enhancer elements (6, 17, 27, 45). Furthermore, in several cases (tk, SV40 early) the orientation of the promoter distal element can be switched relative to the TATA cap site segment without impairing the promoter activity (15, 31). These observations make the previous distinction made between promoter upstream sequences and enhancers somewhat difficult. For the sake of discussion we will maintain the definition of an enhancer as a *cis*-acting element that can stimulate transcription from different basic promoters in an orientation-independent manner when placed 5', 3', or in the middle of a gene. This element can be either a part of promoter distal sequences or located elsewhere in a gene.

TRANSACTIVATION BY VIRAL GENE PRODUCTS

As already mentioned, several DNA viruses show temporal regulation of expression of their genome during infection. The genes transcribed before the onset of massive viral DNA replication are defined as early genes. Those transcribed after DNA replication, mostly viral structural proteins, are defined as late genes. With adeno and herpes virus that are expressed immediately after the infection, one to several proteins, are required for the synthesis of the other early genes that include, among others, enzymes required for DNA replication. A *trans-acting protein* such as Ela of adenovirus is probably not binding directly to the promoter upstream sequences of the activated genes since no common sequence is shared among these genes. Furthermore, Ela activates the transcription of some cellular genes, such as those coding for the 70 kd heat shock protein or the β-globin promoter when present on transfected DNA, but not the endogenous β-globin gene (21). On the other hand, Ela blocks the enhancer function of SV40 (4). It is possible that Ela induces the synthesis of some cellular transcription factors required for the recognition of many different promoters including the viral early promoters. Other cases of transactivation were observed with retroviruses such as HTLV-I, BLV, or LAV (HTLV-III). In these cases a virally coded small protein increases the activity of the viral LTR, one hundred- to a thousandfold. The sequence responding in *cis* to this transactivation overlaps the cap site and includes several dozen nucleotides of the transcribed region. For this reason, it cannot be excluded that the effect occurs here at the level of RNA stabilization or increased efficiency of translation. Whatever the exact mechanism is, the net outcome is an autocatalytic increase in the rate of transcription of the viral genome upon infection (42). A similar observation was made with BPVI non-coding region. This DNA virus contains a segment of DNA that behaves as an enhancer dependent on the presence of viral-coded protein E2 (44).

TRANSCRIPTION FACTORS

One of the major differences between bacterial and higher eukaryotic RNA polymerase II is the inability of the pure eukaryotic enzyme to initiate transcription from promoter sites on double-stranded DNA. The search for a factor similar to the bacterial σ factor, that confers the specificity of initiation to the enzyme, failed. However, RNA polymerase supplied with either a crude cellular extract of Hela cells or a total extract of these cells can recognize some promoters and initiate transcription from the correct cap site (29). Attempts to fractionate the components of the transcription system were partially successful. It seems that some of the factors present in this cell extract are required for initiation at all promoters whereas others are required for initiation only at certain promoters. Roeder and his co-workers (personal communication) partially characterized four factors of the first group. A protein that binds to the TATA box consensus sequence is included among these factors (7, 37). More specific transcription factors that stimulate transcription only from a certain class of promoters were also recently isolated. Tjian and his co-workers isolated a transcription factor, Sp1, that binds the GGGCGG motif found upstream of the SV40 early, tk, and several other viral or cellular promoters (10). This factor stimulates transcription of the SV40 early promoter by partially purified RNA polymerase II in the presence of other general transcription factors. Similarly, this factor and another protein that binds to the CAAT box of the tk promoter are required for the *in vitro* transcription of this gene. Another system where faithful transcription was observed *in vitro* is the *Drosophila* heat shock (hsp 70) gene. Parker and Topol (37) isolated a protein that binds to the heat shock consensus sequence in this promoter and stimulates transcription *in vitro* in the presence of a TATA box-binding protein and partially purified RNA polymerase II.

Proteins that interact with the upstream control sequences were identified for several tissues specific promoters. Immature chicken erythrocytes contain a protein that interacts with the β-globin promoter sequences which is shared among several globin genes (12). A protein (or proteins) that interacts with upstream sequences of the albumin promoter, which is conserved between chicken, mouse, rat, and men, was found in the liver but not the spleen of a rat (M. Raymondjean, S. Cereghini, and M. Yaniv, unpublished observations). These proteins can constitute at least one of the factors that activate such tissue-specific promoters. Their presence will be restricted only to the expressing tissue.

COOPERATIVITY AMONG CONTROL ELEMENTS

The notion that emerges from the preceding paragraphs is that of a multicomponent complex of proteins that act at the level of eukaryotic promoters. Some of these factors are ubiquitous and others are tissue- or stage-specific. Promoters of genes coding for housekeeping functions may require only ubiquitous factors such as TATA box-binding proteins, Sp1 and CAAT box-binding proteins, or only two of these factors. The activity of these genes may be modulated by the number of Sp1 binding sites and the availability of the factors. Tissue-specific promoters, such as globin or albumin, will require upstream factors to increase the affinity for the ubiquitous CAAT- and TATA-binding proteins or to induce a conformational change in the bound factors from a nonfunctional to a functional state. Usually such an action will require the close proximity of the binding sites for these proteins. The difficulty arises when we realize that tissue-specific promoter upstream or far upstream elements are sometimes found quite far from the initiation site and that they can function as tissue-specific enhancers in both possible orientations and in a certain distance. Direct contact can still occur if we permit bending and looping out of DNA sequences introduced between the tissue-specific element and a promoter. However, such looping out may be difficult in the context of chromatin structure and we will therefore need to find other possible mechanisms.

The induction of transcription of promoters regulated by steroid hormones (MMTV, ovalbumin, etc.) or growth factors (*fos*, etc.) will further require the transfer of information from the cytoplasm or cell membrane to the nuclei. In the case of steroid hormone regulation, binding sites for the receptor present on the upstream sequence of the promoter are required for the induction of such promoters (6). In the absence of a receptor, these sequences can behave as negative upstream regulators (P. Chambon, personal communication). For c-*fos* protooncogene regulation, binding of a growth factor to specific receptor on the cell surface will stimulate protein kinase C activity and somehow activate a specific transcription factor that will move to the nucleus and bind to the upstream regulatory sequences present about 300 bp upstream of the *fos* mRNA initiation site (45). In all of these cases the specific regulatory sequences are several hundred bp from the transcription initiation site, thus also raising difficulties in the transmission of the signal to the proximal promoter element.

DNase I HYPERSENSITIVITY IN CHROMATIN

SV40 or polyoma viral genomes are found in the nuclei as minichromosomes formed by the association of viral DNA with the core histones H2A, H2B, H3, and H4. Both biochemical and electron microscopy studies revealed that a segment of the viral genome (including the origin of DNA replication, the promoter, and the enhancer sequences) is excluded from normal nucleosomes. Furthermore, it exhibits a very high degree of sensitivity for endonucleases such as DNase I. Similarly, the immunoglobulin enhancer coincides with a DNase I hypersensitive site in the chromatin. The enhancer behaves as an open window in the chromatin structure that is excluded from the normal nucleosomal repeat. There is a very good correlation between the formation of this open structure and the function of the enhancer. Recent studies have shown that in both cases the enhancer sequences are interacting with cellular nonhistone proteins as shown in Fig. 2B (13, 19, 39, 40, 49). Similarly, many cellular genes harbor DNase I hypersensitive sites in their 5' end. The existence of such sites is usually correlated with gene activity: they are present in tissues that express or are programmed to express a gene but are absent in all other tissues (11). Here again it seems that the promoter sequences are excluded from a normal nucleosomal structure in cells exhibiting DNase I hypersensitivity and that these sequences are occupied by the transcription factors discussed above.

A recent study by Wu (47, 48) of the *Drosophila* hsp 70 gene demonstrates that a DNase I hypersensitive site or region covering 315 bp, extending from +100 to -215 relative to cap site, is already present at low temperature. Exonuclease digestion studies revealed that already before induction the TATA box is occupied by a protein whereas both this sequence and the heat shock responsive element are occupied at high temperatures (Fig. 2A). Less detailed studies of mouse erythroleukemia cells before and after induction of globin synthesis have shown that DNase I hypersensitive sites were already present along this gene before the onset of its synthesis. In essence, DNase I hypersensitive sites can be considered a footmark for the exclusion of some sequences from a uniform nucleosomal structure, probably by the

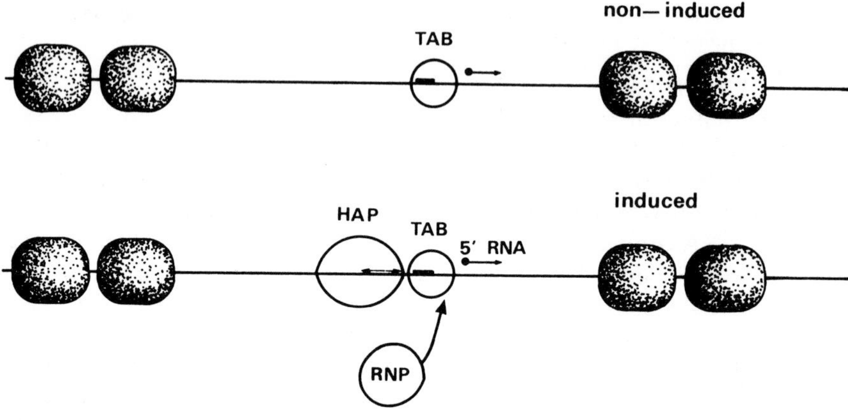

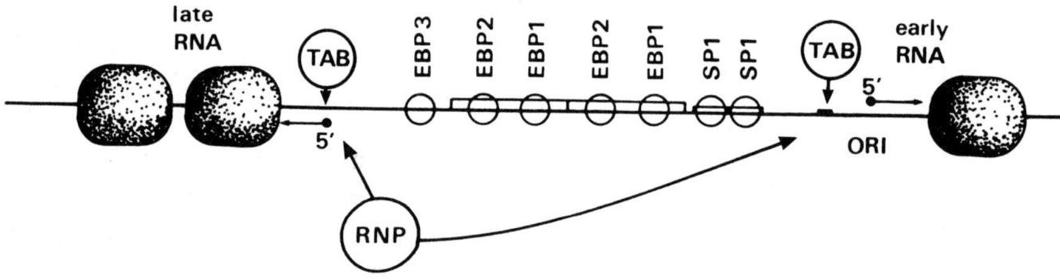

FIG. 2 – Schematic representation of chromatin structure at the promoter enhancer region. The segment of DNA not packed in nucleosomes (dotted ellipsoid bodies) appears histone-free when observed by electron microscopy (SV40) and exhibits a specific pattern of DNase I hypersensitivity (SV40 and hsp 70). The small circles represent proteins interacting with the control sequences. A: *Drosophila* 70 Kd heat shock gene. TAB is the TATA box-binding protein, HAP the heat shock activating protien, and RNP is RNA polymerase II (redrawn with permission from Wu (48)). B: SV40 enhancer-promoter origin region. SP1 is the transcription factor described by Dynan and Tjian (10). EBP1, 2, 3 are hypothetical enhancer binding proteins detected by footprinting *in vivo* of protein DNA contacts along the enhancer region of SV40 (S. Cereghini and M. Yaniv, in preparation). Proteins are not drawn to scale.

binding of a specific protein. Such sites are not limited to promoter or enhancer sequences. They are frequently found far upstream, inside genes, and 3' to genes. It is probable that a certain network of nonhistone protein DNA contacts are formed around a gene. This network excludes a gene that is active or programmed to be active from the mass of inactive chromatin.

COMMITMENT PROTEINS

One can wonder what are the mechanisms that assure a specific pattern of gene expression during development and differentiation. Is the appearance of the specific transcription control factors sufficient to switch on a gene or a group of genes, or are there more complex developmental steps? The fact that genes that are programmed to be expressed, or which have been expressed in a specific cell, conserve some of the DNase I hypersensitive sites and the general DNase I sensitivity characteristic of active genes argues that specific events occur before the final switch of a gene. I would like to suggest that during development a specific set of proteins, or a specific combination of ubiquitous proteins that we define as *commitment proteins*, will bind to a domain that includes a gene programmed to be expressed in a terminally differentiated cell. These proteins will appear during one of the S-phases, occupy sites close to the gene in question, and form a specific chromatin structure. This structure will be transmitted from mother to progeny in stem cells. Induction of terminal differentiation will be coupled with the appearance of a positive transcription control factor(s) and the formation of an active transcription complex. Somatic cell hybridization of differentiated cells with fibroblasts or with micro cells suggests that another factor could be involved in final differentiation. Undifferentiated cells may synthesize a dominant extinguishing function that blocks the expression of genes typical for the fully differentiated cell. This extinguishing factor(s) may inhibit the synthesis of the gene-specific positive regulator, interfere with its function, or block translation of the specific mRNA (14). Such a factor will disappear during final differentiation concomitantly with the appearance of the positive control protein(s).

CONCLUSIONS

This review has attempted to outline the different facets of gene regulation in higher eukaryotes. It has been shown that in addition to the RNA polymerase and several ubiquitous transcription initiation factors, gene, gene group, or cell-specific transcription factors are present in cells. These factors usually interact with the distal upstream sequences of promoters; however, specific control sequences are sometimes present even inside genes. The transcription of genes that are unique to certain types of cells is usually very strictly controlled. It occurs only in a fully differentiated cell. It is possible that during development and commitment a certain set of commitment proteins interact with various sites in a domain surrounding a gene and create an active chromatin conformation that excludes the gene in question from the mass of nonactive chromatin. Upon terminal differentiation, positive transcription factor(s) will be synthesized and switch on the transcription of a gene or a class of genes. The expression of these genes can still be modulated by hormones through the interaction of hormone-receptor complex with the upstream sequences or even with sequences inside the gene. Other external signals can regulate the expression of such genes by inducing covalent modifications in transcription factors, by changing the ion concentration with relation to the rate of transcription, etc. Genes expressed in all cells can also be regulated by the same type of external signals. The human metallothionein gene has a certain level of basal activity in all cells. Its expression is stimulated not only by metals such as Cd or Zn but also by glucocorticoid hormones. Such effects can be additive. The presence of multiple binding sites for the hormone receptor or for metal induction can also graduate the response and create cooperativity in the level of induction. The action of agents such as glucocorticoid hormones can be easily analyzed since the hormone-receptor complex was shown to bind to specific sites in the promoter sequences. It is more difficult to decipher the pathway that involves stimulation by polypeptide hormones or growth factors. In this case the binding to cell surface receptors may induce phosphorylation or other covalent modifications of a transcription factor that will then be activated and/or translocated from the cytoplasm to the nuclei, resulting in the activation of specific genes.

It is clear that both the binding of neurotransmitters to postsynaptic receptors and the ion influx occurring in many cases can result in a modulation of the activity or concentration of transcription factors, perhaps via a cascade of protein kinases or via an increase in cyclic nucleotide concentrations. Such changes can provoke either quantitative or qualitative variations in the pattern of gene expression in neurons. Autocatalytic mechanisms (Kennedy, this volume) or negative feedback loops (Changeux *et al.*, this volume) can sustain these changes in the pattern of gene expression.

REFERENCES

(1) Banerji, J.; Olson, L.; and Schaffner, W. 1983. A lymphocyte specific cellular enhancer is located downstream of the joining region in immunoglobulin heavy chain genes. *Cell* 33: 729-740.

(2) Banerji, J.; Rusconi, S.; and Schaffner, W. 1981. Expression of a β-globin gene is enhanced by remote SV40 DNA sequences. *Cell* 27: 299-308.

(3) Benoist, C., and Chambon, P. 1981. *In vivo* sequence requirements of the SV40 early promoter region. *Nature* 290: 304-310.

(4) Borelli, E.; Hen, R.; and Chambon, P. 1984. Adenovirus 2 Ela products repress enhancer-induced stimulation of transcription. *Nature* 312: 608-612.

(5) Breathnach, R., and Chambon, P. 1981. Organization and expression of eukaryotic split genes coding for proteins. *Ann. R. Biochem.* 50: 349-383.

(6) Chandler, V.L.; Maler, B.A.; and Yamamoto, K.R. 1983. DNA sequences bound specifically by glucocorticoid receptor *in vitro* render a heterologous promoter hormone responsible *in vivo*. *Cell* 33: 489-499.

(7) Davison, B.L.; Egly, J.M.; Mulvihill, E.R.; and Chambon, P. 1983. Formation of stable preinitiation complexes between eukaryotic class B transcription factors and promoter sequences. *Nature* 301: 680-684.

(8) Dierks, P.; Van Ooyen, A.; Cochran, M.D.; Dobkin, C.; Reiser, J.; and Weissmann, C. 1983. Three regions upstream from the cap site are required for efficient and accurate transcription of the rabbit β-globin gene in mouse 3T6 cells. *Cell* 32: 695-706.

(9) Durnam, D.M., and Palmiter, R.D. 1981. Transcriptional regulation of the mouse metallothionein-1 gene by heavy metal. *J. Biol. Chem.* 256: 5712-5716.

(10) Dynan, W., and Tjian, R. 1985. Control of eukaryotic messenger RNA synthesis by sequence specific DNA binding proteins. *Nature* 316: 774-778.

(11) Elgin, S.C. 1981. DNAase I hypersensitive sites of chromatin. *Cell* 27: 413-415.

(12) Emerson, B.M.; Lewis, C.D.; and Felsenfeld, G. 1985. Interaction of specific nuclear factors with the nuclease-hypersensitive region of the chicken adult β-globin gene: nature of the binding domain. *Cell* 41: 21-30.

(13) Ephrussi, A.; Church, G.M; Tonegawa, S.; and Gilbert, W. 1985. B lineage specific interactions of an immunoglobulin enhancer with cellular factors *in vivo*. *Science* 227: 134-140.

(14) Ephrussi, B. 1972. Hybridization of Somatic Cells. Princeton, NJ: Princeton University Press.

(15) Everett, R.D.; Baty, D.; and Chambon, P. 1983. The repeated GC rich motifs upstream from the TATA box are important elements of the SV40 early promoter. *Nucl. Acid Res.* 11: 2447-2464.

(16) Fromm, M., and Berg, P. 1983. SV40 early and late region promoter function are enhanced by the 72 base pair repeat inserted at distant locations and inverted orientations. *Mol. Cell. Biol.* 3: 991-999.

(17) Fujita, T.; Ohno, S.; Yasumitsu, H.; and Tanigushi, T. 1985. Delimitation and properties of DNA sequences required for the regulated expression of human interferon β-gene. *Cell* 41: 489-496.

(18) Gillies, S.D.; Morrison, S.L.; Oi, V.T.; and Tonegawa, S. 1983. A tissue-specific transcription enhancer element is located in the major intron of a rearranged immunoglobulin heavy chain gene. *Cell* 33: 717-728.

(19) Gluzman, Y., editor. 1985. Eukaryotic Transcription: the Role of *Cis* and *Trans* Acting Elements in Initiation. In *Current Comments in Molecular Biology*. Cold Spring Harbor: Cold Spring Harbor Laboratory.

(20) Gorman, C.M.; Moffat, L.F.; and Howard, B.H. 1982. Recombinant genomes which express chloramphenicol acetyltransferase in mammalian cells. *Mol. Cell. Biol.* 2: 1044-1051.

(21) Green, M.R.; Treisman, R.; and Maniatis, T. 1983. Transcriptional activation of cloned human β-globin genes by viral immediate early gene products. *Cell* 35: 137-148.

(22) Gruss, P.; Dhar, R.; and Khoury, G. 1981. Simian virus 40 tandem repeated sequences as an element of the early promoter. *Proc. Natl. Acad. Sci.* 78: 943-947.

(23) Hanahan, D. 1985. Heritable formation of pancreatic β-cell tumors in transgenic mice expressing recombinant insulin/simian virus 40 oncogenes. *Nature* 315: 115-122.

(24) Herbomel, P.; Bourachot, B.; and Yaniv, M. 1984. Two distinct enhancers with different cell specificities coexist in the regulatory region of polyoma. *Cell* 39: 653-662.

(25) Hochschild, A.; Irwin, N.; and Ptashne, M. 1983. Repressor structure and the mechanism of positive control. *Cell* 3: 319-325.

(26) Jacob, F., and Monod, J. 1961. Genetic regulatory mechanisms in the synthesis of proteins. *J. Mol. Biol.* 3: 318-356.

(27) Karin, M.; Haslinger, A.; Holtgreve, H.; Cathala, G.; Slater, E.; and Baxter, J.D. 1984. Activation of a heterologous promoter in response to dexamethasone and cadmium by metallothionein gene 5'-flanking DNA. *Cell* 36: 371-379.

(28) Klarsfeld, A., and Changeux, J.-P. 1985. Activity regulates the levels of acetylcholine receptor α-subunit mRNA cultured chicken myotubes. *Proc. Natl. Acad. Sci.* 82: 4558-4562.

(29) Manley, J.L.; Fire, A.; Cano, A.; Sharp, P.A.; and Gefter, M.L. 1980. DNA dependent transcription of adenovirus genes in a soluble whole cell extract. *Proc. Natl. Acad. Sci.* 77: 3855-3859.

(30) McKnight, S.L., and Kingsbury, R. 1982. Transcriptional control signals of a eukaryotic protein-coding gene. *Science* 217: 316-324.

(31) McKnight, S.L.; Kingsbury, R.C.; Spence, A.; and Smith, M. 1984. The distal transcription signals of the herpes virus tk gene share a common hexanucleotide control sequence. *Cell* 37: 253-262.

(32) Moreau, P.; Hen, R.; Wasylyk, B.; Everett, R.; Gaub, M.B.; and Chambon, P. 1981. The SV40 72 base pair repeat has a striking effect on gene expression both in SV40 and other chimeric recombinants. *Nucl. Acid Res.* 9: 6047-6068.

(33) Neuberger, M.S. 1983. Expression and regulation of immunoglobulin heavy chain gene transfected into lymphoid cells. *EMBO J.* 2: 1373-1378.

(34) Ornitz, D.M.; Palmiter, R.D.; Hammer, R.E.; Brinster, R.L.; Swiff, G.F.; and MacDonald, R.J. 1985. Specific expression of an elastase human growth hormone fusion gene in pancreatic cells of transgenic mice. *Nature* 313: 600-601.

(35) Ott, M.-O.; Sperling, L.; Herbomel, P.; Yaniv, M.; and Weiss, M. 1984. Tissue specific expression is conferred by a sequence from the 5' end of the rat albumin gene. *EMBO J.* 3: 2505-2510.

(36) Parker, C.S., and Topol, J. 1984. A *Drosophila* RNA polymerase II transcription factor binds to the regulatory site of an hsp 70 gene. *Cell* 37: 273-283.

(37) Parker, C.S., and Topol, J. 1984. A *Drosophila* RNA polymerase II transcription factor contains a promoter region specific DNA binding activity. *Cell* 36: 357-369.

(38) Pelham, H.R.B. 1982. A regulatory upstream promoter element in the *Drosophila* hsp 70 heat-shock gene. *Cell* 30: 517-528.

(39) Piette, J.; Cereghini, S.; Kryszke, M.-H.; and Yaniv, M. 1986. Identification of cellular proteins that interact with polyoma or SV40 enhancers. *Cander Cells* 4, in press.

(40) Piette, J.; Kryszke, M.-H.; and Yaniv, M. 1985. Specific interaction of cellular factors with the B enhancer of polyoma virus. *EMBO J.* 4: 2675-2685.

(41) Raibaud, O., and Schwartz, M. 1984. Positive control of transcription initiation in bacteria. *Ann. R. Genet.* 18: 173-206.

(42) Rosen, A.; Sochoski, J.G.; and Haseltine, W. 1985. The location of *cis* acting regulatory sequences in the human T cell lymphotropic virus type III (HTLV.III/LAV) long terminal repeat. *Cell* 41: 813-823.

(43) Rosenberg, M., and Court, D. 1979. Regulatory sequences involved in the promotion and termination of RNA transcription. *Ann. R. Genet.* 13: 319-353.

(44) Spalholz, B.A.; Yang, Y.C.; and Howley, P.M. 1985. Transactivation of a bovine papilloma virus transcriptional regulatory element by the E2 gene product. *Cell* 42: 183-191.

(45) Treisman, R. 1985. Transient accumulation of c-*fos* RNA following serum stimulation requires a conserved 5' element and c-*fos* 3' sequences. *Cell* 42: 889-902.

(46) Walker, M.D.; Edlund, T.; Boulet, A.M.; and Rutter, W.J. 1983. Cell specific expression controlled by the 5' flanking region of insulin and chymotrypsin genes. *Nature* 306: 557-561.

(47) Wu, C. 1984. Activating protein factor binds *in vitro* to upstream control sequences in heat shock gene chromatin. *Nature* 311: 81-84.

(48) Wu, C. 1984. Two protein binding sites in chromatin implicated in the activation of heat-shock genes. *Nature* 309: 229-234.

(49) Yaniv, M., and Cereghini, S. 1986. Structure of transcriptionally active chromatin. *Crit. Rev. Biochem.*, in press.

The Neural and Molecular Bases of Learning,
eds. J.-P. Changeux and M. Konishi, pp. 137–152..
John Wiley & Sons Limited.

Neuronal Biochemical Regulatory Mechanisms

M.B. Kennedy

Division of Biology 216-76
California Institute of Technology
Pasadena, CA 91125, USA

Abstract. Biochemical and cell biological studies of the structure of central nervous system synapses have provided an outline of molecular regulatory mechanisms that are likely to be responsible for transmitter-mediated and activity-dependent alterations in synaptic ion channels, transmitter release, receptor sensitivity, and synaptic structure. Three major classes of second messenger systems are present in synapses. They are the cyclic nucleotide systems, the phosphatidyl inositide/C-kinase systems, and the calcium/calmodulin systems. This paper summarizes our present knowledge of these pathways and discusses ways in which their organization may contribute to synaptic information processing.

INTRODUCTION

Neurons, like all eukaryotic cells, employ networks of cytoplasmic regulatory mechanisms to fine-tune their specialized functions in response to environmental cues (7, 9, 28, 30, 31). The details of these networks are still incompletely understood even in the most thoroughly studied "simple" systems (e.g., control of glycogen breakdown in the liver (9, 21)). However, an explosion of new information about the biochemistry of second messenger systems in the last few years allows us to outline the major regulatory pathways and to begin to understand how they may interact. It seems increasingly clear that most of the cytoplasmic regulatory mechanisms used in the brain have counterparts in other tissues. Therefore, information from studies of nonneural tissues is useful for understanding how brain regulatory mechanisms might work. I will begin this brief review by enumerating some of the changes in neurons induced by their environment which seem likely to be regulated, at least in part, by biochemical second messenger systems. Then I will outline the second messenger systems that are present in the brain and discuss intriguing aspects of their organization that may contribute to synaptic plasticity.

BRAIN REGULATORY MECHANISMS

Brain regulatory mechanisms that may be important for learning include those that alter the properties of synapses and that occur over a relatively long time scale and are controlled by extracellular transmitters and hormones or by electrical activity. They include the following:

a) mechanisms that change the properties of ion channels which govern electrical excitability;

b) mechanisms by which the amount of transmitter released from terminals in response to depolarization is increased or decreased;

c) mechanisms by which the sensitivities of transmitter and hormone receptors are altered;

d) mechanisms by which the shape of the cell or synapse and the extent of dendritic and axonal branching are changed; and

e) mechanisms by which old synapses may be removed or new ones formed in the adult brain.

The best understood of these mechanisms are those that regulate ion channels (39). Long-lasting changes in a variety of K^+ and Ca^{2+} currents can be induced by cAMP- or calcium/diacylglycerol-regulated phosphorylation of the channel itself or of associated proteins (4, 11, 38, 39). Examples of such regulation in a physiological context are discussed by Carew, Alkon, and Baudry *et al.* (all this volume). In contrast to regulation of ion channels, regulation of release and receptor sensitivity are just beginning to be understood. In some cases transmitter release is altered as a consequence of changes in synaptic ion channels ((38); see Carew, this volume), but in others more complex mechanisms, apparently involving regulation of synaptic vesicle function by protein phosphorylation, may come into play (24). It appears that receptor sensitivity can be regulated either by a change in the total number of receptors at a synapse or by alterations in the responses of individual receptor molecules (see Changeux *et al.*, this volume). Finally, mechanisms by which the shape or number of synapses are regulated are very poorly understood. We have only the smallest hints that changes in the structure of synapses occur during learning (e.g., (3, 6, 22)), or that the shape and extent of dendritic branching is dynamic in the healthy adult animal (35). Similarly, we can only guess that removal of old synapses or formation of new ones may be involved in long-term consolidation of learning (see Bear *et al.*, this volume). Thus, very little information is available at the molecular level about how specific reformation of synaptic contacts might occur during learning. Therefore, at this time, studies of the structure of CNS dendrites and synapses and the organization and regulation of their cytoskeleton are important because they could provide clues about the circumstances under which such remodelling may occur.

SECOND MESSENGER SYSTEMS IN THE BRAIN

Neurotransmitters and neurohormones affect the regulation of cells primarily via three second messengers. These are the cyclic nucleotides, phosphatidylinositol, and calcium ion. The concentration of calcium ion can also be altered by electrical activity which opens voltage-gated calcium channels. I will outline the major biochemical pathways for each of these second messengers and discuss briefly what is known about them in the brain.

Cyclic AMP

There are two cyclic nucleotides that function as second messengers: cyclic adenosine monophosphate (cAMP) and cyclic guanosine monophosphate (cGMP). I will focus on the cAMP system. Cyclic AMP is synthesized by hormone-regulated adenylate cyclase, a complex enzyme system composed of three different types of membrane-bound proteins: receptors, "G-proteins," and the catalytic subunit (13). Because many hormones and neurotransmitter receptors can activate the cyclase, it can produce an integrated response to information from several sources. Activation of the cyclase works in the following way. The central catalytic subunit is inactive until it binds the 45 kD α-subunit of the regulatory GTP-binding protein (G-protein) called G_S. In its "resting" state G_S is a complex composed of the α-subunit, a 35 kD β-subunit, and a 10 kD γ-subunit. Hormones that activate the cyclase bind to membrane receptor proteins which then bind to the G_S complex and release the α-subunit. If the free α-subunit has GTP bound to it, it can then bind and activate the cyclase catalyst and stimulate synthesis of cAMP. The activation of the catalyst is terminated by the slow hydrolysis of the α-subunit-bound GTP and the reassociation of the α-subunit with β and γ. G_S is only one member of a family of "G-proteins" (13). Another, called G_i, mediates hormone-regulated inhibition of the cyclase. This protein has the same β-subunit as G_S, but has a different α-subunit (13). Receptor-mediated dissociation of the subunits of G_i

results in inhibition of cAMP synthesis. Much remains to be learned about the roles of other members of the G-protein family, including G_O, a G-protein purified from brain, the function of which is still unknown (40). Potential G-protein functions that are especially intriguing include inhibition of voltage-gated Ca^{2+} channels by GABA and noradrenaline (15) and mediation of receptor-stimulated hydrolysis of phosphatidylinositol (see below) (8, 29, 45). Because all of the G-proteins appear to share the same regulatory β-subunit, activation of any one of them may release free β-subunits and thereby suppress dissociation and activation of the others. The potential for signal integration at the biochemical level is enormous.

Another kind of intergration that may occur at the level of the cyclase has been described by Kandel *et al.* (17) and Ocorr *et al.* (32), who have found that electrical activity can potentiate the activation of adenylate cyclase by serotonin in the *Aplysia* nervous system (see Carew and Baudry *et al.*, both this volume). They postulate that interaction of calcium with the cyclase, perhaps at the level of the G-protein, may mediate this potentiation. There have been reports that a portion of mammalian brain adenylate cyclase is calcium-dependent (2, 46), although this dependence seems to be mediated directly through the catalytic unit and not via the G-protein (2). Potentiation by calcium of the activation of the cyclase by other agents has not been observed in mammalian systems.

Most, if not all, of the regulatory actions of cAMP are caused by activation of the cAMP-dependent protein kinases (21, 28). The predominate form of this enzyme in brain is the Type II cAMP-dependent kinase (5, 12). It is an oligomer of two identical regulatory subunits and two identical catalytic subunits. The regulatory subunits suppress activity of the catalytic subunits. Activation occurs when cAMP binds to the regulatory subunits and causes release of the catalytic subunits. The cAMP-dependent kinase has a broad protein substrate specificity and can thus have many regulatory roles. The spectrum of changes induced in a cell by a rise in cAMP probably depends on the range of substrate proteins that are located near the activated kinase. It has been directly demonstrated that injection of free catalytic subunit into neurons can cause changes in the properties of several types of ion channels (39). The cAMP-dependent kinase may also be involved in changes in the number or sensitivity of transmitter receptors (16) or in regulation of microtubule assembly (28).

Phosphatidylinositol Bisphosphate

Several specific hormones and transmitters initiate receptor-mediated hydrolysis of the phosphoinositides; these include phosphatidylinositol (~5-7% of the total lipid in eukaryotic membranes), phosphatidylinositol phosphate (~1%), and phosphatidylinositol bisphosphate (~0.4%) (25). Binding of these agonists to their receptors activates a phospholipase that catalyzes the lipid hydrolysis. Recent evidence suggests that this activation requires a "G-protein" (see above), one of the family of membrane-bound GTP-binding regulatory proteins. Thus the activation could be linked to other second messenger pathways that involve G-proteins, for example, the cAMP pathway.

Hydrolysis of phosphatidylinositol bisphosphate produces two second messengers: diacylglycerol (the lipid backbone) and inositol triphosphate (the cleaved polar head group). Inositol triphosphate is water-soluble and presumably diffuses into the interior of the cell where it releases calcium ion from internal stores (see section on *Calcium Ion*) (25). Diaclyglycerol is hydrophobic and remains in the membrane where it can activate the calcium- and lipid-dependent protein kinase called C-kinase (a single polypeptide chain of 80 kD) (31). Some evidence suggests that the C-kinase becomes concentrated in the membrane as it is activated (1).

There are many potential consequences of activation of C-kinase in the nervous system. A growing list of ion currents, including a calcium-activated K^+ current in the hippocampus (4) and a voltage-dependent Ca^{2+} current in *Aplysia* bag cells (11), appears to be altered either directly or indirectly following its activation. The selective reduction of the hippocampal K^+ current may be important for generation or maintenance of long-term potentiation (see Alkon and Baudry *et al.*, both this volume). In some nonneuronal systems the C-kinase appears to be involved in regulation of vesicle-mediated release (e.g., (36)), thus it could play an analogous role in the nervous system.

The C-kinase is apparently not uniformly distributed in the mammalian brain (43, 44, 47). It is approximately three times more concentrated in the forebrain than in older brain regions such as the pons or medulla. It appears to be primarily neuronal and within neurons concentrated primarily in dendrites and synaptic terminals rather than cell bodies (47). It location is thus appropriate for its postulated roles in synaptic plasticity.

It may be important to bear in mind that another consequence of the hydrolysis of the phosphoinositides, in addition to the release of inositol triphosphate and diglyceride, may be the increased production of the fatty acid, arachidonic acid, which is the rate-limiting precursor in the production of prostaglandins (25). Prostaglandins are generally released from the cell that produces them and act to regulate neighboring cells. It is possible that prostaglandins may have regulatory functions in the brain that have not yet been recognized.

Calcium Ion

The concentration of calcium ion can be transiently increased within cells or parts of cells by many mechanisms. Electrical activity opens voltage-gated Ca^{2+} channels. Hydrolysis of phosphatidylinositol produces inositol triphosphate which releases Ca^{2+} from internal stores (25). The ion pores of many transmitter-gated receptors, such as the acetylcholine receptor and perhaps the NMDA-type glutamate receptor (26), are large enough to allow the passage of Ca^{2+}. Similarly, within the cell there are many effects of this increased concentration. The C-kinase discussed above can be activated by Ca^{2+} synergistically with its activation by diglyceride (31). In addition, a large list of enzymes and cellular structures can be regulated through the small calcium-binding protein, calmodulin (7).

Calmodulin (CaM) is an 18 kD polypeptide with four Ca^{2+}-binding sites (20). It makes up about 1% of the total brain protein. At resting calcium concentrations (10^{-8}-10^{-7} M) no calcium is bound to CaM, whereas at 10^{-6} M and above the four sites are occupied. In its calcium-bound state CaM regulates several protein kinases (see below), at least one protein phosphatase (41), a cyclic nucleotide phosphodiesterase (7), one form of adenylate cyclase (46), and several cytoskeletal components. Thus, CaM-dependent proteins are likely to enter the regulatory network at several points. Most of the known CaM-regulated proteins are present in the brain and some of them are particularly concentrated there. These include calcineurin (41), a Ca^{2+}-activated protein phosphatase (CaM-activated adenylate cyclase (46)), and Type II CaM-dependent protein kinase (12). The specific roles of the CaM-dependent proteins in synaptic regulation are still largely unknown. However, I will discuss aspects of the structure, location, and regulation of Type II CaM kinase that suggest it may be involved in regulating synaptic plasticity.

Type II CaM Kinase

There are at least five structurally distinct CaM-dependent protein kinases (19). Four of these (phosphorylase kinase, myosin light chain kinase, and CaM kinases I and III) are rather specialized, having a narrow substrate specificity. The fifth kinase is actually a family of structurally related, broad specificity kinases all of which share several characteristics (19). First, they are multimeric proteins composed of clusters of six to twelve homologous subunits with molecular weights of 50-60 K dal. Second, all of the subunits are catalytic, bind CaM, and can be autophosphorylated. Third, each of these kinases has the same relatively broad substrate specificity. For historical reasons we refer to the broad specificity CaM kinase from the brain as Type II CaM kinase. It is a cluster of twelve subunits, ~9 50 kD α-subunits and ~3 60 kD β-subunits.

Type II CaM kinase is 10 to 100 times more concentrated in the brain than in nonneural tissues (12). In contrast, phosphorylase kinase, myosin light chain kinase, and "CaM kinase III" are most concentrated in nonneural tissues, and "CaM kinase I" is present in the brain at about the same level as in other tissues (19). Within the brain, Type II CaM kinase has a highly nonuniform distribution (12). It is extremely concentrated in the hippocampus where it is about 2% of the total protein, slightly less concentrated in cortex where it is 1% of the total, and much less concentrated in lower brain regions where it is approximately 0.1-0.2% of the total protein. Most of the Type II CaM kinase is in neurons where immunocytochemical and biochemical experiments indicate a heterogenous distribution (19, 33). A portion of the kinase appears to be cytosolic and present throughout neurons: in cell bodies, dendrites, axons, and synaptic terminals (5, 33). However, some of it (about half) appears to be associated with particulate structures. The kinase is a major component of isolated postsynaptic densities (18), thus it may be concentrated at the postsynaptic membrane to respond to calcium signals generated in response to electrical activity. It also has been found in isolated synaptic versicles (34), indicating that it may have presynaptic actions. Finally, it has an affinity for microtubules (42) and may thus be involved in aspects of regulation of microtubule function in the brain.

The Type II CaM kinase phosphorylates brain proteins contained in all of the above compartments (5). For example, a particularly robust substrate (high rate, high stoichiometry) is synapsin I, a presynaptic, vesicle-associated protein. There is evidence that the presynaptic kinase may be involved in regulation of transmitter release (24). The microtubule-associated protein MAP_2, which is located in dendrites, is also a good substrate. Several unidentified proteins are phosphorylated in isolated postsynaptic densities (14). Within the cytosol, transmitter-synthesizing enzymes are potential substrates (46), as well as myosin light chain (5). *In vitro*, phosphorylation of nonmuscle myosin by the Type II CaM kinase can activate the actin-dependent ATPase (Edelman, Bennett, Kennedy, and Krebs, submitted). Thus, the Type II CaM kinase can potentially regulate changes in neuronal shape.

A Calcium-triggered Switch

The Type II CaM kinase is regulated by its own autophosphorylation in a way that confers on it the properties of a switch (27, 37). Each subunit can incorporate two to three phosphate groups when the kinase is activated by calcium and CaM, for a total of 30 phosphate groups per dodecameric holoenzyme when the kinase is fully autophosphorylated. Incorporation of a relatively small proportion of these, three to six per holoenzyme (less than one per subunit), alters the requirements for expression of kinase activity. The phosphokinase becomes capable of phosphorylating exogenous substrates in the absence of calcium, although at about one half to one third the rate of that in the presence of calcium. Its maximum activity in the presence of calcium is reduced to ~40-60% of that of native kinase. In addition to the changes in phosphorylation of exogenous substrates, autophosphorylation itself is altered, becoming Ca^{2+}-independent. It can proceed nearly to completion even if Ca^{2+} is removed. The threshold for the shift to a Ca^{2+}-independent state is clearly less than one phosphate per subunit. This suggests that autophosphorylation of a few subunits per holoenzyme produces an allosteric change in the activity of all the subunits. This mechanism could provide an amplification of the intial calcium signal.

Autophosphorylation of the kinase confers on it some of the properties of a molecular switch such as was recently described in a theoretical paper by Lisman (23). The switch would operate as follows. When the kinase is unphosphorylated (state 1), a transient rise in Ca^{2+} concentration would produce an initial burst of high kinase activity accompanied by autophosphorylation. If the Ca^{2+} concentration remained high long enough for the threshold level of autophosphorylation to be reached, the kinase would be switched to a different state (state 2) in which kinase activity would continue after the Ca^{2+} concentration has fallen. A return to the native state would require dephosphorylation by cellular phosphatases. The calcium-independent autophosphorylation, which is characteristic of "state 2," would oppose this dephosphorylation and could prolong the shift in kinase activity. The lifetime of the shifted kinase would be determined by the balance between the rates of Ca^{2+}-

independent autophosphorylation and dephosphorylation by phosphatases. If the rate of autophosphorylation exceeded the rate of dephosphorylation, the shifted state could last as long as the lifetime of the holoenzyme itself.

The rate of autophosphorylation is considerably slower than the rate of phosphorylation of exogenous substrates (27). It appears to take place entirely within each holoenzyme and not across holoenzymes; therefore, the rate would be constant no matter how concentrated the kinase is within the neuron. This allows us to estimate that a rise in calcium concentration of about 10 seconds in a given neuronal compartment would be required to switch most of the kinase to state 2. Thus, the brief millisecond increases in calcium that are caused by single impulses would not be sufficient to switch a significant portion of the kinase. This kinetic behavior is intriguing because it suggests a mechanism by which trains of impulses, like those necessary to produce long-term potentiation, could produce a long-lasting change in kinase activity which would not be produced by a few impulses. We do not yet know whether the kinase assumes state 2 *in vivo*. Nevertheless, the switch model provides a framework in which we can test the hypothesis that autophosphorylation of the kinase might underlie some aspect of the generation of long-term potentiation.

Lisman (23) has pointed out that a kinase which could activate itself by intermolecular autophosphorylation could provide a signal that would outlast molecular turnover. Because autophosphorylation of the Type II CaM kinase appears to be entirely within individual holoenzymes, it does not appear at first glance that the switched state could be perpetuated beyond degradation of the holoenzyme. However, it may be significant that the threshold level of autophosphorylation required for the change to state 2 is considerably less than one phosphate per subunit. Thus, a small number of phosphorylated subunits can cause the entire holoenzyme to switch to the calcium-independent form. Because of this, it is possible that a slow exchange of subunits between holoenzymes, or indiviual degradation and replacement of the subunits, could lead to perpetuation of the switched state beyond the lifetime of single holoenzymes. New subunits added to preexisting phosphoholoenzymes would be rapidly autophosphorylated because of the apparent allosteric effect of the other subunits. This suggestion extends far beyond the limits of the present available data, but it is surprisingly similar to an idea proposed on theoretical grounds a few years ago by Crick (10).

CONCLUSION

We are far from a complete understanding of the molecular details of synaptic regulation and even farther from understanding the molecular changes that encode memories. However, biochemical and structural studies of synapses have provided the first outlines from which the final picture will emerge. A great difficulty encountered in molecular studies of the brain has been its tremendous cellular heterogeneity. Today biochemists and molecular biologists who study the brain are beginning to assemble the tools necessary to overcome this difficulty. We know a great deal about the biochemical characteristics of the major regulatory systems, and we have new immunochemical and immunohistochemical techniques with which to study the expression and alteration of these systems in individual brain regions under controlled physiological circumstances. Only ten years ago the brain was considered too complicated to be studied adequately at the molecular level. Now it has become a last, exciting biochemical frontier.

REFERENCES

(1) Akers, R.F.; Lovinger, D.M.; Colley, P.A.; Linden, D.J.; and Routtenberg, A. 1986. Translocation of protein kinase C activity may mediate hippocampal long-term potentiation. *Science* 231: 587-589.

(2) Andreasen, T.J.; Heideman, W.; Rosenberg, G.B.; and Storm, D.R. 1983. Photoaffinity labeling of brain adenylate cyclase preparations with azido [^{125}I] iodocalmodulin. *Biochemistry* 22: 2757-2762.

(3) Bailey, C.H., and Chen, M. 1982. Morphological basis of long-term habituation and sensitization in *Aplysia*. *Science* 220: 91-93.

(4) Baraban, J.M.; Snyder, S.H.; and Alger, B.H. 1985. Protein kinase C regulates ionic conductance in hippocampal pyramidal neurons: electrophysiological effects of phorbol esters. *Proc. Natl. Acad. Sci.* 82: 2538-2542.

(5) Bennett, M.K.; Erondu, N.E.; and Kennedy, M.B. 1983. Purification and characterization of a calmodulin-dependent protein kinase that is highly concentrated in brain. *J. Biol. Chem.* 258: 12735-12744.

(6) Cheng, F.-L.F., and Greenough, W.T. 1984. Transient and enduring morphological correlates of synaptic activity and efficacy change in the rat hippocampal slice. *Brain Res.* 309: 35-46.

(7) Cheung, W.Y. 1980. Calmodulin plays a pivotal role in cellular regulation. *Science* 207: 19-27.

(8) Cockcroft, S., and Gomperts, B.D. 1985. Role of guanine nucleotide binding protein in the activation of polyphosphoinositide phosphodiesterase. *Nature* 314: 534-536.

(9) Cohen, P. 1982. The role of protein phosphorylation in neural and hormonal control of cellular activity. *Nature* 296: 613-620.

(10) Crick, F. 1984. Memory and molecular turnover. *Nature* 312: 101.

(11) De Riemer, S.A.; Strong, J.A.; Albert, K.A.; Greengard, P.; and Kaczmarek, L.K. 1985. Enhancement of calcium current in *Aplysia* neurones by phorbol ester and protein kinase C. *Nature* 313: 313-315.

(12) Erondu, N.E., and Kennedy, M.B. 1985. Regional distribution of type II Ca^{2+}/calmodulin-dependent protein kinase in rat brain. *J. Neurosci.* 5: 3270-3277.

(13) Gilman, A.G. 1984. G proteins and dual control of adenylate cyclase. *Cell* 36: 577-579.

(14) Grab, D.J.; Carlin, R.K.; and Siekevitz, P. 1981. Function of calmodulin in postsynaptic densities. II. Presence of a calmodulin-activatable protein kinase activity. *J. Cell Biol.* 89: 440-448.

(15) Holz, G.G., IV; Rane, S.G.; and Dunlop, K. 1986. GTP-binding proteins mediate transmitter inhibition of voltage-dependent calcium channels. *Nature* 319: 670-672.

(16) Huganir, R.L., and Greengard, P. 1983. cAMP-dependent protein kinase phosphorylates nicotinic acetylcholine receptor. *Proc. Natl. Acad. Sci.* 80: 1130-1134.

(17) Kandel, E.R.; Abrams, T.; Bernier, L.; Carew, T.J.; Hawkins, R.D.; and Schwartz, J.H. 1983. Classical conditioning and sensitization share aspects of the same molecular cascade in *Aplysia*. *Cold S.H. Quant. Biol.* 48: 821-830.

(18) Kennedy, M.B.; Bennett, M.K.; and Erondu, N.E. 1983. Biochemical and immunochemical evidence that the "major postsynaptic density protein" is a subunit of a calmodulin-dependent protein kinase. *Proc. Natl. Acad. Sci.* 80: 7357-7361.

(19) Kennedy, M.B.; Bennett, M.K.; Erondu, N.E.; and Miller, S.G. 1986. Calcium/calmodulin-dependent protein kinases. *Calcium and Cell Function* 7, in press.

(20) Klee, C.B. 1980. Calmodulin: structure-function relationships. *Calcium and Cell Function* 1: 59-77.

(21) Krebs, E.G., and Beavo, J.A. 1979. Phosphorylation-dephosphorylation of enzymes. *Ann. R. Biochem.* 48: 923-959.

(22) Lee, K.; Schottler, F.; Oliver, M.; and Lynch, G. 1980. Brief bursts of high-frequency stimulation produce two types of structural change in rat hippocampus. *J. Neurophys.* 44: 247-258.

(23) Lisman, J.E. 1985. A mechanism for memory storage insensitive to molecular turnover: a bistable autophosphorylating kinase. *Proc. Natl. Acad. Sci.* 82: 3055-3057.

(24) Llinas, R.; McGuinness, T.L.; Leonard, C.S.; Sugimori, M.; and Greengard, P. 1985. Intraterminal injection of synapsin I or calcium/calmodulin-dependent protein kinase II alters neurotransmitter release at the squid giant synapse. *Proc. Natl. Acad. Sci.* 82: 3035-3039.

(25) Majerus, P.W.; Neufeld, E.J.; and Wilson, D.B. 1984. Production of phosphoinositide-derived messengers. *Cell* 37: 701-703.

(26) Mayer, M.L., and Westbrook, G.L. 1985. Divalent cation permeability of N-methyl-D-aspartate channels. *Soc. Neurosci. Abstr.* 15: 785.

(27) Miller, S.G., and Kennedy, M.B. 1986. Regulation of brain type II Ca^{2+}/calmodulin-dependent protein kinase by autophosphorylation: a Ca^{2+}-triggered molecular switch. *Cell* 44: 861-870.

(28) Nairn, A.C.; Hemmings, H.C.; and Greengard, P. 1985. Protein kinases in the brain. *Ann. R. Biochem.* 54: 931-976.

(29) Nakamura, T., and Ui, M. 1985. Simultaneous inhibitions of inositol phospholipid breakdown, arachidonic acid release, and histamine secretion in mast cells by islet-activating protein, pertussis toxin. *J. Biol. Chem.* 260: 3584-3593.

(30) Nestler, E.J., and Greengard, P. 1984. Protein Phosphorylation in the Nervous System. New York: Wiley.

(31) Nishizuka, Y. 1984. Turnover of inositol phospholipids and signal tranduction. *Science* 225: 1365-1370.

(32) Ocorr, K.A.; Walters, E.T.; and Byrne, J.H. 1985. Associative conditioning analog selectively increases cAMP levels of tail sensory neurons in *Aplysia*. *Proc. Natl. Acad. Sci.* 82: 2548-2552.

(33) Ouimet, C.C.; McGuinness, T.L.; and Greengard, P. 1984. Immunocytochemical localization of calcium/calmodulin-dependent protein kinase II in rat brain. *Proc. Natl. Acad. Sci.* 81: 5604-5608.

(34) Palfrey, H.C.; Rothlein, J.E.; and Greengard, P. 1983. Calmodulin-dependent protein kinase and associated substrates in *Torpedo* electric organ. *J. Biol. Chem.* 258: 9496-9503.

(35) Purves, D., and Hadley, R.D. 1985. Changes in the dendritic branching of adult mammalian neurons revealed by repeated imaging *in situ*. *Nature* 315: 404-406.

(36) Rink, T.J.; Sanchez, A.; and Hallam, T.J. 1983. Diacylglycerol and phorbol ester stimulate secretion without raising cytoplasmic free calcium in human platelets. *Nature* 305: 317-319.

(37) Saitoh, T., and Schwartz, J.H. 1985. Phosphorylation-dependent subcellular translocation of a Ca^{2+}/calmodulin-dependent protein kinase produces an autonomous enzyme in *Aplysia* neurons. *J. Cell Biol.* 100: 835-842.

(38) Siegelbaum, S.A.; Camardo, J.S.; and Kandel, E.R. 1982. Serotonin and cyclic AMP close single K^+ channels in *Aplysia* sensory neurones. *Nature* 299: 413-417.

(39) Siegelbaum, S.A., and Tsien, R.W. 1983. Modulation of gated ion channels as a mode of transmitter action. *Trends Neur.* 6: 307-313.

(40) Sternweis, P.C., and Robishaw, J.D. 1984. Isolation of two proteins with high affinity for guanine nucleotides from membranes of bovine brain. *J. Biol. Chem.* 259: 13806-13813.

(41) Stewart, A.A.; Ingebritsen, T.S.; Manalan, A.; Klee, C.B.; and Cohen, P. 1982. Discovery of a Ca^{2+} and calmodulin-dependent protein phosphatase. *FEBS Lett.* 137: 80-84.

(42) Vallano, M.L.; Goldenring, J.R.; Buckholz, T.M.; Larson, R.E.; and Delorenzo, R.J. 1985. Separation of endogenous calmodulin- and cAMP-dependent kinases from microtubule preparations. *Proc. Natl. Acad. Sci.* 82: 3202-3206.

(43) Walaas, S.I.; Nairn, A.C.; and Greengard, P. 1983. Regional distribution of calcium- and cyclic adenosine 3':5'-monophosphate-regulated protein phosphorylation systems in mammalian brain. I. Particulate systems. *J. Neurosci.* 3.

(44) Walaas, S.I.; Nairn, A.C.; and Greengard, P. 1983. Regional distribution of calcium- and cyclic adenosine 3':5'-monophosphate-regulated protein phorphorylation systems in mammalian brain. II. Soluble systems. *J. Neurosci.* 3: 302-311.

(45) Wallace, M.A., and Fain, J.N. 1985. Guanosine 5'-o-thiotriphosphate stimulates phospholipase C activity in plasma membrane of rat hepatocytes. *J. Biol. Chem.* 260: 9527-9530.

(46) Westcott, K.R.; LaPorte, D.C.; and Storm, D.R. 1979. Resolution of adenylate cyclase sensitive and insensitive to Ca^{2+} and calcium-dependent regulatory protein (CDR) by CDR-sepharose affinity chromatography. *Proc. Natl. Acad. Sci.* 76: 204-208.

(47) Worley, P.F.; Baraban, J.M.; and Snyder, S.H. 1986. Heterogeneous localization of protein kinase C in rat brain: autoradio-

graphic analysis of phorbol ester receptor binding. *J. Neurosci.* 6: 199-207.

(48) Yamauchi, T.; Nakata, H.; and Fujisawa, H. 1981. A new activator protein that activates tryptophan 5-monooxygenase and tyrosine 3-monooxygenase in the presence of Ca^{2+}-, calmodulin-dependent protein kinase. Purification and characterization. *J. Biol. Chem.* 256: 5404-5409.

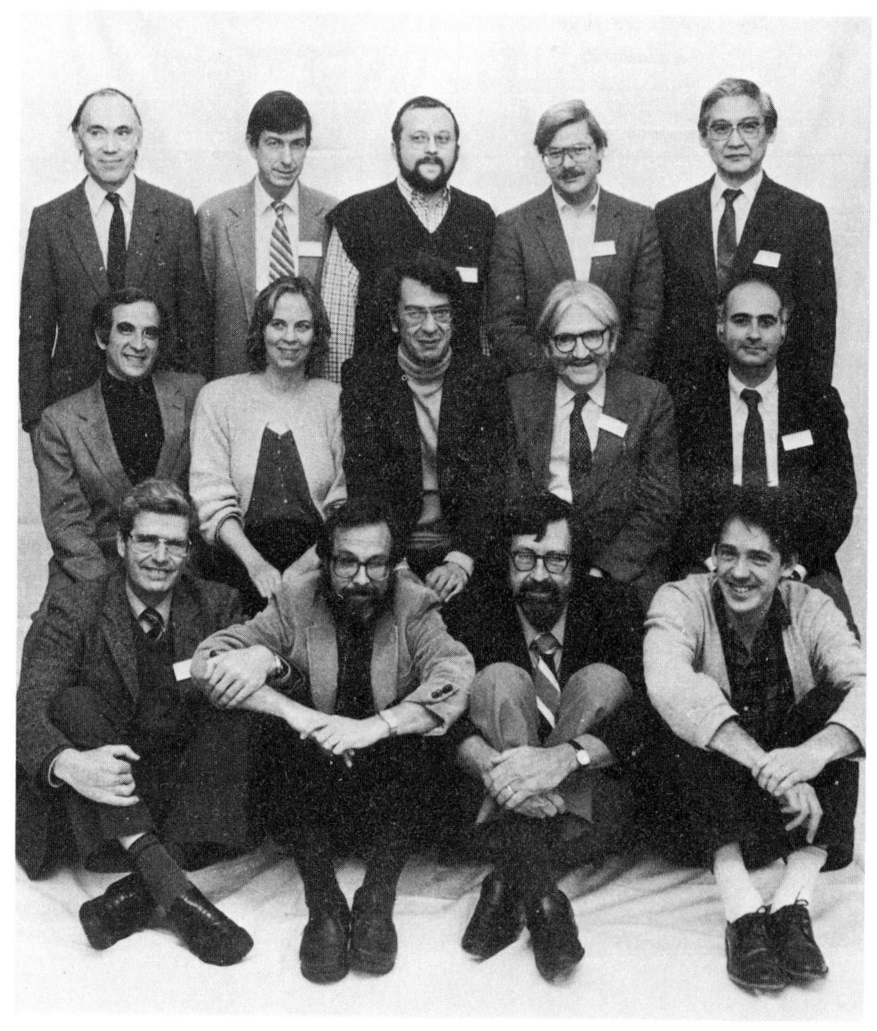

Back row, left to right:
Tim Bliss, Roger Nicoll, Rolf Willmund, Rupert Schmidt, Masao Ito

Middle row, left to right:
Dan Alkon, Mary Kennedy, Michel Baudry, Hersch Gershenfeld, Jack Byrne

Bottom row, left to right:
Per Andersen, Tom Carew, Dick Thompson, Christophe Mulle

The Neural and Molecular Bases of Learning,
eds. J.-P. Changeux and M. Konishi, pp. 153–176.
John Wiley & Sons Limited.

Activity-dependent Regulation of Synaptic Transmission and Its Relationship to Learning
Group Report

M. Baudry, Rapporteur

A.L. Alkon
P.O. Andersen
T.V.P. Bliss
J.H. Byrne
T.J. Carew
H.M. Gerschenfeld
M. Ito
M.B. Kennedy
C. Mulle
R. Nicoll
R. Schmidt
R.F. Thompson
R. Willmund

INTRODUCTION

It is always difficult to evaluate how fast a research field is moving and how much progress has been accomplished since the last review in this field has been written. I could not help, however, but to be struck by a sense of significant progress when I compared the general consensus of our group in the current meeting with the conclusions of the beautiful article by W. Quinn in the previous Dahlem Workshop on The Biology of Learning (54), which was held only two years ago. In our discussions it became clear that the work on *Aplysia* and *Hermissenda* is progressing rapidly and the models derived from these preparations are becoming more and more refined. Moreover, the work with mammalian systems is quickly maturing and the gap between the different so-called simple models is closing at such a fast rate that we are starting to see important points of convergence and divergence. It also seems clear that increased knowledge does not necessarily result in increased complexity (in fact, the greatest discoveries in science are generally revolutionary because they make complex phenomena understandable in relatively simple terms). In this context proof that we are making considerable progress lies in the fact that the different levels of analysis of complex phenomena such as learning and memory (molecular, cellular, neuronal assembly, behavioral levels) are now much closer as a result of the simplifications and generalizations unraveled at every level.

Independent of (and perhaps partially due to) the sometimes animated debate which livened up our discussions, the final conclusions of the group reflected this feeling of convergence and simplifications which, hopefully, is reflected in this report.

DEFINITIONS, SIMPLE MODELS

Because the study of learning evolved from traditional psychology to modern neurobiology, it is often difficult to find an appropriate and unequivocal common language to describe phenomena which relate to behavioral, cellular, and molecular observations. At the current level of our understanding of learning mechanisms it is probably helpful to keep the definition of learning as broad as possible, such as "a change in behavior as a result of experience (excluding damage, disease, or injury)." Experimental psychology has provided a primary subdivision of learning into two main categories: nonassociative and associative learning. The former includes habituation, dishabituation, sensitization, and perhaps some forms of sensory perception learning (such as face recognition), and involves a change in behavior resulting from experiences with *one* kind of stimulus. For example habituation is a decrease in response as a result of repeated experience with one kind of stimulus. Sensitization is an increase in response following (usually strong) stimulation and in most instances dishabituation is simply sensitization and independent of habituation (i.e., if habituation is pronounced, the increased response following sensitization decays back to the habituated level) (64).

Associative learning involves changes in behavior as a result of experiences with *two* kinds of stimuli that have a contingent temporal relationship. In classical or Pavlovian conditioning the conditioned stimulus (CS) is typically (but not always) neutral and precedes the unconditioned stimulus (UCS) which evokes some behavioral response and has reinforcement value, either positive (e.g., food) or negative (e.g., shock). In instrumental or operant learning, presentation of reinforcement (UCS) is made contingent upon the organism's behavior (e.g., pressing a bar to obtain food or avoid shock).

Temporal relationships are critical in associative learning. For both classical and instrumental learning the CS (or emitted behavior) must precede the UCS for learning to occur. Associative learning at its most basic level is learning about cause and effect relationships among stimuli and events in the environment. Backward conditioning (UCS preceding CS presentation) usually does not occur. Visual recognition memory which humans, and to a lesser extent monkeys, do so well is categorized by some workers as associative and by others as nonassociative. Operationally it is inferred from altered responses to a familiar, as opposed to a novel, visual stimulus. Those who view it as associative stress infer that the memory is embedded in, and associated with, existing memory stores, as in an associative network matrix. However, it is important to stress that classical, instrumental, and cognitive associative memory exhibit many similar properties and "laws," i.e., temporal relations, massed vs. spaced practice effects, etc. Thus it is reasonable to consider the possibility that the underlying, neuronal mechanisms of memory storage may be the same in all cases, even though different brain structures and neuronal pathways may be involved.

The simple models which we discussed represent various examples of these different categories of learning. In *Aplysia* two defensive reflexes have been examined in detail: the gill and siphon withdrawal reflex and the tail withdrawal reflex (see Carew, this volume). These behaviors exhibit habituation, sensitization, and associative learning, which have been extensively analyzed on synaptic, biophysical, and molecular levels. In *Hermissenda* light elicits oriented, weakly positive movement and foot lengthening while rotation, a strong aversive stimulus, elicits "clinging" and foot contraction (see Alkon, this volume). In *Hermissenda* paired presentation of light (CS) and rotation of the animal (UCS) produces classical conditioning and its cellular and molecular mechanisms have also been examined in detail. Adaptive modifications of two motor reflexes in mammals were considered: the vestibulo-ocular reflex (VOR) and classical conditioning of the nictitating membrane. Long-term depression (LTD) of the Purkinje cell responses to parallel fiber stimulation was discussed as a potential cellular mechanism underlying this type of adaptation (see Ito and Thompson, both this volume). Long-term potentiation (LTP) of synaptic transmission elicited in various hippocampal pathways by brief bursts of high frequency electrical stimulation was considered as a useful model of activity-dependent changes in synaptic transmission which exhibits associative as well as nonassociative components (see Andersen, this volume).

In all these cases, short-term (minutes) as well as long-term (hours to days or weeks) components have been demonstrated. At this point it should be stressed that the distinction between short term and long term remains relatively arbitrary and does not reflect necessarily the existence of separate mechanisms. It is mainly an operational difference and it is hoped that a better understanding of the underlying mechanisms will permit a more precise definition of these notions (in a few cases there is already some evidence that different molecular mechanisms are responsible for the long-term and short-term effects (see *Aplysia* (50), *Hermissenda* (4,5,6), the differential effects of protein synthesis inhibitors (26,59), and LTP).

CELLULAR MECHANISMS

Although much remains to be discovered concerning the cellular mechanisms underlying the changes in synaptic efficacy in the models discussed above, some general properties and characteristics of these mechanisms are emerging.

Nonassociative Mechanisms

For both habituation and sensitization in *Aplysia* the cellular mechanisms appear to be localized presynaptically and to reflect changes (decrease and increase respectively) in transmitter release resulting in decrease or increase in excitatory postsynaptic potentials (20). Although the precise mechanism underlying habituation is not known, long-term habituation is accompanied by structural changes in the terminals of the neurons exhibiting this phenomenon (decreased number of active zones) (8).

Sensitization is due to the existence of modulatory neurons which act to enhance synaptic transmission between sensory neurons and their target motor neurons. The cellular and molecular mechanisms underlying this enhanced synaptic transmission are well understood and are due to the activation of adenylate cyclase by the facilitatory transmitter, resulting in the stimulation of a cAMP-dependent protein kinase and the phosphorylation of a K^+ channel (S-channel) or of a protein closely associated with this ionic channel(60). This in turn results in the closure of the K^+ channel and in a broader action potential in the sensory neuron leading to a larger Ca^{2+} influx and enhanced transmitter release. Although long-term sensitization has been shown to be accompanied by structural changes opposite to those observed in long-term habituation, the precise molecular mechanisms underlying it are not yet understood. However, recent work using explanted cells in culture seems to indicate that long-term sensitization might require the modification of gene expression and the synthesis of new proteins (50).

Associative Mechanisms

The proposed mechanism for associative leaning in *Aplysia* is activity-dependent enhancement of presynaptic facilitation which is an extension of the cellular mechanism underlying sensitization (32). In this case spike activity in the neurons carrying the CS, and the resulting influx of Ca^{2+} ions, potentiates a calcium-dependent adenylate cyclase which can generate larger levels of cAMP when paired with the UCS than with UCS alone (1). Therefore, more K^+ channels are closed, more Ca^{2+} influx occurs with subsequent test action potentials, and more transmitter is released such that CS alone induces the motor response. In this case the short-term changes reflect the long-lasting (15-30 min) increase in cAMP levels, which have been shown to correlate the changes in behavioral response. The long-term changes are not yet understood, although it has been proposed that protein synthesis is required (50), nor is it known how short-term events trigger the initiation of long-term events.

During acquisition (lasting 1-2 hrs) of classical conditioning in *Hermissenda*, there is prolonged depolarization of the postsynaptic soma compartment (see Alkon, this volume). This depolarization, the result of an integrated response of the visual-vestibular network, accumulates with each paired presentation of the CS and UCS and is accompanied by marked elevation of intracellular Ca^{2+} and reduction of the two K^+ currents, I_A and $I_{Ca^{2+}-K^+}$. During retention (at least 2 days after acquisition) there is no depolarization and no evidence of intracellular Ca^{2+} elevation, but reduction of I_A and $I_{Ca^{2+}-K^+}$ amplitude persists. Furthermore, the rate of K^+ current inactivation is also increased, suggesting that the K^+ channels themselves are modified and not necessarily their density within the soma membrane. The increased sensory cell excitability which results from this K^+ current reduction may account for conditioning-specific differences in the firing of output motor neurons in the visual (CS) pathway. A conditioning-specific biochemical change measured 1-2 hours after acquisition involves a change of Ca^{2+}-dependent phosphorylation of a 20,000 M.W. protein. This and other observations (see Alkon, this volume) suggest that K^+ current reduction is initiated by the pairing of a calcium influx (resulting from CS and UCS presentations) and the resulting activation of a calcium-calmodulin kinase with the activation of the calcium and phospholipid-dependent protein kinase (C-kinase).

Similar biophysical and biochemical mechanisms may contribute to neuronal changes with rabbit conditioning (see Alkon, this volume).

Classical conditioning of the rabbit nictitating membrane produces reduction of post-impulse afterhyperpolarization (AHP) measured in pyramidal cells of hippocampal slices. This AHP reduction, lasting at least 1-2 days and sensitive to C-kinase activation, may be due, at least in part, to modulation of $I_{Ca^{2+}-K^{+}}$ similar to that found for *Hermissenda* conditioning (25).

LTP in the Hippocampus and LTD in the Cerebellum

LTP in the hippocampus represents a long-lasting increase in synaptic efficacy of previously existing excitatory synapses on dendritic spines, while LTD represents a long-lasting depression of transmission from parallel fibers to Purkinje cells as a result of paired activation of parallel and climbing fibers. Local dendritic depolarization appears to be a necessary condition for induction of LTP and LTD (see Andersen, this volume). Coupling in time and space of a sufficient depolarization with activation of synaptic inputs leads to the changes in efficacy of the activated synaptic inputs: enhancement in LTP and decrease in LTD. In both cases there is evidence indicating that influx of Ca^{2+} in the postsynaptic elements plays a critical role for the induction of the changes (see Andersen and Ito, both this volume). In the case of LTP the activation of a voltage- and transmitter-dependent glutamate receptor subtype (the NMDA receptor) seems to provide an amplification mechanism which allows further depolarization and directly or indirectly a larger influx of calcium (22,31). There are also a number of observations suggesting that the activation of protein kinases may play a role in LTP. Long-lasting changes in the phosphorylation of specific proteins have been reported to occur in LTP (3,9,56). It has also been shown that activation of the C-kinase by phorbol esters produces a long-lasting enhancement of synaptic transmission, involving pre- and postsynaptic glutamate mechanisms (53). This is consistent with the observation that activation of the C-kinase stimulates Ca-dependent transmitter release from hippocampal synaptosomes (44). In addition, phorbol esters block a calcium-dependent potassium current and a voltage-dependent chloride current (45). These results suggest that both pre- and postsynaptic mechanisms are involved in the long-term alterations in synaptic efficacy. Increase in transmitter release has been shown to last for several hours after LTP induction. Evidence for postsynaptic changes is provided by the change in the input-output relation reported by several groups (see Andersen, this volume). This means that a given EPSP is able to elicit a spike with greater probability and shorter latency after LTP has been induced. Activation of a calcium-dependent protease (calpain) and the resulting changes in cytoskeletal organization, cell surface receptor distribution, and spine shape have also been proposed to account for the long-term changes in synaptic efficacy (43).

The induction of LTP by repetitive stimulation of afferent fibers requires the stimulus to be above a certain threshold value. This implies that a minimal number of afferent fibers is required (cooperativity) probably operating by reaching a sufficient level of depolarization of the dendrites (see Andersen, this volume). Moreover, it has recently been shown that patterns of stimulation resembling spike discharge patterns of hippocampal neurons in animals in exploratory situations (such as theta rhythm) are optimal to induce LTP (38).

A modulatory role of monoamines mediated by the activation of the cAMP-dependent protein kinase and the resulting reduction of a calcium-dependent K^+ current has been shown to play an important role in LTP (35,46) and is probably best explained by the prolongation of the depolarization induced by the potentiating stimulus.

The precise biochemical and biophysical alterations underlying the long-lasting changes in synaptic efficacy are largely unknown, nor is it known if several forms of LTP can be elicited by the different paradigms of electrical stimulation used by different groups. It is indeed conceivable that in this model variable degrees of pre- and postsynaptic modifications can be achieved, depending on the parameters of electrical stimulation selected. Although LTP has been shown to be irreversible (i.e., no manipulation has been shown to reverse it once established) its duration is also highly variable ranging from several hours in *in vitro* preparations to several weeks in intact animals. Structural changes, such as changes in the number of synaptic contacts and in the shape of dendritic spines, have been reported (21,29,40) but the relationships of these changes to the change in synaptic efficacy are still controversial.

One of the difficulties in attempting to resolve these different experimental results resides in the complex nature of the events elicited by high frequency electrical stimulation. In particular the potentiating stimulus induces a short-term potentiation, generally referred to as post-tetanic (PTP), which lasts 5-15 minutes, superimposed on the development of LTP (see Andersen, this volume). Although PTP and LTP are due to different mechanisms, it was only recently shown that LTP could be elicited in the absence of PTP (66). Thus simultaneous depolarization of the target pyramidal cells by current injection or by glutamate application and weak stimulation of afferent inputs results in

LTP without PTP. Such a paradigm should prove useful in examining the mechanisms underlying LTP.

Also, it was recently shown that the induction of LTP requires the activation of multiple events (37). Using sequential and brief (4 pulses) high frequency trains to two different nonoverlapping sets of inputs, it was found that LTP is observed only in the second sets of synapses and its amplitude is maximal when the interstimulus interval is 200 ms. This suggests that stimulation of the first set of inputs "primes" the target cell, while the stimulation of the second set of inputs triggers the long-lasting changes in synapses which are activated on a "primed neuron." The priming effect requires a delay (ca. 100 ms) and lasts less than 2 seconds (37). A model has been proposed to account for such priming effect (see below).

It should be mentioned that various forms of long-lasting increases in synaptic efficacy, as a result of high-frequency stimulation of afferent fibers, have been reported in peripheral nervous systems as well as in invertebrate preparations. In several of these preparations (13,19,36), though not all (49), the potentiation has been shown to be presynaptically mediated. This strengthens the inherent difficulties in using a single term such as LTP to designate what must obviously reflect multiple cellular mechanisms.

In contrast to LTP, LTD has been discovered rather recently (see Ito, this volume). Technical difficulties make LTD more difficult to analyze than LTP since LTD cannot be studied with the recording of mass field potentials in the cerebellar cortex. LTD can be revealed with unit spike recording or intradendritic recording from Purkinje cells, but it is not an easy task to maintain these recordings stable enough to follow the time course of LTD. The stimulation parameters required for effective induction of LTD in the parallel fibers are critical. Relatively strong stimulation of parallel fibers will activate stellate cells which in turn induce inhibition in Purkinje cell dendrites. The stellate cell inhibition can then prevent the occurrence of LTD, presumably by diminishing the influx of Ca into Purkinje cell dendrites, which normally follows climbing fiber impulses. This complication can be avoided by selecting relatively weak stimuli or by blocking the inhibition by picrotoxin. Finally, stimulation of climbing fibers with too high frequency induces a prolonged silence of Purkinje cell discharge, probably by production of a prolonged membrane hyperpolarization. Low stimulus frequency at 1-4 Hz, which is within the physiological range of climbing fiber discharge, is adequate for driving climbing fibers without such complication. With these precautions, LTD can be reproduced reliably not only *in vivo* but also in *in vitro* slice preparations.

There is still much to investigate about the mechanisms of LTD. Nevertheless, it is now apparent that LTD is caused by the desensitization of quisqualate-specific glutamate receptors in dendritic spines of Purkinje cells as a result of the simultaneous release of the parallel fiber neurotransmitter, presumably L-glutamate, and an increase in Ca concentration inside the spines (see Ito, this volume). Whether Ca ions act directly on glutamate receptors or indirectly through a second messenger process within Purkinje cell dendrites has yet to be determined. If a nucleotide is involved, the most likely candidate is cGMP, as cGMP-dependent protein kinase is specifically high in Purkinje cells (58).

In all these cases it needs to be stressed that the biochemical and biophysical analyses were performed on the cell bodies and not in the terminals or dendrites of the neurons exhibiting the changes in synaptic efficacy. Thus, although it is possible that the alterations measured in the cell body reflect changes directly occuring in the nerve terminals or dendrites, it is conceivable that in some cases the changes are taking place in the cell bodies and may cause changes on the release process because of electrotonic spread. In the case of *Hermissenda*, K^+ current reduction after conditioning was demonstrated in cell bodies which had been isolated by axotomy from all axonal and synaptic membranes. In addition, it has been shown in *Aplysia* that L29, as well as the putative facilitatory serotonergic neurons, projects both on the cell bodies and terminals of the sensory neurons in *Aplysia*, and recent studies using cells in culture indicate that processes and currents in the growth cone are similar to those found in the cell bodies of adult neurons (14).

Common Features

Although much remains to be elucidated in the different models discussed above, it is interesting to extract their general features and common mechanisms. In all cases the observed modifications in synaptic efficacy are the results of changes in preexisting connections. Changes are contingent upon the temporal relationships between various inputs converging on either pre- or postsynaptic common target elements. In most cases they necessitate the conjunction of a spiking activity in one element and the activation of a second messenger system in the common target. In this regard it appears that although several modifiable synapses follow more or less the traditional definition of a Hebb synapse (33), in most cases they rather follow a more general definition of a Hebb synapse in which the conjunction of activity (not necessarily spiking activity) in both elements of the synapse would result in the change in efficacy. The temporal and spatial relationships between two different sets of inputs allow the formation of specific associative elements. Molecular devices integrating various signals provide for the initial aspect of the acquisition process.

MOLECULAR MECHANISMS

Extracellular Signals

So far a variety of neurotransmitters have been shown to mediate the activity-dependent changes in synaptic efficacy (e.g., glutamate, monoamines). In other words, it is the neurotransmitter itself which, as it performs its transmitter function under a "non-learning condition," also initiates the cascade of events that occurs in a "learning condition." Modulators of synaptic efficacy (such as monoamines) might, however, play a sort of general role by their effects on various ionic channels and the resulting changes in cell excitability that they elicit, thus regulating the amplitude of the change in synaptic efficacy. It remains also possible that neuroactive peptides, which could be co-released with traditional neurotransmitters, might play a similar role (34).

Intracellular Signals

Three different second messenger systems have been identified and shown to possess properties ideally suited to represent molecular integrators of multiple input signals. They are ubiquitous in neurons although their relative distributions in various synapses may differ.

The adenylate cyclase system. Several neurotransmitters (biogenic amines in particular) are coupled to adenylate cyclase which catalyzes the production of cAMP (30). This molecule in turn activates a protein kinase by binding to and releasing its regulatory subunit, thus activating the catalytic subunit. As shown in *Aplysia*, such a pathway leads to the phosphorylation of proteins related to a potassium channel (the S-channel) and its closure (60). In addition, recent studies have shown the existence of a calcium-independent and a calcium-dependent form of adenylate cyclase, providing integrative capabilities to this pathway.

The calcium pathway. Calcium ion concentration can be raised intracellularly by several different mechanisms including the opening of voltage-sensitive Ca^{2+} channels, the release of Ca^{2+} from intracellular stores (for instance by inositol-triphosphate, see below), and the influx of calcium through transmitter-gated channels (receptors). Calcium can modulate intracellular biochemistry by at least two different mechanisms:

1. **Activation of calpain.** Two forms of these enzymes have been evidenced in a variety of tissues including brain; a low threshold form is activated by micromolar concentrations of calcium (calpain I) and is present in synaptic membranes while a high threshold form is activated by concentrations of calcium in the range 0.2-0.5 mM (calpain II) which is mainly soluble (52,67). Substrates of these enzymes consist, to a large extent, of the proteins of the cytoskeleton (12), and therefore activation of these enzymes is likely to produce a reorganization of the cytoskeleton and has been shown to participate in stimulus-induced modification of cell shape and cell surface receptor distribution (see (61) for a review).

2. **Activation of calmodulin-dependent enzymes.** Calcium binds to calmodulin and fully activates most of it at calcium concentration of 2-4 μM. Calmodulin, in turn, activates many different enzymes including some forms of adenylate cyclase, a cAMP phosphodiesterase, calmodulin-dependent protein kinases, and calcium-dependent phosphatase. Type II calmodulin-dependent protein kinase is particularly interesting because of its high concentration in hippocampus and cortex where it represents 2% and 1% of total protein respectively ((27) and see Kennnedy, this volume). Although it is present throughout neurons including presynaptic terminals it is concentrated in postsynaptic densities. This kinase phosphorylates synapsin I, a synaptic vesicle protein that may play a role in the regulation of transmitter release. It also phosphorylates myosin light chain and can activate actomyosin contraction. Microtubule-asociated protein II is another substrate and changes in its state of phosphorylation might regulate microtubule polymerization. Type II calmodulin-kinase can be switched into a calcium-independent form by autophosphorylation. Thus once activated by a transient rise in intracellular calcium, an active form of the enzyme could, at least in theory, persist until it is inactivated by phosphatases or by molecular turnover. It has been proposed to participate in changes in synaptic efficacy in *Hermissenda.* Iontophoretic injection of this enzyme was shown to produce the same reduction of I_A and I_{Ca-K} in those neurons which undergo conditioning-specific modification in *Hermissenda* (2, 57).

The phosphatidylinositol-triphosphate pathway. Several neurotransmitters and neuropeptides have been shown to stimulate the hydrolysis of this membrane phospholipid into diacylglycerol and inositol-triphosphate (IP_3) (17). IP_3 diffuses inside the cells and releases calcium from intracellular stores, which thus becomes available for the activation of calcium-dependent enzymes. Diacylglycerol potentiates the activation by calcium of the C-kinase. The C-kinase has been shown to produce increase in calcium-current in *Aplysia* bag neurons and reduction in K+ currents in *Hermissenda* (7) and hippocampal neurons (10, 53) and in Cl currents in hippocampal neurons (45).

All these pathways are thus regulated by multiple signals. In addition, it is clear that they might also regulate similar target proteins, suggesting that the same regulatory processes might be affected by different mechanisms.

Receptor Mechanisms

The rapid progress in the elucidation of receptor structures and functions suggests that, in general, transmitter receptors are regulatory proteins consisting of several subunits with multiple effectors, again providing the expected requirements for integrating multiple signals. A formal model has been proposed which is based on the existence of different states of the receptors (desensitized and active) and on the activity-dependent shift in the equilibrium between these forms (Changeux *et al.*, this volume). The model could account for homosynaptic and heterosynaptic forms of synaptic changes. In particular, the model may account for the LTD observed in the cerebellum. A variant of the model has been proposed to explain some properties of the LTP in the hippocampus. In the latter case, glutamate receptors are supposed to exist in equilibrium between an active and a desensitized state. The priming event induced by the activation of one set of input (or during the initial phase of the activation of a single input) results in the shift of the equilibrium towards the active state, thus increasing the number of receptors in the active state. The executing event elicited by the stimulation of another set of inputs (or by the late phase of the activation of a single input), probably triggered by the large influx of calcium resulting from the activation of the NMDA receptors, is postulated to represent the stabilization of this new equilibrium state mediated by the modification of the membrane interaction with the underlying cytoskeletal structure resulting from the activation of calpain.

It is important to note that the activity-dependent changes in receptor mechanisms applies equally well for receptors coupled to ion channels or for receptors coupled to enzyme activity (adenylate cyclase, PI turnover, etc.).

Transitions from Short-term to Long-term Changes

At the present time, little is known about the mechanisms responsible for the long-term changes in synaptic efficacy observed in various models (except for the cases of *Hermissenda* (6) and *Aplysia* (50) and Carew, this volume) or for the events triggering the long-term changes. Three different types of mechanisms have been proposed to account for the long-term maintenance of modification occuring during the "acquisition procedure."

Covalent modifications of preexisting proteins. This type of modification, although accounting for durable modifications of the functions of key proteins, is not sufficient to explain the formation of very long-lasting or permanent traces of experience in view of the normally occuring protein turnover.

Self-sustaining mechanisms. A model suggesting the triggering by the initial set of events of a positive feedback mechanism maintaining the initial modification has been proposed by various authors ((23, 24, 41) and Changeux *et al.*, this volume). In this regard it is interesting to mention that the autophosphorylation of the type II calmodulin kinase could be viewed as such a self-perpetuating mechanism (Kennedy, this volume).

Change in genomic expression. The initial set of events triggers a modification of gene expression, and the newly synthesized proteins could be directed to the appropriate location (terminals, dendrites) by some type of signaling device. Evidence for such a mechanism has been presented in the long-term changes in synaptic transmission observed in *Aplysia* neurons in cultures (50).

RELATIONSHIPS OF SIMPLE MODELS TO LEARNING AND MEMORY

Invertebrate Preparations

The use of animal preparations with comparatively few neurons has successfully provided the possibility of relating cellular and molecular processes to learning and memory. In *Aplysia*, neural changes (decrease or increase in EPSP) have been directly related both to nonassociative behavioral changes in habituation and sensitization and associative changes in classical conditioning in intact animal (see Carew, this volume). With *Hermissenda*, neural changes (reduction of K^+ currents) have been directly related to retention of associative behavioral changes in intact animals. Moreover, in this latter case the cellular changes were also shown to be sufficient to produce the learning change (28).

When type B photoreceptors were impaled in living organisms, and the K+ current reduction was produced by pairing current injection with light, the behavioral change elicited by presentation of light alone could be measured in days after this manipulation. Thus, in *Hermissenda* at least, it seems that the cellular and biophysical changes proposed by the model are sufficient to account for the behavioral changes.

LTP and LTD

Several lines of evidence suggest that LTP is involved in behavioral learning and memory. In classical conditioning (e.g., of the nictitating membrane (NM) response), pyramidal neurons rapidly increase their frequency of discharges within trials, beginning in the first few trials, and form a predicting "temporal model" of the learned behavioral response (16). When the population spike of dentate granule cells to perforant path stimulation is monitored over the course of learning, it shows an increase that closely parallels the development of the learned behavioral response and persists in time (65). Although the hippocampus is not essential for basic associative learning (e.g., NM conditioning), it becomes essential when greater demands are placed on the memory system, as in discrimination reversal of NM conditioning. However, it has recently been found that if LTP of the perforant path is induced in rabbits, subsequent acquisition of simple NM conditioning is accelerated (15). This result is in apparent contradiction with a similar study in rats, where after maximal potentiation of the perforant path, performance was significantly impaired in a spatial learning task (11).

Recent experiments have taken advantage of the selective blockade of LTP by the NMDA antagonist, aminophosphonovaleric acid (AP-5)(51). Rats receiving a continuous intraventricular perfusion of the drug were tested for their ability to learn a spatial escape task in a swimming pool, a task which has been shown to be severely disrupted by hippocampal lesions. Rats with AP-5 learned the task although their performance was always poorer than control rats. A marked deficit was evidenced when the task was modified to test how much information concerning the spatial location of the escape platform was stored. It is important to stress that under the same conditions rats did not have any problem in learning visual discrimination, excluding the possibility that the drug exerts toxic or damaging nonspecific effects.

Trains of high-frequency stimuli to the perforant path have been used as a CS in a shuttle box paradigm. A correlation was found between development of LTP and learning performance (55). A similar result has been noted in the olfactory system (62). Two-odor smell discrimination can be mimicked by electrical stimulation in two different regions of the olfactory bulb. The patterns of stimulation which produce behavioral learning also cause LTP of responses evoked in the pyriform cortex by single shocks to the olfactory bulb.

Additional correlative evidence pointing to a behavioral role for LTP comes from experiments by Bloch and Laroche (18). Post-trial stimulation of the mesencephalic reticular formation facilitates several forms of learning. Similar stimulation given after a high-frequency train to the perforant path in chronically implanted rats enhances both the degree and the duration of LTP.

In the case of LTD, several lines of evidence also indicate that this cellular change can account for adaptive properties of motor responses. It has now been fairly clearly demonstrated that the LTD in the cerebellum can fully account for the adaptation of the VOR (Ito, this volume). The cerebellar flocculus is inserted in the pathway for this reflex as a modifiable sidepath. LTD will be induced within the flocculus when it is reached by climbing fiber signals representing retinal errors due to inadequate performance of the VOR in conjunction with signals of parallel fibers driven by vestibular mossy fiber signals. The LTD thus induced would have an action such as cutting off wrong wiring responsible for inadequate VOR performance, so that the VOR performance will be improved adaptively. Other current evidence (47,63) demonstrates that the cerebellum is essential for learning and memory of discrete behavioral responses performed to deal with aversive events (e.g., eyelid response, leg-flexion response) and argues strongly that the memory traces are formed in the cerebellum. Normal behavioral learning develops when the CS is electrical microstimulation of the mossy fibers and the UCS is electrical microstimulation of the dorsal accessory olive-climbing fibers (co-stimulation of these same systems, mossy and climbing fibers, produces LTD in decerebrate rabbits or cerebellar slices). In addition, responses of identified Purkinje cells to a tone CS before training seem invariably to exhibit an evoked increase in frequency of discharges. After training, Purkinje cells often show a decreased frequency of discharge within trials that can precede the behavioral conditioned response (CR) by as much as 60 ms or more and predict the form of the learned behavioral response. All these results are at least consistent with a mechanisms such as LTD.

CONCLUSIONS

From Behavior to Molecular Mechanisms

It is fortunate that the search for the molecular mechanisms of learning of specific behavioral tasks or causal relationships is guided and restricted by several constraints. First, anatomical considerations will impose the network in which the learning has to occur and help define the site(s) of convergence (or divergence) of the input signals. Although far from being simple and obvious these considerations have proved to be successfully met in both invertebrate and vertebrate preparations. This will certainly be more difficult for the higher forms of learning, such as found in humans, in view of our limited knowledge and understanding of cortical circuitries. No doubt that the elaboration of models of cortical networks will provide a set of guidelines amenable for experimental testing (42).

The studies of simple models have provided a series of potential cellular and molecular mechanisms which possess enough common features to predict that there are a finite number of biochemical mechanisms which possess the appropriate integrative and adaptive properties required to account for activity-dependent changes in synaptic efficacy. Again improved neuroanatomical techniques might provide maps of the different biochemical mechanisms in different circuitries and brain regions and might permit one to make useful predictions concerning the roles of the different mechanisms in different forms of learning. Second, temporal considerations impose further constraints on the cellular mechanisms involved in the acquisition of causal relationships. Indeed a key question is the extent to which such mechanisms embedded in learning networks in the brain can result in the features characteristic of mammalian learning. To mention only one example here, the most critical and powerful variable in associative learning is time – the CS-UCS onset interval. For discrete stimulus-response learning (i.e., skeletal muscle responses), no learning occurs with backward (UCS first) or simultaneous onset or in fact until the CS precedes the UCS by nearly 100 ms. Learning is best with intervals from 200 to 400 ms and decreases as the interval is lengthened further. In terms of current models, the *Aplysia* system seems to follow this function remarkably well and this seems also to be the case for *Hermissenda* (39). It is not yet clear how LTP and LTD could satisfy this function although the newly described paradigm to obtain LTP also seems to follow this temporal specifity. At the molecular level, it is well known that concerted transitions between states of a molecular system also have embedded in the molecular structure temporal and orderly constraints of interactions of the various effectors (e.g., rates of transition between states, orderly interaction between effectors). These constraints, together with the time delays imposed by the particular networks, must predict the temporal relationships observed at the behavioral level.

There is another aspect of mammalian learning that none of the models and mechanisms under consideration have yet addressed in any obvious way: the control of the temporal properties of the learned response by the CS-UCS interval. At the beginning of learning the CR first appears at about the time of the UCR in CS alone trials. A well learned response has a minimum onset latency of about 10 ms but the maximum amplitude of the learned response has a latency that corresponds closely to the CS-UCS onset interval. In other words, whatever CS-UCS interval is used for training, the learned response is maximal at the time of onset of the UCS. In the case of an aversive UCS, the learned defensive response (eyeblink, limb flexion) is thus most adaptive. It is again hoped that a better knowledge of the cellular mechanisms and circuitries underlying the recall of the learned response will provide answers to this crucial question.

From Molecular Mechanisms to Behavior

Independent of the intrinsic values of understanding what represents one of the greatest challenges to humanity, i.e., understanding the nature and mechanisms of human cognitive processes, it is hoped that this knowledge will provide a variety of tools to manipulate learning processes. We already have drugs which affect more or less selectively various forms of learning. In general, it seems to be easier to prevent the storage of information than to improve it, although manipulations of the catecholaminergic systems have proven effective in some cases (48). A better knowledge of the roles of different modulators and various effector molecules might provide the ability to selectively improve certain forms of learning. Conceivably it might be possible in some distant future to apply this knowledge to improve the conditions of severely learning-impaired humans. Finally, we might also prepare ourselves to face machines built according to principles derived from this knowledge and with learning capabilities matching or even surpassing our own.

REFERENCES

(1) Abrams, T.W.; Bernier, L.; Hawkins, R.D.; and Kandel, E.R. 1984. Possible role of Ca^{++} and cAMP in activity-dependent

facilitation, a mechanism for associative learning in *Aplysia*. *Soc. Neurosci. Abstr.* 10: 269.

(2) Acosta-Urquidi, J.; Alkon, D.L.; and Neary, J.T. 1984. Ca^{2+}-dependent protein kinase injection in a photoreceptor mimics biophysical effects of associative learning. *Science* 224: 1254-1257.

(3) Akers, R.F., and Routtenberg, A. 1985. Protein kinase C phosphorylates a 47 M_r protein (F_1) directly related to synaptic plasticity. *Brain Res.* 334: 147-151.

(4) Alkon, D.L. 1980. Membrane depolarization accumulates during acquisition of an associative behavioral change. *Science* 210: 1375-1376.

(5) Alkon, D.L.; Kubota, M.; Neary, J.T.; Naito, S.; Coulter, D.; and Rasmussen, H. 1986. C-Kinase activation prolongs Ca^{2+}-dependent inactivation of K^+ currents. *Biochem. Biophys. Res. Comm.* 134: 1245-1253.

(6) Alkon, D.L.; Lederhendler, I.; and Shoukimas, J.J. 1982. Primary changes of membrane currents during retention of associative learning. *Science* 215: 693-695.

(7) Alkon, D.L.; Sakakibara, M.; Forman, R.; Harrigan, J.; Lederhendler, I.; and Farley, J. 1985. Reduction of two voltage-dependent K^+ currents mediates retention of a learned association. *Behav. Neural Biol.* 44: 278-300.

(8) Bailey, C.H., and Chen, M. 1983. Morphological basis of long-term habituation and sensitization in *Aplysia*. *Science* 220: 91-93.

(9) Bar, P.R.; Schotman, P.; Gispen, W.H.; Tielen, A.M.; and Lopes da Silva, F.H. 1980. Changes in synaptic membrane phosphorylation after tetanic stimulation in the dentate area of the rat hippocampal slice. *Brain Res.* 198: 478-484.

(10) Baraban, J.M.; Snyder, S.H.; and Alger, B.E. 1985. Protein kinase C regulates ionic conductance in hippocampal pyramidal neurons: electrophysiological effect of phorbol esters. *Proc. Natl. Acad. Sci.* 82: 2538-2542.

(11) Barnes, C.A., and McNaughton, B.C. 1985. Spatial information: how and where is it stored? In *Memory Systems of the Brain*, eds. N.M. Weinberger, J.L. McGaugh, and G. Lynch, pp. 49-61. New York: The Guilford Press.

(12) Baudry, M.; Simonson, L.; Dubrin, R.; and Lynch, G. 1986. A comparative study of soluble calcium-dependent proteolytic activity in vertebrate brain. *J. Neurobiol.* 17: 1, 15-28.

(13) Baxter, D.A.; Bittner, G.D.; and Brown, T.H. 1985. Quantal mechanism of long-term synaptic potentiation. *Proc. Natl. Acad. Sci.* 82: 5978-5982.

(14) Belardetti, F.; Schacher, S.; Kandel, E.R.; and Siegelbaum, S.A. 1985. Serotonin produces a decreased conductance EPSP and broadening of the action potential in growth cones of *Aplysia* sensory neurons. *Soc. Neurosci. Abstr.* **11**: 28.

(15) Berger, T.W. 1984. Long-term potentiation of hippocampal synaptic transmission affects rate of behavioral learning. *Science* 224: 627-632.

(16) Berger, T.W., and Thompson, R.F. 1978. Identification of pyramidal cells as the critical elements in hippocampal neuronal plasticity during learning. *Proc. Natl. Acad. Sci.* 75: 1572-1576.

(17) Berridge, M.J., and Irvine, R.F. 1984. Inositol triphosphate, a novel second messenger in cellular signal transduction. *Nature* 321: 315-321.

(18) Bloch, V., and Laroche, S. 1985. Enhancement of long-term potentiation in the rat dentate gyrus by post-trial stimulation of the reticular formation. *J. Physl.* 360: 215-231.

(19) Brown, T.H., and McAfee, D.A. 1982. Long-term synaptic potentiation in the superior cervical ganglion. *Science* 215: 1411-1413.

(20) Castelluci, V.F., and Kandel, E.R. 1976. Presynaptic facilitation as a mechanism for behavioral sensitization in *Aplysia*. *Science* 194: 1176-1178.

(21) Chang, F.L.F., and Greenough, W.T. 1984. Transient and enduring morphological correlates of synaptic activity and efficacy change in the rat hippocampal slice. *Brain Res.* 309: 35-46.

(22) Collingridge, G.L.; Kehl, S.J.; and McLennan, H. 1983. Excitatory amino acids in synaptic transmission in the Schaffer-collateral-commissural pathway of the rat hippocampus. *J. Physl.* 334: 33-46

(23) Crabtree, B. 1985. A metabolic switch produced by enzymically interconvertible forms of an enzyme. *FEBS Letter* 185: 193-195.

(24) Crick, F. 1984. Memory and molecular turn-over. *Nature* 312: 101.

(25) Disterhoft, J.F.; Coulter, D.A.; and Alkon, D.L. 1986. Conditioning-specific membrane changes of rabbit hippocampal neurons measured *in vitro*. *Proc. Natl. Acad. Sci.* 83, in press.

(26) Dunn, A.J. 1980. Neurochemistry of learning and of memory: an evaluation of recent data *Ann. R. Psych.* 31: 343-390.

(27) Erondu, N.E., and Kennedy, M.B. 1984. Regional distribution of type II Ca^{2+}/calmodulin-dependent protein kinase in rat brain. *J. Neurosci.* 5: 3270-3277.

(28) Farley, J.; Richards, W.G.; Ling, L.; Liman, E.; and Alkon, D.L. 1983. Membrane changes in a single photoreceptor cause associative learning in *Hermissenda*. *Science* 221: 1201-1203.

(29) Fifkova, E., and Van Harreveld, A. 1975. Long-lasting morphological changes in dendritic spines of dentate granular cells following stimulation of the entorhinal area. *J. Neurocyt.* 6: 211-230.

(30) Greengard, P. 1981. Intracellular signals in the brain. *Harvey Lect.* 75: 277-331.

(31) Harris, E.W.; Ganong, A.H.; and Cotman, C.W. 1984. Long-term potentiation in the hippocampus involves activation of N-methyl-D-aspartate receptors. *Brain. Res.* 323: 132-137.

(32) Hawkins, R.D.; Abrams, T.W.; Carew, T.J.; and Kandel, E.R. 1983. A cellular mechanism of classical conditioning in *Aplysia*: activity-dependent amplification of presynaptic facilitation. *Science* 219: 400-405.

(33) Hebb, D.O. 1949. The Organization of Behavior. New York: Wiley.

(34) Hokfelt, T.; Johansson, O.; and Goldstein, M. 1984. Chemical anatomy of the brain. *Science* 225: 1326-1334.

(35) Hopkins, W.F., and Johnston, D. 1984. Frequency-dependent noradrenergic modulation of long-term potentiation in the hippocampus. *Science* 226: 350-352.

(36) Koyano, K.; Kuba, K; and Minota, S. 1985. Long-term potentiation of transmitter release induced by repetitive presynaptic activities in bull-frog sympathetic ganglia. *J. Physl.* 359: 219-233.

(37) Larson, J., and Lynch G. 1986. Induction of synaptic potentiation in hippocampus by patterned stimulation involves two events. *Science* 232: 985-988.

(38) Larson, J.; Wong, D.; and Lynch, G. 1986. Patterned stimulation at the theta frequency is optimal for the induction of hippocampal long-term potentiation. *Brain Res.* 368: 347-350.

(39) Lederhendler, I., and Alkon, D.L. 1986. An optimal, temporally specific, CS-US interval for conditioning in *Hermissenda*. *Soc. Neurosci. Abstr.*, in press.

(40) Lee, K.; Schottler, F.; Oliver, M.; and Lynch, G. 1980. Brief bursts of high-frequency stimulation produce two types of structural change in rat hippocampus. *J. Neurophysl.* 44: 247-258.

(41) Lisman, J.E. 1985. A mechanism for memory storage insensitive to molecular turn-over: a bistable autophosphorylating kinase. *Proc. Natl. Acad. Sci.* 82: 3055-3057.

(42) Lynch, G. 1986. Synapses, Circuits and the Beginnings of Memory. Cambridge, MA: MIT Press.

(43) Lynch, G., and Baudry, M. 1984. The biochemistry of memory: a new and specific hypothesis. *Science* 224: 1057-1063.

(44) Lynch, M.A., and Bliss, T.V.P. 1986. Calmodulin and a diacylglycerol analogue enhance release of preloaded glutamate from normal but not potentiated hippocampus. Abstract for XXX Congress of International Union of Physiological Sciences, in press.

(45) Madison, D.V.; Malenka, R.C.; and Nicoll, R.A. 1986. A voltage-dependent chloride current in hippocampal pyramidal cells is blocked by phorbol esters. *Biophys. J.* 49: 412a..

(46) Madison, D.V., and Nicoll, R.A. 1982. Noradrenaline blocks accommodation of pyrammidal cell discharge in the hippocampus. *Nature* 299: 636-678.

(47) McCormick, D.A., and Thompson, R.F. 1984. Cerebellum: essential involvement in the classically conditioned eyelid response. *Science* 223: 296-299.

(48) McGaugh, J.L.; Martinez, J.L.; Jensen, R.A.; Hannan, T.J.; Vasquez, B.J.; Messing, R.B.; Liang, K.C.; Brenton, C.B.; and Spiehler, V.R. 1982. Modulation of memory storage by treatments affecting peripheral catecholamines. In *Neuronal Plasticity and Memory Formation*, eds. C. Marsan Ajmone and H. Matthies, pp. 311-326. New York: Raven Prėss.

(49) Mochida, S., and Libet, B. 1985. Synaptic long-term enhancement (LTE) induced by a heterosynaptic neural input. *Brain Res.* 329: 360-363.

(50) Montarolo, P.G.; Castelluci, V.F.; Goelet, P.; Kandel, E.R.; and Schacher, S. 1985. Long-term facilitation of the monosynaptic connection between sensory neurons and motor neurons of the gill withdrawal reflex in *Aplysia* in dissociated cell culture. *Soc. Neurosci. Abstr.* 11: 975.

(51) Morris, R.G.M.; Anderson, E.; Lynch, G.; and Baudry, M. 1986. Selective impairment of learning and blockade of long-term potentiation by an N-methyl-D-aspartate receptor antagonist, AP5. *Nature* 319: 774-776.

(52) Murachi, T.; Tanaka, U.; Hatanaka, M.; and Murakami, T. 1981. Intracellular Ca^{++}-dependent protease (calpain) and its high-molecular weight endogenous inhibitor (calpastatin). *Adv. Enzyme Reg.* 19: 407-424.

(53) Nicoll, R.A.; Madison, D.V.; Malenka, R.C.; and Andrade, D. 1985. Actions of phorbol esters on synaptic transmission and membrane currents in hippocampal CA_1 pyramidal neurons. *Neuroscience Abstr.* 11: 150.

(54) Quinn, W.G. 1984. Work in invertebrates on the mechanisms underlying learning. In *The Biology of Learning*, eds. P. Marler and H.S. Terrace, pp. 197-246. Dahlem Konferenzen. Berlin, Heidelberg, New York, Tokyo: Springer-Verlag.

(55) Reymann, K.G.; Ruthrich, H.; Lindenau, L.; Ott, T.; and Matthies H.J. 1982. Monosynaptic activation of the hippocampus as a conditioned stimulus: behavioral effects. *Physl. Behav.* 29: 1007-1012.

(56) Routtenberg, A., and Lovinger, D.M. 1985. Selective increase in phosphorylation of a 47-kDa protein (F_1) directly related to long-term potentiation. *Behav. Neural Biol.* 43: 3-11.

(57) Sakakibara, M.; Alkon, D.L.; DeLorenzo, R.; Goldenring, J.R.; Neary, J.T.; and Heldman, E. 1986. Modulation of calcium-mediated inactivation of ionic currents by Ca^{2+}/calmodulin-dependent protein kinase II. *Biophys. J.*, in press.

(58) Schlichter, D.J.; Detre, J.A.; Aswad, D.W.; Chehrazi, B.; and Greengard, P. 1980. Localization of cyclic GMP-dependent protein kinase and substrate in mammalian cerebellum. *Proc. Natl. Acad. Sci.* 77: 5537-5541.

(59) Shashousa, V.E., and Schmidt, R. 1986. Learning and memory: neurochemical aspects. In *Encyclopedia of Neuroscience*, ed. G. Adelman. Boston: Birkhauser, in press.

(60) Siegelbaum, S.A.; Camardo, J.S.; and Kandel, E.R. 1982. Serotonin and cyclic AMP close single K^+ channels in *Aplysia* sensory neurons. *Nature* 299: 413-417.

(61) Siman, R.; Baudry, M.; and Lynch, G. 1986. Calcium-activated proteases as possible mediators of synaptic plasticity. In *New Insights into Synaptic Function*, eds. G.M. Edelman, W.M. Cowan, and W.E. Gall. New York: John Wiley, in press.

(62) Staubli, U.; Roman, F.; and Lynch, G. 1985. Selective changes in synaptic responses elicited in a cortical network by behaviorally relevant electrical stimulation. *Neuroscience Abstr.* 11: 837.

(63) Thompson, R.F.; McCormick, D.A.; and Lavond, D.G. 1986. Localization of the essential memory trace system for a basic form of associative learning in the mammalian brain. In *One Hundred Years of Psychological Research in America*, eds. S.H. Hulse and B.F. Green, pp. 125-171. Baltimore: John Hopkins University Press.

(64) Thompson, R.F., and Spencer, W.A. 1966. Habituation: a model phenomenon for the study of neuronal substrates of behavior. *Psychol. Rev.* 173:16-43.

(65) Weisz, D.J.; Clark, T.W.; and Thompson, R.F. 1984. Increased activity of dentate granule cells during nictitating membrane response conditioning in rabbits. *Beh. Brain Res.* 12: 145-154.

(66) Wigstrom, H.; Gustafsson, B.; Huang, Y.Y.; and Abraham, W.C. 1986. Hippocampal long-lasting potentiation is induced by pairing single afferent volleys with intracellularly injected depolarizing current pulses. *Acta Physl.* 126: 317-319.

(67) Zimmerman, U.J.P., and Schlaepfer, W.W. 1984. Calcium-activated neutral protease (CANP) in brain and other tissues. *Prog. Neurobiol.* 23: 63-78.

The Neural and Molecular Bases of Learning,
eds. J.-P. Changeux and M. Konishi, pp. 177–204.
John Wiley & Sons Limited.

Cellular and Molecular Advances in the Study of Learning in *Aplysia*

T.J. Carew

Depts. of Psychology and Biology
Yale University
New Haven, CT 06520, USA

Abstract. A tantalizing goal in the study of learning and memory is to directly relate specific molecular changes in the brain to changes in behavior. To even begin to approach this goal first requires preparations that exhibit clear instances of learning. Moreover, the learning should be mediated by a neural circuit that is tractable for cellular investigation. Finally, the elements in the neural circuit that are involved in the learning should be accessible for biochemical analysis. These requirements of course constitute a tall order. However, in recent years several preparations, most of them invertebrate animals, have been developed that meet these requirements (20) and thus these preparations hold considerable promise for molecular approaches to the analysis of learning. In addition, three invertebrate preparations not only hold promise, they have, at least to a limited degree, already delivered. These are the fruit fly *Drosophila* in which a neurogenetic approach has yielded important molecular insights (34, 78), the nudibranch mollusc *Hermissenda*, in which extensive biophysical and biochemical studies of learning have been carried out ((5, 6) and Alkon, this volume), and the marine mollusc *Aplysia*. The purpose of this review is to describe recent developments in cellular and molecular approaches to learning in *Aplysia*.

INTRODUCTION

Aplysia californica is a marine mollusc that has been proven to be an excellent preparation for studying the role that identified nerve cells play in a variety of different behaviors, ranging from elementary reflexes to complex fixed action patterns (48). In addition, many of these behaviors have been shown to be capable of modification by a variety of different forms of learning, ranging in complexity from simple nonassociative forms to more complex forms of associative conditioning.

NONASSOCIATIVE LEARNING

Two forms of nonassociative learning, habituation and sensitization, have been extensively studied in *Aplysia*. Habituation refers to the decrement of a behavioral response that is repeatedly elicited by a mild stimulus, while sensitization refers to an increase in a behavioral response following presentation of a second, novel or noxious stimulus. My goal in this part of the chapter is to provide a brief overview of the analysis of habituation and sensitization in *Aplysia*. Several more detailed reviews have recently been published (for example, see (49,51)).

Many response systems in *Aplysia* exhibit habituation and sensitization. These include the gill and siphon withdrawal reflex (76), the tail withdrawal reflex ((92), see below), inking (17), escape locomotion (93), and the feeding system (60). I will restrict my discussion to studies of the gill and siphon withdrawal reflex as this has been most extensively analyzed.

Behavioral Studies of Habituation and Sensitization

Because of its simplicity and relatively well-delineated neural circuit, the behavior that has received the most experimental attention in *Aplysia* has been the defensive withdrawal reflex of the mantle organs (the gill, siphon, and mantle shelf). This reflex can be elicited by a light tactile stimulus to the siphon which evokes a brisk withdrawal of these organs into the mantle cavity. If the same stimulus is repeatedly delivered, the reflex readily habituates and remains decremented for several minutes to a few hours. However, reflex amplitude can be immediately restored by delivering a strong sensitizing stimulus to another site on the body, such as the head or tail, which produces dishabituation. Dishabituation appears to be simply a specialized case of a more general facilitatory process, sensitization (14). Both habituation and sensitization can be transformed into a long-term form lasting weeks by giving repeated training sessions over several days (18, 75).

Cellular Studies of Habituation and Sensitization

One of the principle advantages of simple systems is that they permit a multilevel analysis of questions of behavioral relevance. The investigation of habituation and sensitization of the gill withdrawal reflex in *Aplysia* has been carried out on three progressively more fundamental levels: synaptic, biophysical, and molecular.

Synaptic analysis. The neural circuit for the gill and siphon withdrawal reflex has been extensively studied and is relatively well understood. It consists of a small population of about 24 identified primary afferent neurons, siphon mechanoreceptors, which make monosynaptic excitatory connections onto identified gill and siphon motor neurons as well as several interneurons. Several lines of evidence indicate that habituation and sensitization are due in large part to homosynaptic depression and heterosynaptic facilitation, respectively, at the synapses from the siphon sensory neurons onto their targets (12, 28). Moreover, a quantal analysis of the sensory neuron synapses during habituation and sensitization showed that both of these processes are presynaptic in origin (24, 25). In addition to short-term changes, these same synaptic connections have been shown to be chronically depressed or enhanced in animals receiving long-term habituation or sensitization training (23, 36). Quite recently, Montarolo and colleagues (64) have found that long-term facilitation of these synaptic connections can be produced by repeated application of serotonin (see below) in dissociated cell culture, and this facilitation is blocked by the protein synthesis inhibitor anisomycin, suggesting that long-term memory at these synapses may involve protein synthesis. Finally, an important anatomical correlate of these observations has been discovered by Bailey and Chen (7) who found that the number of active zones (synaptic release sites) in the sensory neuron terminals are significantly reduced in long-term habituated animals and significantly increased in long-term sensitized animals. Thus these simple forms of learning produce profound ultrastructural as well as functional alterations of the sensory neuron synapses of the gill withdrawal reflex.

Biophysical Analysis. To analyze the ionic currents modulated in the sensory neurons during short-term habituation and sensitization, Klein and Kandel (55, 56) examined the duration of the sensory neuron action potential and found that it was reduced in duration during repeated activation and dramatically prolonged during heterosynaptic facilitation. Accompanying these alterations in spike duration, synaptic transmission was also reduced or enhanced. Voltage clamp studies showed that repeated activation of the sensory neurons was accompanied by a progressive decrease in a voltage-sensitive inward Ca^{2+} current (57). Recent quantitative simulation studies by Gingrich and Byrne (37) suggest however, that Ca^{2+} inactivation may not fully account for habituation and that depletion of neurotransmitter may also play a significant role. Klein and Kandel (56) further found that heterosynaptic facilitation (which underlies sensitization) was produced by a decrease in an outward K^+ current which prolonged the depolarization of the spike and thus enhanced the voltage-sensitive Ca^{2+} current, which in turn enhanced synaptic release. In addition to modulation of Ca^{2+} due to changes in duration of the action potential, a component of Ca^{2+} accumulation independent of spike shape has recently been identified. Boyle *et al.* (11) injected sensory neuron cell bodies with the Ca^{2+}-sensitive dye arsenazo III and found that serotonin enhanced free Ca^{2+} accumulation in response to constant-duration voltage clamp depolarizations, indicating that the Ca^{2+} changes were mediated by some intrinsic change in the handling of Ca^{2+} by the sensory neurons. This intrinsic enhancement of Ca^{2+} accumulation is thought to act synergistically with the reduction in K^+ current to enhance transmitter release. Consistent with this observation, Gingrich and Byrne (37) suggest that in addition to spike broadening, transmitter mobilization may also contribute to heterosynaptic facilitation, a suggestion supported by recent work reported by Hochner and co-workers ((45), see below).

Several lines of evidence suggest that serotonin is one of the facilitating transmitters in *Aplysia*. Immunocytochemical studies indicate that serotonin terminals contact the sensory neurons (53). Moreover, serotonin mimics heterosynaptic facilitation by broadening the action potential, decreasing a K^+ conductance, and enhancing synaptic release from the sensory neurons (55, 56). Recently, it has been shown that similar spike broadening and decreases in conductance in response to serotonin occurs in growth cones of sensory neurons (9) suggesting that spike broadening and an increase in excitability occurs at sensory neuron terminals and contributes to presynaptic facilitation. A voltage clamp analysis of the sensory neurons showed that the K^+ current modulated by serotonin differs from previously described K^+ currents (the delayed K^+, fast K^+, Ca^{2+}-dependent K^+, and muscarine-sensitive K^+) (54). A patch clamp analysis by Siegelbaum and colleagues further characterized the serotonin-sensitive K^+ channel (the "S" channel) in the sensory neurons: it is active at the resting potential, is moderately voltage-dependent and is independent of intracellular Ca^{2+}. Closure of this channel can account for increases in spike duration and Ca^{2+} influx as well as enhanced transmitter release responsible for sensitization (84). Finally, Hochner and co-workers (45) have recently provided evidence in voltage clamped sensory cells in cell culture that serotonin induces presynaptic facilitation by two mechanisms: 1) by closure of S-channels as described above (this predominates when transmitter release is not depressed); and 2) by mobilization of transmitter (which predominates when the synapse is in a depressed state). It is thought that this transmitter mobilization might be related to serotonin modulation of Ca^{2+} handling by the sensory neurons.

Molecular Analysis. At a molecular level most progress has been made in the analysis of short-term sensitization. Based on several independent lines of evidence (for review see (51)) Klein and Kandel (56) proposed a molecular model for sensitization which postulated that serotonin increases adenylate cyclase activity in sensory neuron terminals, thereby increasing intracellular cyclic adenosine monophosphate (cAMP). cAMP in turn stimulates the activity of enzymes (protein phosphokinases) responsible for phosphorylating substrate proteins, one of which is the K^+ channel or a protein closely associated with it. Phosphorylation of the K^+ channel closes it, giving rise to increased duration of the spike, more Ca^{2+} influx and thus more transmitter release. Consistent with this suggestion, Siegelbaum *et al.* (84) found that cAMP closes the S-channel in cell-attached membrane patches, and more recently Shuster *et al.* (83) have found that the catalytic subunit of the cAMP-dependent protein kinase also closes the S-channel in cell-free membrane patches, suggesting that the kinase acts on the internal membrane surface to phosphorylate either the S-channel itself or an associated protein that regulates the channel.

Strong support for the molecular model was obtained by Castellucci *et al.* (26) who found that injection of the catalytic subunit of the cAMP-dependent protein kinase into the sensory neuron broadened its spike and increased its transmitter release. Moreover, facilitation set in motion by serotonin can be blocked by injection of a specific protein inhibitor of the kinase (27) suggesting that the time course of sensitization is due to the persistent activity of the cAMP-dependent kinase (and not, for example, to the stable phosphorylation of the substrate protein). Consistent with this hypothesis, Bernier *et al.* (10) have shown that cAMP is elevated three- to fourfold in single sensory neurons in response to serotonin or stimulation of facilitatory neural pathways, and that the time course of its elevation parallels that of the presynaptic facilitation. Experiments involving the injection of a blocker of adenylate cyclase (GDP beta-S) indicate that the elevation of cAMP during sensitization appears to be due to persistent activity in the adenylate cyclase complex (which has at least three components: a receptor, a regulatory G-protein, and a catalytic subunit) which is thought to be the timekeeping step in short-term sensitization (81).

Recent evidence suggests that multiple facilitatory transmitters may converge on the adenylate cyclase complex in the sensory neurons. Abrams and co-workers (3) have shown that in addition to serotonin, two endogenous neuropeptides in *Aplysia*, the small cardioactive peptides SCP_A and SCP_B, facilitate synaptic transmission from the sensory neurons by a cAMP-dependent closure of the S-channel. Moreover, recent immunocytochemical studies by Ono and McCamman (74) and Kistler *et al.* (52,53) have shown that one class of identified interneurons in *Aplysia*, the L_{29} cells which produce presynaptic facilitation of the sensory neurons and which were originally thought to be serotonergic (41), do not use serotonin as their transmitter. Thus it appears that there are at least three agents which mimic heterosynaptic facilitation, as well as the natural transmitter of L_{29}, that may converge via different receptors on a common molecular cascade in the siphon sensory neurons. A similar idea has also been developed by Ocorr and co-workers who suggest that cAMP may be a common biochemical locus for the effects of 5HT and SCP_B in the tail sensory neurons of *Aplysia* ((68), see below).

Most of the work investigating the cellular and molecular mechanisms of sensitization in *Aplysia* has been focussed on sensory neurons. However, important strides have recently been made in specifying cellular changes that contribute to heterosynaptic facilitation at other loci in the neural circuit for gill and siphon withdrawal. Preliminary studies by Frost, Clark, and Kandel (35) suggest that, similar to sensory neurons, cAMP-dependent molecular changes occur in an identified inhibitory interneuron (36) and in a specific subclass of siphon motor neuron, and that these changes modulate both transmitter release and neuronal excitability, which in turn contribute to the enhancement of reflex output. These findings raise the possibility that sensitization in the gill and siphon withdrawal reflex may involve the coordinated regulation of cellular excitability at several different elements in the circuit, perhaps by means of a common cAMP-dependent molecular mechanisms.

Developmental Studies of Habituation and Sensitization

The behavioral and cellular studies described above have all been carried out in adult *Aplysia*. My colleagues and I have recently undertaken another approach to the investigation of habituation and sensitization by analyzing these simple forms of learning from a developmental perspective (19, 65, 79). The rationale for this approach is that development can provide a powerful analytic tool for studying learning and memory. If different behavioral processes emerge sequentially according to different developmental timetables, this allows the animal to be studied as a "functional mutant," permitting the examination on both behavioral and cellular levels of specific processes that temporarily exist in the absence of others. This approach has already been successfully used to study the development of a variety of forms of synaptic plasticity including PTP (71, 72) and both homosynaptic depression and heterosynaptic facilitation (80). Habituation and sensitization of the defensive withdrawal reflex of the gill and siphon were studied first since so much is known about these processes in the adult. Three questions were examined: 1) How are gill and siphon withdrawal functionally assembled during development? 2) How do habituation, sensitization, and short-term memory emerge during development? 3) Can one establish central neuronal correlates of habituation and sensitization during development?

Functional assembly of gill and siphon withdrawal. In order to study the development of behavioral plasticity in the gill and siphon withdrawal reflex, it was first necessary to understand how this withdrawal system is assembled during development. Kriegstein *et al.* (59) had previously found that development in *Aplysia* occurs in four phases: 1) *embryonic* from fertilized egg to hatching, 2) *larval* from hatching to metamorphosis (days 1-34), 3) *metamorphic* (days 34-37), and 4) *juvenile* (day 37 to sexual maturity, at about day 120). Kriegstein (58) also established external criteria permitting characterization of postembryonic development and maturation into 13 clearly defined stages. The developmental assembly of siphon and gill withdrawal was studied in the four juvenile stages: Stage 9 (lasting 4 days), Stage 10 (lasting 7 days), Stage 11 (lasting about 40 days), and Stage 12 (lasting about 30 days). The siphon first appears in Stage 9, the gill in Stage 10. In the adult the gill and siphon show two kinds of contractions: endogenous ("spontaneous") and elicited. As soon as the siphon develops in Stage 9 it exhibits elicited contractions to brief tactile stimuli; when the gill emerges in Stage 10 it also immediately exhibits siphon-elicited contractions. Thus both the siphon and gill withdrawal components of the reflex are intact as soon as the organs emerge. Both siphon and gill also exhibit spontaneous contractions as soon as they emerge. However, they appear to be independent, occurring synchronously only 20% of the time. This is in marked contrast to adults in which the gill and siphon co-contract during spontaneous contractions. In Stage 12 (about 5-6 weeks later) spontaneous contractions assume the synchronized adult form. These data suggest the hypothesis (19) that early in development there are independent neural oscillators for the siphon and gill (perhaps subcomponents of Interneuron II, an identified oscillatory network subserving respiratory pumping in the adult) which become coupled in Stage 12. In summary, exogenous and endogenous neural control of the gill and siphon appear to have different developmental timetables: exogenous (reflex) control is functional, resembling the adult form as soon as the organs emerge, while endogenous ("spontaneous") control matures more slowly over a period of several weeks.

Habituation, sensitization, and short-term memory. Rankin and Carew (79) have examined habituation and sensitization of siphon withdrawal in early juvenile *Aplysia* (Stages 9-11). Three different inter-stimulus intervals (ISIs: 10, 5, and 1 s) were used to study habituation (adult *Aplysia* will habituate with ISIs as long as 2 min). *Stage 11* animals exhibited clear habituation at all 3 ISIs, with progressively greater decrement with shorter intervals. As in adults, sensitization (produced by tail shock) was evident at this stage. *Stage 10* animals showed little habituation at a 10 s ISI, but clear and progressively greater decrement with 5 and 1 s ISIs. Sensitization was also evident at this stage. Finally, *Stage 9* animals showed no habituation at either 10 or 5 s ISIs; only a 1 s ISI produced decrement. Moreover, in contrast to Stages 10 and 11, sensitization was completely absent at Stage 9. These results show that different forms of learning emerge at different stages of development: habituation is present in the youngest animals tested (Stage 9), while sensitization emerges at a distinct and later stage (stage 10). The ability to store the information that a stimulus has recently occurred, which can be viewed as a rudimentary form of memory, also appears to develop systematically: greater habituation occurs at progressively longer intervals during development, suggesting that at successive stages this simple form of short-term memory is progressively more mature.

Central nervous correlates. Rayport and Camardo (80) had previously shown, by recording from the mucus motor cell R2 in the isolated CNS of juvenile *Aplysia*, that homosynaptic depression is present in its adult form in Stage 9, while heterosynaptic facilitation appears in Stage 10 and reaches maturity in Stages 11 and 12. These results served as an important cellular precedent to the behavioral studies described above since Rayport and Camardo suggested that habituation of the gill and siphon withdrawal reflex (which is mediated by homosynaptic depression) might emerge earlier in development than sensitization (which is mediated by heterosynaptic facilitation), a prediction that we subsequently confirmed (79).

As a first step towards a cellular analysis of the development of learning in the gill and siphon withdrawal reflex, Nolen and colleagues (65) have begun to explore the neural correlates of habituation and sensitization at different stages of development. They examined the central control of the gill and siphon withdrawal reflex in two preparations: semi-intact and the isolated central nervous system (CNS). *Semi-intact:* The gill of Stage 11 animals was removed leaving it attached to the CNS (abdominal ganglion) by the branchial nerve. Electrical stimulation of the afferent siphon nerve reliably evoked a gill contraction which habituated with repeated stimulation and was sensitized by stimulation of a pathway from the tail. These results show that both the centrally projecting siphon afferents and facilitatory inputs make functional connections with gill motor neurons in Stage 11 animals. *Isolated CNS:* Nolen *et al.* then identified neural correlates of habituation and sensitization in the isolated abdominal ganglion by recording the efferent output of the branchial nerve in response to siphon nerve stimulation. Using the same parameters as both the behavior (79) and the semi-intact preparation, the evoked branchial nerve response decremented with repeated stimuli and was facilitated by connective stimulation. These data show that in juvenile *Aplysia* (Stage 11) a component of the withdrawal reflex, as well as its habituation and sensitization, is centrally mediated. These studies, coupled with an intracellular analysis in the CNS of juvenile *Aplysia* at different stages, will permit the investigation of the developmental changes which underlie the emergence of different forms of learning and memory in a neural circuit that has been extensively analyzed on a variety of levels in the adult.

ASSOCIATIVE LEARNING

Associative learning refers to a change in behavior produced by the temporal association of two stimuli: a conditioned stimulus (CS) that serves as a cue or signal, and an unconditioned stimulus (UCS) that serves as reinforcement. In recent years associative learning has been described in a number of behavioral systems in *Aplysia* including: a) the defensive arousal system, b) the withdrawal reflex of the mantle organs, c) the tail withdrawal reflex, d) the feeding system, and e) the head-waving system. I will discuss each of these in turn.

Conditioned Defensive Arousal

In one of the earliest studies of classical conditioning in *Aplysia*, Walters, Carew, and Kandel (94) employed a "conditioned emotional response" (CER) paradigm to examine whether *Aplysia* could learn to associate a chemosensory CS (a shrimp extract) with an aversive UCS (head shock). The behavioral index of conditioning was modulation of escape locomotion by the chemosensory CS. Controls received either unpaired CS-UCS presentations, the CS alone or the UCS alone. Training lasted two days (three trials per day), followed by testing the next day. During testing all animals showed comparable escape locomotion in the *absence* of the CS. However, in the *presence* of the CS, paired animals showed significantly more escape than all controls. Interestingly, the CS by itself did not elicit an obvious conditioned locomotor response after training, leading Walters *et al.* (94) to propose that the CS had come to elicit a central defensive state (analogous to conditioned fear) which modulated escape locomotion To further test this notion, Walters, Carew, and Kandel (95) examined a variety of other behavioral responses in the presence of the shrimp CS following similar training and found these responses modulated by the CS in a motivationally consistent fashion: four defensive responses (head and siphon withdrawal, inking, and escape locomotion) were significantly facilitated in the presence of the CS, while an appetitive response (feeding) was significantly suppressed. These behavioral results thus supported the conditioned fear hypothesis. Further support was obtained by Carew, Walters, and Kandel (21) who recorded intracellularly from motor neurons in the escape locomotion, siphon withdrawal, and inking systems from previously trained and control animals. In the presence of the CS, animals that received paired training showed significant facilitation of synaptic input to all these motor systems while controls showed no facilitation. The CS produced no change in resting potential or input resistance of motor neurons in trained animals, suggesting that the critical changes produced by the CS were presynaptic to the motor neurons. These results, together with the behavioral data, lead these authors to propose that the conditioning exhibited by *Aplysia* in this CER paradigm reflects an association between the CS and a central defensive arousal state resembling conditioned fear in mammals.

Conditioned Withdrawal of the Gill and Siphon

Classical conditioning of gill and siphon withdrawal has been studied in two preparations: 1) a surgically reduced *in vitro* preparation, and 2) intact animals.

***In vitro* conditioning.** Lukowiak and Sahley (63) paired a photic stimulus to the siphon as the CS with a strong tactile stimulus directly to the gill as the UCS. Normally the photic stimulus does not produce gill withdrawal, but after repeated pairing with the UCS, the CS came to elicit gill withdrawl in seven out of ten preparations, whereas it never elicited withdrawal in control preparations that received random CS-UCS presentations. Subsequently Lukowiak (61) described a new paradigm that was more amenable to cellular investigation: a weak tactile stimulus to the siphon served as the CS, while the UCS remained a strong tactile stimulus to the gill. After repeated CS-UCS pairing, the weak siphon CS evoked an enhanced siphon and gill withdrawal response, while a number of controls (random CS-UCS pairing, CS alone, and UCS alone) showed no enhancement. Furthermore, Lukowiak (62) recorded intracellularly from gill motor neurons during paired training and found that the siphon CS evoked larger neuronal responses in these cells as training progressed. Further experiments indicated increased synaptic transmission from siphon sensory neurons contributed to the facilitated input in the gill motor neurons. Thus this *in vitro* preparation provides the opportunity to analyze cellular events in the CNS during the acquisition of a learned response.

Intact animals. Encouraged by the progress made in analyzing sensitization of the gill and siphon withdrawal reflex, Carew, Walters, and Kandel (22) examined whether this reflex might also show associative learning. They paired a weak tactile stimulus to the siphon as the CS with a strong electric shock to the tail as the UCS. After repeated pairing trials the CS came to elicit significantly enhanced gill and siphon withdrawal compared to controls which received random or unpaired CS-UCS presentations, or the CS or UCS alone. Conditioning was rapidly acquired (within 15 trials) and was retained for several days. More recently, using a related paradigm Carew, Hawkins, and Kandel (16) have demonstrated differential classical conditioning of the siphon withdrawal component of this reflex. In differential conditioning two conditioned stimuli are used in the same animal; one (CS+) is paired with the UCS, while the other (CS-) is specifically unpaired. Thus each animal can serve as its own control. Weak tactile stimuli applied to the siphon or mantle shelf served as discriminative stimuli

(CS+ and CS-), and tail shock as the UCS. Differential conditioning could be acquired in a single trial, was retained for more than 24 hours, and increased in strength with increased number of trials. Moreover, siphon conditioning could be produced with two separate sites on the siphon skin as discriminative stimuli. Recently Hawkins, Clark, and Kandel (42) showed that the gill withdrawal component of the reflex can also be differentially conditioned using two sites on the siphon as conditioned stimuli. Finally, Hawkins, Carew, and Kandel (40) found that the interstimulus interval function (which describes the CS-UCS intervals that produced effective conditioning) was quite steep; reliable learning was produced only with a CS-UCS interval of 0.5 s, and to a lesser extent, 1.0 s. No conditioning occurred with intervals of 2, 5, and 10 s, or with backwards (UCS-CS) pairings. Moreover they found that the conditioning depended upon the contingency between the CS and UCS, that is, upon the degree to which the CS *predicted* the UCS. In addition to characterizing essential features of the differential conditioning, these behavioral findings provide important constraints on any cellular model proposed to explain the conditioning.

Two recent important strides in associative learning involving gill and siphon withdrawal have been made. First, Hawkins, Clark, and Kandel (42) have found that gill withdrawal can exhibit an interesting form of operant conditioning. Experimental animals that received siphon shock for relaxing their gills beyond a preset criterion level spent a significantly greater amount of time with their gills contracted beyond that criterion level than yoked controls, during both training and extinction periods. This is a significant advance since so much is already known about the connectivity and plasticity in the gill withdrawal circuit. A second important advance has come from Colwill's (31) recent demonstration that *Aplysia* are capable of forming an association between a shock UCS and the context in which that UCS occurs. This was demonstrated in two ways: 1) animals showed enhanced siphon withdrawal in a shock-associated context compared to a different, non-shock context, and 2) the shock-associated contex was able to interfere with subsequent conditioning of siphon withdrawal. This was the first demonstration of blocking in *Aplysia*, a higher-order form of learning of great importance in theories of Pavlovian conditioning.

Cellular studies of conditioning. To investigate the cellular mechanisms of classical conditioning, Hawkins and colleagues (39) used a differential training procedure in the neural circuit for siphon withdrawal. They recorded from two siphon sensory neurons which both made excitatory monosynaptic connections onto a siphon motor neuron. Tail shock produced significantly greater facilitation of synaptic transmission from a sensory neuron if the shock was immediately preceded by spike activity (produced by intracellular current in the sensory neuron) than if the shock and spike activity were specifically unpaired or if the shock occurred alone. These results suggested that the temporal specificity of the conditioning might be due to an activity-dependent enhancement of facilitation. Further evidence suggested that this enhancement is presynaptic in origin: Hawkins *et al.* (39) examined the duration of the action potential in the sensory neurons (in 50 mM tetraethylammonium) and found that the differential training produced a significantly greater enhancement of spike duration in paired compared to unpaired sensory neurons. Extending these findings, recent voltage-clamp experiments by Hawkins and Abrams (38) suggest that the activity-dependent facilitation involves modulation of the same ionic channel in the sensory neurons (the S-channel) that is involved in sensitization.

These experiments suggest that the mechanism of classical conditioning in *Aplysia* may involve a temporally specific, activity-dependent enhancement of the same cellular process (presynaptic facilitation) that is involved in sensitization. Further evidence that this mechanism can account for the behavioral conditioning has been obtained by Clark (29) who found that just as backward (UCS-CS) pairing does not produce conditioning (40), neither does it produce activity-dependent facilitation of synaptic transmission. Specifically, forward pairing produces significantly greater enhancement of facilitation than backward pairing.

Another model of conditioning emphasizing the importance of activity is that proposed by D.O. Hebb (43), who postulated a critical role for *postsynaptic* activity in synaptic facilitation. Carew and co-workers (15) directly tested this hypothesis in *Aplysia* and found that postsynaptic activity (in siphon motor neurons that mediate the conditioned response) was neither necessary nor sufficient for associative synaptic changes, indicating that at least in this instance, conditioning was not due to a Hebb-type mechanism but rather to activity-dependent enhancement of presynaptic facilitation of transmitter release from sensory neurons onto their follower cells.

The activity-dependent model discussed above emphasizes the relationship between sensitization and its amplified form, classical conditioning. This model thus raises two important questions: 1) How does activity affect the molecular machinery involved in sensitization (specifically, the cAMP cascade)? 2) What aspect of activity is important for the amplification? Preliminary evidence addressing the first question obtained by Abrams and colleagues (1) suggests that the cAMP cascade is directly modulated by spike activity: sensory neurons receiving a brief application of serotonin (as the UCS) immediately after a train of spikes show a fourfold greater level of cAMP than cells exposed to serotonin alone (1, 50). Abrams and co-workers (2) have also addressed the second question. Two lines of evidence suggest that a brief elevation of intracellular Ca^{2+} produced by spike activity in the sensory neurons might serve as the signal for temporal specificity by increasing the cell's normal cAMP response to s rotonin: 1) action potentials paired with serotonin normally enhance the facilitatory (spike broadening) response to serotonin in sensory neurons; but this activity-dependent enhancement does not occur in the *absence* of Ca^{2+} influx (50); and 2) stimulation of adenylate cyclase from *Aplysia* nervous tissue by serotonin is substantially dependent on Ca^{2+}/calmodulin. The ability of serotonin to activate the cyclase is markedly reduced following depletion of calmodulin or following the addition of a calmodulin inhibitor (4). Although these results are preliminary, they suggest that classical conditioning and sensitization in *Aplysia* share at least part of a common molecular cascade and that Ca^{2+} influx during activity may be a critical priming factor for enhancement of that cascade during conditioning.

Classical Conditioning in the Tail Withdrawal Reflex

The tail withdrawal reflex in *Aplysia* is mediated by an identified cluster of mechanoafferent sensory neurons which synapse monosynaptically on tail motor neurons (91) and interneurons (30). Sensitization of the reflex, as well as serotonin, produces an increase in synaptic transmission from these neurons (92). In addition, serotonin produces an increase in input resistance and a concomitant elevation of cAMP in the sensory neurons (13, 67, 69, 77). Walsh and Byrne (87) have shown that the cyclase activator forskolin mimics the 5-HT response in the sensory neurons and blocks subsequent 5-HT responses, suggesting they are acting through a common saturable mechanism. Interestingly, forskolin-modulated currents appear to have two components, one with properties of the S current (54, 84), the other with novel properties (8). Moreover, in the tail sensory neurons serotonin appears to modulate a calcium-activated K^+ current (86) as well as the Ca^{2+}-insensitive S current (84). In biochemical studies, Ocorr and Byrne (67) have shown that, in addition to serotonin, SCP_B (but not tryptamine or FMRF amide) elevates cAMP levels in these neurons, and that serotonin and SCP_B produce an inward current associated with a decrease in input conductance. Taken collectively, these data suggest that sensitization in the tail withdrawal reflex closely resembles that in the gill and siphon withdrawal reflex: both may involve a serotonin-and peptide-sensitive, cAMP-mediated decrease in K^+ conductance.

In addition to the nonassociative effects described above, the sensory neurons of the tail withdrawal reflex also show clear associative plasticity. Walters and Byrne (88) applied a cellular analog of a differential conditioning procedure, recording simultaneously from three sensory neurons and a tail motor neuron. One sensory neuron (CS+) was activated (by intracellular current) paired with tail shock (the UCS), another (CS-) was activated unpaired with the UCS, and the third (sensitization control) was not activated during training. Following five trials, the EPSP from the paired sensory neurons (CS+) was significantly facilitated compared to both the CS- and sensitization controls. Walters and Byrne (89) further observed that CS+ neurons show a slow depolarization after the UCS, while CS- or sensitization control neurons show a hyperpolarization. They suggest that, as a result of this depolarization, a voltage-sensitive Ca^{2+} conductance activated near the resting potential may be modulated by associative training. Based on these results, Walters and Byrne propose that classical conditioning is produced by activity-dependent neuromodulation of synaptic transmission, and that Ca^{2+} could be a major intracellular messenger involved in this process. In a series of recent experiments, Walters and Byrne (90) have suggested that activity-dependent neuromodulation may also be a mechanism of long-term synaptic enhancement similar to long-term potentiation commonly observed in the mammalian CNS.

Recent studies by Ocorr, Walters, and Byrne (69,70) have extended this analysis to a molecular level. They used bilateral clusters of the tail sensory neurons in a biochemical analog of the classical conditioning paradigm: depolarization of an entire cluster by means of a 5 s exposure to high K^+ seawater served as the CS, and a 15 s exposure to serotonin served as the UCS. One cluster received paired CS-UCS presentations, the other specifically unpaired. Following only one trial the paired cluster showed a significantly elevated cAMP content compared to the unpaired cluster. CS alone and UCS alone produced no significant changes. Preliminary studies of phosphodiesterase (PDE) activity by Ocorr and Byrne (66) suggest that the increase in cAMP is due at least in part to stimulation of cyclase activity rather than inhibition of PDE.

Taken together, these results led Ocorr and colleagues (70) to suggest that a pairing-specific enhancement of cAMP levels, perhaps by means of a Ca^{2+}-calmodulin dependent step, may be a biochemical mechanism for associative learning. This hypothesis can now be tested in view of the recent report by Ingram and Walters (46) that the tail withdrawal reflex is capable of differential classical conditioning.

The similarities of the behavioral, cellular, and molecular results of studies of associative conditioning from two systems in *Aplysia* that have been independently analyzed (the reflex withdrawal systems of the mantle and tail) are indeed striking. Results from both systems emphasize the importance of neuronal activity, Ca^{2+} entry, cyclase activation, and reduction of a K^{+} conductance for a pairing mechanism.

Conditioned Cessation of Feeding Responses

Aplysia are herbivores that normally feed on a variety of seaweeds. Susswein and Schwarz (85) have described an interesting form of associative learning in this feeding behavior. They presented animals with seaweed wrapped in a plastic net, allowing the animals to taste the food and attempt to eat it, but not swallow it. Thus, the net-enclosed food became lodged in the buccal cavity. Animals receiving such treatment rapidly learned to cease responding to this inedible food and memory was maintained for at least 24 hours. An essential component of the learning is that the food become stuck within the buccal cavity, which the authors suggest gives rise to stimuli that become paired with lip stimuli from the taste of the food. The learning also displays stimulus specificity: lip stimuli occurring sequentially (rather than paired) with food stuck in the buccal cavity do not produce the conditioned cessation of feeding. Recently Schwarz, Markovich, and Susswein (in preparation) have further specified the parametric features of the learning and shown them to be clearly dissociable from adaptation and satiation. Finally Schwarz and Susswein (82) have found that animals whose esophageal nerves are cut take twice as long to learn as sham controls, suggesting that these nerves carry information for learning that food is inedible. They suggest the hypothesis that gut inputs in these nerves can act as positive or negative reinforcers of feeding. Susswein and colleagues (85) suggest that the learning in their behavioral paradigm resembles operant conditioning since the change in behavior is contingent upon the consequences of the animal's response. Since the neural circuit of feeding has been examined in detail, this preparation offers considerable promise for a cellular analysis of a very interesting form of associative learning.

Operant Conditioning of Head-waving

Aplysia readily show a naturally occurring head-waving behavior in a number of behavioral contexts including searching for a hold-fast, egg laying, and "spontaneously" exploring their environment. Cook and Carew (32, 33) have recently shown that this response can be operantly conditioned. Specifically, *Aplysia* can be operantly trained to rapidly modify their head-waving response (within 10 minutes), increasing the amount of head-waving on one side of their body in order to terminate the presentation of a strong light which the animals find aversive. Yoked controls do not acquire the operant response. Two lines of evidence show that the operant responding is under the control of reinforcement contingencies: 1) when the contingencies are reversed (the original positive side now punished and vice versa), contingent-trained (but not yoked) controls show a significant reduction in their responding, and when the original contingencies are reinstated, contingent animals once again show significant operant responding; and 2) yoked controls do not learn the operant response, yet these same animals readily learn when reinforcement is made contingent upon their responding. Finally, contingent-trained animals do not appear to use external cues (such as visual stimuli) as feedback to determine their body position during acquisition of the operant response. Rather, internally derived cues (e.g., proprioceptive or reafference) appear to play a predominant feedback role during acquisition of the operant task.

Since some of the cellular elements involved in both the operant response and the reinforcement pathways are known (44, 47, 73), this form of associative learning in *Aplysia* may prove to be quite useful in studying the cellular mechanisms of operant conditioning. Moreover, since significant insights into the cellular and molecular mechanisms of classical conditioning have been gained in the gill and tail withdrawal systems in *Aplysia*, it may also be possible in both the head-waving system (33) and the gill withdrawal system (42), as well as the feeding system (85), to compare the relationship between classical and operant conditioning in mechanistic terms.

CONCLUDING REMARKS

It is striking that in an animal such as *Aplysia*, which possesses a seemingly modest behavioral repertoire, a number of different response systems are capable of a wide variety of interesting forms of learning. Among these response systems the two that have provided the greatest gains towards a molecular analysis have been the gill and siphon withdrawal reflex and the tail withdrawal reflex. Taken collectively, work in these two systems suggests several important themes of relevance to molecular mechanisms of learning: endogenous biogenic amines and neuropeptides in *Aplysia* may activate a common molecular cascade in sensory neurons by increasing the activity of an adenylate cyclase complex in the cell's membrane, thereby elevating intracellular cyclic AMP. Cyclic AMP in turn activates specific protein kinases that can phosphorylate a family of substrate proteins, some of which are either K^+ channels themselves or proteins closely associated with them. Additional phosphorylated substrate proteins may have other important functions. For example some might be involved in structural modification of synaptic release sites, and still others might serve as genomic signals to promote long-term cellular changes. Although the work thus far has been predominantly focussed on sensory neurons, similar molecular changes in interneurons and motor neurons could produce modulation of both neuronal excitability and transmitter release at a variety of loci in the neural circuits for these simple reflexes.

Towards General Principles

Because cellular and molecular mechanisms of learning have been analyzed in only a few preparations, it is unrealistic to expect that general principles can be derived at the present time. As yet only two molluscan preparations, *Aplysia* and *Hermissenda*, have yielded detailed models of the biophysical and molecular events that may be involved in the acquisition and storage of learned information. It may be useful, however, as a first step towards searching for general principles, to ask what *Aplysia* and *Hermissenda* may have in common. There are at least four areas in which the models derived from each preparation appear to be on common ground:

1) Learning in both preparations can be localized to individual neurons and involves alteration of previously existing synaptic connections and/or previously existing intrinsic cellular properties.

2) In both *Aplysia* and *Hermissenda* modulation of K^+ conductances appears to be involved in memory storage: in *Aplysia* a unique K^+ current (I_S) is thought to be reduced in cell bodies and terminals of neurons, increasing transmitter release by broadening the action potential; in *Hermissenda* early and Ca^{2+}-dependent K^+ currents (I_A and I_C) are thought to be reduced in a class of photoreceptors, increasing their excitability.

3) In both *Aplysia* and *Hermissenda* protein phosphorylation has been implicated as an important step in the modification of K^+ channels. In

both cases the possibility exists that one of the substrate proteins that is phophorylated is the K^+ channel itself.

4) In both *Aplysia* and *Hermissenda* "second messengers" have been proposed as important for memory because of their role in mediating protein phosphorylation. In *Aplysia* the second messenger is cAMP, whereas in *Hermissenda* both cAMP and Ca^{2+}- calmodulin have been implicated (with Ca^{2+}-calmodulin suggested as the more likely candidate).

Thus it appears that there are several areas of common thinking about mechanisms of memory storage in the models for learning in *Aplysia* and *Hermissenda*. Perhaps the biggest difference in the two models at this point concerns acquisition mechanisms. Acquisition of associative learning in *Aplysia* is thought to involve activity-dependent enhancement of presynaptic facilitation, whereas in *Hermissenda* acquisition is thought to involve cumulative depolarization. Whether these are fundamentally different acquisition mechanisms or whether they may share some features in common remains to be elucidated by further physiological and molecular analysis.

Future Direction

What are some of the important questions and issues that still remain to be examined in *Aplysia*? There are many. For example, one important question concerns the roles of transmitter depletion and transmitter mobilization in habituation, dishabituation, and sensitization respectively. These mechanisms (and the general issue of modulation of Ca^{2+} handling in sensory neurons) will be interesting to explore as complementary mechanisms to the modulation of Ca^{2+} entry that is known to accompany alterations in the duration of the sensory neuron action potential. A second important issue concerns the events occurring at the synaptic terminal of the sensory neuron. Much of the previous work has relied upon current and voltage clamp of sensory neuron cell bodies to provide an indirect estimate or model of the events occurring at the synaptic terminals. Recent technical advances in recording from functional sensory-motor synapses in dissociated cell culture, as well as directly from sensory terminals (growth cones) in cell culture provide a major step toward specifying the cellular and molecular events occurring at sensory neuron terminal release sites during various forms of plasticity. A third major question concerns the pairing mechanism involved in classical conditioning. Although the mechanism is not yet in hand, several leads suggest that Ca^{2+} entry occurring during cellular activity may play a critical role in priming the normal molecular (cAMP) cascade activated by sensitization, thereby enhancing its activity during conditioning. A final question that can now be approached concerns the cellular and, ultimately, the molecular mechanisms underlying operant conditioning. It will be extremely interesting to explore these mechanisms and to compare them to those underlying classical conditioning. In conclusion, it is clear that our understanding of the mechanisms of learning in *Aplysia* is incomplete. Several key issues remain to be elucidated. It is also clear however, that it has been possible in *Aplysia* to begin to forge several important links between specific molecular changes in the central nervous system and changes in behavior produced by learning.

Acknowledgements. In this paper I have drawn heavily from a recent review that my colleague C. Sahley and I have prepared (20). I am very grateful to T. Abrams, J. Byrne, R. Hawkins, E. Kandel, E. Marcus, T. Nolen, and C. Rankin for helpful criticism of this manuscript. I also thank D. Gillespie and E. Marcus for help in preparing the manuscript. This work was supported by NIH Career Development Award 7-KO2-MH00081-09, NIH BRSG Grant 507-RR-07015, and NSF Grant BNS 8311300.

REFERENCES

(1) Abrams, T.W.; Bernier, L.; Hawkins, R.D.; and Kandel, E.R. 1984. Possible roles of Ca^{2+} and cAMP in activity-dependent facilitation, a mechanism for associative learning in *Aplysia*. *Soc. Neurosci. Abst.* 10: 269.

(2) Abrams, T.W.; Carew, T.J.; Hawkins, R.D.; and Kandel. E.R. 1983. Aspects of the cellular mechanism of temporal specificity in conditioning in *Aplysia*: preliminary evidence for Ca^{++} influx as a signal of activity. *Soc. Neurosci. Abstr.* 9: 168.

(3) Abrams, T.W.; Castellucci, V.F.; Camardo, J.S.; Kandel, E.R.; and Lloyd, P.E. 1984. Two endogenous neuropeptides modulate the gill and siphon withdrawal reflex in *Aplysia* by presynaptic facilitation involving cAMP-dependent closure of a serotonin-sensitive potassium channel. *Proc. Natl. Acad. Sci.* 81: 7956-7960.

(4) Abrams, T.W.; Eliot, L.; Dudai, Y.; and Kandel, E.R. 1985. Activation of adenylate cyclase in *Aplysia* neural tissue by Ca^{2+}/Calmodulin, a candidate for an associative mechanism during conditioning. *Soc. Neurosci. Abstr.* 11: 797.

(5) Alkon, D.L. 1983. Learning in a marine snail. *Sci. Am.* 249: 79-84.

(6) Alkon, D.L. 1984. Calcium-mediated reduction of ionic currents: a biophysical memory trace. *Science* 226: 1037-1045.

(7) Bailey, C.H., and Chen, M. 1983. Morphological basis of long-term habituation and sensitization in *Aplysia. Science* 220: 91-93.

(8) Baxter, D.A., and Byrne, J.H. 1985. Forskolin-modulated membrane currents in *Aplysia* tail sensory neurons. *Soc. Neurosci. Abstr.* 11: 789.

(9) Belardetti, F.; Schacher, S.; Kandel, E.R.; and Siegelbaum, S.A 1985. Serotonin produces a decreased conductance EPSP and broadening of the action potential in growth cones of *Aplysia* sensory neurons. *Soc. Neurosci. Abstr.* 11: 28.

(10) Bernier, L.: Castellucci, V.F.; Kandel, E.R.; and Schwartz, J.H. 1982. Facilitatory transmitter causes a selective and prolonged increase in adenosine 3':5'-monophosphate in sensory neurons mediating the gill and siphon withdrawal reflex in *Aplysia. J. Neurosci.* 2: 1682-1691.

(11) Boyle, M.B.; Klein, M.; Smith, S.J.; and Kandel, E.R. 1984. Serotonin increases intracellular Ca^{++} transients in voltage-clamped sensory neurons of *Aplysia californica. Proc. Natl. Acad. Sci.* 81: 7642-7646.

(12) Byrne, J.H.; Castellucci, V.F.; and Kandel, E.R. 1978. Contribution of individual mechanoreceptor neurons mediating defensive gill-withdrawal reflex in *Aplysia. J. Neurophysl.* 41: 418-413.

(13) Byrne, J.H., and Walters, E.T. 1982. Associative conditioning of single sensory neurons in *Aplysia*: II. Activity-dependent modulation of membrane responses. *Soc. Neurosci. Abstr.* 8: 386.

(14) Carew, T.J.; Castellucci, V.F.; and Kandel, E.R. 1971. An analysis of dishabituation and sensitization of the gill-withdrawal reflex in *Aplysia. Int. J. Neurosci.* 2: 79-98.

(15) Carew, T.J.; Hawkins, R.D.; Abrams, T.W.; and Kandel, E.R. 1984. A test of Hebb's postulate at identified synapses which mediate classical conditioning in *Aplysia. J. Neurosci.* 4: 1217-1224.

(16) Carew, T.J.; Hawkins, R.D.; and Kandel, E.R. 1983. Differential classical conditioning of a defensive withdrawal reflex in *Aplysia californica. Science* 219: 397-400.

(17) Carew, T.J., and Kandel, E.R. 1977. Inking in *Aplysia californica*: III. Two different synaptic conductance mechanisms for triggering the central program for inking. *J. Neurophysl.* 40: 721-734.

(18) Carew, T.J.; Pinsker, H.M.; and Kandel, E.R. 1972. Long-term habituation of a defensive withdrawal reflex in *Aplysia. Science* 175: 451-454.

(19) Carew, T.J.; Rankin, C.H.; and Stopfer, M. 1985. Development of learning and memory in *Aplysia*: I. Functional assembly of the gill and siphon withdrawal reflex. *Soc. Neurosci. Abstr.* 11: 643.

(20) Carew, T.J., and Sahley, C.L. 1986. Invertebrate learning and memory: from behavior to molecules. *Ann. R. Neurosci.* 9: 435-487.

(21) Carew, T.J.; Walters, E.T.; and Kandel, E.R. 1981. Associative learning in *Aplysia*: cellular correlates supporting a conditioned fear hypothesis. *Science* 211: 501-504.

(22) Carew, T.J.; Walters, E.T.; and Kandel, E.R. 1981. Classical conditioning in a simple withdrawal reflex in *Aplysia californica*. *J. Neurosci.* 1: 1426-1437.

(23) Castellucci, V.F.; Carew, T.J.; and Kandel, E.R. 1978. Cellular analysis of long-term habituation of the gill-withdrawal reflex of *Aplysia californica*. *Science* 202: 1306-1308.

(24) Castellucci, V.F., and Kandel, E.R. 1974. A quantal analysis of the synaptic depression underlying habituation of the gill-withdrawal reflex in *Aplysia*. *Proc. Natl. Acad. Sci.* 71: 5004-5008.

(25) Castellucci, V.F., and Kandel, E.R. 1976. Presynaptic facilitation as a mechanism for behavioral sensitization in *Aplysia*. *Science* 194: 1176-1178.

(26) Castellucci, V.F.; Kandel, E.R.; Schwartz, J.H.; Wilson, F.D., Nairn, A.C.; and Greengard, P. 1980. Intracellular injection of the catalytic subunit of cyclic AMP-dependent protein kinase simulates facilitation of transmitter release underlying behavioral sensitization in *Aplysia*. *Proc. Natl. Acad. Sci.* 77: 7492-7496.

(27) Castellucci, V.F.; Nairn, A.; Greengard, P.; Schwartz, J.H.; and Kandel, E.R. 1982. Inhibitor of adenosine 3':5'-monophosphate-dependent protein kinase blocks presynaptic facilitation in *Aplysia*. *J. Neurosci.* 2: 1673-1681.

(28) Castellucci, V.; Pinsker, H.; Kupfermann, I.; and Kandel, E.R. 1970. Neuronal mechanisms of habituation and dishabituation of the gill-withdrawal reflex in *Aplysia*. *Science* 167: 1745-1748.

(29) Clark, G.A. 1984. A cellular mechanism for the temporal specificity of classical conditioning of the siphon-withdrawal response in *Aplysia*. *Soc. Neurosci. Abstr.* 10: 268.

(30) Cleary, L.J., and Byrne, J.H. 1985. Interneurons contributing to the mediation and modulation of the tail withdrawal reflex in *Aplysia*. *Soc. Neurosci. Abstr.* 11: 642.

(31) Colwill, R.M. 1985. Context conditioning in *Aplysia californica*. *Soc. Neurosci. Abstr.* 11: 796.

(32) Cook, D.G., and Carew, T.J. 1985. Operant conditioning of head-waving in *Aplysia*. *Soc. Neurosci. Abstr.* 11: 796.

(33) Cook, D.G., and Carew, T.J. 1986. Operant conditioning of head-waving in *Aplysia californica*. *Proc. Natl. Acad. Sci.* 83: 1120-1124.

(34) Dudai, Y. 1985. Genes, enzymes and learning in *Drosophila*. *Trends Neurosci.* 8: 18-22.

(35) Frost, W.N.; Clark, G.A.; and Kandel, E.R. 1985. Changes in cellular excitability in a new class of siphon motor neurons during sensitization in *Aplysia*. *Soc. Neurosci. Abstr.* 11:643.

(36) Frost, W.N., and Kandel, E.R. 1984. Sensitizing stimuli reduce the effectiveness of the L30 inhibitory interneurons in the siphon withdrawal reflex circuit of *Aplysia*. *Soc. Neurosci. Abstr.* 10: 510.

(37) Gingrich, K.J., and Byrne, J.H. 1985. Simulation of synaptic depression, posttetanic potentiation, and presynaptic facilitation of synaptic potentials from sensory neurons mediating gill-withdrawal reflex in *Aplysia*. *J. Neurophysl.* 53: 652-669.

(38) Hawkins, R.D., and Abrams, T.W. 1984. Evidence that activity-dependent facilitation underlying classical conditioning in *Aplysia* involves modulation of the same ionic current as normal presynaptic facilitation. *Soc. Neurosci. Abstr.* 10: 268.

(39) Hawkins, R.D.; Abrams, T.W.; Carew, T.J.; and Kandel, E.R. 1983. A cellular mechanism of classical conditioning in *Aplysia*: activity-dependent amplification of presynaptic facilitation. *Science* 219: 400-405.

(40) Hawkins, R.D.; Carew, T.J.; and Kandel, E.R. 1986. Effects of interstimulus interval and contingency on classical conditioning of the *Aplysia* siphon withdrawal reflex. *J. Neurosci.* 6: 1695-1701.

(41) Hawkins, R.D.; Castellucci, V.F.; and Kandel, E.R. 1981. Interneurons involved in mediation and modulation of gill-withdrawal reflex in *Aplysia*. II. Identified neurons produce heterosynaptic facilitation contributing to behavioral sensitization. *J. Neurophysl.* 45: 315-326.

(42) Hawkins, R.D.; Clark, G.A.; and Kandel, E.R. 1985. Operant conditioning and differential classical conditioning of gill withdrawal in *Aplysia*. *Soc. Neurosci. Abstr.* 11: 796.

(43) Hebb, D.O. 1949. Organization of Behavior. New York: J. Wiley & Sons.

(44) Hening, W.A.; Walters, E.T.; Carew, T.J.; and Kandel, E.R. 1979. Motorneuronal control of locomotion in *Aplysia*. *Brain Res.* 179: 231-253.

(45) Hochner, B.; Schacher, S., Klein, M., and Kandel, E.R. 1985. Presynaptic facilitation in *Aplysia* sensory neurons: a process independent of K+ current modulation becomes important when transmitter release is depressed. *Soc. Neurosci. Abstr.* 11: 29.

(46) Ingram, D.A., and Walters, E.T. 1984. Differential classical conditioning of tail and siphon withdrawal in *Aplysia*. *Soc. Neurosci. Abstr.* 10: 270.

(47) Jahan-Parwar, B., and Fredman, S.M. 1978. Control of pedal and parapodial movements in *Aplysia*. II: Cerebral ganglion neurons. *J. Neurophysl.* 41: 609-620.

(48) Kandel, E.R. 1976. Cellular Basis of Behavior. San Francisco: Freeman.

(49) Kandel, E.R. 1984. Steps towards a molecular grammar for learning: explorations into the nature of memory. In *Medicine, Science and Society*, ed. K.J. Isselbacher, pp. 555-604. New York: J. Wiley & Sons.

(50) Kandel, E.R.; Abrams, T.; Bernier, L.; Carew, T.J.; Hawkins, R.D.; and Schwartz, J.H. 1983. Classical conditioning and sensitization share aspects of the same molecular cascade in *Aplysia*. *Cold S.H. Quant. Biol.* 48: 821-830.

(51) Kandel, E.R., and Schwartz, J.H. 1982. Molecular biology of learning: modulation of transmitter release. *Science* 218: 433-443.

(52) Kistler, H.B., Jr.; Hawkins, R.D.; Koester, J.; Kandel, E.R.; and Schwartz, J.H. 1983. Immunocytochemical studies of neurons producing facilitation in the abdominal ganglion of *Aplysia*. *Soc. Neurosci. Abstr.* 9: 915.

(53) Kistler, H.B., Jr.; Hawkins, R.D.; Koester, J.; Steinbusch, H.W.M.; Kandel, E.R.; and Schwartz, J.H. 1985. Distribution of serotonin-immunoreactive cell bodies and processes in the abdominal ganglion of mature *Aplysia*. *J. Neurosci.* 5: 72-80.

(54) Klein, M.; Camardo, J.; and Kandel, E.R. 1982. Serotonin modulates a specific potassium current in the sensory neurons that show presynaptic facilitation in *Aplysia*. *Proc. Natl. Acad. Sci.* 79: 5713-5717.

(55) Klein, M., and Kandel, E.R. 1978. Presynaptic modulation of voltage-dependent Ca++ current: mechanism for behavioral sensitization. *Proc. Natl. Acad. Sci.* 75: 3512-3516.

(56) Klein, M., and Kandel, E.R. 1980. Mechanism of calcium current modulation underlying presynaptic facilitation and behavioral sensitization in *Aplysia*. *Proc. Natl. Acad. Sci.* 77: 6912-6916.

(57) Klein, M.; Shapiro, E.; and Kandel, E.R. 1980. Synaptic plasticity and the modulation of the Ca++ current. *J. Exp. Biol.* 89: 117-157.

(58) Kriegstein, A.R. 1977. Development of the nervous system of *Aplysia californica. Proc. Nalt. Acad. Sci.* 74: 375-378.

(59) Kriegstein, A.R.; Castellucci, V.; and Kandel, E.R. 1974. Metamorphosis of *Aplysia californica* in laboratory culture. *Proc. Nalt. Acad. Sci* 71: 3654-3658.

(60) Kupfermann, I., and Pinsker, H. 1968. A behavioral modification of the feeding reflex in *Aplysia californica. Comm. Behav. Biol. A* 2: 13-17.

(61) Lukowiak, K. 1982. Associative learning in the isolated siphon, mantle, gill and abdominal ganglion preparation of *Aplysia*: a new paradigm. *Soc. Neurosci. Abstr.* 8: 385.

(62) Lukowiak, K. 1983. Associative learning in an *in vitro Aplysia* preparation: facilitation at a sensory motor neuron synapse. *Soc. Neurosci. Abstr.* 9: 169.

(63) Lukowiak, K., and Sahley, C. 1981. The *in vitro* classical conditioning of the gill withdrawal reflex of *Aplysia californica. Science* 212: 1516-1518.

(64) Montarolo, P.G.; Castellucci, V.F.; Goelet, P.; Kandel, E.R.; and Schacher, S. 1985. Long-term facilitation of the monosynaptic connection between sensory neurons and motor neurons of the gill withdrawal reflex in *Aplysia* in dissociated cell culture. *Soc. Neurosci. Abstr.* 11: 795.

(65) Nolen, T.G.; Marcus, E.; and Carew, T.J. 1985. Development of learning and memory in *Aplysia*: III Central neuronal correlates. *Soc. Neurosci. Abstr.* 11: 643.

(66) Ocorr, K.A., and Byrne, J.H. 1984. Characterization of phosphodiesterase from *Aplysia* pleural ganglia. *Soc. Neurosci. Abstr.* 10: 270.

(67) Ocorr, K.A., and Byrne, J.H. 1985. Membrane responses and changes in cAMP levels in *Aplysia* sensory neurons produced by 5-HT, Tryptamine, FMRF amide and SCP_B. *Neurosci. L.* 55: 113-118.

(68) Ocorr, K.A.; Tabata, M.; and Byrne, J.H. 1985. Cyclic AMP, a common biochemical locus for the effects of 5HT and SCP_B but not FMRF amide in tail sensory neurons of *Aplysia. Soc. Neurosci. Abstr.* 11: 481.

(69) Occor, K.A.; Walters, E.T.; and Byrne, J.H. 1983. Associative conditioning analog in *Aplysia* tail sensory neurons selectively increases cAMP content. *Soc. Neurosci. Abstr.* 9: 169.

(70) Ocorr, K.A.; Walters, E.T.; and Byrne, J.H. 1985. Associative conditioning analog selectively increases cAMP levels of tail sensory neurons in *Aplysia. Proc. Natl. Acad. Sci.* 82: 2538-2552.

(71) Ohmori, H. 1982. Development of posttetanic potentiation at identified inhibitory and excitatory synapses in *Aplysia*. *J. Physl.* 322: 223-240.

(72) Ohmori, H.; Rayport, S.G.; and Kandel, E.R. 1981. Emergence of posttetanic potentiation as a distinct phase in the differentiation of an identified synapse in *Aplysia*. *Science* 213: 1016-1018.

(73) Olson, L., and Jacklet, J.W. 1984. Identification of circadian clock fibers in the CNS of *Aplysia*. *Soc. Neurosci. Abstr.* 9: 624.

(74) Ono, J., and McCaman, R.E. 1984. Immunocytochemical localization and direct assays of serotonin-containing neurons in *Aplysia*. *Neuroscience* 11: 549-560.

(75) Pinsker, H.M.; Hening, W.A.; Carew, T.J,: and Kandel, E.R. 1973. Long-term sensitization of a defensive withdrawal reflex in *Aplysia*. *Science* 182: 1039-1042.

(76) Pinsker, H.; Kupfermann, I.; Castellucci, V.; and Kandel, E.R. 1970. Habituation and dishabituation of the gill-withdrawal reflex in *Aplysia*. *Science* 167: 1740-1742.

(77) Pollack, J.D.; Camardo, J.S.; Bernier, L.; Schwartz, J.H.; and Kandel, E.R. 1982. Pleural sensory neurons in *Aplysia*: a new population for studying the biochemistry and biophysics of serotonin modulation of K^+ currents. *Soc. Neurosci. Abstr.* 8: 523.

(78) Quinn, W.G. 1984. Work in invertebrates on the mechanisms underlying learning. In *The Biology of Learning*, eds. P. Marler and H.S. Terrance, pp. 197-246. Dahlem Konferenzen. Berlin, Heidelberg, New York, Tokyo: Springer-Verlag.

(79) Rankin, C.H., and Carew, T.J. 1985. Development of learning and memory in *Aplysia*: II. Habituation, sensitization and short-term memory. *Soc. Neurosci. Abstr.* 11: 643.

(80) Rayport, S.G., and Camardo, J.S. 1984. Differential emergence of cellular mechanisms mediating habituation and sensitization in the developing *Aplysia* nervous system. *J. Neurosci.* 4: 2528-2532.

(81) Schwartz, J.H.; Bernier, L.; Castellucci, V.F.; Palazzolo, M.; Saitoh, T.; Stapleton, A.; and Kandel, E.R. 1983. What molecular steps determine the time course of the memory for short-term sensitization in *Aplysia*? *Cold S.H. Quant. Biol.* 68: 811-819.

(82) Schwarz, M., and Susswein, A.J. 1984. A neural pathway for learning that food is inedible in *Aplysia*. *Brain Res.* 294: 363-366.

(83) Schuster, M.J.; Camardo, J.S.; Siegelbaum, S.A.; and Kandel, E.R. 1985. Cyclic AMP-dependent protein kinase closes the serotonin-sensitive K^+ channels of *Aplysia* sensory neurons in cell-free membrane patches. *Nature* 131: 392-395.

(84) Siegelbaum, S.A.; Camardo, J.S.; and Kandel, E.R. 1982. Serotonin and cyclic AMP close single K+ channels in *Aplysia* sensory neurones. *Nature* 299: 413-417.

(85) Susswein, A.J., and Schwarz, M. 1983. A learned change of response to inedible food in *Aplysia*. *Behav. Neural Biol.* 39: 1-6.

(86) Walsh, J.H., and Byrne, J.H. 1985. Cyclic AMP and calcium sensitivity of the 5-HT response in tail sensory neurons of *Aplysia*. *Soc. Neurosci. Abstr.* 11: 789.

(87) Walsh, J.H., and Byrne, J.H. 1986. Forskolin mimics and blocks a serotonin-sensitive decreased K+ conductance in tail sensory neurons of *Aplysia*. *Neurosci. L.*, in press.

(88) Walters E.T., and Byrne, J.H. 1983. Associative conditioning of single sensory neurons suggests a cellular mechanism for learning. *Science* 219: 405-408.

(89) Walters, E.T., and Byrne, J.H. 1983. Slow depolarization produced by associative conditioning of *Aplysia* sensory neurons may enhance Ca++ entry. *Brain Res.* 280: 165-168.

(90) Walters, E.T., and Byrne, J.H. 1985. Long-term enhancement produced by activity-dependent modulation of *Aplysia* sensory neurons. *J. Neurosci.* 5: 662-672.

(91) Walters, E.T., Byrne, J.H.; Carew, T.J.; and Kandel, E.R. 1983. Mechanoafferent neurons innervating the tail of *Aplysia*. I. Response properties and synaptic connections. *J. Neurophysl.* 50: 1522-1542.

(92) Walters, E.T.; Byrne, J.H.; Carew, T.J.; and Kandel, E.R. 1983. Mechanoafferent neurons innervating the tail of *Aplysia*. II Modulation by sensitizing stimuli. *J. Neurophysl.* 50: 1543-1559.

(93) Walters, E.T.; Carew, T.J.; and Kandel, E.R. 1978. Conflict and response selection in the locomotor system of *Aplysia*. *Soc. Neurosci. Abstr.* 4: 209.

(94) Walters, E.T.; Carew, T.J.; and Kandel, E.R. 1979. Classical conditioning in *Aplysia californica*. *Proc. Natl. Acad. Sci.* 76: 6675-6679.

(95) Walters, E.T.; Carew, T.J.; and Kandel, E.R. 1981. Associative learning in *Aplysia*: evidence for conditioned fear in an invertebrate. *Science* 211: 504-506.

The Neural and Molecular Bases of Learning,
eds. J.-P. Changeux and M. Konishi, pp. 205–238.
John Wiley & Sons Limited.

Conditioning-specific Modification of Postsynaptic Membrane Currents in Mollusc and Mammal

D.L. Alkon, J. Disterhoft, and D. Coulter

Section on Neural Systems, Laboratory of Biophysics, NINCDS
Marine Biological Laboratory
Woods Hole, MA 02543, USA

Abstract. Classical conditioning of the nudibranch mollusc *Hermissenda crassicornis* was specifically correlated with the reduction of voltage-dependent K^+ current across the soma membrane of identified neurons (the type B cells). This K^+ current reduction has a duration (at least for days) not previously observed for changes of ionic current flux across membranes of differentiated neurons. Conditioning-specific reduction of K^+ currents was shown to be intrinsic to the type B soma membrane, predictive of motoneuron changes, and capable of producing the learned behavioral response in living animals. Other observations indicate that persistent K^+ current reduction results from temporally and stimulus-specific depolarization of the type B cell together with elevation of $Ca^{2+}{}_i$. $Ca^{2+}{}_i$-mediated reduction of K^+ currents appears to involve synergistic interaction of $Ca^{2+}{}_i$-calmodulin and Ca^{2+}- and lipid-dependent phosphorylation of type B cell proteins.

More recently, classical conditioning of the rabbit was specifically correlated with reduction of post-impulse afterhyperpolarization recorded from CA1 neurons in hippocampal slices. The afterhyperpolarization measured arises, at least in part, from activation of a Ca^{2+}-dependent K^+ current, $I_{Ca^{2+}-K^+}$, similar to that reduced in conditioned type B cells of *Hermissenda*. Conditioning-specific reduction of the afterhyperpolarization, and thus $I_{Ca^{2+}-K^+}$, persists for at least 24-32 hours and, because it was measured in hippocampal slices, cannot be explained as simply reflecting conditioning-induced changes elsewhere in the brain.

These molluscan and mammalian K^+ current changes, occurring within a new biophysical temporal domain, were not measured in presynaptic endings, rather they were observed in what can be broadly considered as postsynaptic neuronal compartments. It is suggested that the distribution of such conditioning-induced biophysical transformations can provide a record of associative memory which is recalled by voltage-dependent activation of the involved currents during subsequent conditioned stimulus presentations.

INTRODUCTION

Animal preparations with comparatively few neurons offer the possibility of relating cellular and subcellular processes to learning and memory. A number of such learning preparations have been developed over the last decade including aversive conditioning of *Pleurobranchaea* (31, 49), food aversion of *Limax* (54), habituation and sensitization of *Aplysia* (43), conditioning of *Aplysia* (see Carew, this volume), and Pavlovian conditioning of *Hermissenda* (3, 29, 47). Cellular modifications have been clearly related to long-term (days) behavioral change with the last two preparations. With *Aplysia*, changes in the magnitude of excitatory postsynaptic potentials have been related to retention of the nonassociative behavioral changes, habituation, and sensitization. With *Hermissenda*, increased neuronal excitability and reduction of intrinsic membrane K^+ currents have been related to retention of a learned association between a conditioned (CS) and an unconditioned stimulus (UCS).

At the outset, the usefulness of the nudibranch mollusc *Hermissenda crassicornis* as a model system for analysis of learning behavior (3, 9, 10) and its cellular basis was conceived of in terms of potential relevance to mammalian learning. The question of this possible relevance of molluscan to mammalian learning, in fact, motivated much of the experimental strategies undertaken. It motivated the criteria chosen for what would be considered as learning, the nature of the sensory stimuli to be presented during training, the requirements for establishing mechanisms of acquisition, storage, and recall, and later the approach for demonstrating that such mechanisms were actually shared by a mammalian species (9-11, 33).

CRITERIA FOR LEARNING

Although there is no doubt that nonassociative phenomena (i.e., phenomena elicited by single stimuli) such as sensory adaptation, habituation, and sensitization are important for mammalian experience, the relationship of such phenomena to long-term memory is still unclear. Sensory adaptation is by definition a transient phenomenon: receptors adapt in response to intense and prolonged stimulation, but they lose their adaptation in the absence of such stimulation and thereby regain their sensitivity to less intense stimuli. Similarly, an intense stimulus such as a loud noise can cause generalized arousal but the arousal dissipates and the potential for arousal is restored – this is the adaptive function of arousal. Habituation of limb withdrawal in response to a light touch is also transient or can be eliminated by either an arousing stimulus or stronger touch. For a behaving mammal sensory adaptation, habituation, and sensitization are characteristically reversible while mammalian memory is only initially reversible and is ultimately nonreversible. Mammalian memory usually has another essential feature absent from nonassociative behavioral change: it is predictive. Learned stimulus relationships endow a stimulus with a new meaning for the animal: a single stimulus predicts the occurrence of one or more other stimuli.

Associative learning was therefore sought for a molluscan species in which convergence of two distinct sensory pathways could be demonstrated within a neural system, in this case that of the nudibranch *Hermissenda crassicornis* (2, 4, 5). For *Hermissenda* it was possible to demonstrate an associative behavioral change whose retention is distinct from habituation and/or sensitization and which involves a learned relationship (of stimuli) which is clearly predictive.

Light of weak to moderate intensity (10^1 - 10^4 ergs/cm^2·s) attracts *Hermissenda* (3). This attraction is manifest with a number of behavioral measures. *Hermissenda* move up a gradient of light, i.e, toward the light source (3, 29). During this movement the undersurface of the animal, known as a "foot," elongates (see Fig. 1 and (47)). When the animal initiates movement toward the light the elongation is measurable. *Hermissenda* will also turn toward a light at a light-dark border or edge, i.e., they withdraw and turn away from darkness (42). All of these responses to light will diminish when light is presented repeatedly and/or over a long period of time or when light of great intensity ($> 10^4$ ergs/cm^2·s) is used. None of these responses *remain* diminished hours or days after prolonged exposure to light. Thus, there is no long-lasting sensory adaptation or habituation with light stimuli effective for attracting the animal nor are there any persistent sensitizing or arousing effects of such visual stimulation.

Rotation of *Hermissenda* has an adversive effect. The animal responds to diminish the effect of rotation by moving toward or down a gravitational field. *Hermissenda*, for instance, move toward the center of a rotating table. Also consistent with the adversive quality rotation has for *Hermissenda* is its clinging response (3). At the onset of rotation *Hermissenda* cling to a surface, shortening its "foot" in the process (see Fig. 1 and (47)). Again there is no long-lasting habituation or

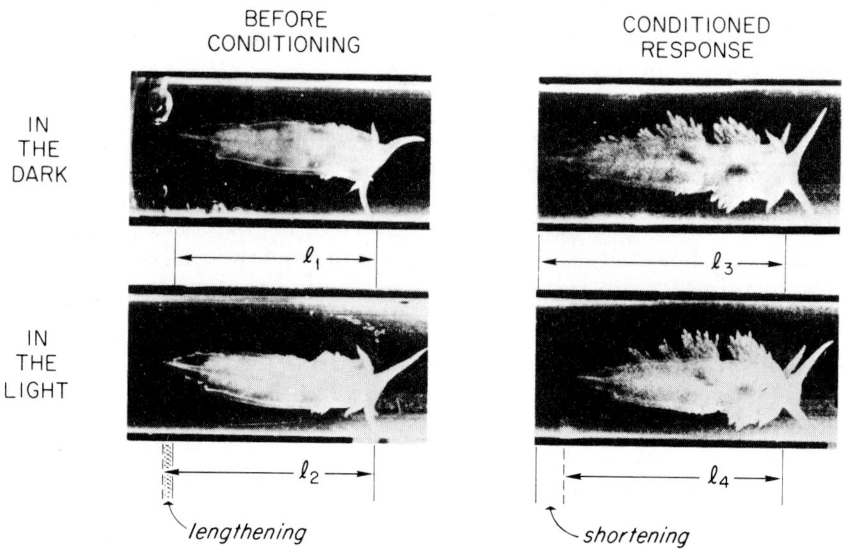

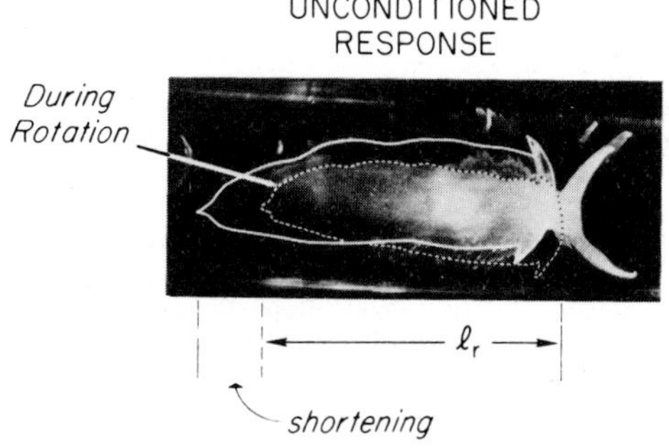

FIG. 1 – Photographic representation of classically conditioned responses of *Hermissenda* foot. Bottom panel is an overlay of two photographs, both taken in the dark; solid white line is the outline of the foot 1 s before rotation; dashed line is the outline of the foot after 3 s of rotation at 97 rpm. Upper panels: comparisons of lengths in the light to lengths in the dark before and after conditioning with paired light and rotation stimuli. l_1: length in the dark before training. l_2: length in the light before training. $l_2 > l_1$ = lengthening. l_3: length in the dark during retention of learned behavior. l_4: length in the light during retention. $l_3 > l_4$ = shortening. l_r: length during rotation was always smaller than before rotation began.

sensitization following rotation of frequencies and durations (2.0 g, 25 s, or 0.5 Hz) used to elicit the responses described or for training (see below).

Repeated presentation of light paired with rotation (whose maximal onset follows that of light by 500 ms and whose offset is simultaneous with that of light) results in a new behavioral response to light: shortening of the foot (see Figs. 1, 2 and (47)). During the first five seconds of light onset, conditioned *Hermissenda* shorten their foot. As described above, before training with paired light and rotation, *Hermissenda* lengthen their foot in response to light. This new response to light closely resembles the old response to rotation, a response not affected by training. As defined behaviorally, as a result of conditioning, light predicts the occurrence of rotation. The meaning of rotation (the UCS) for *Hermissenda*, also defined behaviorally as a result of conditioning, has been transferred to or associated with another stimulus: light (the CS). This learned response to light does not follow training with light and rotation stimuli, which are explicitly unpaired or are presented with a randomly occurring temporal relationship (Fig. 2), nor does the new response follow training with rotation which precedes light. Manifestation of conditioning-specific behavioral change is also apparent with other measures of *Hermissenda* responses to light. Conditioned *Hermissenda* move less readily toward a light source (29) and are less able to withdraw at a light-dark border (46). In addition to pairing specificity and a transfer of meaning from one stimulus to the other, conditioning-specific modification of *Hermissenda* visual responses show other characteristics of vertebrate classical conditioning: stimulus specificity (35), acquisition, retention for at least several weeks (41), a requirement for contingency (34), extinction (53), and savings (29).

NATURE OF TRAINING STIMULI AND RELEVANT NEURAL SYSTEMS

The choice of stimuli used to train *Hermissenda* (light and rotation) was made with the aim of maximizing the possibility that the learning behavior and its cellular mechanisms would be conserved during the course of evolution. We began by hypothesizing that with a sufficiently advanced species (such as a gastropod mollusc) there would be an elementary neural system with the necessary features for learning to associate distinct stimuli. We hypothesized further that these necessary features of the elementary neural system would also appear in much more advanced species, perhaps even mammals.

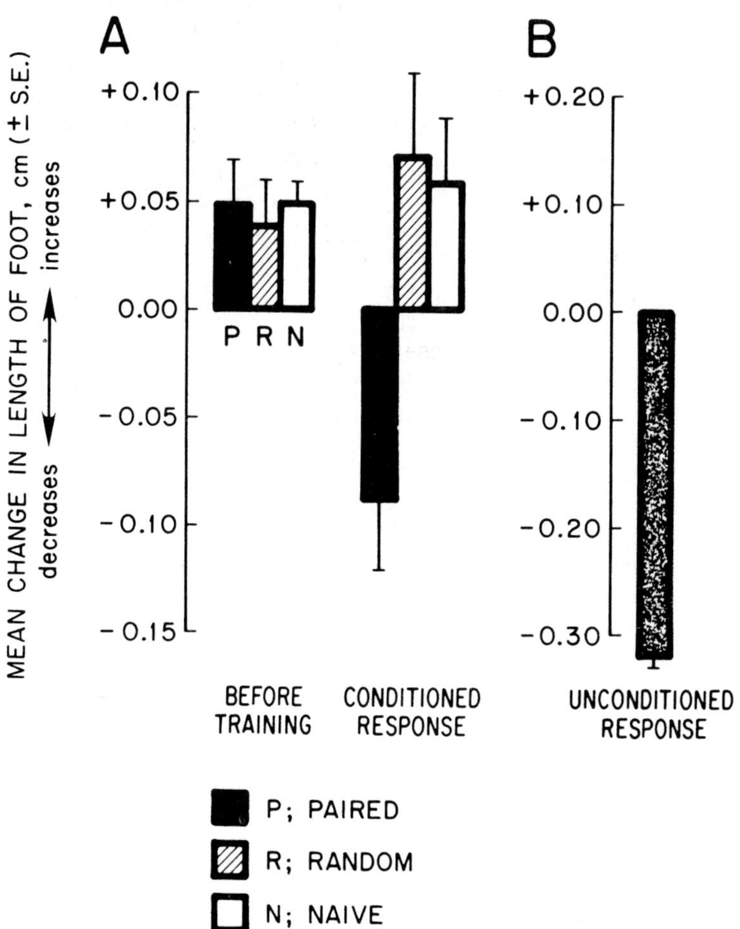

FIG. 2 – Classical conditioning origin of a new response to light in *Hermissenda*. A: Left – before training, foot length increased in response to light onset. Right – after training, Random and Naive groups continue to show light-elicited lengthening but Paired animals have become conditioned to shorten the length of the foot in response to a light stimulus. B: Unconditioned response (UCR) after 6 s of rotation. The conditioned response is about 28% of the UCR. Note the difference in scale between panels A and B (47).

To test these hypotheses it was considered essential to stimulate the neural systems as they had evolved to be stimulated, i.e., training and testing of a gastropod must be accomplished with stimuli which would be transduced and processed by the neural system(s) in a manner at least resembling what occurs in a natural setting. For example, light and rotation are the preferred stimuli of specialized sensory receptors, photoreceptors (14), and "hair cells" (5, 12, 40, 61) in specialized sensory organs (the eyes and statocysts) which send synaptic signals to particular interneurons (2, 38) and motoneurons (38) important for mediating behavioral responses such as turning, foot contraction, etc. In addition, these distinct sensory pathways have well-defined loci of convergence where the two distinct sensory stimuli send signals to the same cells. Intersensory convergence in *Hermissenda* occurs on both the sensory receptors themselves as well as on interneurons (62).

Training with natural stimuli, mediated by an animal's existing sensory pathways and their convergence (Figs. 3A, B), is in contrast to training with stimuli (such as diffuse electric shock) never encountered in the animal's environment and not mediated by discrete well-defined neural pathways. Diffuse electric shock administered to a gastropod appendage or body part can travel through nonneural tissue as well as neural tissue along routes never taken during the animal's natural experience and thus routes not having evolved for their adaptive value. Behavioral and neural change produced with such stimuli do not necessarily require mechanisms which are conserved in evolution and thus which are likely to appear in other more advanced species.

ESTABLISHING MECHANISMS OF ACQUISITION, STORAGE, AND RECALL

The process by which behavioral phenomenology of associative learning is translated into and arises out of biophysical and biochemical phenomena may be able to be conserved over evolutionary time. Although the complexity of neural systems is vastly greater in a mammal, the underlying cell biology involved in storage and recall of learned information may be common to mollusc and mammal. It was thought possible, therefore, that the cellular mechanisms required for a learned association may be first uncovered in a relatively simple system and later sought and found in a mammalian nervous system. The only long-term (days) storage and recall mechanism as yet demonstrated for learning an association involves persistent reduction of voltage-dependent K^+ currents across neuronal membranes. Evidence of such a mechanism, first discovered in *Hermissenda*, has in fact been recently

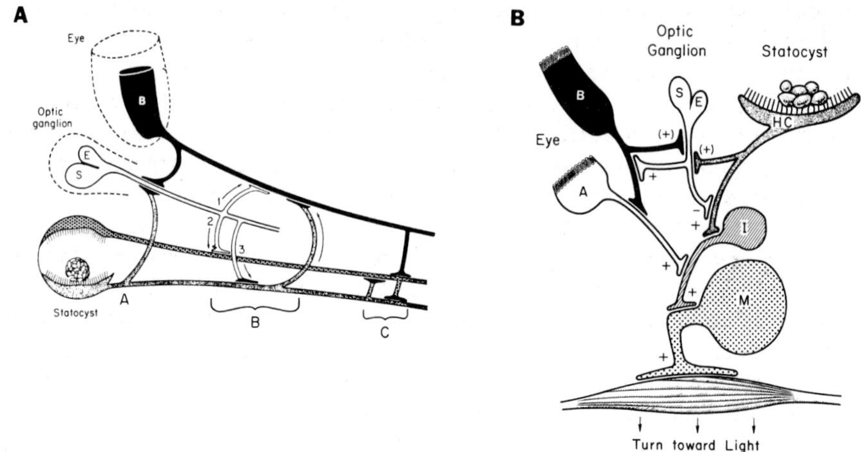

FIG. 3 – A: Intersensory integration by the *Hermissenda* nervous system. A shows convergence of synaptic inhibition from type B and caudal hair cells on S-E cell. B indicates positive synaptic feedback onto type B photoreceptor. 1 indicates direct synaptic excitation; 2 indicates indirect excitation: E-S excites cephalic hair cell that inhibits caudal hair cell and thus disinhibits type B cell. 3 indicates indirect excitation: E-S inhibits caudal hair cell and thus disinhibits type B cell. Indirect excitation where B cell inhibits C cell, and thus disinhibits E cell, is at the bottom. C cell effects are not illustrated. C indicates intra- and intersensory inhibition. Cephalic and caudal hair cells are mutually inhibitory. Type B cell inhibits mainly the cephalic hair cell. All filled endings indicate inhibitory synapses; open endings indicate excitatory synapses. From Tabata and Alkon, 1982.
B: Schematic diagram of visual pathway and its convergence with the statocyst pathway. The type B photoreceptor (B) causes monosynaptic inhibition of the medial type A photoreceptor (A). The medial type A photoreceptor causes monosynaptic excitation of ipsilateral interneurons (I), which are also excited by ipsilateral hair cells (HC). Ipsilateral HC impulses and type B impulses cause a transient inhibition (not shown here) and are followed by long lasting effective excitation (+) of the S/E optic ganglion cell and thereby the type B cell (38).

shown (see below) for CA1 neurons of hippocampal slices obtained from classically conditioned (but not control) rabbits (28, 32, 33). Reduction of a steady-state K^+ current has been implicated as a short-term (many minutes) storage mechanism for nonassociative and associative learning of *Aplysia* (see Carew, this volume).

Before seeking cellular principles in a mammal analogous to those in a gastropod, it was obviously desirable that such principles be shown unequivocally to play a significant role in the lower form. Again, crucial issues for establishing learning mechanisms had to be confronted. Prior to the work on *Hermissenda*, elegant and valuable electrophysiologic correlates had been observed with long-term (days) associative learning of vertebrate species (21-24, 26, 42, 44, 48, 63, 64, 66-69). Specific and clear correlation of neural change with long-term (days) associative learning of behaving animals has been repeatedly found in many different independent studies with *Hermissenda* (17, 19, 30, 35, 39, 53, 65). Neuronal responses to the same light stimuli used for testing intact animals were modified in the conditioned *Hermissenda* at every major stage of sensory, interneuronal, and motoneuron interaction. Conditioning-specific increase of type B photoreceptor excitability, for example, was manifest by a longer light-elicited depolarization, increase of impulse activity, and a larger, voltage change (in darkness) in response to injection of current through a microelectrode. Thus, independent of phototransduction, the resistance of the type B soma membrane to current flow had increased with conditioning. This greater type B input resistance in darkness was later shown to result from conditioning-specific reduction of two commonly encountered voltage-dependent K^+ currents (13, 16-20): an early 4-aminopyridine-sensitive K^+ current known as I_A and a slower K^+ current dependent on intracellular levels of Ca^{2+}, known as $I_{Ca^{2+}-K^+}$. These currents, I_A and $I_{Ca^{2+}-K^+}$, were extensively characterized with macroscopic voltage clamp analysis (e.g., see Figs. 4A, B) and have now been characterized at the level of single channels using cell-attached and inside-out patch clamp techniques (59). A number of observations helped resolve another crucial issue for identifying a learning mechanism, namely whether conditioning-specific neural changes are primary or secondary. Do they result from changes residing within a given neuron (such as the type B cell) or are they simply a passive reflection or consequence of neurohumoral and/or synaptic input from some other neuron(s) which are themselves sites where conditioning-specific changes reside? The type B cell somata were isolated from animals which had on preceding days been conditioned with paired light and rotation or exposed to control procedures. Blind measurements of I_A and $I_{Ca^{2+}-K^+}$ (Figs. 5-8) revealed a conditioning-specific reduction of these currents (in the absence of any change in resting potential). Thus the *Hermissenda* studies provided the first demonstration of learning-induced neuronal changes which were unequivocally *intrinsic* to particular cells and which could not be due of a change to tonic neurohumoral or synaptic input.

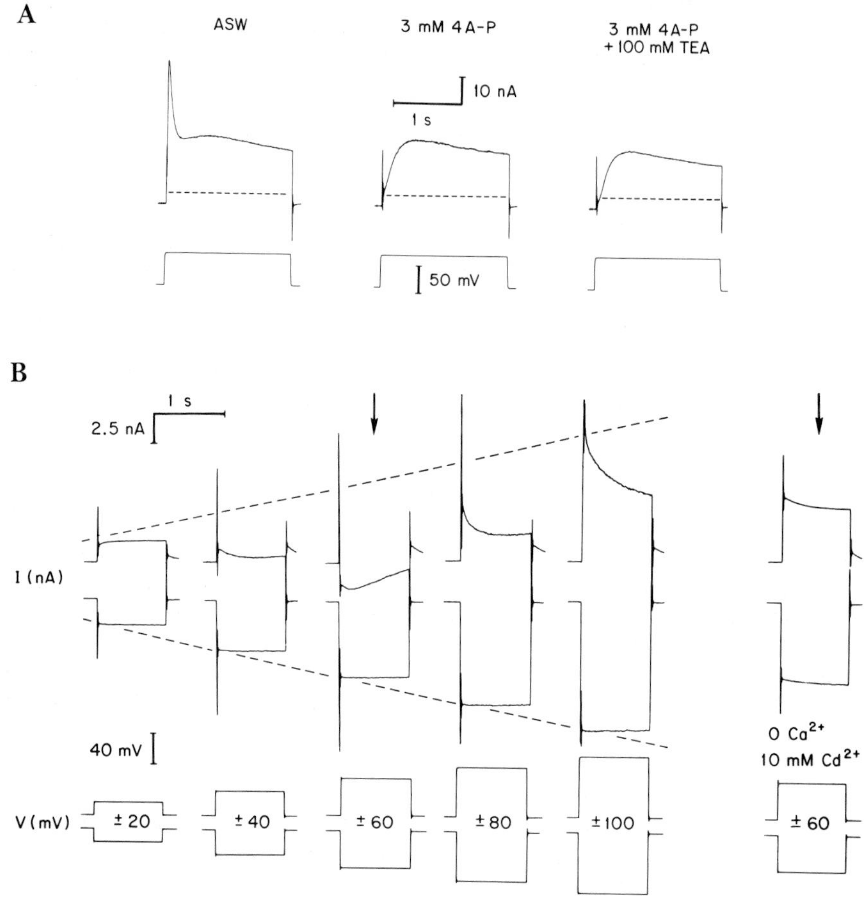

Because the type B cell is presynaptic to all known visual pathway neurons of *Hermissenda*, conditioning-specific reduction of its K+ currents and the consequent increase of excitability are almost certain to have impact on visually guided behavior of the animal. In fact, blind measurements of type B input resistance changes with conditioning predict the degree of conditioning-induced modification of neuronal responses at the output stage of the visual pathway (39). Further evidence of the primary or causal role of type B membrane changes is provided by experiments in which these changes are produced artificially (20, 36, 37). Current injected through a microelectrode

FIG. 4 – A: voltage-dependent outward currents across the membrane of the isolated type B cell soma are shown. The bathing solutions are, from left to right, ASW, 3 mM, 4 A-P added to ASW, and 3 mM 4 A-P and 100 mM TEA added to ASW. Note that addition of 4 A-P and TEA removes only a small portion of the late outward current elicited by command to 0 mV from a holding potential of -60 mV. The dashed lines indicate the level of the nonvoltage-dependent or leak current (13).
B: records of voltage-dependent inward current present in a type B photoreceptor are shown under conditions of 100 mM external Ba^{2+} and K^{+} current blockers (10 mM 4 A-P, 100 mM TEA). From a holding potential of -60 mV, successive command steps in multiples of 20 mV reveal activation of an inward current at potentials more positive than -40 mV. This current increases nonlinearly, reaching its peak value at 0 mV (left arrow) and diminishes thereafter. Note that at 0 mV (absolute) the inward current decreases substantially from its maximum amplitude. Such a decrease was eliminated when substitution of Ba^{2+} for Ca^{2+} in the ASW was preceded by a thorough washing with 0 Ca^{2+}-ASW. From a holding potential of -60 mV, successive commands to potentials less than -60 mV elicit a nonvoltage-dependent leak current, indicated by the lower dashed lines. The upper dashed line is extrapolated from potentials less than or equal to -50 mV. Note than when 10 mM Cd^{2+} is substituted for Ca^{2+} in the external bathing medium the current elicited by the command to 0 mV (absolute) begins to approach the extrapolated leak level (indicated by the dashed line) (13).

---

causes potential changes which simulate the synaptic network effects of paired light and rotation. Appropriate pairing of such current injections with light stimuli will cause enhanced type B cell excitability in living animals, within isolated nervous systems, and as an isolated soma. These artificially induced type B cell changes in li ing animals cause reduction of phototactic behavior similar to that observed with conditioning (37) while unpaired type B cell injection procedures had no effects significantly different from sham-operated animals (i.e., in which type B cells received no current injection).

How do these primary membrane changes of type B cells arise during conditioning, i.e., how are they stored and how are they evoked on subsequent days by CS presentations – how are they recalled? A large number of experimental findings are consistent with the following sequence of underlying cellular events.

In response to a single pairing of light and rotation, the type B cell undergoes greater and more prolonged depolarization (7, 15). This depolarization is the resultant of the integrated visual-vestibular network response to stimulus pairing and is an electrophysiologic expression of pairing-specificity as well as a stimulus specificity of

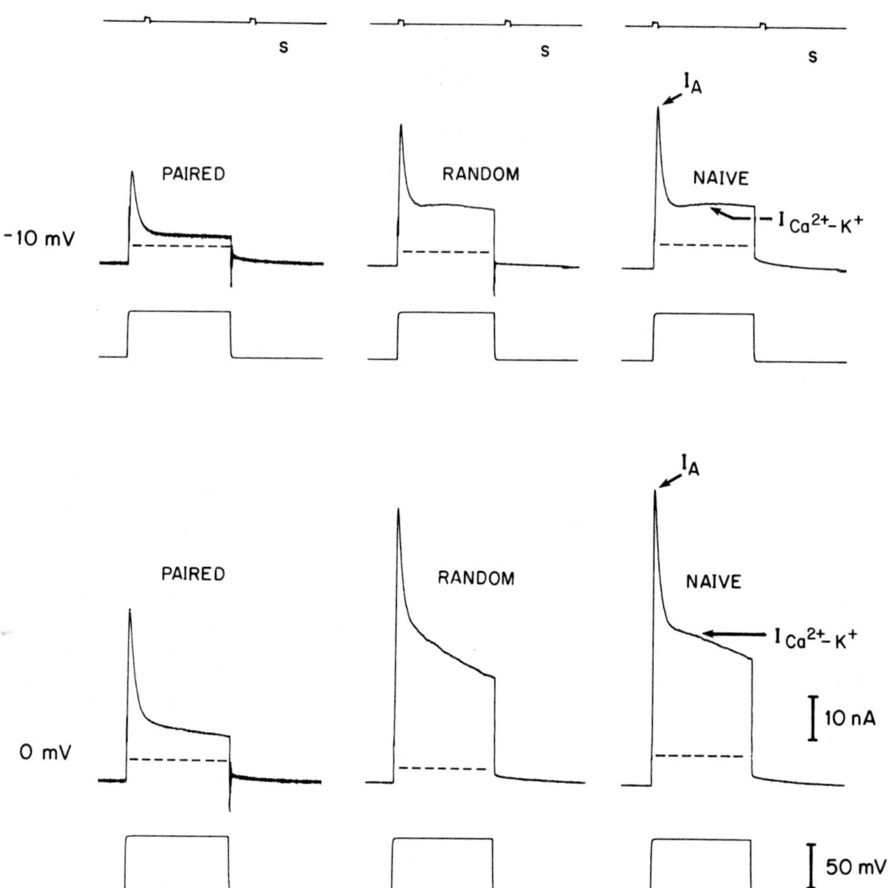

FIG. 5 – Comparison of voltage-dependent K^+ currents measured in type B somata isolated from Paired, Random, and Naive animals one and two days after training experience. The records were chosen to illustrate the reduction of I_A and $I_{Ca^{2+}-K^+}$ for Paired as compared to Random and Naive animals (19).

initial associative learning. In response to repeated pairings of light and rotation, depolarization of the type B cell becomes progressively greater and more prolonged (7, 30). This cumulative type B depolarization, accompanied by prolonged elevation of intracellular Ca^{2+}_i (27) is a cellular expression of the acquisition phase (or increase with practice) of the associative learning. As some evidence suggests, elevated Ca^{2+}_i

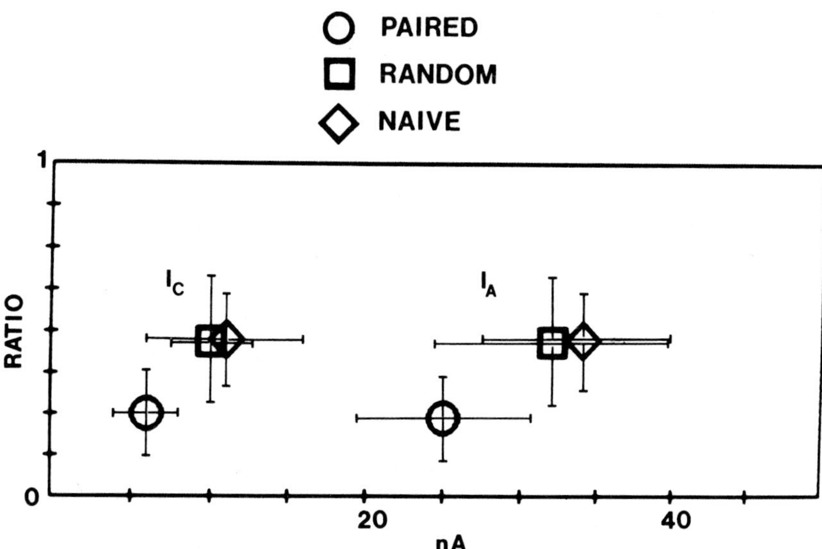

FIG. 6 – Mean phototaxis suppression ratios in relation to ionic current magnitude. For individual animals of each group (Paired:○; Random: □; and Naive:◇) a suppression ratio was obtained and the magnitude of $I_{Ca^{2+}-K^+}$ (on the left) and I_A was measured at – 10 mV (absolute) across the isolated soma membrane of the medial type B cell. The values presented (±S.D.) are the mean ionic currents ($I_{Ca^{2+}-K^+}$ and I_A) measured in relation to the mean suppression ratio for each group. The paired mean ratios and ionic currents are all clearly lower than for the Random and Naive groups (19).

and type B depolarization possibly cause, via Ca^{2+}-dependent phosphorylation of cellular proteins, long-lasting reduction of I_A and $I_{Ca^{2+}-K^+}$ (Figs. 9, 10; (1, 10, 18, 20, 52, 55, 58)). Thus on subsequent days, during which the learned associa ion is retained, I_A and $I_{Ca^{2+}-K^+}$ remain reduced while the type B membrane potential and $Ca^{2+}{}_i$ have returned to normal levels. Persistent reduction of I_A and $I_{Ca^{2+}-K^+}$ is, then, a cellular expression of the behaviorally manifest retention of the associative learning. It should be noted that I_A and $I_{Ca^{2+}-K^+}$ are not significantly activated across the type B membrane at resting levels of potential, i.e., for the unstimulated type B cell. When the type B cell depolarizes, however, in response to subsequent presentations of light stimuli (the CS) I_A and $I_{Ca^{2+}-K^+}$ are significantly activated because of their steep voltage dependence. It is only for the stimulated type B cell, therefore, that the stored learned information becomes expressed, i.e.,

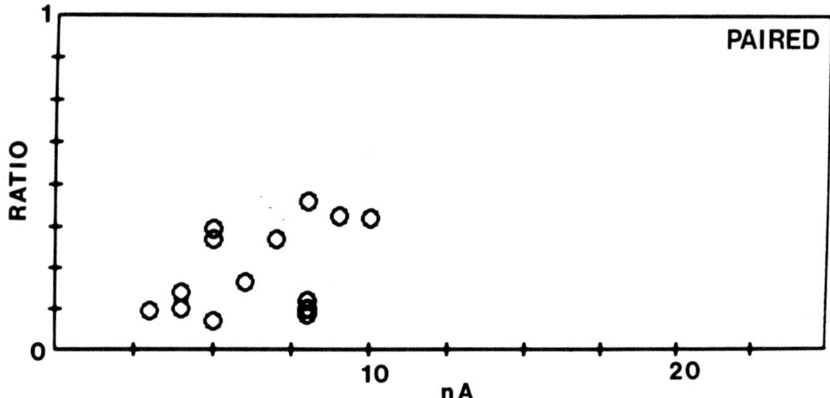

FIG. 7 – Phototaxis suppression ratio in relation to $I_{Ca^{2+}-K^{+}}50$ magnitude for the Paired group. For each animal a suppression ratio was obtained and the magnitude of $I_{Ca^{+}-K^{+}}$ was measured at –10 mV (absolute) across the isolated soma membrane of the medial type B cell. The ratio is significantly correlated with the current magnitude (19).

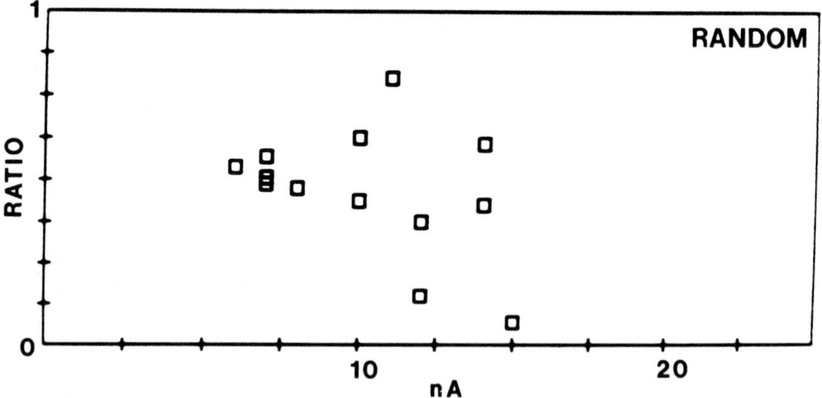

FIG. 8 – Phototaxis suppression ratio in relation to $I_{Ca^{2+}-K}50$ magnitude for the Random group. For each animal a suppression ratio was obtained and the magnitude of $I_{Ca^{2+}-K^{+}}$ was measured at –10 mV (absolute) across the isolated soma membrane of the medial type B cell. The ratio is not significantly correlated with the current magnitude (19).

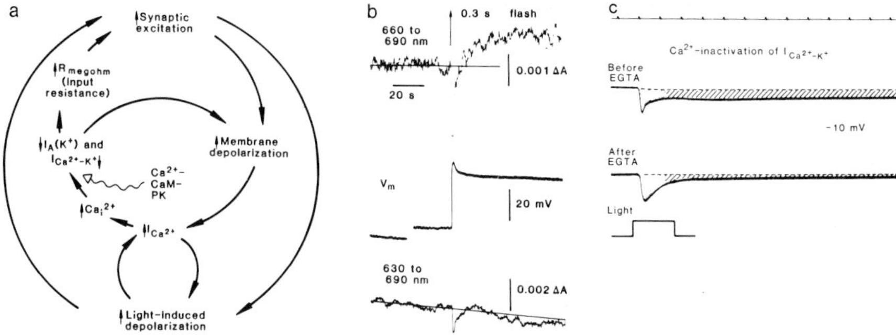

FIG. 9 – a) Regenerative synaptic- and light-induced excitation of the type B photoreceptor. Light-induced depolarization facilitates synaptic excitation and vice versa in response to temporally associated light and rotation. Analyzed in biophysical terms synaptic depolarization causes transient activation, prolonged inactivation of I_A and $I_{Ca^{2+}-K^+}$, and enhancement of a voltage-dependent Ca^{2+} current. Increased intracellular Ca^{2+} causes further inactivation of I_A and $I_{Ca^{2+}-K^+}$ and thus a further increase of effective input resistance. These in turn cause more membrane depolarization. Inactivation of I_A and $I_{Ca^{2+}-K^+}$ by elevated intracellular Ca^{2+} may occur via increased activity of Ca^{2+}-calmodulin-dependent protein kinase (Ca^{2+}-CaM-PK) and C-kinase (10). b) Prolonged elevation of intracellular Ca^{2+} accompanies depolarizing response of isolated type B cell to light. The cell was previously injected with arsenazo III. Absorbance changes at 660- to 690- and 630- to 690- nm wavelength pairs (top and bottom records) and membrane voltage response (middle) after a 0.3 s light flash. Differential absorbance changes at 660 to 690 measure changes of intracellular Ca^{2+} while those at 630 to 690 measure changes of pH (27). c) Ca^{2+} inactivation of $I_{Ca^{2+}-K^+}$. Isolated type B cell soma is placed under voltage clamp at –60 mV in ASW. After 10 minutes' dark adaptation the onset of command depolarizing step to –10 mV (15 seconds) is followed by brief light step ($10^{3.5}$ erg $cm^{-2}s^{-1}$). An apparent long-lasting inward current following the light step results from intracellularly released calcium causing inactivation of steady-state $I_{Ca^{2+}-K^+}$. With the same state of dark adaptation the light-induced decrease of $I_{Ca^{2+}-K^+}$ is reduced after injection (under isopotential conditions) of EGTA (-2.0 nA for 4 min). Calcium inactivation of $I_{Ca^{2+}-K^+}$ occurs in the absence of any inactivation of $I_{Ca^{2+}}$ (18).

recalled. It is the voltage-dependent activation of I_A and $I_{Ca^{2+}-K^+}$ which is the cellular expression of the behavioral phenomenon of recall of the learned association.

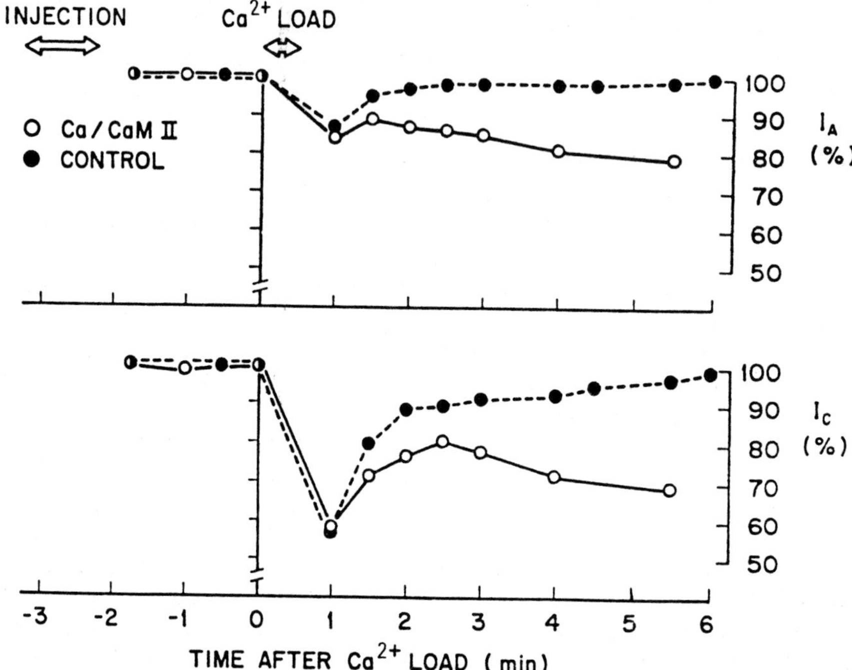

FIG. 10 – Time course of I_A (upper panel) and I_C (lower panel) reduction by CaM kinase II following a Ca^{2+} load. I_A and I_C were measured as the peak outward currents 20 ms (I_A) and 300-400 ms (I_C) from the onset of a command depolarization to -5mV absolute (holding potential = -60 mV). Ca^{2+} loads were given before (closed circles) and after iontophoretic injection of CaM kinase II. I_A and I_C amplitudes before the Ca^{2+} load are normalized as 100%. Note that CaM kinase II injection prevents recovery of I_A and I_C reduction after a Ca^{2+} load (55).

A METHODOLOGIC ASIDE

The biophysical translations of the behavioral phenomenology of learning just described were made possible by direct measurements of the parameters involved. The measurements were made in the type B cell body (an egg-shaped structure with a long diameter of ~40 μm and a short diameter of ~25 μm) which had been axotomized. Since the axon is < 1 μm diameter its removal causes no significant leakage of cellular contents or current and probably seals after axotomy. There are no synaptic endings nor is there an impulse-generating membrane on the cell body. Two and three microelectrodes could then be used to effect voltage-clamp and iontophoretic injection of substances such as Ca^{2+} or

Ca^{2+}-dependent kinases. The learning-specific reduction of ionic currents observed in *Hermissenda* were in the type B cell body, not in its presynaptic endings. This is not to say that similar modification of ionic currents could not also occur in these endings but these would be difficult to directly demonstrate with existing methodology.

MOLECULAR MECHANISMS OF MEMORY STORAGE

Differential absorption spectrophotometry allowed monitoring of the $Ca^{2+}{}_i$ within the cell body (27) and application of microgel techniques provided assessment of protein phosphorylation within *Hermissenda* eyes (each of which contains only five photoreceptors). Conditioning-specific changes (lasting at least 2-3 hours) of Ca^{2+}-dependent phosphorylation of a 20,000 M.W. protein within the eyes (52) suggested a biochemical pathway which might contribute to the transition of short-term to persistent modification of membrane currents during learning. Subsequently, a large number of biochemical manipulations of the cell body yielded results consistent with the hypothesis that Ca^{2+}-calmodulin-dependent phosphorylation acts in synergy with Ca^{2+}- and lipid-dependent phosphorylation to bring about persistent conditioning-specific K^+ current changes. These manipulations included iontophoretic injection of the Ca^{2+}-calmodulin-dependent protein kinase, phosphorylase kinase (1), the type II Ca^{2+}-calmodulin-dependent protein kinase from brain (Fig. 10; (55, 58)), and ionositol triphosphate (58). Other protocols involved activation of the Ca^{2+}- and lipid-dependent kinase (C-kinase) with such agents as phorbol ester (water soluble) (16) and inhibition of phosphorylation with trifluoperazine or calmidazolium. In each case the appropriate control substances (e.g., heat-inactivated enzymes, inositol monophosphate, nonimmune sera, etc.) were always tested in parallel, and in each case the reduction of I_A and $I_{Ca^{2+}-K^+}$ were shown to depend on the elevation of $Ca^{2+}{}_i$ and the consequent activation of Ca^{2+}-dependent phosphorylating enzymes.

Finally, in more recent studies, learning-induced conditions (e.g., prolonged depolarization and elevation of $Ca^{2+}{}_i$) were simulated by exposing whole *Hermissenda* nervous systems to elevated external K^+, veratradine, or activators of the phospholipid and Ca^{2+}-dependent C-kinase (50). Activation of the C-kinase with phorbol ester caused translocation of this enzyme from cytosolic to membrane loci and increased sensitivity to calcium stimulation of low-molecular-weight protein phosphorylation, most notable the 20,000 M.W. protein which showed phosphorylation differences with conditioning. Depolarization conditions (high K^+_o, veratradine) cause phosphorylation differences of the 20,000 M.W. protein as well as a 25,000 M.W. protein (previously shown to be sensitive to an I_A channel blocker, 4-aminopyridine; see (51)). A marked hysteresis in Ca^{2+}-dependent phosphorylation of the 25,000 M.W. protein appeared when the simulating conditions were removed. Thus the nervous systems were only exposed to high K^+_o for a brief period (10 to 30 minutes) but changes of Ca^{2+}-dependent phosphorylation persisted for hours after normal external K^+ was restored.

Although we have some insight as to how storage may be initiated during learning and memory, little is known about the molecular basis for long-term (days) or permanent memory records. In *Hermissenda*, a calcium load after activation of Ca^{2+}/CaM-II kinase together with the C-kinase can reduce I_A and $I_{Ca^{2+}-K^+}$ currents, the same currents changed with conditioning, for 1-3 hours. Thus, initiating biochemical steps involving protein phosphorylation are consistent with the previously observed conditioning-specific difference in phosphorylation of a 20,000 M.W. protein in the *Hermissenda* eyes. In *Aplysia*, serotonin-like substances cause adenylate cyclase activation which is related to reduction of the soma ("S") K^+ current, at least for many minutes.

A molecular mechanism for long-term storage could involve relatively irreversible pre- or posttranslational or a regenerative (positive feedback) process. An example of a biochemical reaction which could participate in a regenerative process involving Ca^{2+}-dependent K^+ current inactivation was proposed some years ago for *Hermissenda* conditioning (8, 9). At that time it was known that Ca^{2+}/CaM-dependent kinases were capable of phosphorylating themselves (autophosphorylation) with very little reversibility. Such autophosphorylation might keep the enzyme in a relatively permanent activated state which in turn could be responsible for further self-activation (and K^+ current reduction) and would persist despite cellular turnover of the enzyme itself. Such regenerative or "self-sustaining" posttranslational processes have really not been demonstrated, though they have been considered plausible by several investigators (see Changeux and Kennedy, both this volume).

MECHANISMS SHARED BY MOLLUSCS AND MAMMALS

Although of some interest to the comparative biologist, the observations on *Hermissenda* learning and its physiology are, in themselves, not of great import. The potential significance of these findings lies in what they may indicate about our own ability to learn and remember. Many differences between the physiology of molluscan and mammalian learning are intuitively obvious. Given that distinct sensory modalities rarely interact in the retina, let alone on retinal receptor cells, we would not expect intrinsic storage of a learned association in rods and cones similar to Ca^{2+}-mediated reduction of K^+ currents in *Hermissenda* type B photoreceptors (where distinct sensory modalities do interact). Given the vast number of neurons in mammalian systems and the clinically evident redundancy with which sensory information can be represented, we would not expect the degree of localization of storage apparent with the *Hermissenda* type B (and more recently type A) cells. Rather we would expect, for even fairly simple associations, representation in a number of brain regions affording a variety of reference frames (e.g., visual, auditory, positional, emotional, etc.) for particular stimulus relationships. We would not expect that production of membrane changes in single neurons (as was shown with the type B cells) could result in the same behavioral change produced by conditioning a mammal. On the contrary, it would seem necessary to stimulate a whole *set* of neuronal changes which were distributed across mammalian brain regions to recreate a learning experience and expression of its recall.

There is also reason, however, to expect some similarity for the physiology of molluscan and mammalian learning. The most common sites of convergence known in mammalian brain are postsynaptic (as described above for the *Hermissenda* type B cell). A myriad of presynaptic inputs converge on the dendritic branches and cell body, for example, of each hippocampal pyramidal cell. It is also known that the ionic currents identified for the type B cell soma membrane also occur on central mammalian neurons such as the pyramidal cells. The two voltage-dependent K^+ currents which are reduced with *Hermissenda* learning (I_A and $I_{Ca^{2+}-K^+}$), as well as other currents such as a sustained inward Ca^{2+} current, ($I_{Ca^{2+}}$) a delayed outward K^+ current, I_{K^+} (the delayed rectifier), and an early inward Na^+ current (I_{Na^+}), have all been identified in hippocampal pyramidal cells, known as CA1 cells (25, 60). Prolonged elevation of $Ca^{2+}{}_i$ (as was measured in the type B somata) was also observed in CA1 cell bodies in response to electrical stimulation of afferent input (45).

Thus, although the geometry and location within the nervous system of convergence sites are radically different in the mammal and the mollusc the biophysical properties of these sites are remarkably similar. The way these convergence sites may change to store learned information might also have considerable similarity. In our studies of rabbit hippocampal slices and conditioning of the nictitating membrane response we asked whether there was any evidence for such similarity. Was there any evidence that neurons undergo intrinsic membrane changes which persist after classical conditioning and resemble those found in *Hermissenda*? Given the intuitive expectation of a distributed set of neuronal changes representing a learned association in a mammal, we were not seeking a conditioning-specific change which had a clearly demonstrable causal relation to a learned behavior (as was possible for *Hermissenda*), nor did we believe that lesion experiments would resolve such an issue. When a lesion eliminates a CR the affected brain area need not be a storage site but simply essential for expresison of learned behavior. Conversely, when a lesion does not eliminate a CR the affected brain area may still store learned information which is expressed in a behavioral change not observable with a particular behavioral assay (such as nictitating membrane closure or eyeball retraction).

Berger and Thompson previously obtained clear changes of extracellular recorded activity of hippocampal pyramidal cells during classical conditioning of the rabbit nictitating membrane (21-23, 63). In this paradigm a tone (CS) is paired with eyeball shock or an air puff to the corneal surface (UCS). During acquisition the tone begins to elicit the same nictitating membrane response as that elicited by the UCS prior to conditioning, and tone also begins to elicit increased impulse activity from CA1 and CA3 hippocampal cells. Was this conditioning-specific increase of impulse activity a manifestation of increased excitability (as was observed for the type B cell), i.e., did it represent a change of membrane currents intrinsic to the hippocampal cells or was it a reflection of augmented synaptic input? If synaptic input was augmented, was this a result of primary or causal modification of neurons presynaptic to the hippocampus?

To address these questions intracellular recordings were made from CA1 cells (now from approximately 1500 cells in three separate studies) within hippocampal slices taken from animals which had one of three training histories (28, 32, 33). Twenty-four to thirty-four hours prior to recording, rabbits had finished three days of classical conditioning (reaching at last 90% successful CRs), pseudoconditioning (with randomized explicitly unpaired tone and shock), or maintenance (i.e., no training). No conditioning-specific differences of membrane potential, input resistance, or impulse amplitude were observed. There was, however, an unequivocal conditioning-specific reduction of the afterhyperpolarization (AHP) in both amplitude and duration, which followed 1-4 impulses elicited by a positive current injection (Figs. 11, 12). For instance, in one study (28) the conditioned AHP ($X = 2.98$ mV $\pm$ S.D. 1.514 ($N = 43$)), following a 100 ms positive pulse eliciting four impulses, was significantly lower ($P < .002$ two-tailed t-test) than the pseudoconditioned AHP ($X = 5.15$ mV $\pm$ S.D. 2.178 ($N = 38$)) as well as the naive AHP ($X = 4.32 \pm$ S.D. 1.92 ($N = 36$)). The magnitude of the conditioning-specific difference increased with the increasing number of preceding impulses ((28) and in preparation). This would not be the case if the AHP differences were simply due to a difference in the K^+ equilibrium potential. The maximum AHP, measured within 300-400 ms of the current pulse onset, is a manifestation of the Ca^{2+}-dependent K^+ current, $I_{Ca^{2+}-K^+}$, previously identified in CA1 cells. Oberservations in other laboratories as well as our own indicate that afterhyperpolarization (measured in this way) is eliminated or drastically reduced by intracellular iontophoresis of EGTA (to buffer $Ca^{2+}{}_i$), replacement of external Ca^{2+} with Ba^{2+}, and/or perfusion with blockers of $I_{Ca^{2+}}$ such as Ca^{2+} or Cd^{2+}. All of these results are consistent with $I_{Ca^{2+}-K^+}$ as the major ionic current underlying the afterhyperpolarization. Thus conditioning-specific reduction of afterhyperpolarization indicates conditioning-specific reduction of the CA1 $I_{Ca^{2+}-K^+}$ just as was observed for *Hermissenda* type B cells. Changes of other currents which might contribute to this conditioning-specific reduction of the AHP cannot yet be ruled out.

Several points of clarification need emphasis. First, since lesions of the hippocampus do not eliminate the CR (see Thompson *et al.*, this volume) the reduction of $I_{Ca^{2+}-K^+}$ within hippocampal CA1 cells cannot bear a causal relation to the acquisition and retention of this response. What has been demonstrated is that training with paired tone and shock (but not unpaired stimuli) produces a modification of $I_{Ca^{2+}-K^+}$ which *is* manifest 1 – 1 1/2 days later. This modification, strikingly similar to $I_{Ca^{2+}-K^+}$ reduction in type B cells (for which there is evidence of a causal role in learning), indicates a new temporal domain of biophysical phenomena – a temporal domain lasting at least days rather than milliseconds, seconds, or minutes. This new temporal domain could be peculiar to the physiology of learning and may represent either a permanent storage mechanism itself or a crucial step toward such a mechanism. Although conditioning-induced reduction of CA1 $I_{Ca^{2+}-K^+}$ does not bear a causal relation to the CR measured here, it

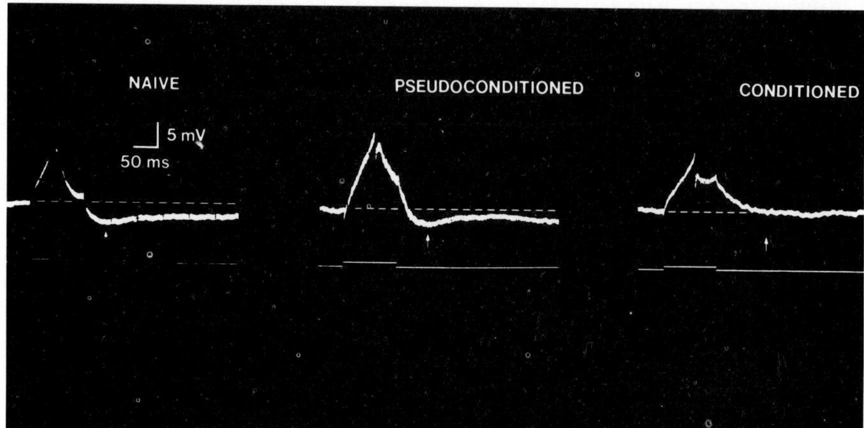

FIG. 11 - AHP after one spike in a naive, pseudoconditioned, and conditioned neuron. A 100 ms depolarizing current pulse sufficient to elicit one action potential was injected into the cell. The AHP can be seen by comparing the voltage response following the depolarizing pulse to the baseline (indicated by the dashed white line in the figure to facilitate comparison). The point where it was measured in these traces is indicated by the arrow. Note that AHP is considerably reduced in the conditioned as compared to the naive and pseudoconditioned neuron. One trace is illustrated for each neuron (33).

could still have such a role in generating another learned response or aspect of learning such as sensory preconditioning which might be assayed with other measuring techniques.

Additional questions to be answered concern both the locus on the CA1 cell of the $I_{Ca^{2+}-K^+}$ modification and the possible contribution of other conditioning-induced changes of ionic currents. For instance, a conditioning-specific reduction of $I_{Ca^{2+}}$, which is indirectly responsible for $I_{Ca^{2+}-K^+}$ (via elevation of $Ca^{2+}{}_i$) cannot yet be ruled out. One approach to resolve this issue consists of iontophoretic injection of Ca^{2+} into CA1 cells from the three groups. If $I_{Ca^{2+}-K^+}$ elicited by such injection were lower for conditioned animals, it would have to be independent of any changes of $I_{Ca^{2+}}$.

It is not at all clear where $I_{Ca^{2+}-K^+}$ is modified on the CA1 cell. The change in afterhyperpolarization is recorded from the cell body but it may arise elsewhere, for example, on the CA1 dendritic branches. Most of this afterhyperpolarization appears to be a function of the number of

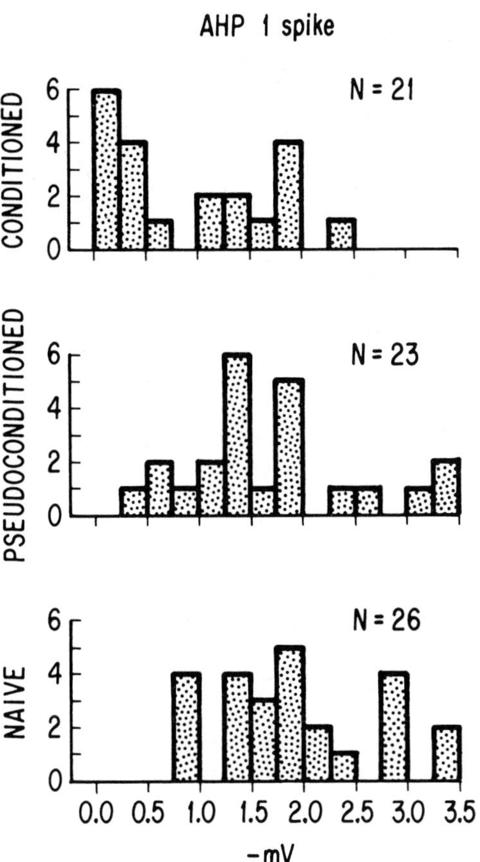

FIG. 12 – A histogram of the AHP response to one spike for the conditioned, pseudoconditioned, and naive cell groups. The distribution of AHPs for the conditioned neurons overlaps the other two groups except for the responses of 0.5 mV and less (33).

impulses which precede it. Observations on other central vertebrate neurons (e.g., cerebellar Purkinje cells) indicate that the voltage-dependent Na^+ current responsible for fast-action potential flows across the soma membrane and not that of the dendrites, whereas a voltage-dependent Ca^{2+} current responsible for more sustained-action potentials flows across dendritic membranes. If conditioning-induced reduction of $I_{Ca^{2+}-K^+}$ occurs on dendrites and not on the soma membrane the sustained depolarization during a Ca^{2+}-action potential may be larger and thus, by spreading passively to the soma, cause greater depolarization during the period following the soma action potentials when the afterhyperpolarization is measured. By this reasoning soma action potentials, elicited by injection of positive current into the soma, would spread to dendrites where Ca^{2+}-action potentials would be triggered. These, in turn, would spread passively back to the soma and, if larger as a result of conditioning-specific reduction of dendritic $I_{Ca^{2+}-K^{+}}$, would be associated with an apparent reduction of afterhyperpolarization of the soma. This is only one of many hypothetical explanations based on assumed loci for conditioning-induced reduction of $I_{Ca^{2+}-K^{+}}$. Simultaneous intracellular recording from CA1 somata and dendrites may eventually help determine the actual loci of the learning-induced current changes.

A final question raised by our CA1 findings concerns the information processing capability of the hippocampus. Forty to fifty percent of CA1 recordings in conditioned animals showed a reduction of ther afterhyperpolarization. At first glance only 50 to 60% of CA1 cells remain for neural integration and other associations unrelated to the learned association of tone and periorbital shock. Of course this need not be the case at all. Another association could, for example, also involve 40 to 50% of CA1 cells many of which, but not all, are shared with the first association. Specificity for encoding each association could be provided by the particular combination of cells involved. Furthermore, the degree of afterhyperpolarization reduction could differ for a given CA1 cell depending on which association was learned.

It is nevertheless surprising, if not counterintuitive, that so many CA1 cells did show conditioning-induced reduction of the afterhyperpolarization. Such a finding, which is consistent with *in vivo* recordings obtained previously, suggests that many cells may even participate in storing very discrete associations. It would seem important, therefore, to compare which *set* of neurons changed with one association to that set changed with a second association. Such a comparison might be achieved with techniques which surveyed excitability of large numbers of cells within a slice, such as through the use of voltage-sensitive dyes or extracellular field potential measurements. Alternatively, careful relation of CA1 intracellular recordings to the geometric location of each CA1 cell within the hippocampus might reveal association-specific distributions of afterhyperpolarization changes.

A critical aspect of the way the CS and the UCS are associated by the nervous system involves their initial and subsequent interaction along preexisting neuronal pathways. Observations from *Hermissenda* indicate that the genetically specified visual-vestibular networks provide for synaptic interaction both at the level of sensory receptors and second-order neurons (or interneurons). Actual interaction at the soma of the type B cell (where conditioning-specific modifications were measured) at least begins by electrical spread (see Fig. 13) from the synaptic compartment to the soma compartment. The electrical events (e.g., depolarization) then elicit voltage-dependent currents (e.g., an inward Ca^{2+} current) which in turn can participate in the generation of long-lasting biochemical consequences (e.g., via Ca^{2+}/CaM and C-kinase activation) and biophysical changes (K^{+} current reduction at least for many days).

The role of electrical spread from the postsynaptic UCS locus to the CS locus does not exclude other types of interaction (e.g., via diffusion of an intracellular second messenger). These other modes of interaction would be slower and might not provide the temporal resolution characteristic of vertebrate conditioning. Neurochemical modulation of postsynaptic membrane currents at the UCS locus could, in addition, facilitate electrical spread. α_2-receptor agonists, for example, reduce postsynaptic K^{+} currents of the type B cell and thereby increase input resistance (56, 57). The postsynaptic excitatory current (probably carried by Na^{+} ions) will thus be associated with a larger voltage change and cause more depolarizatiopn at the CS locus.

Serotonin-like substances in *Aplysia*, however, are thought to directly modify membranes, at least during short-term learning (see Carew, this volume). Serotonin, for example, causes little voltage change but reduces a steady-state "S" current. In addition, serotonin activates adenylate cyclase and elevates intracellular Ca^{2+}. All of these effects were measured in the presence of serotonin although the biochemical effects last some minutes after serotonin removal. Tail shock, which produces sensitization of the *Aplysia* gill withdrawal reflex, also produces reduction of the "S" current (again for many minutes) measured in the sensory cell soma. Associative enhancement of the gill withdrawal reflex has been proposed to involve interaction of Ca^{2+} elevation and adenylate cyclase activation. Although these observations more directly involve the *Aplysia* sensory cell soma, changes within terminal synaptic endings have been suggested based on monitoring of postsynaptic potentials. The relationship of all these

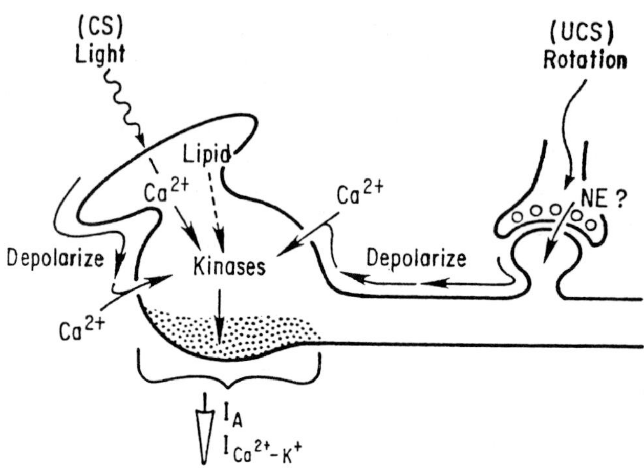

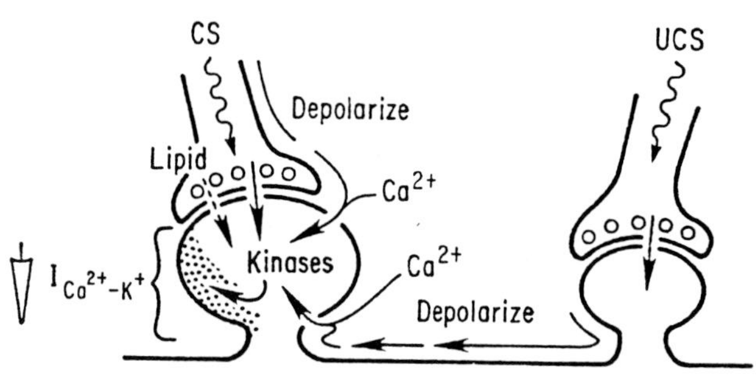

FIG. 13 – Schematic summary for cellular interaction of CS and UCS *Hermissenda* and hippocampus.

effects, lasting many minutes, to persistent nonassociative and associative behavioral change of *Aplysia*, lasting many days, has not yet been established but is now being explored with cell culture techniques.

Short-term changes during long-term potentiation (LTP) (see Andersen, this volume) and long-term depression (LTD) (see Ito, this volume), as well as during modification of visual cortical cells (see Singer, this volume), appear to share some essential features with the initiating events during *Hermissenda* classical conditioning (see Table 1). All appear to involve postsynaptic compartments, prolonged depolarization, and elevation of intracellular Ca^{2+}. In the case of LTP the postsynaptic modifications may be even closer to the *Hermissenda* changes in that there is preliminary evidence of reduced AHP (and thus possibly $I_{Ca^{2+}-K^{+}}$ reduction) as well as regulation of postsynaptic $I_{Ca^{2+}-K^{+}}$ by C-kinase activation (see Andersen, this volume).

Table 1 - Common model features

	LTP	LTD	Eyeblink conditioning	*Aplysia*	*Hermissenda*	Visual cortex *
Postsynaptic	±	+	+	–	+	+
Initial depolarization and ↑ Ca^{2+}_i	±	+	?	?	+	+
C-kinase implicated	+	?	+	–	+	?
Initial K^+ current reduction	?	?	?	+	+	?
Altered cell geometry	+	?	?	?	?	+
Persistent K^+ current reduction	?	?	?	?	+	–
Monamine amplification	+	+	?	+	?	+

* See Singer, this volume

CONCLUSION

Our data indicate that classical conditioning of either *Hermissenda* or the rabbit results in a biophysical record. Reduction of voltage-dependent K^+ currents persists days after repeated temporal association of distinct sensory stimuli. Biochemical evidence suggests that such K^+ current reduction could arise, via pairing-specific depolarization and Ca^{2+}_i elevation, as a consequence of a synergistic interaction of Ca^{2+}-calmodulin-dependent and Ca^{2+}-and lipid-dependent phosphorylation of neuronal proteins. Thus, at the level of cellular physiology, we have a basis for associative memory lasting for days or longer. The relationship of this basis to mechanisms for permanent associative memory (e.g., lasting for years), however, will have to be determined.

A knowledge of cellular physiology, of course, does not necessarily reveal the integrative function of neural systems in the learning process. Much of the important integration, as it relates to the defining features of associative learning, has been uncovered for *Hermissenda*. Much less of such integration is understood for even the well-circumscribed nictitating membrane conditioning of the rabbit. The insights into cellular storage mechanisms in *Hermissenda* and rabbit may, however, suggest experimental techniques by which a record of learning might be traced through a neural system. Biochemical markers (e.g., monoclonal antibodies to critically involved enzymes) might indicate neuronal loci preferentially activated and thereby transformed by a training paradigm. In brain slices, and perhaps ultimately in an intact brain, the pattern of environmental stimuli which is remembered might be revealed as a pattern of neural alterations – a pattern which represents and recreates an image of prior experience.

REFERENCES

(1) Acosta-Urquidi, J.; Alkon, D.L.; and Neary, J.T. 1984. Ca^{2+}-dependent protein kinase injection in a photoreceptor mimics biophysical effects of associative learning. *Science* 224: 1254-1257.

(2) Alkon, D.L. 1973. Neural organization of a molluscan visual system. *J. Gen. Phys.* 61: 444-461.

(3) Alkon, D.L. 1974. Associative training of *Hermissenda*. *J. Gen. Phys.* 64: 70-84.

(4) Alkon, D.L. 1974. Sensory interactions in the nudibranch mollusc *Hermissenda crassicornis*. *Fed. Proc.* 33: 1083-1090.

(5) Alkon, D.L. 1975. Responses of hair cells to statocyst rotation. *J. Gen. Phys.* 66: 507-530.

(6) Alkon, D.L. 1979. Voltage-dependent calcium and potassium ion conductances: a contingency mechanism for an associative learning model. *Science* 205: 810-816.

(7) Alkon, D.L. 1980. Membrane depolarization accumulates during acquisition of an associative behavioral change. *Science* 210: 1375-1376.

(8) Alkon, D.L. 1983. Regenerative changes of voltage-dependent Ca^{2+} and K^{+} currents encode a learned stimulus association. *J. Physl. Paris* 78: 700-706.

(9) Alkon, D.L. 1983. Learning in a marine snail. *Sci. Am.* 249: 70-84.

(10) Alkon, D.L. 1984. Calcium-mediated reduction of ionic currents: a biophysical memory trace. *Science* 226: 1037-1045.

(11) Alkon, D.L. 1984. Persistent calcium-mediated changes of identified membrane currents as a cause of associative learning. In *Primary Neural Substrates of Learning and Behavioral Change*, eds. D.L. Alkon and J. Farley, pp. 291-324. New York: Cambridge University Press.

(12) Alkon, D.L., and Bak, A. 1973. Hair cell generator potentials. *J. Gen. Phys.* 61: 619-637.

(13) Alkon, D.:, Farley, J.; Sakakibara, M.; and Hay, B. 1984. Voltage-dependent calcium and calcium-activated potassium currents of a molluscan photoreceptor. *Biophys. J.* 46: 605-614.

(14) Alkon, D.L., and Fuortes, M.G.F. 1972. Responses of photoreceptors in *Hermissenda*. *J. Gen. Phys.* 60: 631-649.

(15) Alkon, D.L., and Grossman, Y. 1978. Long-lasting depolarization and hyperpolarization in eye of *Hermissenda*. *J. Neurophysl.* 41: 1328-1342.

(16) Alkon, D.L.; Kubota, M.; Neary, J.T.; Naito, S.; Coulter, D.; and Rasmussen, H. 1986. C-kinase activation prolongs Ca^{2+} dependent inactivation of K^{+} currents. *Biochim. Biophys. Acta* 134: 1245-1253.

(17) Alkon, D.L.; Lederhendler, I.; and Shoukimas, J.J. 1982. Primary changes of membrane currents during retention of associative learning. *Science* 215: 693-695.

(18) Alkon, D.L., and Sakakibara, M. 1985. Calcium activates and inactivates a photoreceptor soma K^{+} current. *Biophys. J.* 48: 983-995

(19) Alkon, D.L.; Sakakibara, M.; Forman, R.; Harrigan, J.; Lederhendler, I.; and Farley, J. 1985. Reduction of two voltage-dependent K^{+} currents mediates retention of a learned association. *Behav. Neur. Biol.* 44: 278-300.

(20) Alkon, D.L.; Shoukimas, J.; and Heldman, E. 1982. Calcium-mediated decrease of a voltage-dependent potassium current. *Biophys. J.* 40: 245-250.

(21) Berger, T.W.; Alger, B.E., and Thompson, R.F. 1976. Neuronal substrate of classical conditioning in the hippocampus. *Science* 192: 483-485.

(22) Berger, T.W., and Thompson, R.F. 1977. Limbic system interrelationships: functional division among hippocampal-septal connections. *Science* 197: 587-589.

(23) Berger, T.W., and Thompson, R.F. 1978. Identification of pyramidal cells as the critical elements in hippocampal neuronal plasticity during learning. *Proc. Natl. Acad. Sci.* 75: 1572-1576.

(24) Brons, J., and Woody, C.D. 1980. Long-term changes in excitability of cortical neurons after Pavlovian conditioning and extinction. *J. Neurophysl.* 44: 605-615.

(25) Clark, R.B., and Wong, R.K.S. 1983. Three components of outward current in isolated mammalian cortical neurons. *Soc. Neurosc. Abstr.* 9: 601.

(26) Cohen, D.H., and MacDonald, R.L. 1976. Involvement of the avian hypothalamus in defensively conditioned heart rate change. *J. Comp. Neur.* 167: 465-480.

(27) Connor, J.A., and Alkon, D.L. 1984. Light- and voltage-dependent increases of calcium ion concentration in molluscan photoreceptors. J. *Neurophysl.* 51: 745-752.

(28) Coulter, D.A.; Kubota, M.; Moore, J.W.; Disterhoft, J.F.; and Alkon, D.L. 1985. Conditioning-specific reduction of CA1 afterhyperpolarization amplitude and duration in rabbit hippocampal slices. Soc. *Neurosc. Abstr.* 11: 981.

(29) Crow, T.J., and Alkon, D.L. 1978. Retention of an associative behavioral change in *Hermissenda crassicornis. Science* 201: 1239-1241.

(30) Crow, T.J., and Alkon, D.L. 1980. Associative behavioral modification in *Hermissenda*: cellular correlates. *Science* 209: 412-414.

(31) Davis, W.J.; Villet, J.; Lee, D.; Rigler, M.; Gillette, R.; and Prince, E. 1980. Selective and differential avoidance learning in the feeding and withdrawal behavior of *Pleurobranchaea californica. J. Comp. Physl. A Sens. Neural Behav. Physiol.* 138: 157-176.

(32) Disterhoft, J.F.; Coulter, D.A.; and Alkon, D.L. 1985. Biophysical alterations of rabbit hippocampal neurons studied *in vitro* after conditioning. *Soc. Neurosc. Abstr.* 11:

(33) Disterhoft, J.F.; Coulter, D.A.; and Alkon, D.L. 1986. Conditioning-specific membrane change of rabbit hippocampal neurons measured *in vitro*. *Proc. Natl. Acad. Sci.* 83: 2733-2737.

(34) Farley, J. 1985. Contingency learning and causal detection in *Hermissenda*: behavioral and cellular mechanisms. *Behav. Neuro.*, in press.

(35) Farley, J., and Alkon, D.L. 1982. Associative neural and behavioral change in *Hermissenda*: consequences of nervous system orientation for light and pairing specificity. *J. Neurophysl.* 48: 785-807.

(36) Farley, J., and Alkon, D.L. 1985. Cellular mechanisms of learning, memory and information storage. *Ann. R. Psych.* 36: 419-494.

(37) Farley, J.; Richards, W.G.; Ling, L.J.; Liman, E.; and Alkon, D.L. 1983. Membrane changes in a single photoreceptor cause associative learning in *Hermissenda. Science* 221: 1201-1203.

(38) Goh, Y., and Alkon, D.L. 1984. Sensory, interneuronal and motor interactions within the *Hermissenda* visual pathway. *J. Neurophysl.* 52: 156-169.

(39) Goh, Y.; Lederhendler, I.; and Alkon, D.L. 1985. Input and output changes of an identified neural pathway are correlated with associative learning in *Hermissenda. J. Neurosc.* 5: 536-543.

(40) Grossman, Y.; Alkon, D.L.; and Heldman, E. 1979. A common origin of voltage noise and generator potentials in statocyst hair cells. *J. Gen. Physl.* 73: 23-48.

(41) Harrigan, J.F., and Alkon, D.L. 1985. Individual variation in associative learning of the nudibranch mollusc *Hermissenda crassicornis. Biol. Bull.* 168: 222-238.

(42) Horn, G. 1981. Neural mechanisms of learning: an analysis of imprinting in the domestic chick. *P. Roy. Soc. Lon.* B 213: 101-137.

(43) Kandel, E.R. 1976. Cellular Basis of Behavior: An Introduction to Behavioral Neurobiology. San Francisco: Freeman Press.

(44) Kraus, N., and Disterhoft, J.F. 1982. Response plasticity of single neurons in rabbit auditory association cortex during tone-signalled learning. *Brain Res.* 246: 205-215.

(45) Krnjevic, K.; Morris, M.E.; Reifenstein, R.J.; and Ropert, N. 1982. Depth distribution and mechanism of changes in extracellular K^+ and Ca^{2+} concentrations in the hippocampus. *Can. J. Physl. Pharm.* 60: 1658-1671.

(46) Lederhendler, I.; Gart, S.; and Alkon, D.L. 1983. Reduced withdrawal from shadars: an expression of primary neural changes of associative learning in *Hermissenda. Soc. Neurosci. Abstr.* 10: 270.

(47) Lederhendler, I.; Gart, S.; Alkon, D.L. 1986. Classical conditioning of *Hermissenda*: origin of a new response. *J. Neurosc.*

(48) Moore, J.W.; Desmond, J.E.; and Berthier, N. 1982. The metencephalic basis of the conditioned nictitating response. In *Conditioning: Representation of Involved Neural Functions*, ed. C.D. Woody, p. 459. New York: Plenum Press.

(49) Mpitsos, G.J., and Collins, S.D. 1975. Learning: rapid aversive conditioning in the gastropod mollusc *Pleurobranchaea*. *Science* 188: 954-956.

(50) Naito, S.; Neary, J.; Sakakibara, M.; and Alkon, D.L. 1985. Elevated external potassium causes persistent change of specific protein phosphorylation in *Hermissenda* nervous system. *Soc. Neurosc. Abstr.*, 11: (Part I) 746.

(51) Neary, J.T., and Alkon, D.L. 1983. Protein phosphorylation/-dephosphorylation and the transient, voltage-dependent potassium conductance in *Hermissenda crassicornis*. *J. Biol. Chem.* 258: 8979-8983.

(52) Neary, J.T.; Crow, T.J.; and Alkon, D.L. 1981. Change in a specific phosphoprotein band following associative learning in *Hermissenda*. *Nature* 293: 658-660.

(53) Richards, W.G.; Farley, J.; and Alkon, D.L. 1984. Extinction of associative learning in *Hermissenda*: behavior and neural correlates. *Beh. Brain Res.* 14: 161-170.

(54) Sahley, C.; Rudy, J.W.; and Gelperin, A. 1984. Associative learning in a mollusk: a comparative analysis. In *Primary Neural Substrates of Learning and Behavioral Change*, eds. D.L. Alkon and J. Farley. New York: Cambridge University Press.

(55) Sakakibara, M.; Alkon, D.L.; DeLorenzo, R.; Goldenring, J.R.; Neary, J.T.; and Heldman, E. 1986. Modulation of calcium-mediated inactivation of ionic currents by Ca^{2+}/calmoldulin-dependent protein kinase II. *Biophys.* J. 50: 319-327.

(56) Sakakibara, M.; Alkon, D.L.; Heldman, E.; Naito, S.; and Lederhendler, I. 1986. Effects of α_2-adrenergic agonists and antagonists on photoreceptor membrane currents. *J. Neurochem.*, in press.

(57) Sakakibara, M.; Alkon, D.L.; Lederhendler, I.; and Heldman, E. 1984. α_2-receptor control of Ca^{2+}-mediated reduction of voltage-dependent K^+ currents. Soc. *Neurosc. Abstr.* 10: 950.

(58) Sakakibara, M.; Alkon, D.L.; Neary, J.T.; DeLorenzo, R.; Gould, R.; and Heldman, E. 1986. Ca^{2+}-mediated reduction of K^+

currents is enhanced by injection of IP_3 or neuronal Ca^{2+}/calmodulin kinase type II. *Biophy. J.*, in press.

(59) Sakakibara, M.; Hopp, H.P.; and Alkon, D.L. 1986. Light-induced calcium dependent K^+ channels recorded from patches of non-rhabdomeric soma membrane of photoreceptors. *Biophys. J. Abstr.*

(60) Segal, M., and Barker, J. 1984. Rat hippocampal neurons in culture: potassium conductances. *J. Neurophysl.* 51: 1409-1433.

(61) Stommel, E.W.; Stephens, R.E.; and Alkon, D.L. 1980. Motile statocyst cilia transmit rather than directly transduce mechanical stimuli. *J. Cell Biol.* 87: 652-662.

(62) Tabata, M., and Alkan, D.L. 1982. Positive synaptic feedback in visual system of nudibranch mollusk *Hermissenda crassicornis*. *J. Neurophysl.* 48: no. 1.

(63) Thompson, R.F.; Barchas, J.D.; Clark, G.A.; Donegan, N.; Kettner, R.E.; Lavond, D.G.; Madden, J., IV; Mauk, M.D.; and McCormick, D.A. 1984. Neuronal substrates of associative learning in the mammalian brain. In *Primary Neural Substrates of Learning and Behavioral Change*, eds. D.L. Alkon and J. Farley, pp. 71-99.

(64) Tsukahara, N.; Oda, Y.; and Notsu, T. 1981. Classical conditioning mediated by the red nucleus in the cat. *J. Neurosc.* 1: 72-79.

(65) West, A.; Barnes, E.S.; and Alkon, D.L. 1982. Primary changes of voltage responses during retention of associative learning. *J. Neurophysl.* 48: 1243-1255.

(66) Woody, C.D., Yarowsky, P.; Owens, J.; Black-Cleworth, P.; and Crow, T. 1974. Effect of lesions of cortical motor areas on acquisition of eyeblink in the cat. *J. Neurophysl.* 37: 385-394.

(67) Yeo, C.H.; Hardiman, M.J.; and Glickstein, M. 1985. Classical conditioning of the nictitating membrane response of the rabbit. I. Lesions of the cerebellar nuclei. *Exp. Brain Res.* 60: 87-98.

(68) Yeo, C.H.; Hardiman, M.J.; and Glickstein, M. 1985. Classical conditioning of the nictitating membrane response of the rabbit. II. Lesions of the cerebellar cortex. *Exp. Brain Res.* 60: 99-113.

(69) Yeo, C.H.; Hardiman, M.J.; and Glickstein, M. 1985. Classical conditioning of the nictitating membrane response of the rabbit. III. Connections of cerebellar lobule HVI. *Exp. Brain Res.* 60: 114-126.

The Neural and Molecular Bases of Learning,
eds. J.-P. Changeux and M. Konishi, pp. 239–262.
John Wiley & Sons Limited.

Long-term Potentiation - Outstanding Problems

P. Andersen

Institute of Neurophysiology
University of Oslo
0162 Oslo 1, Norway

Abstract. Long-term potentiation is a particular type of synaptic plasticity which has many features that make it an interesting model of learning. It is induced by a short train of afferent impulses at physiological frequencies and has a duration of several hours. Both presynaptic and postsynaptic changes are involved. Presynaptically there is an increased release of the presumed physiological transmitter glutamate. Postsynaptically one sees an increased tendency toward spike discharge and reduced latency when responses are released by a given EPSP.

The induction of the process requires participation of a critical number of synapses, the presence of calcium ions, and can be blocked by the NMDA receptor blocker APV. An essential link in the induction seems to be a prolonged dendritic depolarization above a certain value, possibly related to the NMDA channel. Entry of calcium ions may serve as a signal for further biochemical changes, probably involving the activation of protein kinases. Possible substrates for such kinases are several potassium channels, the partial closure of which would explain some of the enhanced postsynaptic excitability seen during LTP.

Three major classes of explanation for postsynaptic effects have been offered: unmasking of receptors, thickening of the spine neck by a contractile process, and alteration of the membrane characteristics of the spine head. The evidence bearing upon these theories are discussed. For the most durable changes, protein synthesis seems necessary.

TYPES OF SYNAPTIC PLASTICITY

Following activation many synapses show alterations of their efficiency. Thus, in neuromuscular endplates in mammals, frog, and crayfish facilitation and depression of the synaptic transmission are seen after a single previous impulse (65, 67). Facilitation is seen within a few tens of milliseconds after activation, whereas depression may follow after longer conditioning test intervals. Following short tetanic stimulation there is an enhancement taking two forms: augmentation, with a time course of decay of about 7 s, followed by potentiation lasting a few minutes (66, 67).

All these forms of changed synaptic transmission are seen in several pathways in the hippocampal formation (4, 70). However, in addition, short periods (seconds) of tetanic stimulation, above a certain strength, give rise to an entirely new form of synaptic improvement: a very long-lasting enhancement of transmission (hours to weeks), long-term potentiation (LTP) (20, 57). A similar phenomenon has since been found in many other systems (see below). However, much work is needed to see whehther they may be related, or indeed identical.

REASONS FOR INTEREST IN LTP

There are several reasons for the considerable interest neurobiologists have shown for this type of enhanced transmission. First, the long duration of the enhancement is such that it may be a useful model for learning and memory. Second, the initiating tetanic stimulation is relatively short (from 200 ms to a few seconds) and well within the physiological range of the donor cells. Third, it occurs in many synapses including parts of the brain which seem essential for storage of permanent memory traces (72, 80-82).

Another cause for interest is that the enhancement appears to depend upon a certain critical strength of stimulation. With weak tetanic stimulation only facilitation, augmentation, and post-tetanic potentiation are seen. However, above a certain strength LTP appears as well (71). This phenomenon, which has been termed *cooperativity*, has been interpreted to mean that collaboration of several afferent fibers is necessary to produce LTP. This *associative element* of LTP make it even more interesting from a theoretical point of view since it may form a basis for a conditioning learning paradigm.

Recently many reports of LTP in areas outside the hippocampal formation have been published. The phenomenon has now been demonstrated in the visual cortex, rostral colliculus, the striatum and sympathetic ganglion of rats, the medial part of the medial geniculate body in cats, and in the optic tectum in teleosts (21, 38, 49, 52, 74, 92, 103). Although LTP so far has been most thoroughly investigated in the hippocampal formation, these reports suggest that LTP may be a general phenomenon.

FEATURES OF LTP

The enhancement of synaptic transmission during LTP is expressed in several ways (Fig. 1). There is an enhanced field excitatory postsynaptic potential (EPSP) signifying an increased inward current at, or near, the tetanized synapses (20,29). There is also an enhanced amplitude and a reduced latency of the extracellularly recorded population spike (20) (see Fig. 1A). Correspondingly, there is an enhanced probability of discharge of individual single units recorded intra- or extracellularly and a greatly reduced discharge latency of individual cells to a given strength of the afferent input (10) (see Fig. 1B).

The LTP effect is cumulative with the number and the duration of tetanic periods delivered (20). The process needs synaptic transmission during its induction (33). Blocking of the quisqualic acid type of glutamate receptor with diglutamic-diethyl ester (DGEE) does not prevent LTP unless the synaptic transmission is completely abolished. Conversely, blocking of the NMDA receptor by 2-amino-5-phosphono-valerate (APV) effectively blocks the LTP process with no obvious alteration of normal synaptic transmission (25, 64, 100).

LTP may be induced even when the target cell is prevented from firing during the tetanic stimulation by hyperpolarization (101). This observation and the fact that LTP does not follow antidromic activation (20) argues against coactivation as an essential requirement for its induction.

SITE AND DURATION OF LTP CHANGES

Changes take place at or close to the excitatory synapses on the dendrites since no change can be seen in the soma membrane potential, the input resistance, or the response to depolarizing pulses (9). The duration of the LTP depends upon the state of the preparation, notably the degree of anesthesia and certain stimulation parameters. In hippocampal slices the process usually lasts from half an hour up to a few hours. In anesthetized but otherwise intact preparations the process may last for several hours. In intact and awake animals the time course may last for weeks (18) and seems to depend on two processes. The exact duration is disputed. Barnes (13) found two components with decay time constants of 5.3 days and 37 days, whereas Racine *et al.* (83) have given 1.5 hours and 5 days.

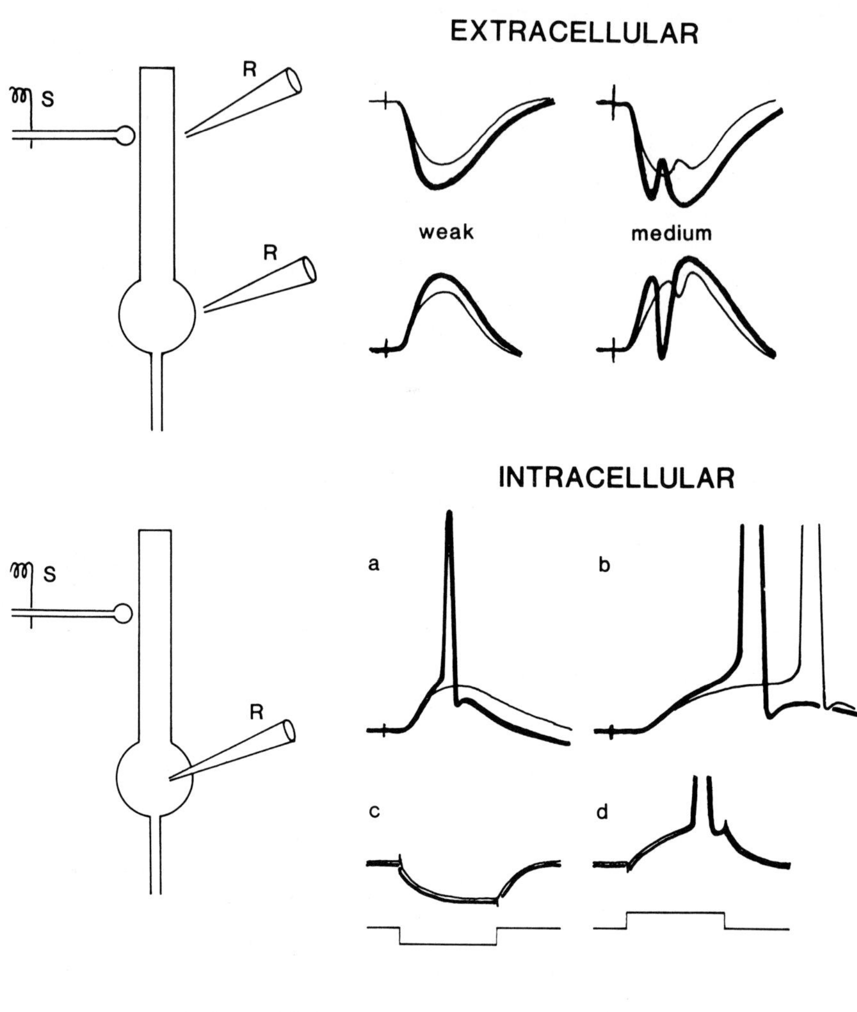

FIG. 1 – Diagram of electrophysiological features of LTP. Upper part shows records before (thin lines) and after (thick lines) establishment of LTP when recorded from the layers of activated dendrites (upper row) or cell bodies (lower row). S - stimulus electrode, R - recording electrode. Lower part shows a) how the EPSP is moderately increased but may give rise to discharge. b) shows the large decrease in discharge latency while c) and d) show that the responses to hyperpolarizing and depolarizing pulses, respectively, are not changed (slightly offset for clarity).

HOMOSYNAPTIC OR HETEROSYNAPTIC EFFECT?

In the CA1 area the LTP effect is homosynaptic. This term refers to a group of fibers and not to individual axons. Whether tetanization of a single axon can induce LTP at its boutons remains to be seen. So far, all experiments have been made with groups of axons, probably in the range of hundreds or thousands. Using two separate inputs (isolated fiber bundles) to the same cell or group of cells, LTP developed only in those synapses which were tetanically activated (9, 10, 60). There are claims to a heterosynaptic mechanism in that a coupling of crossed and ipsilateral afferents from the entorhinal area to the dentate region is necessary to produce potentiation of the crossed pathway (54). Also in the mossy fiber/CA3 synapse, heterosynaptic effects have been reported (73, 105). However, in this case there is some difficulty with regard to the input control since the experiments have only relied upon monitoring stimulation strength for this purpose. For a clarification of these situations direct measurements of the size of the input volley and restriction of alternative impulse routes are needed. Recently, Goddard's group (1, 2) found that tetanization of the lateral perforant path gives a long-lasting depression of responses to the medial perforant path. This heterosynaptic depression, however, was compensated for by an increased excitability of the spike initiating mechanism. Wigström and Gustafsson (98) made observations which they interpreted as heterosynaptic modulation of LTP, although an unknown amount of occlusion introduced some uncertainty.

Following the tetanus there is a transient and general depression of the synaptic transmission. By intracellular recording many cells show a moderate hyperpolarization, associated with a conductance increase which is strongest in the first five minutes after the tetanization (39), which might explain part of the post-tetanic depression.

A trivial explanation for the increase of the intra- and extracellularly recorded EPSPs would be an alteration of the number of activated afferent fibers. However, by comparing the threshold stimulus current and the size of the presynaptic afferent volley before and after the tetanization this factor can be controlled. Furthermore, through the use of separate tetanizing and test cathodes, tetanus-induced excitability changes at the test cathode (e.g., polarization) may be prevented. The supernormal excitability period which has been described for hippocampal fibers (96) lasts so short that it will probably have no relevance. On the other hand, Sastry (88) has reported reduced antidromic field potentials in the entorhinal area with a time course like LTP. Although these data may be given alternative interpretation, Sastry claims that there is a reduced excitability of the perforant path fibers during LTP.

Neither recurrent nor forward inhibition is changed during LTP (40,41).

OUTSTANDING PROBLEMS

There are three major problem areas associated with our understanding of the LTP phenomenon. These concern the *locus of change*, the *mechanisms* underlying these changes, and, finally, the *initiation process*.

There is now considerable evidence for a *double locus* for LTP in that both presynaptic and postsynaptic processes are involved. The presynaptic boutons deliver increased amounts of transmitter, at least for the first two hours of LTP. This increase may well be a necessary process for a proper induction of the postsynaptic processes. Postsynaptic changes are indicated by greatly improved spike initiation which is clearly above what can be explained by the amplitude of the EPSP. The postsynaptic changes may represent a cascade of events, the dissimilar development of which may explain the variation of the observed intensity and duration of LTP in different situations. Furthermore, postsynaptic changes allow associative coupling between several inputs to take place. In this way activation of neighboring synapses may be mutually reinforcing.

Presynaptic Mechanisms

The action potential in the afferent fibers depolarizes the *en passage* boutons and opens voltage-gated Ca^{2+} channels, giving a large increase of the calcium concentration in the bouton (47, 55, 56). Calcium ions are required for the exocytotic release of transmitter. The increased concentration of ionic calcium in the bouton is rapidly reduced by binding to proteins and by uptake into membrane cisterns and mitochondria. In the perforant path/granule cell and radiatum fiber/CA1 pyramidal cell synapses, in which LTP has been studied most extensively, there is good evidence that the excitatory synapses use glutamate (glu) and/or aspartate (asp) as transmitters (17, 27, 42, 76, 85).

Evidence for a presynaptic locus for LTP can be sought either by measurement of an increased release of transmitter, quantal analysis of the postsynaptic response, or recording of an increased excitatory synaptic potential without changes in either the sensitivity or number of receptors or in the input resistance or membrane potential of the target cell.

The first example of an increased transmitter release post-tetanically was given by Skrede and Malthe-Sørenssen (90) who preloaded hippocampal slices with [^{3}H] D-aspartate. This radiolabelled analogue of glutamate is taken up by the same high affinity uptake system which transports L-glutamate but is not metabolized in nervous tissue (11). Following LTP induction there was an increased resting release of [^{3}H]-aspartate. Using a more direct approach, Dolphin *et al.* (28) loaded hippocampal slices with hot glutamine (34). The glutamine was taken up by presynaptic boutons and deaminated to glutamate by glutaminase. Following high frequency stimulation to induce LTP there was an increased release of [^{3}H]-glutamate in parallel with the changes of the synaptic potential and population spike. Similar results were seen for endogenous glu and asp release during tetanus-induced LTP and potentiation triggered by high extracellular calcium (34, 35) and by K^+ -induced Ca^{2+} -dependent release of preloaded glu and/or asp (35).

The increased release of transmitter in response to orthodromic activation is in accord with the increased extra- and intracellularly recorded EPSPs without any change in the input resistance and resting potential of the soma membrane (Fig. 1B) (9). The increased EPSP could, however, be due to the effect of an unaltered amount of transmitter if either the number or the affinity of the glutamate receptors were increased. However, no LTP-associated increase of glutamate sensitivity to iontophoretic application has been seen in spite of an adequate electrode localization as judged from the fast and near constant depolarizing responses to glutamate application (44, 61, 89, 94).

Unfortunately, no convincing quantal analysis of the release of transmitter from hippocampal synapses is available. Such an analysis is eagerly awaited because of the strong evidence this technique could provide for or against a presynaptic locus for LTP. Voronin (95) has claimed such a quantal analysis, but the high noise level, inadequate calculation of the noise contribution, and apparent greatly variable number of fibers involved make this claim somewhat uncertain. Some of the variability could represent Cl^- inverted inhibitory postsynaptic potentials (IPSPs) which is a common finding in such experiments unless GABA receptors have been blocked. Furthermore, the presumed quantal size appears considerably larger than when found with a deconvolution technique after severe reduction of the number of afferent fibers (8).

A possible mechanism underlying the increased transmitter release during LTP could be an enhanced concentration of calcium ions inside the presynaptic terminal. This would be similar to what has been observed during facilitation, augmentation, and post-tetanic potentiation in the frog and rat neuromuscular junction (48, 65-67). However, if an increased level of calcium ion should also be responsible for the LTP effect, it probably represents a different mechanism, due to the much longer time course of the effect. Here an interesting possibility is the involvement of a protein, synapsin I. This has been proposed to be an anchoring device for the vesicles by linking the vesicle membrane to the cytoskeleton. It may alter the mobility of the vesicles by its degree of phosphorylation (77). Verification of this idea requires a correlation between the level of synapsin I and the degree of LTP.

Other proteins presumed to be presynaptically located also show changes in phosphorylation after induction of LTP (75, 93) although the molecular weights differ in these two investigations. Routtenberg's group found a selective increase in phosphorylation of a 47 KD protein (58, 86, 87) whereas the Dutch group found enhanced phosphorylation of a 52 KD protein, with weak changes in a 43 KD amd a 48 KD band.

A final possibility for the enhanced release of transmitter during LTP is a change in the number or action of autoreceptors on the boutons. Such receptors have been inferred by the interference of glutamate receptor agonists with the calcium-dependent, potassium-induced glutamate and aspartate release in the olfactory cortex (26) and hippocampus (69). It is unknown by which mechanism the autoreceptors might operate during LTP. One theoretical possibility is that release glutamate depolarizes the bouton such that voltage-dependent inward calcium currents may increase.

Postsynaptic Mechanisms

There is a striking discrepancy between the large changes in spike latency and probability of discharge on one hand and the modestly increased EPSP recorded intracellularly on the other (9). Even in extracellular records there is often a discrepancy between the clear changes of the population spike and the small or moderate increases of the associated field EPSP (19, 20, 104). Therefore, it is likely that the process involves an enhancement of the spike generating mechanism in addition to the EPSP changes (1, 9, 20). In the following sections, three major classes of theories for possible postsynaptic LTP mechanisms are discussed.

Morphological changes of spines were reported by Fifkova and van Harreveld (37) and Fifkova and Anderson (36) based upon electron microscopic studies of material fixed by a freeze substitution method (Fig. 2A). The tissue showed considerable enlargement and swelling of

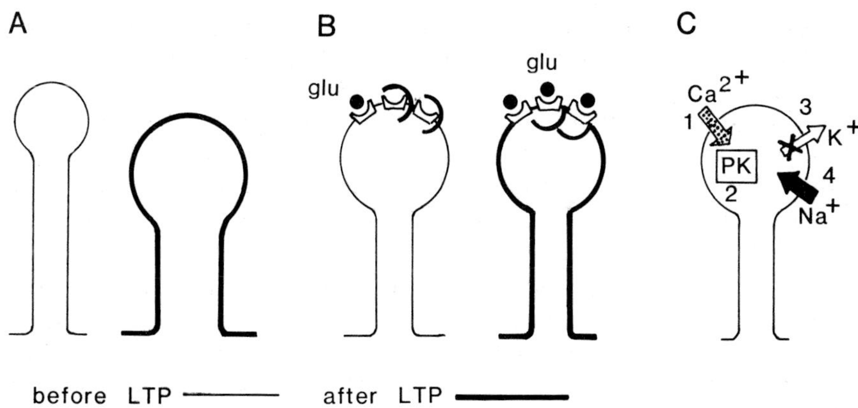

FIG. 2 – Three models for postsynaptic changes during LTP. A) Morphological changes may include enlargement of the whole spine, increased stalk diameter, and reduced stalk length. B) Receptors for glutamate (glu) may be unmasked giving increased binding. C) Calcium entry (1) may activate a protein kinase (PK) (2) which reduces the current through a potassium channel (3). The resulting increased depolarization may give potentiation of the spike-related slow prepotentials or dendritic spikes due to sodium entry (4).

spines in areas subjected to high frequency synaptic activation. However, freeze substitution does not seem to be the method of choice for preservation of membranes and similar changes have not been reported in aldehyde-fixed material. In such material Lee *et al.* (53) could not see any large changes in the size or shape of the spines apart from a small tendency for ovoid spine heads to attain a more globular form. In addition, they reported (53) a 30 per cent increase of symmetrical synapses on shafts of neuronal elements, the majority of which seems to be pyramidal cells. Recently, Chang and Greenough (24) have reported similar findings but attribute the localization to interneurons based upon indirect evidence. If substantiated this surprisingly fast and large alteration might be of critical importance in explaining the LTP change. Since the synapses are symmetric and on the shafts of small dendrites, they are probably of GABA nature; GAD positive material has been found in such synapses (84).

Receptor changes. Baudry and G. Lynch (14) proposed that the LTP process is associated with an enhanced binding of glutamate to synaptic membranes. Browning *et al.* (23) found an increased phosphorylation of a 40 KD protein to follow high frequency synaptic stimulation (tested after two minutes). This was first believed to be a protease (16) but was later found to be the alpha subunit of pyruvate dehydrogenase (22). This enzyme could be involved in presynaptic changes during LTP, but it is less certain whether it also may play a role postsynaptically.

Later, G. Lynch and Baudry (59) proposed that the increased N+-independent binding is due to an unmasking of glutamate receptors at the postsynaptic site of the trained synapses (Fig. 28). This theory implies that there is a calcium-dependent protease, calpain, which uses fodrin as a substrate. A proteolytic alteration of the submembranous filamentous fodrin molecules could lead both to changes of the spine configuration and to an unmasking of receptor molecules at binding sites. Intriguing as this theory is, a major difficulty remains in that no groups have been able to show increased glutamate-induced responses (depolarization, spike discharges) of the time course in question. Either no change or reduced responses have been observed (44, 60, 61, 89, 94). Two groups, one employing the same biochemcial technique as Baudry and G. Lynch, have been unable to verify the increased glutamate binding associated with LTP (64, 89).

Local postsynaptic excitability changes. A common observation during LTP is the great increase in the probability of synaptically activated discharge of individual units and the remarkable reduction in their activation latency without a comparable increase of the EPSP amplitude. Consequently, there may be a change in the excitability of the postsynaptic membrane close to the tetanized synapses, possibly in the spines themselves. The occurrence of an increased probability of occurrence of small all-or-nothing spike (5), earlier called dendritic spikes (7), suggests such an increased dendritic regenerative activity. This increased excitability could either be due to augmented depolarizing prepotentials similar to those seen in the soma membrane (51) or to a prolonged local depolarization because of removal of processes of suppression. It is interesting to note that the afterhyperpolarization, following both EPSPs and spikes, reduced in parallel with the LTP-initiating depolarization. Since the slow afterhyperpolarization is due to a calcium-sensitive potassium current (43), it is possible that this channel may be partly turned off, a process similar to that which occurs during plastic presynaptic changes in *Aplysia* (46). A candidate for this mechanism may be the calcium-dependent protein kinase C (Fig. 2C), which has a K-channel protein as its substrate. Application of phorbol ester, which activates this kinase, has been shown to block the slow afterhyperpolarization in hippocampal pyramidal cells (12). On the other hand, Haas and Rose (40, 41) could not find LTP in cells recorded with CsCl-filled electrodes and suggested that K+ channels must operate to sustain LTP. Further studies seem necessary to verify this observation.

If LTP is associated with a slow turn-off of voltage-sensitive potassium channels, synaptic activation will give a larger and more prolonged spine depolarization, which in turn would increase the probability for spike activation. This idea presupposes the presence of regenerative channels, either in the spine head itself or in its immediate vicinity. Such channels could also explain the earlier described conduction along the dendrites (7) and the presence of large spikes within dendrites (16). Membrane alterations of this type require insertion of new channels and protein synthesis, for example of the kind reported in the hippocampal formation by Duffy *et al.* (31). Protein synthesis blockers have been reported to abolish the later parts of LTP (50).

Requirement for LTP Induction

Cooperativity. In an important paper, McNaughton *et al.* (71) showed that the LTP effect has a definite stimulus threshold. This stimulus strength, when delivered as a single shock, seems to be close to the cell discharge threshold. McNaughton *et al.* (71) interpreted this finding to mean that a minimum number of afferent fibers must be activated for LTP to occur. This could either be due to a signal betwen neighboring fibers or some local postsynaptic process which may influence neighboring synapses.

Calcium ions are necessary for LTP to develop, as seen by altering the extracellular calcium level during the inducing tetanus (32, 33, 102) or by injecting chelating agents intracellularly (62). In most granule cells in which EGTA was injected (23/28) no LTP was seen, although surrounding cells showed clear signs of LTP as judged by extracellular recordings. Treatment by high calcium levels alone also leads to long-lasting synaptic enhancement, similar or identical to LTP (94).

Another requirement for LTP production is the presence of *monoamines*, particulary serotonin. By reducing the tissue serotonin level by more than 70 per cent Bliss *et al.* (19) blocked the major part of LTP in dentate granule cells. Reduction of the noradrenaline level by more than 90 per cent also reduced the LTP, although less so than serotonin reduction.

Blocking of synaptic transmission with GDEE does not effect LTP provided the synaptic transmission is not blocked completely (33). In contrast, blockade of the NMDA receptor with APV completely abolishes LTP production in spite of a retained synaptic transmission (25, 63). Intracellular recording showed that such NMDA application gave rise to a well developed and long-lasting depolarization followed by a profound reduction of synaptic transmission. After the depression, however, there was recovery and an enhanced transmission for several minutes ((25), Andersen and Hvalby, unpublished observations). Thus the NMDA receptor may be critically involved in LTP, possibly by causing depolarization and subsequent opening of voltage-sensitive calcium channels.

Although *inhibition* itself does not seem to be critically involved in establishing LTP (40,41), picrotoxin enhances LTP (97, 99). Application of an inhibitory process immediately in front of the tetanizing stimuli will negate the later development of LTP (30). The inhibition probably operates by shunting (3, 6) and prevents depolarization from taking place, thus removing the initiating process.

Initiation of LTP

In an intracellular study, coupled with recordings from the dendritic level of the activated synapses, Andersen *et al.* (5) showed that tetanic stimulation is associated with a local dendritic depolarization plateau at the site of tetanized synapses due to summation of EPSPs. The depolarization plateau had to reach a certain amplitude and duration to induce subsequent LTP. The necessary level of depolarization varied somewhat from cell to cell. It appeared as the algebraic sum of facilitation and depression (caused by depletion), varied with the frequency and duration of the tetanus. The threshold seemed to be associated, however, with the ability to create a slowly growing depolarizing potential on top of the summated EPSP, similar to the slow prepotentials in response to long depolarizing or glutamate pulses (51, 91). This late depolarization showed cumulative behavior from one tetanic period to the next, even when these were separated by several seconds. Involvement of a dendritic depolarization in LTP induction was also found by Wigström and Gustafsson (100).

In a test of the idea that dendritic depolarization is an essential inducive element, cells were simultaneously depolarized and activated synaptically at low frequency (44). The depolarization was produced in three different ways: a) depolarization of the soma by current injection through the intracellular electrode, b) dendritic depolarization through the application of longitudinal currents by external, nonpolarizing electrodes, and c) local glutamate iontophoresis at a "hot spot" at the level of the orthodromically activated synapses. Neither of the two first procedures led to any LTP-like change of the synaptic transmission when coupled to low frequency synaptic activation. However, conjunction of low frequency synaptic activation and glutamate-induced depolarization gave rise to an enhancement of the synaptic efficiency in 16 of 23 cells tested. The time course of the effect was from 15 to 60 minutes after only 10 to 50 pairings of a 200-800 ms glutamate pulse and a single orthodromic volley near it end. The effect was only seen for synapses in the glutamate-influenced part of the dendritic tree and only during conjunctive stimulation. Control synapses in other parts of the dendrites did not show any systematic changes after the pairings. No effect was seen after the same number of glutamate pulses was given alone, neither did responses of the soma membrane to hyperpolarizing or depolarizing pulses show any alterations. In the remaining cells, neither a change nor an unspecific slow depression was seen, probably due to an action of glutamate on the release properties of the afferent fibers (69). Recently, Wigström *et al.* (102) and Kelso *et al.* (48a) have found similar enhancement following conjunction with strong depolarizing pulses and synaptic activation.

These data support the idea that local depolarization of the dendrites, most likely of the spines themselves, is a requirement for establishment of LTP changes. However, conjunctive synaptic stimulation is also necessary. During tetanically induced LTP the afferent volley provides both types of signals, depolarization due to the summated EPSPs, and the signal delivered by synaptic transmission *per se*.

The situation is reminiscent of the plastic changes of parallel fiber synapses on cerebellar Purkinje cells, where conjunction of climbing fiber or glutamate-induced depolarization and synaptic activation through parallel fibers led to an hour-long decrease in synaptic transmission (45).

During sustained depolarization the NMDA receptor may be activated by glutamate or aspartate, or both. As a consequence, Na^{+} and/or Ca^{2+} enters the cell through Mg^{2+}-sensitive channels (68, 79) reinforcing the depolarization so that voltage-sensitive calcium channels open more. The amount of calcium which enters will thus be dependent both upon the duration of the depolarization (EPSP plateau) and upon the degree of NMDA receptor involvement. The latter is determined by the amount of transmitter release and extracellular Mg^{2+} concentration. Therefore, according to this view, the presynaptic changes are acting as a trigger for the postsynaptic alterations. The increase in ionized calcium may act as a second messenger to activate enzymatic reactions, either proteases (59) or protein kinase C, itself Ca dependent, which has been shown to have a calcium-sensitive potassium channel protein as its substrate (12). The consequent slow depolarization could give a local enhancement of regenerative processes, either due to the activation of promotional processes such as slow prepotentials or to the insertion into the membrane of more channels of importance for local dendritic regenerative activity. In this way a mechanism for associative enhancement of neighboring synapses emerges. It rests upon the idea that the LTP-instrumental depolarization will only be felt by participating and neighboring synapses. Only active synapses will be changed and only if the local dendritic depolarization is above a certain threshold level. This represents a reinterpretation of the cooperativity concept (71) which solely uses the number of afferent fibers as variable. Modulatory compounds could work by allowing high frequency afferent discharges to occur, either by reducing accommodation or by altering the size and duration of the local dendritic depolarization.

CONCLUSION

Long-term potentiation serves as an interesting model for learning and memory processes. The long duration of the synaptic potentiation is of particular interest. Following a short tetanic stimulation, well inside the physiological range for discharge of the participating neurons, the synaptic transmission may be improved for hours, days, or even weeks (13, 18).

The duration of sensory (iconic) memory has a time constant of decay of about 100 ms, whereas the duration of primary memory has a time constant of decay in the order of 10-15 s (78). Because LTP process has a much longer time course, it is likely to be a member of the family of secondary memory processes. LTP could either be the initial part of the secondary memory itself or a process necessary for the induction of the changes which are responsible for secondary memory processes. It need not be a general event but could be an elementary change that takes place at certain strategic synapses in a neuronal network necessary for the memory process to form. For this purpose it is interesting that LTP can both develop gradually and regress if the system is left unstimulated.

The LTP process seems to be one in which both presynaptic and postsynaptic changes take place. At the moment the evidence does not allow an estimation of the relative importance of the presynaptic versus the postsynaptic processes. To the contrary, several observations suggest that the enhanced presynaptic delivery of transmitter acts as an essential element in triggering the postsynaptic changes.

REFERENCES

(1) Abraham, W.C.; Bliss, T.V.P.; and Goddard, G.V. 1985. Heterosynaptic changes accompany long-term but not short-term potentiation of the perforant path in the anaesthetized rat. *J. Physl. Lon.* 363: 335-349.

(2) Abraham, W.C., and Goddard, G.V. 1983. Asymmetric relationships between homosynaptic long-term potentiation and heterosynaptic long-term depression. *Nature* 305: 717-719.

(3) Alger, B.E., and Nicoll, R.A. 1982. Pharmacological evidence for two kinds of GABA receptor on rat hippocampal pyramidal cells studied *in vitro*. *J. Physl. Lon.* 328: 125-141.

(4) Andersen, P. 1960. Interhippocampal impulses. II. Apical dendritic activation of CA1 neurons. *Acta Physl. Scand.* 48: 178-208.

(5) Andersen, P.; Avoli, M.; and Hvalby, ø. 1984. Evidence for both pre- and postsynaptic mechanisms during long-term potentiation in hippocampal slices. *Exp. Brain Res. Suppl.* 9: 315-324.

(6) Andersen, P.; Dingledine, R.; Gjerstad, L.; Langmoen, I.A.; and Mosfeldt-Laursen, A. 1980. Two different responses of hippocampal pyramidal cells to application of gamma-amino-butyric-acid (GABA). *J. Physl. Lon.* 305: 279-296.

(7) Andersen, P., and Lømo, T. 1966. Mode of activation of hippocampal pyramidal cells by excitatory synapses on dendrites. *Exp. Brain Res.* 2: 47-260.

(8) Andersen, P.; Sayer, R.J.; and Redman, S. 1985. Fluctuations in the amplitude of excitatory postsynaptic potentials evoked in hippocampal CA1 pyramidal cells *in vitro*. *P. Aus. Physl. Soc.* 16: 100P.

(9) Andersen, P.; Sundberg, S.H.; Sveen, O.; Swann, J.N.; and Wigström, H. 1980. Possible mechanisms for long-lasting potentiation of synaptic transmission in hippocampal slices from guinea pigs. *J. Physl. Lon.* 302: 463-482.

(10) Andersen, P.; Sundberg, S.H.; Sveen, O.; and Wigström, H. 1977. Specific long-lasting potentiation of synaptic transmission in hippocampal slices. *Nature* 266: 736-737.

(11) Balcar, V.J., and Johnston, G.A.R. 1972. The structural specificity of the high affinity uptake of L-glutamate and L-aspartate by rat brain slices. *J. Neurochem.* 19: 2657-2666.

(12) Baraban, J.M.; Snyder, S.H.; and Alger, B.E. 1985. Protein kinase C regulates ionic conductance in hippocampal pyramidal neurons: electrophysiological effects of phorbol esters. *Proc. Natl. Acad. Sci.* 82: 2538-2542.

(13) Barnes, C.A. 1979. Memory deficits associated with senescence: a neurophysiological and behavioral study in the rat. *J. Comp. Physl. Psych.* 93: 74-104.

(14) Baudry, M., and Lynch, G. 1980. Hypothesis regarding the cellular mechanisms responsible for long-term synaptic potentiation in the hippocampus. *Exp. Neurol.* 68: 202-204.

(15) Baudry, M., and Lynch, G. 1980. Regulation of hippocampal glutamate receptors: evidence for the involvement of a calcium-activated protease. *Proc. Nat. Acad. Sci.* 77: 2298-2302.

(16) Benardo, L.S.; Masukawa, L.M; and Prince, D.A. 1982. Electrophysiology of isolated hippocampal pyramidal dendrites. *J. Neurosci.* 2: 1614-1622.

(17) Biscoe, T.J., and Straughan, D.W. 1966. Micro-electrophoretic studies of neurones in the cat hippocampus. *J. Physl. Lon.* 183: 341-359.

(18) Bliss, T.V.P., and Gardner-Medwin, A.R. 1973. Long-lasting potentiation of synaptic transmission in the dentate area of the unanaesthetized rabbit following stimulation of the perforant path. *J. Physl. Lon.* 232: 357-374.

(19) Bliss, T.V.P.; Goddard, G.V.; and Riives, M. 1983. Reduction of long-term potentiation in the dentate gyrus of the rat following selective depletion of monoamines. *J. Physl. Lon.* 334: 475-491.

(20) Bliss, T.V.P., and Lømo, T. 1973. Long-lasting potentiation of synaptic transmission in the dentate area of the anaesthetized rabbit following stimulation of the perforant path. *J. Physl. Lon.* 232: 331-356.

(21) Brown, T.H., and McAfee, D.A. 1982. Long-term synaptic potentiation in the superior cervical ganglion. *Science* 215: 1411-1413.

(22) Browning, M.; Bennett, W.F.; Kelly, P.; and Lynch, G. 1981. Evidence that the 40,000 Mr phosphoprotein influenced by high frequency synaptic stimulation is the alpha subunit of pyruvate dehydrogenase. *Brain Res.* 218: 255-266.

(23) Browning, M.; Dunwiddle, T.; Bennett, W.; Gispen, W.; and Lynch, G. 1979. Specific changes after repetitive stimulation of the hippocampal slice. *Science* 203: 60-62.

(24) Chang, F.-L.F., and Greenough, W.T. 1984. Transient and enduring morphological correlates of synaptic activity and efficacy change in the rat hippocampal slice. *Brain Res.* 309: 35-46.

(25) Collingridge, G.L.; Kehl, S.J.; and McLennan, H. 1983. Excitatory amino acids in synaptic transmission in the Schaffer collateral-commissural pathway of the rat hippocampus. *J. Physl. Lon.* 334: 33-46.

(26) Collins, G.G.S.; Anson, J.; and Surtees, L. 1983. Presynaptic kainate and N-methyl-D-aspartate receptors regulate excitatory amino acid release in the olfactory cortex. *Brain Res.* 265: 157-159.

(27) Cotman, C.W., and Hamberger, A. 1978. Glutamate as a CNS neurotransmitter: properties of release, inactivation and biosynthesis. In *Amino Acids as Chemical Transmitters*. NATO Advanced Study Institutes Series A16, ed. F. Fonnum, pp.379-412. New York: Plenum Press.

(28) Dolphin, A.C.; Errington, M.L.; and Bliss, T.V.P. 1982. Long-term potentiation of the perforant path *in vivo* is associated with increased glutamate release. *Nature* 297: 496-498.

(29) Douglas, R.M., and Goddard, G.V. 1975. Long-term potentiation of the perforant path-granule cell synapse in the rat hippocampus. *Brain Res.* 86: 205-215.

(30) Douglas, R.M.; Goddard, G.V.; and Riives, M. 1982. Inhibitory modulation of long-term potentiation: evidence for a post-synaptic locus of control. *Brain Res.* 240: 259-272.

(31) Duffy, C.; Teyler, T.J.; and Shashoua, V.E. 1981. Long-term potentiation in the hipppocampal slice: evidence for stimulated secretion of newly synthesized proteins. *Science* 212: 1148-1151.

(32) Dunwiddie, T.V, and Lynch, G. 1979. The relationship between extracellular calcium concentrations and the induction of hippocampal long-term potentiation. *Brain Res.* 169: 103-110.

(33) Dunwiddie, T.; Madison, D.; and Lynch, G. 1978. Synaptic transmission is required for initiation of long-term potentiation. *Brain Res.* 150: 413-417.

(34) Feasey, K.J.; Lynch, M.A.; and Bliss, T.V.P. 1985. Ca^{2+}–induced long-term potentiation in CA3 region of hippocampus is associated with an increased release of aspartate: an *in vivo* study in the rat. *Neurosci. L. Suppl.* 21: 545.

(35) Feasey, K.J.; Lynch, M.A.; and Bliss, T.V.P. 1986. Long-term potentiation is associated with an increase in Ca-dependent, K-stimulated release of [^{14}C]-glutamate from hippocampal slices: an *ex-vivo* study in the rat. *Brain Res.* 364: 39-44.

(36) Fifkova, E., and Anderson, C.L. 1981. Stimulation-induced changes in dimensions of stalks of dendritic spines in the dentate molecular layer. *Exp. Neurol.* 74: 621-627.

(37) Fifkova, E., and van Harreveld, A. 1977. Long-lasting morphological changes in dendritic spines of dentate granular cells following stimulation of the entorhinal area. *J. Neurocyt.* 6: 211-230.

(38) Gerren, R.A., and Weinberger, N.M. 1983. Long-term potentiation in the magnocellular medial geniculate nucleus of the anesthetized cat. *Brain Res.* 265: 138-142.

(39) Gustafsson, B., and Wigström, H. 1983. Hyperpolarization following long-lasting tetanic activation of hippocampal pyramidal cells. *Brain Res.* 275: 159-163.

(40) Haas, H.L., and Rose, G. 1982. Long-term potentiation of excitatory synaptic transmission in the rat hippocampus: the role of inhibitory processes. *J. Physl. Lon.* 329: 541-552.

(41) Haas, H.L., and Rose, G. 1984. The role of inhibitory mechanisms in hippocampal long-term potentiation. *Neurosci. L.* 47: 301-306.

(42) Herz, A., and Nacimiento, A. 1965. Über die Wirkung von Pharmaka auf Neurone des Hippocampus nach mikroelektrophoretischer Verabfolgung. *Naunyn-Schmiedeberg's Arch. Exp. Pat. Pharm.* 251: 295-314.

(43) Hotson, J.R., and Prince D.A. 1980. A calcium-activated hyperpolarization follows repetitive firing in hippocampal neurons. *J. Neurophysl.* 43: 409-419.

(44) Hvalby, Ø.; Lacaille, J.-C.; Andersen, P.; and Hu, G.-Y. 1986. Coupling of glutamate-induced dendritic depolarization with synaptic activation causes long-lasting potentiation of CA1 hippocampal synapses. *Acta Physl. S.* 127: 4A.

(45) Ito, M.; Sakurai, M.; and Tongroach, P. 1982. Climbing fibre induced depression of both mossy fibre responsiveness and glutamate sensitivity of cerebellar Purkinje cells. *J. Physl. Lon.* 324: 113-134.

(46) Kandel, E.R., and Schwartz, J.H. 1982. Molecular biology of learning: modulation of transmitter release. *Science* 218: 433-422.

(47) Katz, B., and Miledi,R. 1965. The effect of calcium on acetylcholine release from motor nerve terminals. *P. Roy. Soc. Lon. B* 161: 496-503.

(48) Katz, B., and Miledi, R. 1968. The role of calcium in neuromuscular facilitation. *J. Physl. Lon.* 195: 481-492.

(48a) Kelso, S.R.; Ganong, A.H.; and Brown, T.H. 1986. Hebbian synapses in hippocampus. *Proc. Natl. Acad. Sci.* 83: 5326-5330.

(49) Komatsu, Y.; Toyama, K.; Maeda, J.; and Sakakuchi, H. 1981. Long-term potentiation investigation in a slice preparation of striate cortex in young kittens. *Neurosci. L.*26: 269-274.

(50) Krug, M.; Lössner, B.; and Ott, T. 1984. Anisomycine blocks the late phase of long-term potentiation in dentate gyrus of freely moving rats. *Brain Res. Bull.* 13: 39-42.

(51) Lanthorn, T.; Storm, J.; and Andersen, P. 1984. Current-to-frequency transduction in CA1 hippocampal pyramidal cells: slow prepotentials dominate the primary range firing. *Exp. Brain Res.* 53: 431-443.

(52) Lee, K.S. 1982. Sustained enhancement of evoked potentials following brief, high-frequency stimulation of the cerebral cortex *in vitro*. *Brain Res.* 239: 617-623.

(53) Lee, K.S.; Schottler, F.; Oliver, M.; and Lynch, G. 1980. Brief bursts of high-frequency stimulation produce two types of structural change in rat hippocampus. *J. Neurophysl.* 44: 247-258.

(54) Levy, W.B., and Steward, O. 1979. Synapses as associative memory elements in the hippocampal formation. *Brain Res.* 175: 233-245.

(55) Llinàs, R.; Steinberg, I.Z.; and Walton, K. 1981. Presynaptic calcium currents in squid giant synapse. *Biophys. J.* 33: 289-322.

(56) Llinàs, R.; Steinberg, I.Z.; and Walton, K. 1981. Relationship between presynaptic calcium current and postsynaptic potential in squid giant synapse. *Biophys. J.* 33: 323-352.

(57) Lømo, T. 1966. Frequency potentiation of excitatory synaptic activity in the dentate area of the hippocampal formation. *Acta Physl. Scand. Suppl.* 277, 68: 128.

(58) Lovinger, D.M.; Akers, R.F.; Nelson, R.B.; Barnes, C.A.; McNaughton, B.L.; and Routtenberg, A. 1985. A selective increase in phosphorylation of protein F1, a protein kinase C substrate, directly related to three day growth of long term synaptic enhancement. *Brain Res.* 343: 137-143.

(59) Lynch, G., and Baudry, M. 1984. The biochemistry of memory: a new and specific hypothesis. *Science* 224: 1057-1063.

(60) Lynch, G.S., Dunwiddie, T. and Gribkoff, V. 1977. Heterosynaptic depression: a postsynaptic correlate of long-term potentiation. *Nature* 266: 737-739.

(61) Lynch, G.S.; Gribkoff, V.K.; and Deadwyler, S.A. 1976. Long term potentiation is accompanied by a reduction in dendritic responsiveness to glutamic acid. *Nature* 264: 151-153.

(62) Lynch, G.; Larson, J.; Kelso, S.; Barrionuevo, G.; and Schottler, F. 1983. Intracellular injections of EGTA block induction of hippocampal long-term potentiation. *Nature* 305: 719-721.

(63) Lynch, M., Errington, M.L.; and Bliss, T.V.P. 1985. Long-term potentiation and the sustained increase in glutamate release which follow tetanic stimulation of the perforant path are both blocked by D(-) aminophosphonovaleric acid. *Soc. Neurosc.* 11A: 834.

(64) Lynch, M.A.; Feasey, K.; and Bliss, T.V.P. 1985. Long-term potentiation in the hippocampus: increased release of preloaded glutamate and aspartate without increase in glutamate receptor binding. *Neurosci. L. Suppl.* 22: 48.

(65) Magleby, K.L. 1973. The effect of tetanic and post-tetanic potentiation on facilitation of transmitter release at the frog neuromuscular junction. *J. Physl. Lon.* 234: 353-371.

(66) Magleby, K.L., and Zengel, J.E. 1976. Augmentation: a process that acts to increase transmitter release at the frog neuromuscular junction. *J. Physl. Lon.* 257: 449-470.

(67) Magleby, K.L., and Zengel, J.E. 1976. Long term changes in augmentation, potentiation and depression of transmitter release as a function of repeated synaptic activity at the frog neuromuscular junction. *J. Physl. Lon.* 257: 471-494.

(68) Mayer, M.L.; Westbrook, G.L.; and Guthrie, P.B. 1984. Voltage-dependent block by Mg^{2+} of NMDA responses in spinal cord neurones. *Nature* 309: 261-263.

(69) McBean, G.J., and Roberts, P.J. 1981. Glutamate-preferring receptors regulate the release of D-[^{3}H]aspartate from rat hippocampal slices. *Nature* 291: 593-594.

(70) McNaughton, B.L. 1982. Long-term synaptic enhancement and short-term potentiation in rat fascia dentata act through different mechanisms. *J. Physl. Lon.* 324: 249-262.

(71) McNaughton, B.L.; Douglas, R.M.; and Goddard, G.V. 1978. Synaptic enhancement in fascia dentata: cooperativity among coactive afferents. *Brain Res.* 157: 277-293.

(72) Milner, B.; Corkin, S.; and Teuber, H.-L. 1968. Further analysis of the hippocampal amnesic syndrome: 14-year follow-up study of H.M. *Neuropsychologia* 6: 215-234.

(73) Misgeld, U.; Sarvey, J.M.; and Klee, M.R. 1979. Heterosynaptic postactivation potentiation in hippocampal CA3 neurons: long-term changes of the postsynaptic potentials. *Exp. Brain Res.* 37: 217-229.

(74) Mochida, S., and Libet, B. 1985. Synaptic long-term enhancement (LTE) induced by a heterosynaptic neural input. *Brain Res.* 329: 360-363.

(75) Morgan, D.G., and Routtenberg, A. 1981. Brain pyruvate dehydrogenases: phosphorylation and enzyme activity altered by a training experience. *Science* 214: 470-471.

(76) Nadler, J.V.; Vaca, K.W.; White, W.F.; Lynch, G.S.; and Cotman, C.W. 1976. Aspartate and glutamate as possible transmitters of excitatory hippocampal afferents. *Nature* 260: 538-540.

(77) Nestler, E.J., and Greengard, P. 1984. Protein Phosphorylation in the Nervous System, pp. 398. New York: John Wiley & Sons.

(78) Norman, D.A. 1982. Learning and Memory, pp. 129. San Francisco: W.H. Freeman and Company.

(79) Nowak, L.; Bregestovski, P.; Ascher, P.; Herbet, A.; and Prochiantz, A. 1984. Magnesium gates glutamate-activated channels in mouse central neurones. *Nature* 307: 462-465.

(80) O'Keefe, J., and Nadel, L. 1978. The Hippocampus as a Cognitive Map, pp. 570. Oxford: Clarendon Press, Oxford University Press.

(81) Olton, D.S., and Feustle, W.A. 1981. Hippocampal function required for nonspatial working memory. *Exp Brain Res.* 41: 380-389.

(82) Olton, D.S.; Walker, J.A.; and Wolf, W.A. 1982. A disconnection analysis of hippocampal function. *Brain Res.* 233: 241-254.

(83) Racine, R.J.; Milgram, N.W.; and Hafner, S. 1983. Long-term potentiation phenomena in the rat limbic forebrain. *Brain Res.* 260: 217-231.

(84) Ribak, C.E.; Vaughn, J.E.; and Saito, K. 1978. Immunocytochemical localization of glutamic acid decarboxylase in neuronal somata following colchicine inhibition of axonal transport. *Brain Res.* 140: 315-332.

(85) Roberts, P.J.; Storm-Mathisen, J.; and Johnston, G.A.R. 1981. Glutamate Transmitter in the Central Nervous System, pp. 226. Chichester, New York, Boston, Toronto: John Wiley & Sons.

(86) Routtenberg, A.; Lovinger, D.; Cain, S.; Akers, R.; and Steward, O. 1983. Effects of long term potentiation of perforant path-dentate gyrus synapses in the intact hippocampus on *in vitro* phosphorylation of a 47 KD protein (F1). *Fed. Proc.* 42: 755.

(87) Routtenberg, A.; Lovinger, D.; and Steward, O. 1985. Selective increase in phosphorylation of a 47 KD protein (F1) directly related to long-term potentiation. *Behav. Neurol. Biol.* 43: 3-11.

(88) Sastry, B.R. 1982. Presynaptic change associate with long-term potentiation in hippocampus. *Life Sci.* 30: 2003-2008.

(89) Sastry, B.R., and Goh, J.W. 1984. Long-lasting potentiation in hippocampus is not due to an increase in glutamate receptors. *Life Sci.* 34: 1497-1501.

(90) Skrede, K.K., and Malthe-Sørenssen, D. 1981. Increased resting and evoked release of transmitter following repetive electrical tetanization in hippocampus: a biochemical correlate to long-lasting synaptic potentiation. *Brain Res.* 208: 436-441.

(91) Storm, J., and Hvalby, Ø. 1985. Repetitive firing of CA1 hippocampal pyramidal cells elicited by dendritic glutamate: slow prepotentials and burst-pause pattern. *Exp. Brain Res.* 60: 10-18.

(92) Teyler, T.J., and Discenna, P. 1984. Long-term potentiation as a candidate mnemonic device. *Brain Res. Rev.* 7: 15-28.

(93) Tielen, A.M.; Degraan, P.N.E.; Mollevanger, W.J.; Lopes Da Silva, F.H.; and Gispen, W.H. 1983. Quantitave relationship bewteen post-tetanic biochemical and electrophysiological changes in rat hippocampal slices. *Brain Res.* 277: 189-192.

(94) Turner, R.W.; Baimbridge, K.G.; and Miller, J.J. 1982. Calcium-induced long-term potentiation in the hippocampus. *Neuroscience* 7: 1411-1416.

(95) Voronin, L.L. 1983. Long-term potentiation in the hippocampus. *Neuroscience* 10: 1051-1069.

(96) Wigström, H., and Gustafsson, B. 1981. Increased excitability of hippocampal unmyelinated fibres following conditioning stimulation. *Brain Res.* 229: 507-513.

(97) Wigström, H., and Gustafsson, B. 1983. Facilitated induction of hippocampal long-lasting potentiation during blockade of inhibition. *Nature* 301: 603-604.

(98) Wigström, H., and Gustafsson, B. 1983. Heterosynaptic modulation of homosynaptic long-lasting potentiation in the hippocampal slice. *Acta Physl. Scand.* 119: 455-458.

(99) Wigström, H., and Gustafsson, B. 1983. Large long-lasting potentiation in the dentate gyrus *in vitro* during blockade of inhibition. *Brain Res.* 275: 153-158.

(100) Wigström, H., and Gustafsson, B. 1984. A possible correlate of the postsynaptic condition for long-lasting potentiation in the guinea pig hippocampus *in vitro*. *Neurosci. L.* 4: 327-332.

(101) Wigström, H.; McNaugton, B.L.; and Barnes, C.A. 1982. Long-term synaptic enhancement in hippocampus is not regulated by postsynaptic membrane potential. *Brain Res.* 233: 195-199.

(102) Wigström, H.; Swann, J.W.; and Andersen, P. 1979. Calcium dependency of synaptic long-lasting potentiation in the hippocampal slice. *Acta Physl. Scand.* 105: 126-128.

(103) Wilson, D.A., and Racine, R.J. 1983. The post-natal development of post-activation potentiation in the rat neocortex. *Dev. Brain Res.* 7: 271-276.

(104) Wilson, R.C.; Levy, W.B.; and Steward, O. 1981. Changes in translation of synaptic excitation to dentate granule cell discharge accompanying long-term potentiation. II. An evaluation of mechanisms utilizing dentate gyrus dually innervated by surviving ipsilateral and sprouted crossed temporodentate inputs. *J. Neurophysl.* 46: 339-355.

(105) Yamamoto, C., and Chujo, T. 1978. Long-term potentiation in thin hippocampal sections studied by intracellular and extracellular recording. *Exp. Neurol.* 58: 242-250.

The Neural and Molecular Bases of Learning,
eds. J.-P. Changeux and M. Konishi, pp. 263–280.
John Wiley & Sons Limited.

Characterization of Synaptic Plasticity in the Cerebellar and Cerebral Neocortex

M. Ito

Dept. of Physiology, Faculty of Medicine
University of Tokyo
Bunkyo-ku, Tokyo 113, Japan

Abstract. Current knowledge of synaptic plasticity in the cerebellar cortex and cerebral neocortex is reviewed. The existence of a special type of synaptic plasticity, earlier suggested theoretically, has now been substantiated by the discovery of long-term depression (LTD). LTD occurs in the synaptic transmission from parallel fibers to Purkinje cells under conjunctive activation of parallel fibers and climbing fibers. It lasts at least one hour, and probably over many hours, following conjunctive stimulation for only 30 s. Plateau potentials induced by climbing fiber impulses in Purkinje cell dendrites play a key role in induction of the LTD, presumably through Ca influx associated with the plateau potentials. The direct cause of LTD is the lowering of sensitivity of Purkinje cell dendrites to glutamate, the putative neurotransmitter of parallel fibers. The pharmocological subtype of the glutamate receptors involved in LTD is quisqualate-specific. Functional implications of LTD have been demonstrated in studies of the remarkable adaptiveness of the vestibulo-ocular reflex (VOR), and data from both lesion experiments and recording of neuronal signals of cerebellar neurons supports the view that LTD plays the essential role in the learning processes of the cerebellum. In contrast to the LTD in the cerebellum and LTP in the hippocampus, evidence is scarce for the existence of synaptic plasticity operating functionally in the motor or visual areas of the normal adult neocortex, but it would be important to explore the association cortex which may have higher learning potentiality.

INTRODUCTION

While classic lesion experiments have long suggested learning capability of the cerbellar cortex (11, 30), our knowledge of underlying synaptic plasticity is rather new. Heterosynaptic interaction in cerebellar Purkinje cells was first suggested theoretically as representing such cerebellar synaptic plasticity (1, 4, 16, 31). In spite of the early failure of experimental investigations, long-term depression (LTD) has eventually been discovered as its physiological substrate (19). Recent efforts have been devoted to characterize LTD in more detail and to investigate its mechanisms (9, 19, 20). Roles of LTD in cerebellar learning have also been investigated both experimentally (8, 14, 38) and theoretically (12, 13). Classic lesion experiments suggested learning capability of the cerbral neocortex (25, 34). Efforts have been devoted to specify synaptic plasticity inherent to the cerebral neocortex yet cerebral synaptic plasticity does not seem to be characterized satisfactorily, and its molecular mechanisms and functional roles are largely obscure.

SYNAPTIC PLASTICITY IN THE CEREBELLAR CORTEX

Theoretical Postulates of the Heterosynaptic Interaction in the Purkinje Cells

Each Purkinje cell in the cerebellar cortex receives two morphologically distinct synaptic inputs: one from numerous parallel fiber axons of granule cells in the cerebellar cortex and the other from a single climbing fiber originating from the inferior olive (Fig. 1). This unique structural arrangement of dual synaptic inputs to Purkinje cells provoked theorists' speculation of its functional meaning. As climbing fiber impulses exert powerful postsynaptic excitatory action on Purkinje cells, Brindley (4) pointed out the possibility that the climbing fiber-induced postsynaptic excitation of Purkinje cells interacts with presynaptic impulses of parallel fibers in the manner of Hebb synapse. Marr (31) suggested an additional possibility that a "change" factor is released from climbing fiber terminals to modify efficacy of synaptic transmission from parallel fibers to Purkinje cells. He took the view that conjunctive activation of a parallel fiber and a climbing fiber, both converging onto a Purkinje cell, leads to sustained enhancement of synaptic efficacy from that parallel fiber either through the Hebb type of mechanisms or release of a "change" factor. Albus (1), however, preferred sustained depression of the synaptic efficacy for practical reasons. Grossberg (16) proposed another interpretation: climbing fibers convey unconditioned stimulus signals while parallel fibers carry conditioned stimulus signals; parallel fiber-Purkinje cell synapses could be intensified in the manner of classical conditioning.

LTD as a Physiological Substrate of the Heterosynaptic Interaction

Heterosynaptic interaction in Purkinje cells can be examined by conjunctive stimulation of parallel fibers and climbing fibers. Even

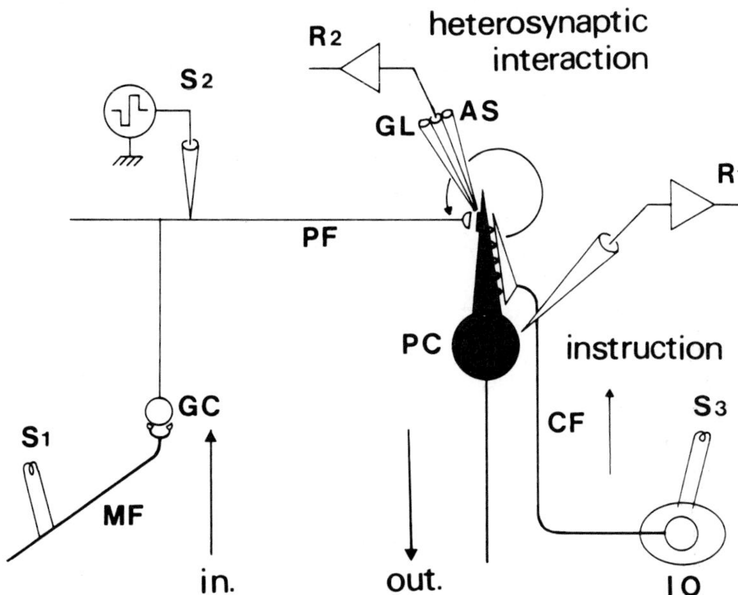

FIG. 1 – Cerebellar cortical circuit and stimulating and recording arrangements for testing the heterosynaptic interaction. PC: Purkinje cells; GC: granule cell; MF: mossy fiber; CF: climbing fiber; IO: inferior olive; PF: parallel fiber; S_1, S_2, S_3: stimulating electrodes; R_1, R_2: amplifier; GL: glutamate; AS: aspartate; in.: input to the cerebellar cortex; out.: output of the cerebellar cortex.

though earlier experiments failed to support their existence, we (17) finally succeeded in finding that conjunctive activation of parallel fibers and climbing fibers did induce an LTD in the transmission from the conjunctively stimulated parallel fibers to Purkinje cells. In the initial experiment (16), stimulation of a vestibular nerve was adopted to activate the mossy fiber-parallel fiber pathway to the cerebellar flocculus. Floccular Purkinje cells respond to vestibular nerve stimuli with latencies of several milliseconds through this mossy fiber-parallel fiber pathway. Conjunctive stimulation of a vestibular nerve and the inferior olive, the source of climbing fibers, was thus shown to induce a depression in the responsiveness of floccular Purkinje cells to stimulation of the vestibular nerve; the depression has an early phase lasting for 10 min followed by a later slow phase lasting over one hour (Fig. 2). Involvement of synapses other than parallel fiber-Purkinje cell synapses was excluded in this depression through careful control experiments. Occurrence of LTD has now been investigated through direct stimulation of a parallel fiber beam instead of mossy fibers (9, 18) and also by replacing parallel fiber stimulation with iontophoretic application of glutamate, a putative neurotransmitter of parallel fibers ((19), see also Fig. 1). In addition to these *in vivo* studies on rabbit cerebellum, intracellular recording from Purkinje cells *in vitro* slice preparations of guinea pig cerebellum successfully revealed the LTD in the amplitude of parallel fiber-induced excitatory postsynaptic potentials (EPSPs) in Purkinje cell dendrites (35).

Earlier failure in detecting the LTD might have been due to the following three reasons. First, climbing fibers might have been stimulated at too high of a frequency; general depression might have been induced in Purkinje cells and disturbed observations of parallel fiber excitation of Purkinje cells. Second, intensity for parallel fiber stimulation was possibly too strong so that stellate cell inhibition might have been evoked and prevented occurrence of LTD (see below). Third, recording of mass field potentials could have been used for monitoring Purkinje cell excitation. However, the mass field potentials provide only a poor index of LTD (18), presumably because of contamination by potentials generated from cerebellar cortical neurons other than Purkinje cells. To induce prominent LTD, parameters for stimulating parallel fibers (both frequency and intensity) should be cautiously selected and the transmission from parallel fibers to Purkinje cells should be monitored with unit spike recording or intradendritic recording from individual Purkinje cells.

FIG. 2 – Effect of conjunctive stimulation of a vestibular nerve and the inferior olive. A: strip chart record of simple spike discharge from a floccular Purkinje cell. Bin width, 0.5 s. The chart runs left to right. Between the open and filled triangles is a gap of 3 min. Horizontal dashed line: period of 2/s stimulation of the ipsilateral vestibular nerve. Horizontal continuous line: period of conjunctive 4/s stimulation of the inferior olive and 20/s stimulation of the ipsilateral vestibular nerve. B and C: peristimulus histograms constructed during the period b and c in A. Upward arrows mark times of vestibular nerve stimulation. Calibration for b and c: 10 impulses/bin/100 sweeps. D, ordinate: values of the firing index of Purkinje cells in response to vestibular nerve stimulation. The average values of 2-3 trials performed during each 5 min period are plotted. Note that plotted values of the firing index were normalized by control values before conjunctive stimulation. D: spontaneous discharge rate, averaged for each 5 min period. Measurements from five different Purkinje cells are superposed in C and D (19).

Time course of LTD. In the above tests conjunctive stimulation of parallel fibers and climbing fibers at the rates of 1-4 Hz for 0.5 up to 8 min effectively induced LTD, which usually consisted of an initial phase for about 10 min followed by a later phase lasting for one hour or more. Because of technical difficulties inherent to extracellular recording from

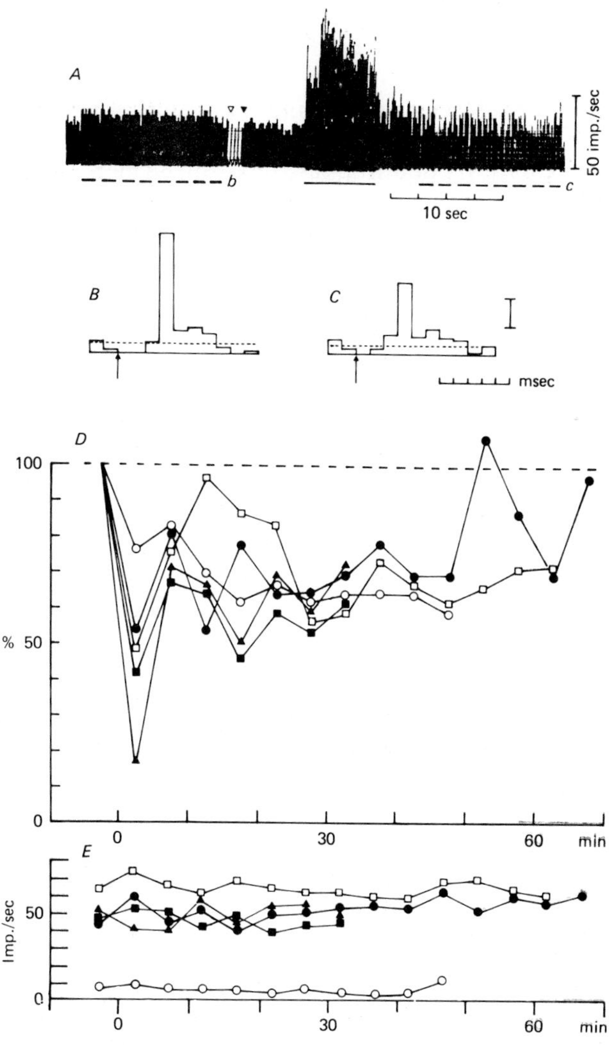

single Purkinje cells it is difficult to follow the time course of LTD over an hour. In several cases, though, LTD has been observed to sustain over three hours (M. Kano and M. Kato, personal communication).

Efforts should be made to follow the whole time course of LTD and estimate its dependence on stimulus conditions. For the present it is certain that conjunctive activation of parallel fibers and climbing fibers of 0.5 to 8 min at a physiological range of frequency for climbing fiber firing (1-4 Hz) produces LTD lasting for an hour or more (9, 19, 35). Depression in a time scale of hours would be long enough to explain motor adaptation (see below). However, it is uncertain whether LTD lasts longer under rigorous stimulating conditions or whether it eventually turns to be permanent. Such permanent persistence would be necessary for explaining maintenance of acquired motor skills if it is due entirely to LTD.

Timing of conjunctive stimulation. The timing of parallel fiber and climbing fiber stimulations to induce effectively LTD has been found to be allowed a relatively wide latitude. Stimulation of parallel fibers during the period between 20 ms prior and 150 ms subsequent to the stimulation of climbing fibers is nearly equally potent in inducing the LTD. Even those occurring 250 ms after a climbing fiber impulse induced the LTD, though with less probability (C.-F. Ekerot and M. Kano, personal communication). Therefore, as contrasted with the critical timing postulated by Marr (31), the conjunctive stimulation does not need to be critically timed; rather, the LTD may depend on some variable factor such as enhanced correlation between the firing of parallel fibers and that of climbing fibers as theoretically postulated (12). The idea of critical timing of collision with parallel fiber discharges seems to be unrealistic also in view of the characteristically slow, irregular pattern of climbing fiber discharge (see (17)).

Mechanisms of LTD

Involvement of glutamate receptors. Involvement in the LTD of postsynaptic chemosensitivity of Purkinje cells to L-glutamate was first demonstrated by our finding that conjunctive iontophoretic application of L-glutamate with electrical stimulation of climbing fibers induces a sustained depression of L-glutamate sensitivity of Purkinje cells (19). The depression of L-glutamate sensitivity displayed two phases similar to those of LTD. Since L-glutamate is a putative neurotransmitter of parallel fibers (see (17)), it is postulated that the LTD in parallel fiber-Purkinje cell transmission is underlaid by the decreased L-glutamate sensitivity of Purkinje cells, presumably at synaptic sites on dendritic spines.

Involvement of postsynaptic glutamate sensitivity in LTD has also been evidenced by testing parallel fiber-Purkinje cell transmission after conjunctive application of L-glutamate with electrical stimulation of climbing fibers (20). Parallel fiber-Purkinje cell transmission at Purkinje cell dendritic synapses, where L-glutamate was applied in conjunction with climbing fiber stimulation, underwent indeed a long-lasting depression equivalent to the LTD in time course and magnitude.

Several glutamate analogues were similarly tested. When applied in conjunction with electrical stimulation of climbing fibers, quisqualate was the most effect in inducing LTD of parallel fiber-Purkinje cell transmission, even more effective than L-glutamate (20). By contrast, kainate, NMDA (N-methyl-D-aspartate), or aspartate had no such effect at all. Therefore, quisqualate-selective glutamate receptors appear to be specifically involved in the mechanism of LTD.

Involvement of Ca influx. Another important finding as to mechanisms of LTD is that LTD is abolished by conditioning climbing fiber impulses with postsynaptic inhibiton of Purkinje cell dendrites (9). The inhibition is induced by stimulation of off-beam parallel fibers for a Purkinje cell, which excites stellate cells supplying inhibitory synapses to dendrites of that Purkinje cell. Since stellate cell inhibition depresses the plateau potential induced in Purkinje cell dendrites by climbing fiber impulses (5, 10), and since the plateau potential is presumed to represent influx of Ca ions into Purkinje cell dendrites (29), it is suggested that Ca influx during plateau potentials play a key role in the induction of LTD. This postulate is in accordance with the observation that antidromic activation of Purkinje cells, which is not accompanied with plateau potentials, is never effective in inducing LTD when paired with parallel fiber stimulation (M. Sakurai, personal communication).

The dependence of LTD on the climbing fiber-evoked plateau potentials is consistent with the relatively wide latitude for timing of parallel fiber-climbing fiber conjunction (see above), as the plateau potential has a long duration of up to 1 s (10). The above observation would exclude the possibility that LTD is caused by a "change" factor released from climbing fiber terminals (31) because it is then difficult to explain why LTD is abolished by postsynaptic inhibiton in Purkinje cell dendrites. Nevertheless, the possibility would remain that a "change" factor is released from Purkinje cell dendrites subsequent to generation of plateau potentials.

The most likely mechanisms of LTD at molecular levels would thus be that the climbing fiber-induced Ca influx cooperates with the neurotransmitter of parallel fibers and acts to desensitize quisqualate-selective glutamate receptors in the postsynaptic membrane (Fig. 3). Ca may act directly on receptor molecules, but considering that cyclic GMP and related substances are abundant in Purkinje cells, it is possible that second messenger processes are intercalated between the Ca entry and desensitization of glutamate receptors. Contribution of Ca to desensitization of acetylcholine receptors has been suggested (32) and discussed in connection with allosteric properties of the acetylcholine receptor protein (6).

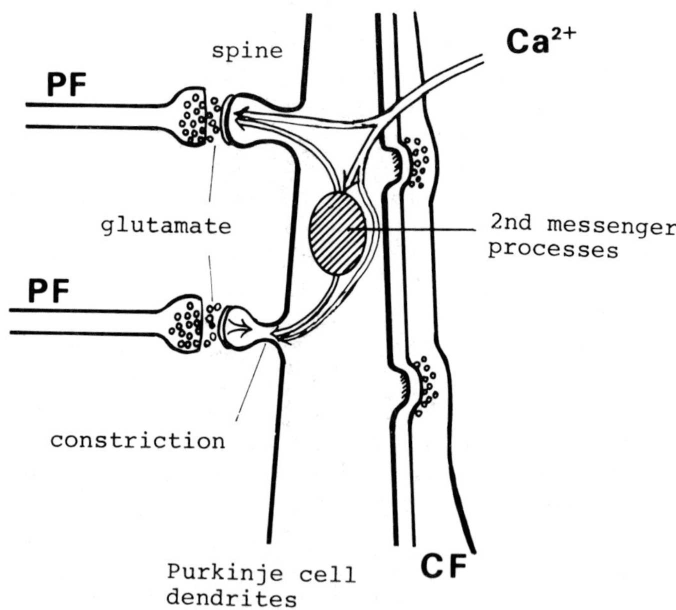

FIG. 3 – Possible mechanisms of LTD. PF: parallel fiber; CF: climbing fiber; constriction of the spine neck is illustrated only as a possibility.

Roles of LTD in Motor Adaptation

Behavior of Purkinje cells has been examined in alert animals performing certain tasks of motor adaptation.

In hand movement. Gilbert and Thach (14) reported that, when a monkey held a lever with an arm in a central position against load perturbations, Purkinje cells in lobules III through V exhibited an increased occurrence of complex spikes (representing activation by climbing fiber impulses) and a concurrent decrease in simply spikes (sign of activation by parallel fiber impulses). As the hand movement was adapted to a new load the occurrence of complex spikes returned to control level, whereas the occurrence of simple spikes was maintained at a reduced level. These observations suggest that load perturbation induces climbing fiber impulses and thereby depresses parallel fiber-Purkinje cell transmission by induction of LTD. The link from LTD to the adaptive adjustment of hand movement, however, has not yet been dissected.

In VOR. We adopted adaptive modification of the VOR as an experimental paradigm for testing cerebellar learning mechanisms (17). The gain of the horizontal VOR is modified under mismatched visual-vestibular stimulating conditions, as first demonstrated by Gonshor and Melvill Jones (15). It either increases or decreases toward minimization of retinal error signals under given stimulating conditions. This adaptiveness of the VOR is abolished by ablation of the flocculus and also by severance of the visual climbing fiber pathway to the flocculus. Purkinje cells specifically involved in the control of the horizontal VOR can be recorded in floccular areas where local stimulation through the recording microelectrode induces abduction of the ipsilateral eye. These H-zone Purkinje cells, as they may be called, responded to optokinetic stimulation with modulation of complex spikes and head rotation with modulation of simple spikes. Under sustained visual-vestibular stimulating conditions, complex spikes were kept modulated, and simple spike modulation altered gradually, reciprocally to complex spike modulation (8, 38). For example, when complex spikes were modulated in phase with head movement, simple spike modulation became less and less in-phase, or more and more out-phase. These observations can be explained by assuming that LTD occurred in parallel fibers mediating vestibular signals when they were conjunctively activated with visual climbing fiber signals.

The modified behavior of floccular Purkinje cells can be related to adaptive adjustment of the horizontal VOR based on the known neuronal connections of the flocculus and the VOR arc (Fig. 4). The flocculus forms a sidepath of the major VOR arc with mossy fiber afferents mediating vestibular signals to the flocculus and with floccular Purkinje cells supplying inhibitory signals to relay cells of the VOR. Vestibular responses of floccular Purkinje cells thus imply additional signals generated in the VOR arc, and these additional signals account for a modifiable component of the VOR dynamics. When visual climbing fiber signals representing retinal errors reach the flocculus, the LTD would occur in parallel fiber-Purkinje cell connections which are active at that moment when the VOR performs erroneously. Inappropriate connections in the flocculus would thus be depressed, and the performance of the VOR would be modified toward minimization of retinal error signals.

Performance of the entire flocculo-VOR system has been computer-simulated (13). Fujita's adaptive filter model (12) of the cerebellum utilizes a learning principle similar to Marr-Albus' model and it can manipulate frequency modulated time analogue signals similar to nerve impulses occurring in actual nervous systems. With the adaptive filter

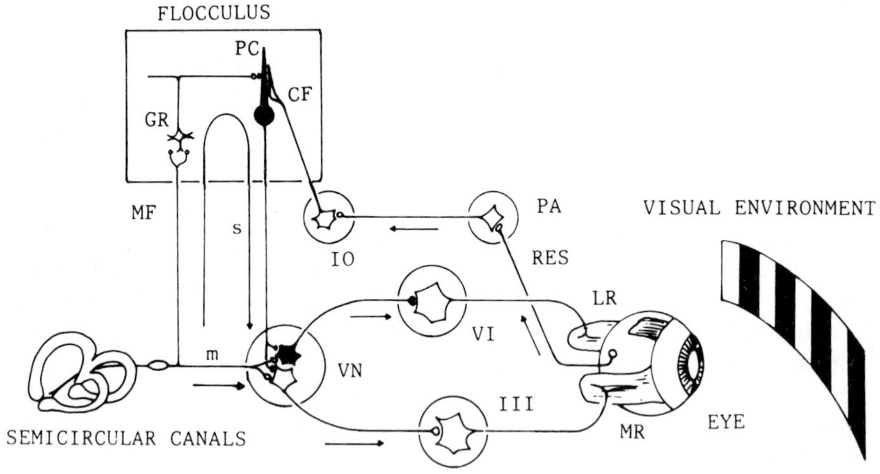

FIG. 4 – Major connections in the flocculo-VOR system. VN: vestibular nuclei; PA: pretectal area; RES: retinal error signal; MR: medial rectus muscle; LR: lateral rectus muscle; III and IV: oculomotor and abducens motoneurons; m: major pathway for the VOR; s: floccular sidepath (17).

model in place of the flocculus, the model of the whole flocculo-VOR system successfully reproduced the performance of human horizontal VOR adapted to the reversal of visual fields with dove prism goggles.

Problems to be Solved

Is there any long-term facilitation? So far, evidence is available only for LTD, but not for any facilitatory effect of the heterosynaptic interaction in Purkinje cells. The facilitatory process introduced in Fujita's (12) adaptive filter model of the cerebellum is such that it occurs when the incidence of simultaneous activation of a climbing fiber and a parallel fiber is reduced below the background level, opposite to the LTD which occurs when the incidence is enhanced above the background level. In slice preparations of the cerebellum, some long-lasting facilitation has indeed been seen to occur after repetitive stimulation of parallel fibers alone (M. Sakurai, personal communication). However, it is yet uncertain if this facilitation represents reactivation of desensitized glutamate receptors.

Do other synapses also undergo a long-term change? Heterosynaptic interaction has been assumed to occur also in those synapses supplied by parallel fibers to basket cells and stellate cells (1, 12). However, no evidence has so far substantiated this assumption (19).

Is there any presynaptic event involved in LTD? Evidence is available only for postsynaptic events involved in LTD, but the possibility that LTD also involves a long-term presynaptic event such as decreased transmitter release has not yet been excluded.

Is spine morphology involved in LTD? As the parallel fiber-Purkinje cell synapses are formed on the top of dendritic spines, constriction of the spine neck would prevent postsynaptic currents generated at the subsynaptic membrane from spreading to dendritic shafts. A possibility thus emerges that such morphological changes account for LTD, or at least a part of it, as hypothetically illustrated in Fig. 3. This situation is analogous, though opposite in the direction, to the shortening of spines postulated to occur in cerebral cortical neurons (7, 21, 23). So far, no evidence is available for a morphological change of Purkinje cell spines to be related to LTD.

Does the climbing fiber serve only for plasticity? In addition to the role in conveying instruction signals for plastic reorganization of the cerebellar cortical network, some other roles have been suggested (see (17)). For example, climbing fibers appear to exert trophic influences on Purkinje cell morphology and function. Climbing fibers may also be a source of impulse signals that exert certain short-term effects on the ongoing impulse traffics in the cerebellar cortex (see (17)). It is important to know how these suggested multiple roles are interrelated to each other.

Are monoaminergic afferents involved in production of LTD? The cerebellar cortex receives noradrenaline- and serotonin-containing afferent fibers. Depletion of noradrenaline from the brain has been claimed to abolish the VOR adaptation (22), but a later study suggests that serotonin is the key factor of this effect (33). A likely possibility is that the monoaminergic afferents act on induction of LTD by affecting climbing fiber-induced plateau potentials or second messenger processes in Purkinje cell dendrites. Another possibility to be entertained is that monoamines interfere with glutamate receptors in Purkinje cells, as serotonin effectively depresses glutamate sensitivity of Purkinje cells (27).

Can the role of the cerebellum in classically conditioned reflexes be explained by LTD? Very recently, it was shown that the cerebellum plays a key role in acquisition and maintenance of the classically conditioned eyelid and nictitating membrane response (28). If a cerebellar nuclear pathway is able to mediate the classically conditioned responses, unless it is depressed by the inhibitory action of a cerebellar cortical sidepath, the occurrence of the conditioned reflex can be explained to be due to the removal of the cerebellar inhibition (disinhibition) by LTD. LTD would be induced in the cerebellar sidepath through conjunction of conditioned stimuli conveyed by mossy fiber afferents and unconditioned stimuli conveyed by climbing fiber afferents. Recent data seem to conform to this scheme ((41), see also Thompson, this volume).

Does LTD represent universal memory processes in cerebellar learning? Studies of the VOR have lead to a general scheme of adaptive control systems which are capable of modifying its dynamic characteristics according to environmental changes in a trial. Adaptive control systems, however, have no ability to learn control in order to improve their dynamic characteristics according to experiences in prior trials. Learning control requires a second memory for previous experiences. I would like to point out that the LTD also accounts for the second memory owing to the structure called the dentato-rubro-olivery triangle (17).

SYNAPTIC PLASTICITY IN THE CEREBRAL NEOCORTEX

Efforts devoted to demonstrate an LTP in the neocortex similar to that found in the hippocampus yielded controversial results (see (37)).

Positive evidence has been available in rat neocortex (26, 39) and also in striate cortex of young kittens (24). LTP is postulated as a candidate mnemonic device (36).

Efforts to test synaptic plasticity in the neocortex have also been made by pairing antidormic and orthodromic stimulation. Paired tetanization of pyramidal tract axons and thalamocortical fibers has been claimed to produce sustained facilitation in the thalamocortical EPSPs in pyramidal tract neurons (2). However, since stimulating currents were not well controlled in this experiment, confirmation is still needed.

Synaptic efficacy could be modified not only by changes of synaptic mechanisms themselves but also by a change of postsynaptic membrane excitability. The excitability of pyramidal tract cells has been shown to increase in association with classical eye blink conditioning (40). Tetanic antidromic stimulation (100/s for 5 min) has also been shown to induce an increase of excitability of pyramidal tract neurons for direct cortical stimulation (3). In contrast, repetitive transsynaptic activation induced decreases in excitability of pyramidal tract neurons.

Open Problems

Neocortical synaptic plasticity could, in fact, be heterogeneous and could vary from cortical area to area. So far the motor area and visual area have been investigated, but in view of learning potentiality an emphasis should be placed on association cortices.

Neocortical synaptic plasticity may also be age-dependent. For example, the LTP in the visual cortex has been demonstrated only during a limited period of time between 3 and 7 postnatal weeks (24). Such critical period may be area-dependent and presumably the longest in association cortices.

In addition to these problems at synaptic levels, there are numerous problems at system levels which will have to be solved before we are able to understand the entire processes of cognitive memory and learning. These processes, apparently going on in the cerebrum (including the hippocampus and amygdala), would be totally different from those dedicated to adaptive control of motor and autonomic functions in the cerebellum. New network and system models, representing mechanisms of cognitive memory and learning, are invaluable for the heuristic discovery of experimental approaches to them.

REFERENCES

(1) Albus, J.S. 1971. A theory of cerebellar function. *Math. Biosci.* 10: 25-61.

(2) Baranyi, A., and Fehér, O. 1978. Conditioned changes of synaptic transmission in the motor cortex of the cat. *Exp. Brain Res.* 33: 283-298.

(3) Bindman, L.J.; Lippold, O.C.J.; and Milne, A.R. 1979. Prolonged changes in excitability of pyramidal tract neurones in the cat: a postsynaptic mechanism. *J. Physl.* 286: 457-477.

(4) Brindley, G.S. 1964. The use made by the cerebellum of the information that it receives from sense organ. *IBRO Bull.* 3: 80.

(5) Campbell, N.C.; Ekerot, C.-F.; and Hesslow, G. 1983. Interaction between responses in Purkinje cells evoked by climbing fibre impulses and parallel fiber volleys. *J. Physl.* 340: 225-238.

(6) Changeux, J.-P.; Bon, F.; Cartaud, J.; Deniller-Thiéry, A.; Giraudat, J.; Heidmann, T.; Holton, B.; Nghiem, H.-O.; Popot, J.-L.; Van Rapenbusch, R.; and Tzartos, S. 1983. Allosteric properties of the acetylcholine receptor protein from *torpedo marmorata. Cold S.H. Quant. Biol.* 48: 35-52.

(7) Crick, F. 1982. Do dendritic spines twitch? *Trends Neurosci.* 5: 44-46.

(8) Dufossé, M.; Ito, M.; Jastreboff, P.J.; and Miyashita, Y. 1978. A neuronal correlate in rabbit's cerebellum to adaptive modification of the vestibulo-ocular reflex. *Brain Res.* 150: 611-616.

(9) Ekerot, C.-F., and Kano, M. 1985. Long-term depression of parallel fibre synapses following stimulation of climbing fibres. *Brain Res.* 342: 357-360.

(10) Ekerot, C.-F., and Oscarsson, O. 1981. Prolonged depolarization elicited in Purkinje cell dendrites by climbing fibre impulses in the cat. *J. Physl.* 318: 207-221.

(11) Flourens, P. 1842. Recherches Expérimentalles sur les Propriétés et les Fonctions du Système Nerveux dans les Animaux Vertebrés, édition 2. Paris: Baillière.

(12) Fujita, M. 1982. Adaptive filter model of the cerebellum. *Biol. Cybern.* 45: 195-206.

(13) Fujita, M. 1982. Simulation of adaptive modification of the vestibulo-ocular reflex with an adaptive filter model of the cerebellum. *Biol. Cybern.* 45: 207-214.

(14) Gilbert, P.F.C., and Thach, W.T. 1977. Purkinje cell activity during motor learning. *Brain Res.* 128: 309-328.

(15) Gonshor, A., and Melvill Jones, G. 1966. Extreme vestibulo-ocular adaptation induced by prolonged optical reversal of vision. *J. Physl.* 256: 381-414.

(16) Grossberg, S. 1969. On learning of spatiotemporal patterns by networks with ordered sensory and motor components. I. Excitatory components of the cerebellum. *Stud. Appl. Math.* 48: 105-132.

(17) Ito, M. 1984. The Cerebellum and Neural Control. New York: Raven Press.

(18) Ito, M., and Kano, M. 1982. Long-lasting depression of parallel fiber-Purkinje cell transmission induced by conjunctive stimulation of parallel fiber and climbing fibers in the cerebellar cortex. *Neuroscience* 33: 253-258.

(19) Ito, M.; Sakurai, M.; and Tongroach, P. 1982. Climbing fibre induced depression of both mossy fibre responsiveness and glutamate sensitivity of cerebellar Purkinje cells. *J. Physl.* 324: 113-134.

(20) Kano, M., and Kato, M. 1985. Specific glutamate sensitivity involved in the long-term depression of parallel fiber-Purkinje cell transmission in rabbit cerebellar cortex. *Neurosci. L.* 22: S26.

(21) Kawato, M.; Hamaguchi, T.; Murakami, F.; and Tsukahara, N. 1985. Quantitative analysis of electrical properties of dendritic spines. *Biol. Cybern.* 50: 447-454.

(22) Keller, E.L., and Smith, A. 1983. Suppressed visual adaptation of the vestibulo-ocular reflex in catecholamine-depleted cats. *Brain Res.* 258: 323-327.

(23) Koch, C., and Poggio, T. 1983. A theoretical analysis of electrical properties of spines. *P. Roy. Soc. Lon. B* 218: 455-477.

(24) Komatsu, Y.; Toyama, K.; Maeda, J.; and Sakaguchi, H. 1981. Long-term potentiation investigated in a slice preparation of striate cortex of young kittens. *Neurosci. L.* 26: 269-274.

(25) Lashley, K.S. 1943. Studies of cerebral function in learning, XII. Loss of the maze habit after occipital lesions in blind rats. *J. Comp. Neur.* 79: 431-462.

(26) Lee, K.S. 1982. Sustained enhancement of evoked potentials following brief, high-frequency stimulation of the cerebral cortex *in vitro*. *Brain Res.* 239: 617-623.

(27) Lees, M.; Strahlendorf, J.C.; and Strahlendorf, H.K. 1986. Modulatory actions of serotonin on glutamate-induced activation of cerebellar Purkinje cells. *Brain Res.* 361: 107-113.

(28) Lincoln, J.S.; McCormick, D.A.; and Thompson, R.F. 1982. Ipsilateral cerebellar lesions prevent learning of the classically conditioned nictitating membrane/eyelid response. *Brain Res.* 242: 190-193.

(29) Llinás, R., and Sugimori, M. 1980. Electrophysiological properties of *in vitro* Purkinje cell dendrites in mammalian cerebellar slices. *J. Physl.* 305: 197-213.

(30) Luciani, L. 1981. Il Cervelletto: Nuovi Studi di Fisiologia Normale et Pathologica. Florence: Le Monnier.

(31) Marr, D. 1969. A theory of cerebellar cortex. *J. Physl.* 202: 437-470.

(32) Miledi, R. 1980. Intracellular calcium and desensitization of acetylcholine receptors. *P. Roy. Soc. Lon. B* 209: 443-452.

(33) Miyashita, Y., and Watanabe, E. 1984. Loss of vision-guided adaptation of the vestibulo-ocular reflex after depletion of brain serotonin in the rabbit. *Neurosci. L.* 51: 177-182.

(34) Pavlov, I.P. 1927. Conditioned reflexes. Oxford: Oxford Univ. Press.

(35) Sakurai, M. 1985. Long-term depression of parallel fiber-Purkinje cell synapses *in vitro*. *Neurosci. L.* 22: S26.

(36) Teyler, T.J., and Discenna, P. 1984. Long-term potentiation as a candidate mnemonic device. *Brain Res. R.* 7: 15-28.

(37) Voronin, L.L. 1983. Long-term potentiation in the hippocampus. *Neuroscience* 10: 1051-1069.

(38) Watanabe, E. 1984. Neuronal events correlated with long-term adaptation of the horizontal vestibulo-ocular reflex in the private flocculus. *Brain Res.* 297: 169-174.

(39) Wilson, D.A., and Racine, R.J. 1983. The postnatal development of post-activation potentiation in the rat neocortex. *Dev. Brain Res.* 7: 271-276.

(40) Woody, C.D., and Black-Cleworth, P.A. 1973. Differences in excitability of cortical neurons as a function of motor projection in conditioned cats. *J. Neurophysl.* 36: 1104-1116.

(41) Yeo, C.H.; Hardiman, M.J.; and Glickstein, M. 1985. Classical conditioning of the nictitating membrane response of the rabbit. III. Connections of cerebellar lobule HVI. *Exp. Brain Res.* 60: 114-126.

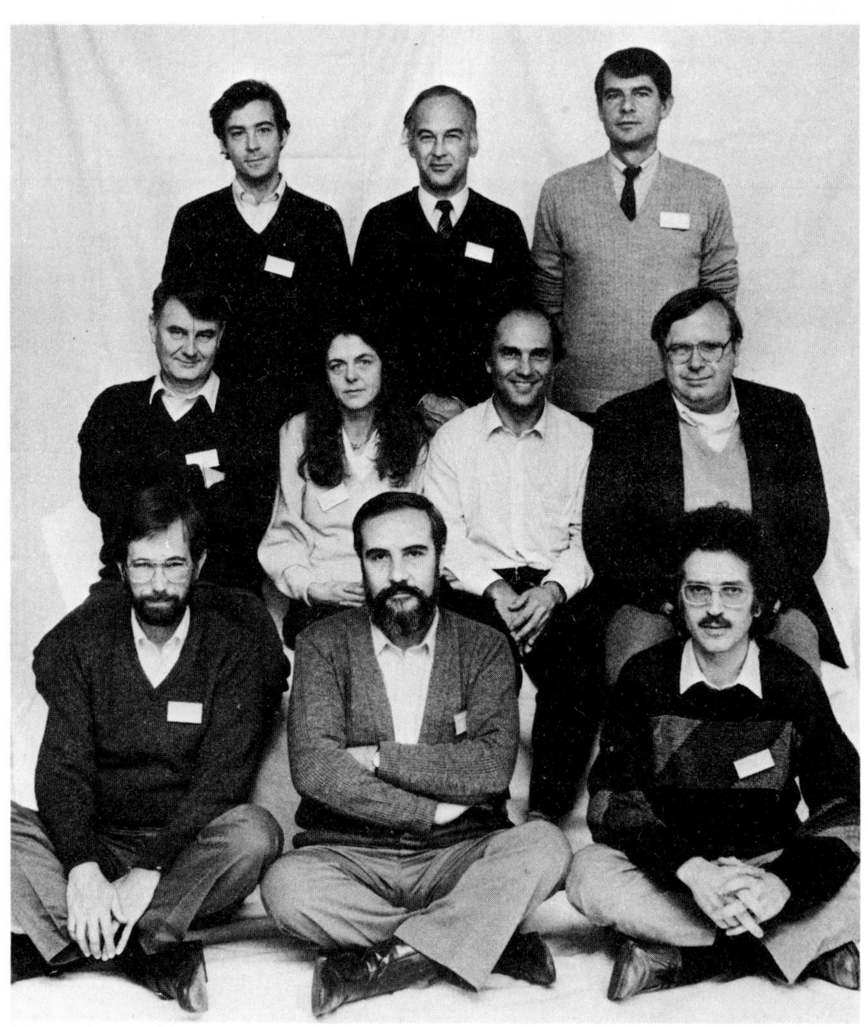

Back row, left to right:
Mark Bear, Carl Cotman, Wolf Singer

Middle row, left to right:
Terje Lømo, Claudia Stürmer, Giorgio Innocenti, Mike Merzenich

Bottom row, left to right:
Ron Meyer, Constantino Sotelo, Wilfried Seifert

Not Shown: P. Rakic

The Neural and Molecular Bases of Learning,
eds. J.-P. Changeux and M. Konishi, pp. 281–300.
John Wiley & Sons Limited.

Activity-dependent Modification of Functional Circuitry as a Possible Basis for Learning
Group Report

M.F. Bear, Rapporteur

C.W. Cotman, G.M. Innocenti, T. Lømo, M.M. Merzenich, R.L. Meyer, P. Rakic, W. Seifert, W. Singer, C. Sotelo, C.A.O. Stürmer

INTRODUCTION

It is becoming increasingly clear that brain circuitry is not "hard-wired." Rather accumulated evidence indicates that synaptic connections may be modified considerably both during development and in adulthood. The group discussion was aimed at examining the hypothesis that such modifications of neural circuits are a substrate for adult learning. This report is focused on the following questions:

1. Which types of modification are most likely to resemble processes that contribute to adult learning?
2. What are the rules of activity-dependent changes in excitatory circuitry?
3. Which mechanisms are feasible to explain these changes?
4. Are these mechanisms sufficient to account for any forms of adult learning?

The first task of our group was to determine which of the demonstrated types of circuit modification might realistically resemble a neural basis of learning. To be related to learning, it was reasoned, the modifications must be activity-dependent and demonstrable in the adult nervous system. Parameters that could not fulfill these requirements were considered to represent constraints on learning-related changes in functional circuitry.

The group next made an attempt to determine the rules which govern the activity-dependent modification of neural circuits. The main strategy here was to examine the evidence supporting the hypothesis that activity plays a role in the development and/or regeneration of neural circuits in several model systems. The models discussed were primarily the vertebrate neuromuscular junction, the mammalian visual cortex, and the retino-tectal projection of fish and amphibia. While the specific changes observed in these systems may not underlie any form of adult learning, it is reasonable to assume that common principles may guide activity-dependent modifications both during development and in adulthood.

As it turned out, some basic rules were found to be compatible with the neural mechanisms that have been proposed to account for synaptic modifications in several invertebrate and *in vitro* vertebrate models. However, it also became obvious that there are some differences and that many important questions remain unanswered. For example, the relative significance of structural vs. functional changes in synapses during learning is an unsettled issue. Such areas were identified as highly promising targets for further research.

Finally, we asked whether the rules for activity-dependent changes in developing and/or regenerating circuits could also apply to learning-related changes in the adult. For a modification to be considered relevant to adult learning, it not only must be activity-dependent and demonstrable in adults but must also be induced by changes in activity (as opposed to changes induced by cutting a nerve, for example). Recent work by Merzenich and colleagues (see Merzenich, this volume) suggests that shifts in the adult somatic-sensory cortical map fulfill all these criteria and may be guided by similar rules. Moreover, the changes observed in the organization of the somatotopic map are consistent with a model for recognition memory, which depends on the cerebral cortex. This discussion resulted in a suprisingly coherent synthesis of a possible neural basis of one form of learning.

APPARENT CONSTRAINTS ON ACTIVITY-DEPENDENT MODIFICATIONS OF CIRCUITRY

Axonal Topography

Under the appropriate conditions, neurons in the adult mammalian CNS can extend axons for considerable distances. One compelling demonstration of this comes from the grafting experiments of Aguayo and colleagues (see (1) for a review). They have shown that CNS neurons of adult rodents have the capacity to project axons into peripheral nerve grafts for distances of several centimeters. Furthermore, lesion experiments have shown that some widespread projection systems (for example, the noradrenergic locus coeruleus and the cholinergic basal forebrain projections) have the capacity for extensive growth even in the environment of the mature CNS. Thus, the question arises of whether the large-scale remodelling of neural circuits by axonal growth should be considered as a candidate for a substrate of learning.

One system in which axonal growth and navigation has been extensively investigated is the optic projection of amphibia and fish. In these animals, retinal ganglion cell axons will regenerate after nerve crush, grow to the optic tectum, and assume their appropriate laminar and topograhical relationships. For such large-scale remodelling to be relevant to learning, it should be dependent on activity. The activity-dependence of circuit formation has been examined by Harris (12). He transplanted the eye bud from the axolotl into the head of a species of salamander that produced endogenous tetrodotoxin (TTX). In spite of being electrically silenced and initially misrouted by the surgical procedure, optic fibers from the axolotl eye grew into the correct parts of the brain to innervate the appropriate nuclei and lamina of the visual centers. Moreover, the projection to the tectum was topographically organized. A similar analysis has also been done for regeneration in the goldfish by making repeated intraocular injections of TTX during optic nerve regeneration. When the optic nerve is crushed (23, 29), or when optic fibers are surgically misrouted into the wrong part and/or layer of the tectum (21, 22), fibers still manage to grow to the appropriate visual centers, the correct layer of the tectum, and into the topographically appropriate part of the tectum. Also, in anophtalmic mice lateral geniculate neurons project to cortex in topograhical order (16). Likewise in monkeys in which both eyes were enucleated at early embryonic stages, topograhically correct geniculo-cortical and cortico-geniculate connections are made in the absence of any information from the periphery (Rakic, unpublished). These sorts of data suggest that the growth and rough topography of axonal projections is not dependent on activity. Thus, intrinsic topographical cues appear to provide one constraint on the possible modification of an anatomical map by activity.

This, of course, is not to say that activity plays no role in determining (and maintaining) the final organization of such maps. After initial synapse formation, activity appears to be crucial for the refinement of axonal topograhy. For example, while the gross organization of regenerating retino-tectal axons in the goldfish is unaffected by TTX, the fine topography is entirely disrupted, both anatomically (23) and functionally (29). Likewise, visual input appears to be a critical determinant of the final orientation of the developing isthmo-tectal projection in frogs (33). Nonetheless, the extent to which axonal arbors may be pruned by activity appears to decrease rapidly after topography is formed. This has been shown convincingly for developing geniculo-cortical (30) and callosal (15) connections in cats, to name only two examples. This same observation applies to axonal sprouting in the mature brain. With the exception of certain "global" systems, such as the central noradrenergic and cholinergic projections, the capacity for axonal growth appears to be severely limited in the environment of the adult brain. For example, the most extensive growth of non-cholinergic axons in the dentate gyrus after lesions of the entorhinal cortex is on the order of 30-40 microns (see Cotman, this volume). These considerations suggest that major translocations of axonal terminal arbors are not a likely basis for learning-related changes in the adult mammalian nervous system. This limits the degrees of freedom available for learning-related circuit modifications and focuses attention on small changes in arbor size and/or changes occurring strictly at the synaptic level.

Synapse Density

It is no surprise that changes in synaptic junctions are a likely substrate for learning. However, it is remarkable that despite large inter-individual differences in experience the total synapse density in several areas of the adult brain, including the cerebral cortex, remains nearly constant (3, 28). The number of synapses formed within a structure may be thought to define its available repertoire for learning-related modifications. Thus, an important consideration is how total synapse density and number is regulated.

There are a number of indications that the postsynaptic target cell controls synapse density. For example, experimentally doubling the number of afferent axons to the superior cervical ganglion decreases the number of synapses per axon but does not change the total synapse density. Similarly, the deafferentation of a dendritic field results in a rapid replacement by nearby synapses until the normal synapse density is reestablished (see Cotman, this volume, for further discussion).

Insights into the mechanism of synapse density regulation have come from the study of muscle (see Lømo, this volume). Doubling the number of axons by transplanting two foreign nerves into a previously denervated muscle results in a corresponding decrease in motor unit size. The fact that ectopic neuromuscular junctions tend to be spaced at least 1 mm apart suggests the existence of zones that are refractory to synapse formation. Such zones on the dendrites of CNS neurons would serve to space synapses evenly on a target, which would yield a constant synapse density.

Is total synapse density a relevant parameter for learning-related changes in functional circuits? One intriguing observation suggests that it might be: there is a striking increase in cortical synapse density during early postnatal development. In the cat visual cortex, for example, the density of synapses exceeds the adult value from three weeks until approximately four months of age (34). This coincides with the "critical period" during which connections are most readily modified by visual experience. Surprisingly, this exuberant synapse density appears simultaneously in all cortical areas examined in the monkey including frontal, motor, somatosensory, visual, and limbic areas (28). Thus if the high synapse density plays a crucial role in defining the visual critical period, these results would predict that "critical periods" in association areas would occur at the same ages.

What is the activity dependence of synapse density? Rakic and colleagues have addressed this question by examining the effects of premature exposure to light on the course of synaptogenesis in the monkey striate cortex (5). The results indicate that the onset, tempo, and sequence of synaptogenesis in all cortical layers proceeds according to conceptual age regardless of the time of the animal's birth. They then performed the opposite experiment by removing both eyes at an early embryonic age and quantifying synapses at various postnatal ages. Remarkably, the synapse density in visual cortex achieves the normal adult level (Bourgeois and Rakic, unpublished). However, there are indications from experiments in the visual cortex of cats that sensory deprivation does slow the rate of synapse formation, particularly for the axo-spinous contacts (34). Furthermore, in rats it has been shown that depletion of brain norepinephrine will actually accelerate synapse formation slightly in the visual cortex (25). Thus, the synapse density "ceiling" at a given age may be modulated by activity-dependent processes. However, this type of slow modulation is an unlikely basis for a learning-related change. Rather, the data seem to indicate that in the time frame of a learning paradigm, the nervous system operates within a rather narrowly defined range of synapse density.

Tentative Conclusions and Outstanding Problems

To summarize, the preceeding discussion suggests two conclusions for the normal mature brain. First, much of the available axonal infrastructure is relatively fixed; second, the total density of synapses within a given structure remains relatively constant. It follows then that the changes in these parameters are an unlikely basis for adult learning.

Before these conclusions are accepted, however, several qualifications need to be made. For example, while we can say with confidence that in several well-characterized systems, such as the geniculo-cortical projection in cats, activity-dependent changes are not detectable in the normal adult, this does not mean that no such changes occur. Our measures may simply not be sensitive enough to pick up small changes in terminal arbors, and one would expect that any changes would necessarily be small in order to maintain proper function. Furthermore, the possibility remains open that certain connections, such as the associational fibers of the cerebral cortex, might have the potential for considerable activity-dependent axonal growth under conditions that have not yet been discovered. The anatomical limits on activity-dependent changes in the axonal infrastructure of point-to-point projections in the adult nervous system still need further study.

The conclusion that learning-related changes in the nervous system are constrained by a narrowly defined range of available synaptic sites also needs to be qualified. A constant synapse *density* translates into constant synapse *number* only if the volume does not also change. The interindividual variation in the cortical volume of randomly selected adult cats appears to be slight, suggesting a relatively low variation in the total number of synapses within this structure (3). On the other hand, cats reared in controlled, impoverished environments (4) display a significant decrease in the surface area (but not thickness) of the cerebral cortex and therefore must also have fewer cortical synapses (since the total synapse density is not changed significantly). Moreover, whereas the total number of synapses within a structure may remain constant this is not to say that the relative percentage of synapses from different sources does not change. Indeed, there is evidence for major rearrangements of this sort (i.e., synapse turnover, see Cotman, this volume). For example, while the total number of geniculo-cortical terminals (as seen using LM autoradiography) seems to be unaffected by monocular deprivation in kittens, the relative proportion of terminals from the lateral geniculate (LGN) lamina subserving the two eyes is dramatically altered. Finally, the low coefficient of variation for *total* synapse density does not exclude large differences within a single class of synapse. This has been clearly shown by Colonnier and colleagues in the cat striate cortex (3, 4). They found the coefficient of variation of total synapse density to be less than 10%. The variation among Gray's type I synapses, the major class in the cerebral cortex, was even lower. However, Gray's type II synapses, which constitute only about 15% of the synapses in visual cortex, were found to vary greatly between individuals (coefficient of variation, about 30%). This raises the important point that the rules which govern experience-dependent changes are likely to be different for different types of circuitry.

RULES FOR THE MODIFICATION OF EXCITATORY CIRCUITS

The role of activity during the development and/or regeneration of neural circuits has been extensively investigated in several model systems including the retino-tectal projection in lower vertebrates, the geniculo-cortical connections in mammals, and the vertebrate neuromuscular junction (reviewed in papers by Singer and Lømo, both this volume). These studies have revealed some striking similarities in the ways in which excitatory circuitry in different locations is modified according to use. From this analysis it is possible to formulate certain rules that appear to guide activity-dependent changes in functional circuitry. In this section we will highlight some of these modification rules, and in a subsequent section we will examine how well these rules fit the activity-dependent changes that have recently been demonstrated in the adult cerebral cortex (see Merzenich, this volume).

Homosynaptic Regulation

In most circuits of the central nervous system it is difficult to selectively manipulate pre- and postsynaptic activity in a controlled way due to the complexities imposed by reciprocal connections and convergence of multiple pathways onto single neurons. These same complexities do not exist at the vertebrate neuromuscular synapse, hence this preparation has proven to be a valuable model for the role of activity in synapse formation and maintenance. The principles of activity-dependent regulation of neuromuscular junctions are described in the background paper by Lømo (this volume). Many of these principles have obvious relevance to the activity-dependent regulation of more complex neural circuits in the CNS. Some of these include:

1. The level of postsynaptic activity determines the receptivity of the cell to synapse formation: an inactive target is receptive, an active one is not.
2. The maturation of an immature junction requires evoked postsynaptic activity.
3. Vacated endplates are more receptive to reinnervation than are adjacent regions of the cell membrane.

From these principles it may be concluded that the target cell plays a crucial role in the regulation of the synapses impinging upon it. In particular, point number 2 has important implications for the activity-dependent stabilization of circuits in the CNS. Unlike the muscle, whose activity monotonically follows that of the afferent axon, most neurons in the CNS require spatial or temporal summation of synaptic potentials in order to be activated above threshold. This means that converging afferents to a neuron, be they from the same source (homosynaptic input) or from multiple sources (heterosynaptic input), might be expected to be maintained preferentially if they were synchronously active. In fact, this phenomenon is observed in both the retino-tectal and the geniculo-cortical model systems (see below). More importantly in the context of learning, however, is that this same principle appears to apply to adult models of activity-dependent circuit modifications, such as long-term potentiation (LTP) in the hippocampus (see Andersen, this volume), and use-dependent shifts in the somatic sensory cortical map (see Merzenich, this volume). Because synchronously active inputs "work together toward a common end" (the definition of "cooperate") – that "end" being synaptic stabilization or strengthening – this phenomenon has been termed *cooperativity* (see also Andersen, this volume).

Heterosynaptic Regulation

From the preceeding discussion it is clear that activity evoked in a cell by stimulation of one afferent input could potentially have profound effects on the synapses of a second input from another source. One good model used to study this problem is the segregation of geniculo-cortical axons into ocular dominance columns. Early in development, projecting axons from the LGN, relaying information from the contralateral and ipsilateral eyes, respectively, are intermingled within cortical layer IV (27). Normal visual experience leads to the segregation of these axon terminals into ocular dominance columns (14). However, Stryker has shown in kittens that if the two optic nerves are stimulated *synchronously* then the mixed geniculate terminals in layer IV are maintained and presumably mature (32). The maintenance of overlapping inputs from two eyes by synchronous activation is an instructive example of heterosynaptic cooperativity.

When the two eyes are stimulated *asynchronously*, however, the mixed afferents segregate into ocular dominance (OD) columns. An analogous activity-dependent segregation of axons occurs in lower vertebrates when two eyes are made to innervate the optic tectum during development (8) or during regeneration (21). These results argue for the action of a second activity-dependent process involved in circuit selection, *competition*. This process is illustrated by comparing the effects of monocular and binocular deprivation on visual cortical circuitry (see Singer, this volume, for a more detailed discussion). While brief periods of binocular deprivation (BD) have only mild consequences on geniculo-cortical circuitry, comparable periods of monocular deprivation (MD) lead to a striking disconnection of the inactive afferents. The concept that has evolved to explain these findings is that geniculate afferents compete with each other for a finite amount of synaptic space in layer IV. The closure of one eye put its afferents at a competitive disadvantage. Hence, these synapses are lost and replaced by synapses of open-eye afferents. There is no imbalance of presynaptic activity after BD so no competitive disconnection occurs.

The available evidence suggests, however, that competition cannot depend solely on presynaptic activity levels. In order to be at a competitive advantage an afferent must also apparently be effective in driving the target neuron. Thus, stimulus conditions that are sufficient to activate the geniculate afferents, but do not drive visual cortical cells, will not cause shifts in OD. This means that both the stabilization of active synapses and the weakening of inactive synapses require postsynaptic activity (see Singer, this volume, for further discussion).

Neuromodulatory Regulation

While postsynaptic activation, as measured by soma spikes, appears to be a necessary condition for synaptic gain changes in the visual cortex, it is not sufficient. For example, no OD changes are normally observed in anesthetized or paralyzed animals even though monocular visual stimulation elicits action potentials in cortical neurons. However, if cortical excitability is raised in anesthetized kittens by pairing the visual stimulation with electrical activation of the midbrain reticular formation (MRF), synaptic modifications can be induced (Singer, this volume). These observations suggest that the postsynaptic depolarization must exceed some critical level before synaptic modification will occur, and this modification threshold is higher than the threshold for Na+ spikes. There is evidence in the visual cortex suggesting that this modification threshold is normally achieved only if cholinergic and noradrenergic projections are present (2). Thus, "global" systems potentially can exert a profound effect on synaptic modifiability by regulating cortical excitability.

Tentative Conclusions and Outstanding Problems

To summarize, many activity-dependent changes in functional circuitry require the depolarization of postsynaptic cells beyond a certain threshold. At most locations in the CNS, activation above this threshold minimally requires the synchronous discharge of converging afferents. Under these conditions the active synapses will be stabilized at the expense of the inactive. These considerations suggest that *selection of afferents according to their coincidence of activation* may be the basic algorithm of activity-dependent changes in excitatory circuitry.

It is encouraging that converging lines of inquiry have led to similar conclusions regarding the modification of excitatory circuitry. However, one must resist the temptation to generalize too broadly. Different types of excitatory circuitry use different transmitters and synapses upon different types of target. It is reasonable to expect significant variation in the ways these circuits are modified. To cite just one example, there is physiological evidence that geniculo-cortical synapses on inhibitory interneurons are more resistant to MD than are synapses on pyramidal cell dendrites (31). Moreover, it should be stressed that these rules at best apply only to excitatory circuits. The effects of activity on inhibitory connections are not yet understood.

The role of neuromodulation is becoming clear, at last, in the synaptic modifications which occur in the kitten visual cortex. This may be a special case unique to the cerebral cortex or it may be a more universal phenomenon. It would be of great interest to know whether "global" systems can regulate synaptic modifications at other locations and in different species.

Finally, while the pivotal role of the postsynaptic cell in regulating synaptic modifications is well established, many characteristics of the neuromuscular synapse appear to be dependent on the *pattern of presynaptic activity* as well (see Lømo, this volume). For example, an endplate with a "fast" morphology (many round, discrete boutons connected by thin axon branches) may be transformed in the direction of a "slow" appearance (irregular terminal branches with fewer boutons per unit endplate area) by stimulating the nerve with a slow pattern. This transformation is never complete and appears to occur within a finite adaptive range. Nonetheless, these data indicate that presynaptic patterns of activity can be an important determinant of synaptic properties. This may have important consequences for the interpretation of data from certain CNS model systems in which artificial patterns of activity are imposed experimentally.

POSSIBLE MECHANISMS

Due to the complexity of *in vivo* vertebrate models it has been difficult to approach the neural mechanisms which underlie activity-dependent changes in circuitry. However, considerable progress in this direction has been made using invertebrate and *in vitro* vertebrate models (see Carew, Alkon, Andersen, Ito, and Baudry *et al.*, all this volume). It is of interest to see how well these mechanisms fit the rules that appear to account for the modification of functional circuits.

Activation Threshold

The induction of LTP in the hippocampus requires activation of NMDA receptors, (7, 11) and the postsynaptic entry of Ca^{2+} ions (19). These and many other observations (Andersen, this volume) have led to the concept that cooperativity among converging afferents is required to depolarize the target dendrite beyond the threshold for postsynaptic Ca^{2+} entry presumably through gates linked to the NMDA receptor. Elevated postsynaptic Ca^{2+} may trigger intracellular changes which lead to enhanced synaptic efficacy.

Likewise, postsynaptic Ca^{2+} entry has been implicated in the acquisition of a classically conditioned response in *Hermissenda* (Alkon, this volume). The type B photoreceptor is both depolarized by light and synaptically activated by inputs from the vestibular system. The pairing of light with rotation of the animal depolarizes the cell beyond the threshold for Ca^{2+} entry. Elevated intracellular Ca^{2+} leads to a long-term decrease in K^+ conductance, thus leaving the cell more excitable to light than before conditioning.

In these two examples, homosynaptic and heterosynaptic cooperativity, respectively, are necessary for the strengthening of active inputs apparently due to a requirement for postsynaptic Ca^{2+} entry to effect a change in synaptic efficacy. These data suggest that the modification threshold hypothesized above for circuit modifications may relate to voltage-dependent Ca^{2+} entry. There are two indications that this may be the case in the visual cortex. First, the intracortical infusion of the

NMDA receptor blocker 2-amino-5-phosphonovalerate (APV) will interfere with OD changes after MD. Second, the conditions needed to evoke OD changes in anesthetized kittens (the pairing of MRF and visual stimulation) lead to measurable decreases in extracellular Ca^{2+} (Singer, this volume).

Neuromodulation

Most structures in the forebrain receive a diffuse innervation from several widely projecting systems in addition to the specific, topographically organized excitatory afferents. Two such systems are the noradrenergic projection from the locus coeruleus and the cholinergic projection from the basal forebrain. Until recently it has been unclear how these "global" projections influence information processing. The pioneering work of Kasamatsu and Pettigrew (17) first suggested that the noradrenergic system might play a role in regulating synaptic modifications in the visual cortex. Specifically, they showed that the cortical infusion of 6-hydroxydopamine, a catecholamine neurotoxin which depletes norepinephrine (NE), would prevent the OD shift after MD. Recent work suggests that the cortical cholinergic projection also facilitates synaptic modifications in the visual cortex (2). Interestingly, it appears that NE and acetylcholine (ACh) might actually be substitutive in their modulation of cortical modifiability (see Singer, this volume).

One plausible mechanism by which NE and ACh might regulate synaptic modifications comes from work done in the hippocampal slice preparation by Nicoll and colleagues (6, 20). They found that both ACh and NE decrease the Ca^{2+}-dependent K^+ current which underlies the afterhyperpolarization in pyramidal cells. This current may be thought of as a brake to prevent excessive postsynaptic Ca^{2+} entry. Hence, the blockade of this conductance by ACh and NE can be expected to facilitate voltage-dependent Ca^{2+} entry into dendrites. In addition, both ACh and NE stimulate the production of intracellular second messengers which activates kinases. Thus it is conceivable that these modulators may regulate certain phosphoproteins involved in the modification of synapses.

Locus of Change

One issue that appears to be unresolved even in simple model systems is how information, once acquired, is stored in the nervous system (see Baudry *et al.*, this volume). However, it does appear certain that memory is a structural change, not a reverberating pattern of activity. The structural changes that have been proposed to store information have ranged from covalent modification of intrinsic membrane proteins to subtle adjustments of the cytoskeleton, to the growth of new synapses. These mechanisms are not mutually exclusive, of course, and may even reflect transitions from short-term to long-term storage.

There is evidence suggesting that learning can induce changes in the pattern or number of synapses (reviewed by Cotman *et al.*, this volume). For example, Tsukahara and co-workers have shown that cortical inputs to neurons in the red nucleus (RN) will redistribute after lesions of the cerebellar input. This sprouting of new synapses causes measurable changes in the excitatory postsynaptic potential (EPSP) evoked in RN cells by cortical stimulation. Importantly, a similar change in the EPSP can be produced in a classical conditioning paradigm that does not involve direct lesions (although EM confirmation of ultrastructural changes is still lacking). Similarly, Larson and Greenough (18) have reported changes in the dendritic branching of cortical pyramidal cells as a result of training the animal to reach for food with its nonpreferred paw. Because cortical synapse density is not changed (recall above discussion), these dendritic changes presumably reflect alterations in the number of synapses impinging nto these cells.

Cotman and colleagues have introduced the concept of synapse *turnover* which they envisage to occur continuously throughout the lifetime of the animal (see Cotman *et al.*, this volume). One of the most compelling examples of this is the changes observed in the synapses formed by supraoptic hypothalamic neurons onto the fenestrated capillaries of the neurohypophysis (13). These synapses may be induced to form or withdraw by simply changing the animal's state of hydration.

Several important questions need to be addressed before we can assess the contribution of naturally occuring synapse turnover to learning mechanisms. For example, what is the stimulus for synapse elimination? How do new synapses replace old synaptic contacts? Are these processes dependent on activity? One preparation that promises to be useful in this inquiry is the retino-tectal projection in fish.

Both the retina and tectum continue to grow throughout most of the fish's life. However, while the retina adds new ganglion cells at its peripheral margin, the tectum adds new cells at its caudal pole (26). Despite this differential growth simple retinotopy is preserved in the tectum through all stages of growth. That is, ganglion cell axons from the center of the retina always project to the geometrical center of the tectum, and the ganglion cell axons from the periphery of the retina project to the periphery of the tectum. This implies the translational movement of axon terminals across the tectum as new axons are added at the periphery. There is direct experimental evidence for such a shifting of terminals in the goldfish optic tectum (10). Thus, newly arriving axons at the tectal periphery force the preexisting arbors to move to new sites. This sort of continuous formation and loss of synapses is, by definition, synapse turnover.

Despite abundant experimental evidence for the continuous displacement and relocation of terminal arbors in the fish optic tectum, the mechanisms which govern this process remain obscure. While it does appear that newly arriving axons are at a competitive advantage over their older predecessors, it is unknown at present whether this process is dependent on activity. Thus, the importance of synapse turnover as a mechanism for the activity-dependent modification of functional circuitry is not yet proven. This question clearly needs further study.

Tentative Conclusions and Outstanding Problems

In summary, mechanisms involving postsynaptic Ca^{2+} entry can account for activity-dependent modifications of functional circuitry at many locations. Ca^{2+} entry requires dendritic depolarization beyond a threshold level; this level is achieved only by synaptic coactivation. The amount of synaptic excitation needed to reach this threshold depends on target excitability which may be regulated by neuromodulators. The processes that follow Ca^{2+} entry, and which lead to the storage of learned information, are largely unknown.

At this time perhaps the greatest problem with these conclusions is that for most systems they are based purely on speculation! Clearly, direct tests of this "Ca^{2+} hypothesis" are necessary. The combined use of *in vitro* brain slices with the traditional *in vivo* preparations, as has already been done in the hippocampus, promises to be one particularly useful approach to the neural mechanisms underlying changes in circuitry in other systems.

RELEVANCE TO ADULT LEARNING

The evidence reviewed above suggests that activity-dependent modifications of excitatory circuitry in a number of developing and/or regenerating systems are guided by common principles and may be explained by similar mechanisms. Until recently, however, we were left to speculate about whether similar types of circuitry changes could actually contribute to adult learning, the fundamental problem being that similar modifications had not been demonstrated in the brain of an adult mammal. However, an exciting new avenue of research has been opened by the finding that topographical representations of the body surface in the cerbral cortex may be substantially altered by peripheral nerve lesions and, more importantly, by differential use. The evidence for shifts in the cortical map is discussed in detail by Merzenich (this volume) and will not be repeated here. Instead we shall briefly examine some of the principles that appear to govern these changes and compare them with the rules already established for other model systems.

Activity-dependent Changes in the Adult Cerebral Cortex

Shifts in the somatotopic map of the body surface in area 3b can be elicited by a number of manipulations including differential behavioral use of restricted skin surfaces. Several features of this functional remapping are listed individually below:

1) Shifts in representational topography do not exceed one millimeter. This suggests that the spatial constraints of remapping are likely to be determined by the available axonal infrastructure. This fits with the conclusion reached above, i.e., that major translocation of terminal arbors is not a likely basis for activity-dependent changes in the adult. The important implication here is that circuit selection is achieved by an alteration of synaptic effectiveness, not selective growth of axons.

2) Synchronously activated skin regions show a high probability of sharing representational topography. This result is exactly what would be predicted if synaptic coactivation were required for the stabilization of converging excitatory afferents. This supports the principle of contingency-matching in the selection of neural circuits.

3) Effecting a change in the map depends on the state of the animal. State-dependent signals are likely to be conveyed to the cortex along the modulatory pathways from the brain stem and basal forebrain. Thus, these projections are implicated in the regulation of map adjustments in the adult somatic sensory cortex as well as of ocular dominance changes in the immature visual cortex.

4) Representational topography is shared by neuronal groups that have sharp borders. The sharpness of group borders suggests a threshold phenomenon which determines whether a pattern of activation will cause a strengthening of connections. It is tempting to speculate that this threshold relates to postsynaptic Ca^{2+} entry as we discussed above.

Thus, the rules which appear to govern the activity-dependent changes in the adult somatic sensory map are largely consistent with those proposed to explain the circuit modifications that occur during development or regeneration. A final issue that needs to be raised is whether such changes occur within the time frame of learning. This has been shown unequivocally to be the case in the auditory cortex. Diamond and Weinberger (9) have demonstrated tonotopic shifts that are context-dependent and which occur within the time frame of a classical conditioning paradigm.

Cortical Learning in the Adult Primate

The activity-dependent changes in the functional circuitry of the cerebral cortex still need to be related to learning. One form of learning that appears to depend on the cerebral cortex, particularly the associational areas, has been called "recognition memory" by Mishkin (24). It differs from stimulus-response learning in two important ways. First, it lacks the same requirement for reinforcement. Second, it is more easily forgotten. Lesions of the amygdala and hippocampus severely interfere with recognition memory. Mishkin's working hypothesis is that the "gluing" of neurons into an ensemble which stores sensory information requires the appropriately timed activation, via limbic structures, of the cholinergic basal forebrain projections to the cerebral cortex.

It is too early to determine the relationship of this hypothesis to the observed alterations in the functional circuitry of the somatic sensory cortex. However, a striking similarity between recognition memory and visual cortical plasticity does emerge. Recognition memory recovers after lesions of either the hippocampus or the amygdala. However, the combined destruction of these structures causes a profound memory deficit (24). In an analogous fashion, OD plasticity appears to recover after lesions of either the noradrenergic or cholinergic projections; combined depletion of cortical ACh and NE reliably retards this type of plasticity (2). In this context it is interesting to note that a major target of the amygdala appears to be the nucleus basalis of Meynert.

Tentative Conclusions

In summary, the activity-dependent shifts of topographical maps in the adult cerebral cortex and the changes in excitatory circuitry observed in other systems appear to be guided by fundamentally similar rules. These rules call for the strengthening of synchronously active inputs if they drive the target neuron beyond a certain threshold. There is evidence in the adult somatic sensory and auditory cortex, and in the immature visual cortex, that modifications of circuitry are also influenced by cholinergic and noradrenergic mechanisms. One similarity between these types of circuit modification and cortical learning mechanisms appears to be this dependence on extrathalamic modulation. A high priority for future research in this area will be to determine whether cortical circuitry changes and recognition memory generally share the same requirements.

CONCLUDING REMARKS

Activity-dependent modifications of functional circuitry appear to occur within an adaptive range that constricts with age. Early in development, circuit modifications can include demonstrable changes in axonal arbors, while the modifications appear to be limited to synaptic gain changes in the adult. Nevertheless, the guiding priniciples of activity-dependent circuit selection appear to be similar regardless of age. The basic algorithm, by which excitatory afferents are selected by their coincidence of activation, allows for the associative specificity required of a learning mechanism.

Using the developmental models where changes are easier to induce and detect, we can now begin to approach the molecular mechanisms of activity-dependent circuit selection. In the adult we now have the tools to ask whether classical learning paradigms can be used to induce changes in functional circuitry. Then we can ask whether these changes are essential for different types of learning to occur. Thus, there is good reason for being optimistic that we are close to uncovering the neural basis of at least some forms of learning.

REFERENCES

(1) Aguayo, A.J. 1986. Axonal regeneration from injured neurons in the adult mammalian central nervous system. In *Synaptic Plasticity*, ed. C.W. Cotman, chap. 15. New York: The Guilford Press.

(2) Bear, M.F., and Singer, W. 1986. Modulation of visual cortical plasticity by acetylcholine and noradrenaline. *Nature* 320: 172-175.

(3) Beaulieu, C., and Colonnier, M. 1985. A laminar analysis of the number of round-asymmetrical and flat-symmetrical synapses on spines, dendritic trunks, and cell bodies in area 17 of the cat. *J. Comp. Neur.* 231: 180-189.

(4) Beaulieu, C., and Colonnier, M. 1985. The differential effect of impoverished and enriched environments on the number of "round asymmetrical" and "flat symmetrical" synapses in the visual cortex of the cat. *Neurosci. Abstr.* 11: 68.5.

(5) Bourgeois, J.-P., and Rakic, P. 1984. Premature exposure to light does not alter the course of synaptogenesis in the primate striate cortex. *Neurosci. Abstr.* 10: 1078.

(6) Cole, A.E., and Nicoll, R.A. 1984. Characterization of a slow cholinergic postsynaptic potential recorded *in vitro* from rat hippocampal pyramidal cells. *J. Physl. Lon.* 352: 173-1188.

(7) Collingridge, G.L.; Kehl, S.J.; and McLennan, H. 1983. Excitatory amino acids in synaptic transmission in the Schaffer collateral-commissural pathway of the rat hippocampus. *J. Physl. Lon.* 334: 33-46.

(8) Constantine-Patton, M., and Law, M.I. 1978. Eye-specific segregation requires neural activity in three-eyed frogs. *Science* 202: 639-641.

(9) Diamond, D.M., and Weinberger, N.M. 1985. The expression of learning-induced plasticity of single neurons in the auditory cortex is context-dependent. *Neurosci. Abstr.* 11: 245.4.

(10) Easter, S.S., and Stürmer, C.A.O. 1984. An evaluation of the hypothesis of shifting terminals in the goldfish optic tectum. *J. Neurosci.* 4: 1052-1063.

(11) Harris, E.W.; Ganong, A.H.; and Cotman, C.W. 1984. Long-term potentiation in the hippocampus involves activation of N-methyl-D-aspartate receptors. *Brain Res.* 323: 132-137.

(12) Harris, W.A. 1980. The effects of eliminating impulse activity on the development of the retinotectal projection in salamanders. *J. Comp. Neur.* 194: 303-317.

(13) Hatton, G.I. 1985. Reversible synapse formation and modulation of cellular relationships in the adult hypothalamus under physiological conditions. In *Synaptic Plasticity*, ed. C.W. Cotman, chap. 3. New York: Gilford Press.

(14) Hubel, D.H.; Wiesel, T.N.; and LeVay, S. 1977. Plasticity of ocular dominance columns in monkey striate cortex. *Phil. Trans. R. Soc. Lon. B.* 278: 377-409.

(15) Innocenti, G.M., and Frost, D.O. 1979. Effects of visual experience on the maturation of the efferent system to the corpus callosum. *Nature* 280: 231-234.

(16) Kaiserman-Abramof, R.I.; Graybiel, A.M.; and Nauta, W.J.H. 1980. The thalamic projection to cortical area 17 in a congenitally anophtalmic mouse strain. *Neuroscience* 5: 41-52.

(17) Kasamatsu, T., and Pettigrew, J.D. 1979. Preservation of binocularity after monocular deprivation in the striate cortex of kittens treated with 6-hydroxydopamine. *J. Comp. Neur.* 185: 153-162.

(18) Larson, J.R., and Greenough, W.T. 1981. Effects of handedness training on dendritic branching of neurons in forelimb area of rat motor cortex. *Soc. Neurosci. Abstr.* 7: 65.

(19) Lynch, G.; Larson, J.; Kelso, S.; Barrionuevo, G.; and Schottler, F. 1983. Intracellular injections of EGTA block induction of hippocampal long-term potentiation. *Nature* 305: 719-721.

(20) Madison, D.V., and Nicoll, R.A. 1982. Noradrenaline blocks accomodation of pyramidal cell discharge in the hippocampus. *Nature* 299: 636-638.

(21) Meyer, R.L. 1979. Extra optic fibers exclude normal fibers from tectal regions in goldfish. *J. Comp. Neur.* 183: 883-902.

(22) Meyer, R.L. 1982. Tetrodotoxin inhibits the formation of ocular dominance columns in goldfish. *Science* 218: 589-591.

(23) Meyer, R.L. 1983. Tetrodotoxin inhibits the formation of refined topography in goldfish. *Dev. Brain Res.* 6: 293-298.

(24) Mishkin, M. 1982. A memory system in the monkey. *Phil. Trans. R. Soc. Lon. B* 298: 85-95.

(25) Parnavelas, J.G., and Blue, M.E. 1982. The role of the noradrenergic system in the formation of synapses in the visual cortex of the rat. *Dev. Brain Res.* 3: 140-144.

(26) Raymond, P.A., and Easter, S.S. 1983. Postembryonic growth of the optic tectum in goldfish. I. Location of germinal cells and number of neurons produced. *J. Neurosci.* 3: 1077-1051.

(27) Rakic, P. 1976. Prenatal genesis of connections subserving ocular dominance in the rhesus monkey. *Nature* 261: 467-471.

(28) Rakic, P.; Bourgeois, J.-P.; Eckenhoff, M.E.; Zecevic, N.; and Goldman-Rakic, P.S. 1986. Concurrent overproduction of synapses in diverse regions of the primate cerebral cortex. *Science* 232: 232-235.

(29) Schmidt, J.T., and Edwards, D.L. 1983. Activity sharpens the map during the regeneration of the retinotectal projection in goldfish. *Brain Res.* 269: 29-39.

(30) Shatz, C.J., and Stryker, M.P. 1978. Ocular dominance in layer IV of the cat's visual cortex and the effects of monocular deprivation. *J. Physl. Lon.* 281: 267-283.

(31) Singer, W. 1977. Effects of monocular deprivation on excitatory and inhibitory pathways in cat striate cortex. *Exp. Brain Res.* 134: 508-578.

(32) Stryker, M.P. 1981. Late segregation of genicular afferents to the cat's visual cortex after recovery from binocular impulse blockade. *Neurosci. Abstr.* 7: 842.

(33) Udin, S.B. 1983. Abnormal visual input leads to development of abnormal axon trajectories in frogs. *Nature* 301: 336-338.

(34) Winfield, D.A. 1983. The postnatal development of synapses in the different laminae of the visual cortex in the normal kitten and in kittens with eyelid suture. *Dev. Brain Res.* 9: 155-169.

The Neural and Molecular Bases of Learning,
eds. J.-P. Changeux and M. Konishi, pp. 301–336.
John Wiley & Sons Limited.

Activity-dependent Self-organization of Synaptic Connections as a Substrate of Learning

W. Singer

Max-Planck-Institut für Hirnforschung
6000 Frankfurt 71, F.R. Germany

INTRODUCTION

Learning can be defined operationally as a stimulus- and, hence, activity-dependent neuronal process that leads to a consistent and long-lasting change of behavioral responses. The formation of a memory trace may thus be considered as a modification of the neuronal program that specifies stimulus-response relations. In the CNS the program which determines such relations is stored by the architecture of interneuronal connectivity and by the differential weighting of the transfer functions of these connections. Thus, any activity-dependent process that modifies, in a sufficiently stable and long-lasting way, the excitatory or inhibitory interactions between pairs of neurons could serve as a mechanism of learning, and any long-lasting alteration of intercellular communication can be considered as an engram.

Activity-dependent long-term changes of neuronal connectivity are a ubiquitous phenomenon during early ontogeny and a constituent factor in the self-organization of the brain. During postnatal development these shaping processes become increasingly subtle and dependent on a growing number of variables. In the following paragraphs I shall review examples of such activity-dependent processes whereby I shall follow the chronological order by which these phenomena emerge during ontogeny. One of the conclusions from this review will be that neuronal mechanisms mediating adult learning might be derived from the very processes of neural plasticity that serve as mechanisms for self-organization during development.

AXONAL SEGREGATION AND RETRACTION

In most structures of the peripheral and central nervous system the selectivity of neuronal connectivity is the result of a developmental process that has two stages. During the first stage connections are established in excess and with rather limited precision. During the second stage this coarse connectivity pattern is pruned by selective elimination of "ectopic" pathways (for review of the extensive literature see (17, 80, 106, 130)). Evidence is available that these elimination processes are influenced by neuronal activity. In the central nervous system most of the data on such activity-dependent modifications of connectivity patterns have been collected in the visual system. The reason is that in this system neuronal activity can be manipulated very easily by sensory deprivation. Since reviews of the extensive literature on the structural and functional effects of visual deprivation are available (36), only selected issues are discussed here.

In adult cats and monkeys and a variety of other mammalian species with overlapping binocular visual fields, the afferents from the two eyes terminate in different laminae of the visual relay of the thalamus, and the corresponding thalamo-cortical afferents terminate, in turn, within well segregated alternating patches or bands in layer IV of striate cortex (54). A segregation of afferents from the two eyes into alternating ocular dominance stripes is also seen in the optic tectum of mammals and under certain conditions even in the tectum of fish and frogs, suggesting a very basic principle of organization (24, 56, 104). In the cat thalamus segregation of the afferents from the two eyes is completed shortly after birth (105, 106). In the visual cortex the pattern of ocular dominance (OD) columns develops shortly before birth in monkeys and shortly after birth in cats (69, 70, 93, 94). The evidence is compelling that this pattern results from retraction of previously overlapping connections rather than from selective growth into prespecified territories. Initially, the afferents from the two eyes are intermingled completely and at least for the cat there is evidence that at this stage the fibers of the two eyes possess functional connections with common target cells both at the thalamic (106) and cortical level (108). Experiments in which the spontaneous activity of the eyes has been blocked with repeated application of tetrodotoxin (TTX) indicate that the segregation of afferents is promoted by neuronal activity. Archer (5) observed persistence of binocularly driven cells in the cat LGN after prolonged postnatal blockade of retinal activity with TTX injections. A retardation of the segregation of thalamo-cortical fibers into ocular dominance patches has been observed with binocular deprivation (89,

128) and an accentuation of segregation has been seen in cats in which the activity patterns arriving from the two eyes had been made dissimilar by alternating occlusion or the induction of squint (4, 107, 13). This latter finding suggested that the pattern, rather than activity *per se*, might be an important parameter for axonal segregation. Support for this hypothesis comes from experiments with TTX blockade of the retina. In the kitten visual cortex the terminal fields of the two eyes remain overlapping when the two retinae are silenced (125) and they segregate despite TTX blockade if the optic nerves are continuously stimulated electrically. Interestingly, however, it turned out that segregation occurred only when stimulation of the two nerves was asynchronous. When the two nerves were activated always simultaneously, columns did not form (126).

These findings suggest that the selection process which sorts fibers according to their ocular provenance identifies the afferents on the basis of their activation pattern. There is evidence in the cat retina that adjacent ganglion cells show some correlation of their spontaneous activity (81) and Rodieck and Smith (98) have shown that in the dark the retinae of the two eyes generate slow rhythmical activities which are synchronous within the same eye but not phase-locked between the eyes. There is thus the possibility that fibers can be identified at the cortical level as coming from the same or different eye by evaluating the correlation between their respective firing patterns. This interpretation is attractive because, if correct, it would imply interesting parallels between the processes mediating axonal segregation during early stages of development on the one hand and processes that serve to optimize functional binocularity during later postnatal development on the other. As discussed below, the correlation between neuronal activity patterns is an important parameter for these later developmental stages. However, while during early development self-generated activity of the retina and the subsequent visual relays appear to be sufficient to promote the segregation of OD columns, the selection processes occurring during later postnatal phases appear to require that the retina is stimulated with contours.

Similar observations have been made in the optic tectum of frogs and fish in which the formation of OD columns had been induced by transplanting eye grafts whose efferents compete with those of the original eyes for target space in the optic tectum (24, 56). Here, too, segregation follows overlap and can be prevented by silencing the retinae (16, 83). In this case the interesting observation has been made that segregation does still occur even if only one of the competing eyes remains active (83).

PLASTICITY OF OCULAR DOMINANCE COLUMNS

It is a well established fact that asymmetries in the activation of afferents from the two eyes cause corresponding asymmetries in the geometry of OD columns (11, 55, 69, 95, 129). In both cats and monkeys monocular deprivation leads to a shrinkage of the territories innervated by the deprived eye and to an expansion of the domains occupied by afferents from the normal eye (11, 69, 108, 129). This malleability of the width of columns is restricted to a critical period of early postnatal development. During this period reversal of eye closure can lead to a reversal of the previously induced asymmetries (11). While it is clear that these morphological modifications are caused by the imbalance between the activity patterns provided by the two eyes, little is known about the border conditions of these changes. It has been suggested that the system of ocular dominance bands remains susceptible to activity-dependent modifications until the afferents from the two eyes have segregated completely (69). Indeed, in the cat there is a fairly good correlation between the time course of column formation on the one hand and column plasticity on the other. In the monkey, however, there seems to be a dissociation. The segregation of OD columns is nearly complete at birth (94, 95) but modifiability of the columns persists postnatally (11, 129).

The development of cell sizes in the lateral geniculate reflects these changes of right and left eye territories in the visual cortex. Cells in laminae corresponding to the deprived eye shrink while cells innervating the expanding territories may show a hypertrophy (43, 45). These changes of LGN cell sizes are considered to be secondary to the shrinkage and expansion of their terminal arborizations in the visual cortex. However, recent data have shown that the hypertrophy of the nondeprived LGN neurons is only transient (43, 123). With prolonged monocular deprivation the cell sizes in the laminae connected to the normal eye also drop below normal levels although not as drastically as those in the deprived laminae. This raises the interesting possibility that the interactions between the pathways from the two eyes are not only competitive (43) but have also a synergistic component. This point will be discussed further in the context of the functional correlates of early deprivation.

The extent to which neuronal response properties reflect the segregation of afferents from the two eyes and the sizes of the territories occupied by these afferents varies in the different cortical laminae. The correlation is very close in layer IV, the principal target layer of thalamic afferents (68), but it is loose at best in nongranular layers. In layer IV neurons tend to become monocular as the afferents from the two eyes segregate (108) and the frequency of right and left eye dominated cells reflects approximately the deprivation-induced asymmetries of right and left eye territories. Under normal developmental conditions, however, cells in nongranular layers remain excitable from both eyes despite axonal segregation in layer IV (39) and with deprivation their ocularity may become skewed much more than one would expect from the asymmetries in the termination pattern of thalamic afferents. This emphasizes the importance of intracortical circuitry for the formation of binocular receptive fields, a point that will be dealt with in more detail below.

ACTIVITY-DEPENDENT REFINEMENT OF TOPOGRAPHIC MAPS

Other examples for an activity-dependent rearrangement of axonal patterns come from the development and refinement of topographic maps. A well investigated model system in the mammalian brain is the callosal connections between visual areas. In the striate cortex of the normal adult cat, callosal connections are strictly confined to the cortical representation of the vertical meridian. In the kitten, cells projecting through the callosum are found scattered throughout area 17 and their axons are directed towards cortical territories normally not innervated by callosal fibers (58). These ectopic connections disappear during the first postnatal weeks and there is evidence that this rearrangement, too, is to some extent influenced by neuronal activity. When kittens are dark-reared the elimination of callosal fibers proceeds beyond the level attained with normal visual experience and there is evidence for a critical period during which visual signals have a consolidating effect on normotopic callosal fibers (37, 59, 61). When kittens are made strabismic the retraction of ectopic callosal connections remains incomplete with the effect that pathways persist between territories of the visual cortex that are normally devoid of callosal connections (60, 76). It has been proposed that this persistence is related to the incongruency of the activation patterns arriving from the two eyes. It remains unclear, however, whether the ectopic fibers have a functional role in linking those areas in the cortex which possess corresponding pairs of receptive fields in the visual space. An alternative explanation is that the callosal fibers take over synaptic space that is freed by strabismus-induced competition between the afferents from the two eyes. Cynader *et al.* (28) have shown that callosal and retinal afferents compete with each other during early postnatal development, disruption of the retinal input enhancing the efficacy of callosal connections.

Very similar experience-dependent processes have been observed for the tangential connections within striate cortex. Shortly after birth and prior to visual experience these form an exuberant network of distinct lattice-like projections. With normal visual experience the spread of these intrinsic connections is reduced to adult levels, whereas in the absence of visual experience this network of horizontal connections disappears almost completely (75). In analogy to the callosal connections this indicates that neuronal activity does not only promote segregation and disruption of axonal projections but may also have a stabilizing effect on certain, presumably the functionally well-adapted, pathways.

An activity-dependent shaping of projection patterns has also been observed in the optic tectum of goldfish and of *Xenopus*. In the former, blockade of retinal activity prevented the refinement of the retinotopic order of retinal afferents both during development and regeneration (84, 102). In the latter, visual deprivation impeded the development of precise correspondence between the representations of the two eyes (65, 135, 136).

Another activity-dependent selection process has recently been observed in the cat LGN and does not result in topographical but in functional specification. In the adult animal LGN relay cells receive excitatory input exclusively either from on- or off-center retinal ganglion cells (115) while shortly after birth on- and off-center fibers still converge onto the same relay cells. Experiments with TTX blockade of retinal activity indicate that in this case, too, segregation does depend on neuronal activity (5), raising the interesting possibility that the coherency of firing patterns is higher among the respective on- and off-channels than between them.

PLASTICITY OF ORIENTATION PREFERENCES IN THE VISUAL CORTEX

An experience-dependent pruning of functional properties and a rearrangement of columnar organizations occurs also in the domain of orientation selectivity. In the primary visual cortex of normal adult cats and monkeys, cells with preferences for vertical, horizontal, and oblique orientations are encountered with about equal frequency whereby cells with similar preferences are grouped in slabs or bands which extend throughout all cortical layers (52). When cats are deprived of contour vision from birth, numerous cortical cells fail to develop orientation selectivity and many cells stop responding to activation of retinal afferents (119). When visual experience is restricted to a narrow range of orientations, the large majority of cortical neurons assumes a preference for this orientation (10, 48). Visualization of orientation columns with the deoxyglucose method reveals that in this case columns encoding the experienced orientations expand on the expense of columns corresponding to the deprived orientations (116). As with monocular deprivation the changes are more pronounced in superficial and deep layers than in layer IV. In the latter, regularly spaced islands are preserved which can be assumed to contain neurons encoding nonexperienced orientations. This suggests that within layer IV cells are capable of developing selectivities for orientations that have not been experienced previously. Data from very young or dark-reared animals support this notion. A fraction of simple cells in layer IV develop orientation selectivity despite the lack of contour vision (13, 19, 47, 71, 109, 127) and the sequence regularity of the columnar arrangement is maintained (51, 141). Whether this skeleton of orientation columns within layer IV requires self-generated activity for its expression as it is the case for the OD columns is not known yet. As the deprivation experiments indicate, activity is indispensable for the development of orientation selectivity outside layer IV. Moreover, in this case activity has to be structured by contour vision, self-generated activity patterns not being sufficient. This issue will be elaborated further in the discussion of experience-dependent modifications of receptive field properties.

ACTIVITY-DEPENDENT CONSOLIDATION AND DISRUPTION OF FUNCTIONAL BINOCULARITY

In the preceding paragraphs evidence has been reviewed indicating that neuronal activity influences the segregation of axonal arborizations, the refinement of topographic projections, and the expression of columnar patterns. In this section I shall concentrate on activity-dependent modifications of excitatory connections that are required for the development of binocular receptive fields and presumably also for the sharpening of orientation selectivity.

Before visual experience becomes effective in influencing the ocularity of cortical neurons, most cells in the visual cortex of cats and monkeys respond to stimulation of both eyes. This condition is maintained with normal experience but also with dark rearing. With monocular deprivation, however, the large majority of cortical cells loses the ability to respond to the deprived eye (12, 139). The cells which continue to respond to the deprived eye are located preferentially within layer IV in the center of the shrunken termination fields of the deprived eye (108). This suggests that only those cells continue to respond to the deprived eye which have been monocularly driven by this eye right from the beginning. With reverse suture, if it occurs early enough, the previously closed eye may recover control over most cortical neurons while the previously open eye in turn becomes ineffective (12, 140).

When induced early in development, at times when axonal segregation is not yet completed, these functional changes go in parallel with the retraction and expansion of thalamic afferents within layer IV and reflect to some extent the formation and withdrawal of synaptic connections between thalamic afferents and cortical target cells. However, these modifications of ocular dominance most certainly also include changes in the efficacy of intracortical synaptic connections, this latter mechanism becoming relatively more prominent at later stages of development when axonal segregation is already in an advanced stage. This has to be inferred from the evidence that marked changes in the ocularity of cortical neurons can occur without or with only minor modifications of the termination patterns of thalamic afferents in layer IV (for review see (132)). One example is the late changes of ocular dominance in dark-reared kittens. In normally reared kittens monocular deprivation is only effective during a critical period that lasts about 3 months (92). In dark-reared kittens, by contrast, monocular deprivation induces changes of ocular dominance even after the end of this period (27). These late changes of ocularity are, however, not associated with changes of columnar patterns in layer IV (87, 88). Another example for such a dissociation is the modifications occurring with strabismus. Here the morphological pattern of ocular dominance columns in layer IV is nearly unchanged (70), while the functional ocularity of cortical neurons is drastically altered. Most cells are monocular and driven either by the right or the left eye (53). Finally, there is evidence from single cell recording and deoxyglucose mapping in monocularly deprived cats that activity is still present within the deprived eye's columns but is confined to layer IV, indicating transmission failure at the level of intracortical connections (15, 108). It is these latter changes in excitatory transmission rather than the macroscopic rearrangements of columnar patterns that will be dealt with in the following section.

MECHANISMS OF ACTIVITY-DEPENDENT MODULATION OF EXCITATORY TRANSMISSION

A primary cause for the loss of responses to the deprived eye is most probably reduced efficacy of excitatory transmission since current source density analysis reveals a dramatic reduction of EPSP-related inward currents (85). During early phases of deprivation, however, interocular inhibition also appears to contribute since some responses to the deprived eye can be recovered by blocking intracortical GABAergic inhibition (110).

As long as ocular dominance changes are associated with structural changes of the terminal arborizations of geniculate afferents, stabilization and removal of connections are certainly one cause of modifications of excitatory transmission (55, 131, 132). The reduction in the number of dendritic spines with deprivation is direct support for such numerical changes in synaptic connections (25, 40, 132, 137, 143). However, there are also more subtle ultrastructural modifications of synaptic complexes following manipulations of visual experience. With monocular deprivation the size and the organelle content of presynaptic boutons, the number of perforated synapses, and the dimensions of the postsynaptic spines are abnormal (131). This suggests that the efficacy of synaptic transmission may be also regulated through mechanisms other than simple changes in the number of connections ((90), for review see (132, 138)).

Recently, activity-dependent changes of response properties including ocular dominance have been observed to occur within intervals ranging from minutes to a few hours ((18, 38, 99), Mioche and Singer, in preparation) suggesting the action of processes with relatively fast time constants. We ignore the exact turnover rates of synapse formation and elimination during development but it would seem unlikely that these processes alone could account for the fast changes that can occur in response to visual stimulation. Whether the ultrastructural changes are the *cause* for the fast activity-dependent modifications of synaptic gain or the *consequence* of a long-lasting reduction of synaptic activity in the deprived pathway is unknown. Clearly, changes in spine geometry could be fast enough to account for the fastest of the modifications observed to date (31, 32).

CONDITIONS REQUIRED FOR THE INDUCTION OF OCULAR DOMINANCE CHANGES

In contrast to the fragmentary data on the neuronal mechanisms mediating activity-dependent modifications of ocular dominance, detailed information is available on the conditions that need to be fulfilled for their induction.

The Role of Postsynaptic Activation

It has become clear that changes in ocular dominance do not solely depend on the level of activity in the afferent connections. It appears, rather, that the critical variable is the state of activation of the postsynaptic neuron and, in particular, the degree of temporal correlation between pre- and postsynaptic activation. This is illustrated by the following examples. First, if in 4-week-old kittens one eye is closed light-tight and the other exposed to diffuse light whose intensity is continuously modulated, the ocular dominance of cortical neurons does not shift towards the stimulated eye (118). In this case the afferents from the stimulated eye are more active than those from the deprived eye, but most cortical cells cannot respond to the activity conveyed by the stimulated eye because their receptive fields are selective for spatial contrast gradients. Another indication for the relevance of postsynaptic activation comes from experiments in kittens which were monocularly deprived for a few days and then had the previously open eye occluded and the previously closed eye exposed to contours of a single orientation (96, 97). During this second phase of exposure differential gain changes occurred only for pathways connecting to those cortical cells whose orientation preference matched the experienced orientations and hence could respond to the signals conveyed by the open eye. For these cells the efficacy of afferents from the stimulated eye increased while that of afferents from the deprived eye decreased. These cells became monocular and excitable only from the newly open eye. Cells whose orientation preference did not correspond to the orientations seen by the stimulated eye and hence could not respond to activity from this eye remained connected to the previously open eye. Thus, even though the geniculo-cortical pathways from the stimulated eye conveyed normally patterned activity and were more active than those from the deprived eye, they did not repress the latter from those postsynaptic cells which could not respond.

From a series of related experiments it was concluded that these modifications of excitatory transmission follow rules which closely resemble those postulated by Hebb (46), Stent (124), and Changeux (22, 23) for adaptive neuronal connections (97). These rules are summarized in Table 1. The basic assumptions are that changes of synaptic efficacy require the activation of the postsynaptic structure and that the direction of the change – increase or decrease of efficacy – depends on the

TABLE 1 – Rules for activity-dependent modification of synaptic transmission.

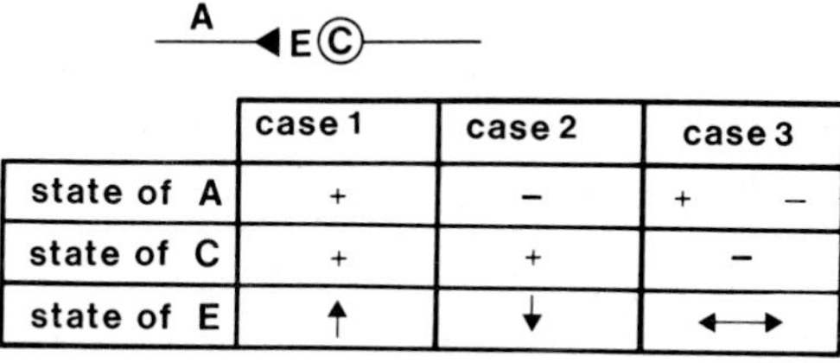

	case 1	case 2	case 3
state of A	+	–	+ –
state of C	+	+	–
state of E	↑	↓	↔

Consequences on convergent pathways.

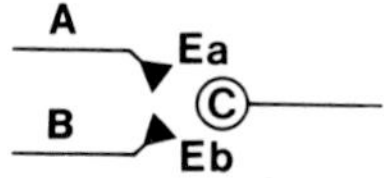

Correlation between A and B	positive	negative	negative
Initial efficacy of Ea and Eb	Ea ≥ Eb or Ea ≤ Eb	Ea > Eb	Ea < Eb
Resulting changes of Ea and Eb	Ea ↗ Eb ↗	Ea ↗ Eb ↘	Ea ↘ Eb ↗
Resulting circuitry	Association of A and B	Competitive disconnection of A or B	

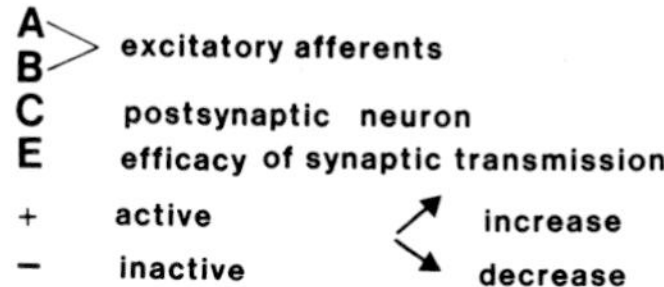

correlation between pre- and postsynaptic activation. The efficacy of excitatory transmission appears to increase when presynaptic afferents and the postsynaptic cell are active in temporal contiguity and to decrease when the postsynaptic target is active while the presynaptic terminal is silent. These rules, when applied to circuits where two (or more) afferent pathways converge onto a common postsynaptic target cell, have the effect to stabilize selectively and hence associate pathways that convey correlated activity. The only requirement is that the conveyed activity patterns are capable of driving the postsynaptic neuron. Likewise, these selection criteria lead to competition between converging pathways if these convey uncorrelated activity. In that case there is always one subset of afferents inactive while the other is driving the postsynaptic cell. Hence one subset will increase its gain at the expense of the respective other. Eventually, those afferents will win which have the highest probability of being active in temporal contiguity with the postsynaptic target cell. So far these rules have predicted correctly the results of the numerous studies in which vision has been manipulated in a way that interferes with the correlation between the responses arriving from the two eyes. However, a direct demonstration in identified pairs of neurons of the validity of these modification rules is still lacking. Recent evidence in support of such a Hebbian process comes from experiments in which the cortical cells were act vated directly by iontophoretic application of K^+ ions (Frégnac, personal communication) or excitatory amino acids (42). If strong postsynaptic activation was repeatedly made contingent with a particular pattern of afferent activity, the cell's responses to this pattern increased. This increase outlasted conditioning by up to 1 h and was selective for the pattern of activation used during conditioning.

Further support for the crucial role of the correlation between pre- and postsynaptic activation in ocular dominance plasticity comes from experiments in which selective ocular dominance changes were prevented by continuous infusion of glutamate into striate cortex (28).

Indications for the participation of the postsynaptic neurons in activity-dependent reorganization of excitatory connections are also available for the fish optic tectum (100, 101, 103). In regions where postsynaptic responses were abolished with local application of α-bungarotoxin, retinal terminals appeared to retract suggesting a stabilizing action of postsynaptic activity.

The Duration of Hebbian Simultaneity in the Visual Cortex

The modification rules predict that pathways consolidate only when they are active in contingency with the postsynaptic cell. For converging pathways (e.g., those arriving from the two eyes), this implies that they have to be active simultaneously if they are to remain connected to a common target cell. As soon as they get out of phase they will compete with each other and one pathway will become repressed. The cutoff point, beyond which asynchrony between the activity patterns from the two eyes leads to disruption of binocularity, has now been determined using high-speed liquid crystal shutters which allowed for rapidly alternating monocular occlusion in freely behaving kittens (3). The maximal interval of asynchrony still compatible with the maintenance of binocular connections was in the order of 200 to 400 ms.

This suggests that the signal which is generated by one eye persists, presumably in the postsynaptic cell, for a few hundred ms. This seems to exclude action potentials as the relevant signal and even conventional EPSPs are probably not capable of bridging such long intervals. It is known from psychophysical work, however, that the visual system integrates over such time spans and that the neuronal representation of a stimulus persists for 300 to 400 ms.

The Role of Nonretinal Signals in Ocular Dominance Plasticity
The evidence reviewed above suggests that the activation of postsynaptic target cells is a necessary prerequisite for the induction of experience-dependent modifications. However, it has now become clear that the generation of action potentials in the postsynaptic cell is not sufficient to produce a change. Even when contour vision is unrestricted and retinal signals readily elicit responses in the neurons of the visual cortex, vision-dependent modifications of excitatory transmission fail to occur in a variety of rather different conditions. Thus, neurons of the kitten's striate cortex may remain binocular despite monocular deprivation when the open eye is surgically rotated within the orbit (121), when large angle squint is induced in both eyes (122), or when strabismus is induced by bilateral cyclotorsion (26). In this case contour vision *per se* is unimpaired but the abnormal eye position and motility leads to massive disturbances of the kittens' visuo-motor coordination. Initially the inappropriate retinal signals cause abnormal visuo-motor reactions and during this period they are effective in influencing cortical ocular dominance. Subsequently, however, the kittens rely less and less on visual cues and develop a near complete neglect of the visual modality. In this phase retinal signals no longer modify ocular dominance. They also fail to support the development of orientation-selective receptive fields.

These latter results suggest that retinal signals only influence the development of cortical functions when the animal uses them for the control of behavior. This view is compatible with two lines of evidence. First, independent results from several laboratories indicate that retinal signals do not lead to changes of cortical functions when the kittens are paralyzed and/or anesthetized while exposed to visual patterns. Even though the light stimuli undoubtedly drives cortical cells they fail to bring about changes of ocular dominance (35, 112, 117) or to develop orientation selectivity (18). Further evidence comes from experiments in which a sensory hemineglect was induced in dark-reared kittens by placing unilateral lesions in the intralaminar nuclear complex of the thalamus (113). In addition, in order to instigate changes of ocular dominance these kittens had one eye sutured closed before they were exposed to light. Later electrophysiological analysis revealed that the neurons in the visual cortex of the normal hemisphere had become monocular as is usual with monocular deprivation. However, neurons in the visual cortex of the hemisphere with the lesion had remained binocular. In addition, the vigor of the neuronal responses and the selectivity of the receptive fields were nearly as low as if this hemisphere had been deprived of vision altogether. Thus, although both hemispheres had received identical signals from the open eye, these signals induced the expected modifications only in the normal hemisphere and remained rather ineffective in the hemisphere which – because of the diencephalic lesion – "attended" less to retinal stimulation. A further consequence of the diencephalic lesion was that it diminished the typical effects of reticular arousal in the lesioned hemisphere.

Another manipulation which prevents retinal signals from inducing cortical modifications is the abolition of proprioceptive signals from the extraocular muscles. When this input is disrupted by bilaterally severing the ophthalmic branch of the IIIrd cranial nerve, retinal signals neither stimulate the development of orientation selectivity (134) nor do they induce changes of ocular dominance (20). In this case eye movements are virtually normal (33) and the uptake of visual signals is not hindered at all. Thus, nonretinal signals about eye position and/or motility appear also to be involved in gating vision-dependent modifications. In agreement with this conclusion is the finding that changes in ocularity can be induced in anesthetized preparations when the eyes are passively moved while the retina is stimulated with contours (35).

Stimulation experiments support the notion that central core structures, which are related to the ascending arousal system, have a permissive role in cortical plasticity. By pairing monocular light stimulation with electrical activation of central core structures it proved possible to induce changes of ocular dominance in kittens that were anesthetized and paralyzed (117). Effective sites for the electrical conditioning stimuli were the mesencephalic reticular formation and the thalamic region whose destruction had prevented cortical modifications in the lesion study. Significant modifications of ocular dominance were observed in the population of cortical cells sampled after 8-12 h of conditioning stimulation (117). More recently it became possible to observe the effects of such conditioning in individual continuously recorded cells.

This revealed that measurable changes of ocular dominance and orientation preference can be induced within 30-60 min (38).

Ca^{2+} Ions as Possible Messengers for the Induction of Activity-dependent Modifications

The lesion and stimulation experiments reported above indicated that the central core activation system has a permissive effect on cortical plasticity. Electrical activation of central core structure markedly enhances the excitability of visual pathways. It facilitates the transmission of retinal signals through the lateral geniculate nucleus. Furthermore, it raises cortical excitability, enhancing dramatically transmission along intracortical pathways (for reviews see (11, 112)). From this the hypothesis was inferred that the process mediating cortical plasticity has a threshold which is reached only when retinal signals are coincident with additional facilitatory input. Because of the indication that postsynaptic activation is required for a modification to occur it was assumed that this threshold process should operate on the postsynaptic side, i.e., in the cortical neurons in which both retinal and nonretinal inputs converge. As a possible substrate for such a threshold process the high threshold voltage-dependent Ca^{2+} channels were considered. Their voltage threshold is higher than that of the Na^{+} channels which mediate the regenerative action potential, and they appear to be located in dendritic rather than in somatic membranes (73). Moreover, there is evidence from developing Purkinje cells that these channels are particularly numerous in the membranes of developing neurons (74). An attempt was made, therefore, to determine with ion-selective electrodes whether stimuli known to modify cortical response properties also led to an activation of Ca^{2+} channels (38).

The results revealed a close correlation between the occurrence of changes in neuronal response properties and the activation of Ca^{2+} fluxes from extra- to intracellular compartments. When light stimuli were coincident with central core stimulation – a condition sufficient to induce modifications of cortical response properties – the extracellular Ca^{2+} concentration decreased. With light or central core stimulation alone (conditions which do not lead to adaptive changes) the extracellular Ca^{2+} concentration was not measurably altered. In addition to the correlation between Ca^{2+} channel activation and change-inducing stimulus combinations there were a number of interesting covariations between Ca^{2+} fluxes and changes of single cell activity, the latter having been measured simultaneously with the Ca^{2+} signal. Repeated application (once every 20 s) of stimulus combinations that led to a decrease of Ca^{2+} led to gradually increasing Ca^{2+} responses. This enhancement of stimulus-contingent Ca^{2+} decreases built up over approximately 1 h and persisted for a considerable time after the end of stimulation, control levels being reached only after 30-60 min. The enhancement of the Ca^{2+} response went in parallel with an enhancement of the single cell responses to light. This facilitation of light responses was not due to a global increase of excitability but was specific to the stimulus configuration that was used during conditioning. When the light stimulus used during conditioning did not match the initial preferences of the receptive fields of the units, the selective enhancement of the neurons' responses to this stimulus appeared as a modification of the neurons' receptive field. The cells came to respond best to the stimulus configuration used during conditioning.

These correlations between the activation of Ca^{2+} fluxes and the occurrence of activity-dependent modifications of cortical response properties do not prove a causal relation between the two phenomena. Furthermore, the available data does not allow one to conclude that the decrease of extracellular Ca^{2+} concentration is actually due to Ca^{2+} entry into neuronal somata or dendrites. The possibility that Ca^{2+} fluxes responsible for the measured signals go into other compartments, in particular into presynaptic endings, should not be dismissed. Yet, it appears that less unproven assumptions are required if one assumes that the Ca^{2+} channels, which are responsible for the stimulus-dependent decrease, are located in the membranes of the postsynaptic neurons.

Such a postsynaptic mechanism could well account for the heterosynaptic control of adaptive changes. The direction of the change, increase or decrease of the efficacy of excitatory transmission, would be determined by the correlation between the activation of the pre- and postsynaptic elements whose coupling is modifiable. Whether a change does occur, however, would be determined by Ca^{2+} entry in the postsynaptic element and hence would depend on the activation of additional afferents. This model could account for the evidence that a global rise of excitability (such as follows central core stimulation) facilitates the occurrence of adaptive changes and that manipulations that decrease excitability (such as anesthesia, paralysis, and central core lesions) reduce the chances to obtain modifications in response to retinal stimulation. If the relevant postsynaptic event in the Hebbian modification were a Ca^{2+}-dependent process rather than an action potential the long duration of the "simultaneity interval" could also be accounted for more easily. The time constants of Ca^{2+} currents are longer than those of conventional action potentials and the intracellular processes triggered by Ca^{2+} can all be assumed to be slow compared to synaptically induced membrane potential changes.

The Chemical Nature of Permissive Gating Signals

Kasamatsu and Pettigrew (63) have shown that neurons of the kitten striate cortex remain binocular despite monocular deprivation when cortical norepinephrine (NE) is depleted by local infusion of the neurotoxin 6-hydroxydopamine (6-OHDA). Since they could demonstrate that microperfusion of the depleted cortical tissue with NE reinstalls ocular dominance plasticity (64), these authors have proposed that normal NE levels are a necessary prerequisite for ocular dominance plasticity. Subsequently, however, several independent investigations have indicated that ocular dominance changes can be induced despite NE depletion. In these investigations 6-OHDA was either injected prior to monocular deprivation or the noradrenergic input to cortex was blocked by means other than local 6-OHDA application (1, 7, 8, 29, 30). This apparent controversy may now have been resolved by the demonstration that ocular dominance plasticity is influenced *both* by noradrenergic and cholinergic mechanisms (9). Ocular dominance plasticity is abolished only if *both* the noradrenergic pathway from locus coeruleus and the cholinergic projection from the basal forebrain are lesioned. Disruption of either system alone is not sufficient to arrest plasticity. The initial finding that intracortical or intraventricular application of 6-OHDA blocked ocular dominance plasticity can probably be attributed to an unexpected pharmacological property of 6-OHDA. This drug, in addition to its neurotoxic effect, antagonizes the effects of acetylcholine (9, 114). These results suggest that both neuromodulators acetylcholine and norepinephrine have a permissive function in cortical plasticity, either system being capable of substituting the other.

At the present stage we can only speculate on the mechanisms by which the two systems could facilitate plasticity. Established effects of both modulators are that they close K^{+} channels (44, 66, 79). This has two consequences which could both promote plasticity: first, the length constant of the dendrites increases and, second, the depolarization in response to EPSPs is enhanced. Increasing the length constants can be expected to enhance cooperative (but also competitive) interactions between pathways converging onto the same dendrite because the

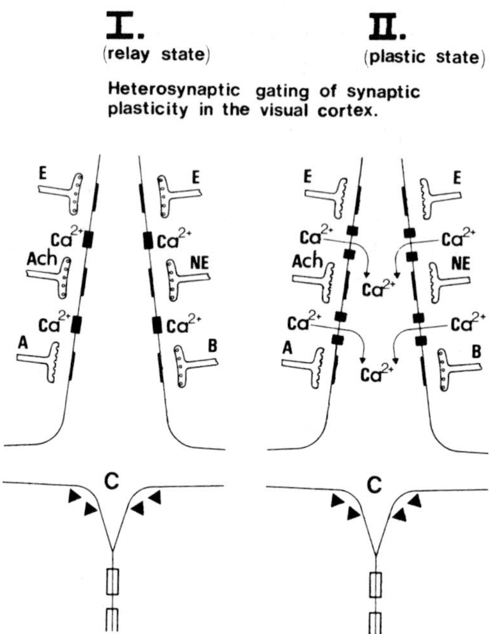

FIG. 1 – Schematic representation of conditions likely to be involved in activity-dependent modifications of synaptic connections in the visual cortex. It is proposed that cortical neurons can assume two states of activation: a relay state and a plastic state. In the former, neurons are activated by a subset of input connections (A) and relay this activity by means of Na^+-dependent action potentials. In this case the involved neuronal activities do not induce any modifications of synaptic transmission. In the latter state, the subset of excitatory afferents (A) is again active but, in addition, modulatory cholinergic (ACh) and noradrenergic (NE) afferents and further, presumably recurrent, excitatory inputs (E) are supposed to be active. This cooperative interaction between specific and modulatory input systems is assumed to entrain an activation of calcium channels, the surge of intracellular free calcium serving as a trigger for the adaptive change. In accordance with the rules listed in Table 1 we assume that in the plastic state an intracellular signal is generated which stabilizes active and destabilizes inactive synaptic connections.

membrane potential changes induced by synaptic action would spread over greater distances. The enhanced depolarization following K^+ channel closure is likely to increase the probability of Ca^{2+} channel activiation. Another mode of action of the two modulators is via second messenger systems. NE stimulates via a ß-receptor coupled with cyclase intracellular cAMP production while ACh via the inositol pathway enhances intracellular Ca^{2+} levels (for review see (91)). Synergistic interactions between both second messengers Ca^{2+} and cAMP are known to occur and hence NE and ACh could substitute each other also at this level. These interpretations imply cooperativity at the postsynaptic side and hence locate the "decision process" for the occurrence of a change in the postsynaptic neuron. However, it should be emphasized that this by no means excludes presynaptic modifications as a mechanism for long-term changes of synaptic efficiency. As suggested in Fig. 1, it is certainly conceivable that a chemical signal is generated postsynaptically when all requirements for the occurrence of an adaptive change are fulfilled, and that this signal is then made available to the respective presynaptic terminals. Indeed, the retrograde changes in the LGN after monocular deprivation suggest that such retrograde transneuronal signalling systems exist in the CNS.

FUNCTIONAL IMPLICATIONS OF OCULAR DOMINANCE PLASTICITY

The benefits of binocular vision are stereopsis and improved figure-ground distinction. For the realization of these functions, connections have to be developed between the two eyes and the visual cortex which assures that cortical neurons possess *two* corresponding receptive fields, one in each eye. This implies that the pathways which relay signals from the two eyes to binocular target cells in visual cortex have to originate from precisely corresponding retinal loci. Retinal correspondence depends on parameters such as the size of the eyes, the position of the eyes in the orbit, and the interocular distance. These parameters are obviously influenced by epigenetic factors. Hence, it is in principle impossible to anticipate with any great precision which retinal loci will actually be corresponding in the mature system. This raises problems for the developmental process which establishes binocular connections. One solution is to use functional criteria to identify corresponding connections. Per definition, corresponding afferents convey identical activity patterns when the animal is fixating a target with both eyes. A mechanism is needed, therefore, which selectively stabilizes pathways conveying correlated activity patterns. Activity-dependent modifications of connections that follow the rules listed above have such an effect. The requirements for the initial connectivity are that the projections from the two eyes establish a coarse retinotopic order and overlap sufficiently to allow for selection. The large receptive fields of cortical cells in visually inexperienced kittens suggest that there is such exuberancy in initial excitatory connections (120). However, there is an important additional condition which needs to be fulfilled to assure the success of such selection by functional criteria. Selection should only occur when the kitten is actually fixating an unambiguous target with both eyes. Since in the other instances the activity patterns from the two eyes do not contain any systematic correlations, all afferents, even those originating from actually corresponding retinal loci, would compete with each other. Binocularity would become destroyed rather than optimized. Hence, the selection process needs to be gated and must not solely depend on retinal activity.

Obviously, the proprioceptive signals from extraocular muscles are ideally suited to participate in this gating process. They could allow modifications to occur only when the eyes are at rest. Moreover, for the selection to become successful some coarse alignment of the eyes needs to be assured. Since binocular connections – although rather imprecise – are established already by genetic instructions, coarse alignment of the eyes can be achieved by correlating the patterns arriving from the two eyes. This, however, requires processing and hence an awake and "attentive" brain. From these considerations it becomes plausible that modulatory systems such as the noradrenergic and cholinergic projections are involved in ocular dominance plasticity, too. These systems modulate the excitability of thalamic and cortical target areas in a state-dependent way (for review see (34, 86)). Thus, they can very effectively assure that activity-dependent modifications occur only when sensory signals are processed and dentified as appropriate in the respective behavioral context.

Similar functions have been attributed to the activity-dependent modifications of retinal maps in the tectum of *Xenopus*. Visual deprivation (65) and blockade of retinal activity both abolished the readjustment of correspondence between the representations of the two eyes in the tectum (135, 136). In *Xenopus* the positions of the eyes are changing throughout development and hence binocular correspondence is even less predictable than in kittens. Whether this experience-dependent adjustment of connections in the tectum is influenced by modulatory systems, such as ocular dominance plasticity in the visual cortex, has not yet been investigated.

SELF-ORGANIZATION AND LEARNING

On a formal level the activity-dependent refinement of projection patterns shares the characteristic features of a learning process. Two sets of variables (in the case of the kitten visual cortex and the afferents from the two eyes) become permanently associated with a common effector, the cortical target cell. The criterion for this association is coherency of activation, just as in classical or operant conditioning. Furthermore, in order for this association to occur, activity patterns must match some predispositions of the learning organism. In our case the minimal requirement appears to be that the retinal signals conform with the response properties of cortical neurons, i.e., the visual stimuli have to contain spatial contrast gradients. Moreover, as with normal learning, selective associations occur only when the stimulus patterns are processed by an awake and attentive brain. Finally, in our case the associations tend to be very stable once they are established. In this respect similarities exist at least with certain forms of procedural learning and classical conditioning. The only marked difference between developmental plasticity and adult learning seems to be the existence of a critical period for the expression of the former. In this respect the refinement of binocular correspondence resembles a special form of learning, namely imprinting. Here, too, associations are formed during early ontogeny and these become fixed and irreversible after the end of a critical period (for review see (50, 57)). The adaptive value of such a critical period is obvious in our case. Once binocular correspondence is established this variable must become fixed to serve as a reference frame for higher level processes which compute distance from retinal disparities.

ARE THERE SIMILARITIES BETWEEN NEURONAL MECHANISMS MEDIATING OCULAR DOMINANCE PLASTICITY AND ADULT LEARNING?

As far as vertebrates are concerned, the knowledge about neuronal correlates of learning is still fragmentary. This contrasts the situation in invertebrates where the molecular correlates of associative conditioning are nearly understood (cf. Baudry *et al.* and Dudai *et al.*, this volume). Despite the possibility that the generality of invertebrate mechanisms may be limited and despite the still rather indirect conclusions reached from vertebrate work, I want to draw attention to a few phenomena that seem to be common to the various forms of activity-dependent neuronal plasticity.

The Involvement of Ca^{2+} Ions

In all cases where long-term changes of excitability and/or synaptic efficacy can be induced by neuronal activity, Ca^{2+} ions appear to serve as messengers translating membrane depolarization into biochemical signals. Both in *Aplysia* and *Hermissenda* the surge of free Ca^{2+} in the cytosol appears to function as the molecular equivalent of the conditioned stimulus (2, 21). The same is likely to be the case in the cerebellum since the complex spike of Purkinje cells which follows climbing fiber activation is associated with the activation of high threshold Ca^{2+} channels (62). Long-term potentiation (LTP) in the hippocampus also appears to require free Ca^{2+} ions in the cytosol of postsynaptic dendrites (77, 78). Finally, a Ca^{2+}-dependent process has also been implicated in activity-dependent long-term modifications of excitability of motor cortex neurons (144). The evidence suggesting an involvement of Ca^{2+} ions in ocular dominance plasticity has been reviewed above. Recently, evidence has been obtained that hippocampal LTP is reduced when NMDA receptors are blocked with 7-APV. In the visual cortex it could be demonstrated that local infusion of 7-APV reduces ocular dominance plasticity and impairs experience-dependent maturation of receptive field properties (65a). Since activation of NMDA receptors promotes Ca^{2+} entry, both findings may be related to a messenger function of Ca^{2+} ions in neuronal plasticity.

Considering this evidence for a ubiquitous involvement of Ca^{2+} ions in mediating activity-dependent long-term modifications, the phylogenetic development of an additional Na^{+} spike mechanism may be seen as a well adapted process to dissociate information processing from information storage.

The Involvement of Neuromodulators and Receptor-dependent Second Messenger Systems

In *Aplysia*, serotonin has been suggested as the molecular signal mediating the response to the conditioned stimulus. It activates a membrane-bound cyclase and causes a surge of intracellular cAMP (for review see (21)). An increase of cAMP also appears as a necessary step in hippocampal LTP (77). In this case it is unclear whether the rise of cAMP is due to activation of a receptor-coupled cyclase or whether it is secondary to activation of a Ca^{2+}-dependent cyclase. Since NE facilitates LTP, the former possibility deserves consideration (14, 49). Finally, NE has also been shown to facilitate the experience-dependent reorganization of templates in the rabbit olfactory bulb (41). The evidence for a permissive role of NE and ACh in ocular dominance plasticity has been reviewed above.

Threshold Phenomena, Temporal Contiguity, and Cooperativity

There are indications from all vertebrate model systems that adaptive modifications have a threshold which is trespassed only if a sufficiently strong activation is achieved. Available evidence suggests that this threshold process is located at the postsynaptic side. In neurons of the motor cortex, changes in response to synaptic activation are facilitated when the postsynaptic neuron is depolarized by intracellular current injection, by antidromic stimulation, or by activation of additional excitatory inputs (6, 144, 145). In the cerebellum, changes in the efficiency of parallel fiber synapses required concomitant activation of Purkinje cells by climbing fibers (62). In the hippocampus, LTP is facilitated if converging excitatory inputs are coactivated simultaneously (67, 72, 82), if glutamate is applied directly, or if postsynaptic inhibition is reduced while the afferents that are to be potentiated are stimulated (for references on cooperativity in LTP see (142)). All these manipulations are likely to enhance local dendritic depolarization. The evidence for threshold processes in ocular dominance plasticity has been reviewed above.

CONCLUDING REMARKS

Despite the relatively few data on the molecular basis of plasticity in the vertebrate brain some similarities are recognizable between the mechanisms of adaptive processes in the different model systems. This suggests that nature may have been conservative in preserving mechanisms that make nerve nets adaptive and hence can be used for the storage of information. While the basic molecular machinery that mediates these adaptive processes may have remained the same throughout phylogeny, the systems controlling this machinery seem to have become increasingly sophisticated. In *Aplysia* and *Hermissenda*, rather undifferentiated activity patterns suffice to induce changes and they do so reliably and rather independently of the animal's central state. Moreover, the mechanism of plasticity is implemented in the synaptic terminal of the sensory neuron which is postsynaptic to the pathway mediating the unconditioned response and at the same time is presynaptic in the circuit relaying the conditioned response. This limits the variables which can influence the modification process. As illustrated by the example of ocular dominance plasticity a more complex set of requirements has to be met in order to bring about long-term modifications in the vertebrate neocortex. Here the interactions between the various input systems that induce and modulate adaptive changes occur most likely at the level of a common postsynaptic dendrite. This allows for a much higher degree of combinatory complexity and compartmentalization of interactions. In principle, any excitatory, inhibitory, and/or modulatory input to the dendrite could influence the probability *and* the direction of an adaptive change. Moreover, because the adaptive process appears to be independent of the postsynaptic Na^+ spike, activity can be relayed without inducing changes providing the option of having adaptive processes gated by internally generated "now print" signals.

The phylogenetic trend to subject long-term modifications of neuronal transmission to an increasingly sophisticated and global control appears to be repeated during ontogeny. The activity-dependent selection processes that serve to enhance the order and specificity of neuronal connections can be subdivided into at least two classes. One occurs early during embryogenesis and depends mainly, if not exclusively, on self-generated patterns of neuronal activation. These early adaptive processes seem to depend on local interactions. In the case of the neuromuscular junction where multiple innervations are reduced by activity-dependent competition, superimposed control systems are obviously not required since they are absent (130). In the case of axonal segregation in the visual cortex and tectum, the role of nonlocal control systems is unknown. Since this segregation can occur already *in utero* or in complete darkness it must depend on self-generated activity. It is interesting in this context that the early electrical events in the CNS are probably based mainly on Ca^{2+} currents, Na^+-dependent processes developing only in more mature neurons (74). One might speculate that this is one of the reasons why relatively unstructured activity seems to suffice to promote plasticity and why additional "print" signals are not required. The second class of adaptive processes starts after birth and is influenced by sensory signals. Here, as reviewed above, multiple constraints are imposed by both local and global requirements for stimulus adequacy. For this class of adaptive processes it becomes difficult, if not impossible, to distinguish between self-organization and learning. My bias is that even adult learning might be considered as the continuation of the self-organizing processes that serve at first to adopt the building blocks of our nervous system to each other and that subsequently serve to adapt the whole system to its environment. This view point predicts that there should be a continuity between early self-organization and adult learning not only at the level of formal description but also at the level of molecular mechanisms.

REFERENCES

(1) Adrien, J.; Blanc, G.; Buisseret, P.; Frégnac, Y.; Gary-Bobo, E.; Imbert, M.; Tassin, J.P.; and Trotter, Y. 1985. Noradrenaline and functional plasticity in kitten visual cortex: a reexamination. *J. Physl. Lon.* 367: 73-98.

(2) Alkon, D.L. 1983. Learning in a marine snail. *Sci. Am.* 249: 70.

(3) Altmann, L.; Luhmann, H.J.; Singer, W.; and Greuel, J. 1985. Ocular dominance distribution in the striate cortex of kittens raised with rapidly alternating monocular occlusion. *Neurosci. L. Supp.* 22: S353.

(4) Anderson, P.A.; Olavarria, J.; and Van Sluyters, R.C. 1983. The pattern of ocular dominance columns in areas 17 and 18 of normal and visually deprived cats as revealed in tangential sections of unfolded cortex. *Neurosci. Abstr.* 9: 910.

(5) Archer, S.M.; Dubin M.W.; and Stark, L.A. 1982. Abnormal development of kitten retinogeniculate connectivity in the absence of action potentials. *Science* 217: 743-745.

(6) Baranyi, A., and Feher, O. 1981. Long-term facilitation of excitatory synaptic transmission in the single cortical neurones of the cat produced by repetitive pairing of synaptic potentials following intracellular stimulation. *Neurosci. L.* 23: 303-308.

(7) Bear, M.F., and Daniels, I.D. 1983. The plastic response to monocular deprivation persists in kitten visual cortex after chronic depletion of norepinephrine. *J. Neurosci.* 3: 407-416.

(8) Bear, M.F.; Paradiso, M.A.; Schwartz, M.; Nelson, S.B.; Carnes, K.M.; and Daniels, J.D. 1983. Two methods of catecholamine depletion in kitten visual cortex yield different effects on plasticity. *Nature* 302: 245-247.

(9) Bear, M.F., and Singer, W. 1986. Modulation of visual cortical plasticity by acetylcholine and noradrenaline. *Nature* 320, No. 6058: 172-176.

(10) Blakemore, C., and Cooper, G.F. 1970. Development of the brain depends on the visual environment. *Nature* 228: 477-478.

(11) Blakemore, C.; Garey, L.J.; Henderson, Z.B.; Swindale, N.V.; and Vital-Durand, F. 1980. Visual experience can promote rapid axonal reinnervation in monkey visual cortex. *J. Physl.* 307: 25P-26P.

(12) Blakemore, C.; Garey, L.J.; and Vital-Durand, F. 1978. The physiological effects of monocular deprivation and their reversal in the monkey's visual cortex. *J. Physl.* 282: 223-262.

(13) Blakemore, C., and Van Sluyters, R.C. 1975. Innate and environmental factors in the development of the kitten's visual cortex. *J. Physl.* 248: 663-716.

(14) Bliss, T.V.P.; Goddard, G.V.; and Riives, M. 1983. Reduction of long-term potentiation in the dentate gyrus of the rat following selective depletion of monoamines. *J. Physl.* 334: 475-491.

(15) Bonds, A.B.; Silverman, M.S.; Sclar, G.; and Tootell, R.B. 1980. Visually evoked potentials and deoxyglucose studies of monocularly deprived cats. *ARVO* 1980: 225.

(16) Boss, V.C., and Schmidt, J.T. 1984. Activity and the formation of ocular dominance patches in dually innervated tectum of goldfish. *J. Neurosci.* 4: 2891-2905.

(17) Brown, M.C.; Jansen, J.K.S.; and VanEssen, D.C. 1976. Polyneuronal innervation of skeletal muscle in newborn rats and its elimination during maturation. *J. Physl.* 261: 387-422.

(18) Buisseret, P.; Gary-Bobo, E.; and Imbert, M. 1978. Ocular motility and recovery of orientational properties of visual cortical neurones in dark-reared kittens. *Nature* 272: 816-817.

(19) Buisseret, P., and Imbert, M. 1976. Visual cortical cells: their developmental properties in normal and dark reared kittens. *J. Physl.* 255: 511-525.

(20) Buisseret, P., and Singer, W. 1983. Proprioceptive signals from extraocular muscles gate experience-dependent modifications of receptive fields in the kitten visual cortex. *Exp. Brain Res.* 51: 443-450.

(21) Carew, T.J.; Hawkins, R.D.; Abrams, T.W.; and Kandel, E.R. 1984. A test of Hebb's postulate at identified synapses which mediate classical conditioning in *Aplysia*. *J. Neurosci.* 4: 1217-1224.

(22) Changeux, J.-P., and Danchin, A. 1976. Selective stabilization of developing synapse as a mechanism for the specification of neuronal networks. *Nature* 264: 705-712.

(23) Changeux, J.-P.; Heidmann, T.; and Patter, P. 1984. Learning by selection. In *The Biology of Learning*, eds. P. Marler and H.S. Terrace, pp. 115-133. Dahlem Konferenzen. Berlin, Heidelberg, New York, Tokyo: Springer-Verlag.

(24) Constantine-Paton, M., and Law, M.I. 1978. Eye-specific termination bands in tecta of three-eyed frogs. *Science* 202: 639-641.

(25) Cragg, B.G. 1967. Changes in visual cortex on first exposure of rats to light. *Nature* 215: 251-253.

(26) Crewther, S.G.; Crewther, D.P.; Peck, C.K.; and Pettigrew, J.D. 1980. Visual cortical effects of rearing cats with monocular or binocular cyclotorsion. *J. Neurophysl.* 44: 97-118.

(27) Cynader, M. 1983. Prolonged sensitivity to monocular deprivation in dark-reared cats: effects of age and visual exposure. *Dev. Brain Res.* 8: 155-164.

(28) Cynader, M.; Leporé, F.; and Guillemot, J.P. 1981. Interhemispheric competition during postnatal development. *Nature* 290: 139.

(29) Daw, N.W.; Robertson, T.W.; Rader, R.K.; Videen, T.O.; and Cosica, C.J. 1984. Substantial reduction of noradrenaline by lesions of adrenergic pathway does not prevent effects of monocular deprivation. *J. Neurosci.* 4: 1354-1360.

(30) Daw, N.W.; Videen, T.O.; Parkinson, D.; and Rader, R.K. 1985. DSP-4 depletes noradrenaline in kitten visual cortex without altering the effects of monocular deprivation. *J. Neurosci.* 5: 1925-1933.

(31) Fifková, E. 1985. A possible mechanism of morphometric changes in dendritic spines induced by stimulation. *Cell. Mol. Neurobiol.* 5: 47-63.

(32) Fifková, E., and Van Harreveld, A. 1977. Long-lasting morphological changes in dendritic spines of granular cells following stimulation of the entorhinal area. *J. Neurocytol.* 6: 211-230.

(33) Fiorentini, A., and Maffei, L. 1977. Instability of the eye in the dark and the proprioception. *Nature* 269: 330-331.

(34) Foote, S.L.; Bloom, F.E.; and Aston-Jones, G. 1983. Nucleus locus coeruleus: a new evidence of anatomical and physiological specificity. *Physiol. Rev.* 63: 844-914.

(35) Freeman, R.D., and Bonds, A.B. 1979. Cortical plasticity in monocularly deprived immobilized kittens depends on eye movement. *Science* 206: 1093-1095.

(36) Frégnac, Y., and Imbert, M. 1984. Development of neuronal selectivity in primary visual cortex of cat. *Physiol. Rev.* 64: 325-434.

(37) Frost, D.O, and Innocenti, G.M. 1986. Effects of sensory experience on the development of visual callosal connections. In Two Hemispheres - One Brain, ed. F. Lepore. New York: Alan Liss Inc., in press.

(38) Geiger, H., and Singer, W. 1986. A possible role of Ca^{++}-currents in developmental plasticity. Exp. Brain Res. Suppl., in press.

(39) Gilbert, C.D. 1977. Laminar differences in receptive field properties of cells in cat primary visual cortex. *J. Physl.* 268: 391-421.

(40) Globus, A.; Rosenzweig, M.R.; Bennett, E.L.; and Diamond, M.C. 1973. Effects of differential experience on dendritic spine counts in rat cerebral cortex. *J. Comp. Physl. Psych.* 82: 175-181.

(41) Gray, C.M.; Freeman, W.J.; and Skinner, E. 1984. Associative changes in the spatial amplitude patterns of rabbit olfactory EEG are norepinephrine dependent. *Neurosci. Abstr.* 10: 121.

(42) Greuel, J.; Luhmann, H.J.; and Singer, W. 1986. Persistent changes of single cell responses in kitten striate cortex produced by pairing sensory stimulation with iontophoretic application of neurotransmitters and neuromodulators. In *Cellular Mechanisms of Conditioning and Behavioral Plasticity*, ed. C.D. Woody. Plenum Press, in press.

(43) Guillery, R.W. 1972. Binocular competition in the control of geniculate cell growth. *J. Comp. Neurol.* 144: 117-127.

(44) Halliwell, J.V., and Adams, P.R. 1982. Voltage-clamp analysis of muscarinic excitation in hippocampal neurons. *Brain Res.* 250: 71-92.

(45) Headon, M.P.; Sloper, J.J.; and Powell, T.P.S. 1984. Simultaneous hypertrophy of cells related to each eye in the lateral geniculate nucleus of the infant monkey following short-term reverse suture. *Dev. Brain Res.* 15: 295-297.

(46) Hebb, D.O. 1949. The Organization of Behavior. New York: John Wiley & Sons.

(47) Hirsch, H.V.B.; Leventhal, A.G.; McCall, M.A.; and Tieman, D.G. 1983. Effects of exposure to lines of one or two orientations on different cell types in striate cortex of cat. *J. Physl.* 337: 241-255.

(48) Hirsch, H.V.B., and Spinelli, D.N. 1970. Visual experience modifies distribution of horizontally and vertically oriented receptive fields in cats. *Science* 168: 869-871.

(49) Hopkins, W.F., and Johnston, D. 1984. Frequency dependent noradrenergic modulation of long-term potentiation in the hippocampus. *Science* 226: 350-351.

(50) Horn, G. 1981. Neural mechanisms of learning: an analysis of imprinting in the domestic chick. *P. Roy. Lon. B* 213: 101-137.

(51) Hubel, D.H., and Wiesel, T.N. 1963. Receptive fields of cells in striate cortex of very young, visually inexperienced kittens. *J. Neurophysl.* 26: 994-1002.

(52) Hubel, D.H., and Wiesel, T.N. 1963. Shape and arrangement of columns in cat's striate cortex. *J. Physl.* 160: 106-154.

(53) Hubel, D.H., and Wiesel, T.N. 1965. Binocular interaction in striate cortex of kittens reared with artificial squint. *J. Neurophysl.* 28: 1041-1059.

(54) Hubel, D.H., and Wiesel, T.N. 1972. Laminar and columnar distribution of geniculo-cortical fibers in the macaque monkey. *J. Comp. Neur.* 146: 421-450.

(55) Hubel, D.H.; Wiesel, T.N.; and LeVay, S. 1977. Plasticity of ocular dominance columns in monkey striate cortex. *Phil. Trans. Roy. Soc. Lon. B* 278: 377-409.

(56) Ide, C.F.; Fraser, S.E.; and Meyer, R.L. 1983. Eye dominance columns formed by an isogenic double-nasal frog eye. *Science* 221-295.

(57) Immelmann, K. 1984. The natural history of bird learning. In *The Biology of Learning*, eds. P. Marler and H.S. Terrace, pp. 271-288. Dahlem Konferenzen. Berlin, Heidelberg, New York, Tokyo: Spinger-Verlag.

(58) Innocenti, G.M., and Clarke, S. 1984. The organization of immature callosal connections. *J. Comp. Neur.* 230: 287-309.

(59) Innocenti, G.M., and Frost, D.O. 1979. Effects of visual experience on the maturation of the efferent system to the corpus callosum. *Nature* 280: 231-234.

(60) Innocenti, G.M., and Frost, D.O. 1980. The postnatal development of visual callosal connections in the absence of visual experience or of the eyes. *Exp. Brain Res.* 39: 365-375.

(61) Innocenti, G.M.; Frost, D.O.; and Illes, J. 1985. Maturation of visual callosal connections in visually deprived kittens: a challenging critical period. *J. Neurosci.* 5: 255-267.

(62) Ito, M.; Sakurai, M.; and Tongroach, P. 1982. Climbing fibre induced depression of both mossy fibre responsiveness and glutamate sensitivity of cerebellar Purkinje cells. *J. Physl.* 324: 113-134.

(63) Kasamatsu, T., and Pettigrew, J.D. 1979. Preservation of binocularity after monocular deprivation in the striate cortex of kittens treated with 6-hydroxydopamine. J. *Comp. Neur.* 185: 139-161.

(64) Kasamatsu, T.; Pettigrew, J.D.; and Ary, M.-L. 1979. Restoration of visual cortical plasticity by local microperfusion of norepinephrine. *J. Comp. Neur.* 185: 163-182.

(65) Keating, M.J. 1975. The time course of experience dependent synaptic switching of visual connections in *Xenopus laevis*. *P. Roy. Soc. Edinburgh B* 189: 603-610.

(65a) Kleinschmidt, A.; Bear, M.F.; and Singer, W. 1986. Effects of the NMDA-receptor antagonist APV on visual cortical plasticity in monocularly deprived kittens. *Neurosci. Lett. Supp.* 26: 558.

(66) Krnjevic, K.; Pumain, R.; and Renaud, L. 1971. The mechanism of excitation by acetylcholine in the cerebral cortex. *J. Physl.* 215: 247-268.

(67) Lee, K.S. 1983. Cooperativity among afferents for the induction of long-term potentiation in the CA1 region of the hippocampus. *J. Neurosci.* 3: 1369-1372.

(68) LeVay, S., and Gilbert, C.D. 1976. Laminar patterns of geniculocortical projection in the cat. *Brain Res.* 113: 1-19.

(69) LeVay, S., and Stryker, M.P. 1979. The development of ocular dominance columns in the cat. *Soc. Neurosci. Symp.* 4: 83-98.

(70) LeVay, S.; Stryker, M.P.; and Schatz, C.J. 1978. Ocular dominance columns and their development in layer IV of the cat's visual cortex: a quantitative study. *J. Comp. Neur.* 179: 223-244.

(71) Leventhal, A.G., and Hirsch, H.V.B. 1980. Receptive-field properties of different classes of neurons in visual cortex of normal and dark-reared cats. *J. Neurophysl.* 43: 1111-1132.

(72) Levy, W.B., and Steward, O. 1983. Temporal contiguity requirements for long-term associative potentiation/depression in the hippocampus. *Neuroscience* 8: 791-797.

(73) Llinas, R. 1979. The role of calcium in neuronal function. In *The Neurosciences Fourth Study Program*, 4th, eds. F.O. Schmitt and F.G. Worden, pp. 555-571. Cambridge, MA: MIT Press.

(74) Llinas, R., and Sugimori, M. 1979. Calcium conductances in Purkinje cell dendrites: their role in development and integration. *Prog. Brain Res.* 51: 323-334.

(75) Luhmann, H.J.; Martínez Millán, L.; and Singer, W. 1986. Development of horizontal intrinsic connections in cat striate cortex. *Exp. Brain Res.* 63: 443-448.

(76) Lund, R.D.; Mitchell, D.E.; and Henry, G.H. 1978. Squint-induced modification of callosal connections in cats. *Brain Res.* 144: 169-172.

(77) Lynch, G., and Baudry, M. 1984. The biochemistry of memory: a new and specific hypothesis. *Science* 224: 1057-1063.

(78) Lynch, G.; Larson, J.; Kelso, S.; Barrionuevo, G.; and Schottler, F. 1983. Intracellular injections of EGTA block induction of hippocampal long-term potentiation. *Nature* 305: 719-721.

(79) Madison, D.V., and Nicoll, R.A. 1982. Noradrenaline blocks accommodation of pyramidal cell discharge in the hippocampus. *Nature* 299: 636-638.

(80) Mariani, J. 1983. Elimination of synapses during the development of the central nervous system. *Prog. Brain Res.* 58: 383-392.

(81) Mastronarde, D.N. 1983. Correlated firing of cat retinal ganglion cells. I. Spontaneously active inputs to X and Y cells. *J. Neurophysl.* 49: 303-324.

(82) McNaughton, B.L.; Douglas, R.M.; and Goddard, G.V. 1978. Synaptic enhancement in fascia dentata: cooperativity among coactive afferents. *Brain Res.* 157: 277-293.

(83) Meyer, R.L. 1982. Tetrodotoxin blocks the formation of ocular dominance columns in goldfish. *Science* 218: 589-591.

(84) Meyer, R.L. 1983. Tetrodotoxin inhibits the formation of refined retinotopography in goldfish. *Dev. Brain Res.* 6: 293-298.

(85) Mitzdorf, U., and Singer, W. 1980. Monocular activation of visual cortex in normal and monocularly deprived cats: an analysis of evoked potentials. *J. Physl.* 304: 203-220.

(86) Moore, R.Y., and Bloom, F.E. 1979. Central catecholamine neuron system: anatomy and physiology of the norepinephrine and epinephrine systems. *Ann. Rev. Neurosci.* 2: 133-168.

(87) Mower, G.D.; Caplan, C.J.; Christen, W.G.; and Duffy, F.H. 1985. Dark rearing prolongs physiological but not anatomical plasticity of the cat visual cortex. *J. Comp. Neur.* 235: 448-466.

(88) Mower, G.D., and Christen, W.G. 1985. Role of visual experience in activating critical period in cat visual cortex. *J. Neurophysl.* 53: 572-589.

(89) Mower, G.D.; Christen, W.G.; and Caplan, C.J. 1984. Absence of ocular dominance columns in binocularly deprived cats. *Inv. Ophth. Vis. Sci. Suppl.* 25: 214 (ARVO abstr.).

(90) Müller, L.; Pattiselanno, A.; and Vrensen, G. 1981. The postnatal development of the presynaptic grid in the visual cortex of rabbits and the effect of dark-rearing. *Brain Res.* 205: 39 -48.

(91) Nestler, E.J.; Walaas, S.J.; and Greengard, P. 1984. Neuronal phosphoproteins: physiological and clinical implications. *Science* 225: 1357-1364.

(92) Olson, C.R., and Freeman, R.D. 1980. Profile to the sensitive period for monocular deprivation in kitten. *Exp. Brain Res.* 39: 17-21.

(93) Rakic, P. 1976. Prenatal genesis of connections subserving ocular dominance in the rhesus monkey. *Nature* 261: 467-471.

(94) Rakic, P. 1977. Prenatal development of the visual system in rhesus monkey. *Phil. Trans. Roy. Soc. Lon.* 278: 245-260.

(95) Rakic, P. 1981. Development of visual centers in the primate brain depends on binocular competition before birth. *Science* 214: 928-931.

(96) Rauschecker, J.P., and Singer, W. 1979. Changes in the circuitry of the kitten's visual cortex are gated by postsynaptic activity. *Nature* 280: 58-60.

(97) Rauschecker, J.P., and Singer, W. 1981. The effects of early visual experience on the cat's visual cortex and their possible explanation by Hebb synapses. *J. Physl.* 310: 215-239.

(98) Rodieck, R.W., and Smith, P.S. 1966. Slow dark discharge rhythms of cat retinal ganglion cells. *J. Neurophysl.* 29: 942-953.

(99) Schechter, P.B., and Murphy, E.H. 1976. Brief monocular visual experience and kitten cortical binocularity. *Brain Res.* 109: 165-168.

(100) Schmidt, J.T. 1985. Apparent movement of optic terminals out of a local postsynaptically blocked region in goldfish tectum. *J. Neurophysl.* 53: 237-251.

(101) Schmidt, J.T. 1985. Formation of retinotopic connections: selective stabilization by an activity-dependent mechanism. *Cell. Mol. Neurobiol.* 5: 65-84.

(102) Schmidt, J.T., and Edwards, D.L. 1983. Activity sharpens the map during the regeneration of the retinotectal projection in goldfish. *Brain Res.* 269: 29-39.

(103) Schmidt, J.T., and Eisele, L.E. 1985. Stroboscopic illumination and dark rearing block the sharpening of the retinotectal map in goldfish. *Neuroscience* 14: 535-546.

(104) Schmidt, J.T., and Tieman, S.B. 1985. Eye-specific segregation of optic afferents in mammals, fish, and frogs: the role of activity. *Cell. Mol. Neurobiol.* 5: 5-34.

(105) Shatz, C.J. 1983. The prenatal development of the cat's retinogeniculate pathway. *J. Neurosci.* 3: 482-499.

(106) Shatz, C.J., and Kirkwood, P.A. 1984. Prenatal development of functional connections in the cat's retinogeniculate pathway. *J. Neurosci.* 4: 1378-1397.

(107) Shatz, C.J.; Lindström, S.; and Wiesel, T.N. 1977. The distribution of afferents representing the right and left eyes in the cat's visual cortex. *Brain Res.* 131: 103-116.

(108) Shatz, C.J., and Stryker, M.P. 1978. Ocular dominance in layer IV of the cat's visual cortex and the effects of monocular deprivation. *J. Physl.* 281: 267-283.

(109) Sherk, H., and Stryker, M.P. 1976. Quantitative study of cortical orientation selectivity in visually inexperienced kittens. *J. Neurophysl.* 39: 63-70.

(110) Sillito, A.M.; Kemp, J.A.; and Blakemore, C. 1983. The role of GABAergic inhibition in the cortical effects of monocular deprivation. *Nature* 291: 318-322.

(111) Singer, W. 1977. Control of thalamic transmission by corticofugal and ascending reticular pathways in the visual system. *Physiol. Rev.* 57: 386-420.

(112) Singer, W. 1979. Central core control of visual cortex functions. In *The Neurosciences Fourth Study Program*, eds. F.O. Schmitt and F.G. Worden, pp. 1093-1109. Cambridge, MA: MIT Press.

(113) Singer, W. 1982. Central core control of developmental plasticity in the kitten visual cortex: I. Diencephalic lesions. *Exp. Brain Res.* 47: 209-222.

(114) Singer, W., and Bear, M.F. 1985. Acetylcholine, norepinephrine and the extrathalamic control of visual cortical plasticity. *Neurosci. Abstr.* 141: 10.

(115) Singer, W., and Creutzfeldt, O.D. 1970. Reciprocal lateral inhibition of on- and off-center neurons in the lateral geniculate body of the cat. *Exp. Brain Res.* 10: 311-330.

(116) Singer, W.; Freeman, B.; and Rauschecker, J. 1981. Restriction of visual experience to a single orientation affects the organization or orientation columns in cat visual cortex: a study with deoxyglucose. *Exp. Brain Res.* 41: 199-215.

(117) Singer, W., and Rauschecker, J. 1982. Central core control of developmental plasticity in the kitten visual cortex. II. Electrical activation of mesencephalic and diencephalic projections. *Exp. Brain Res.* 47: 223-233.

(118) Singer, W.; Rauschecker, J.; and Werth, R. 1977. The effect of monocular exposure to temporal contrasts on ocular dominance in kittens. *Brain Res.* 134: 568-572.

(119) Singer, W., and Tretter, F. 1976. Receptive field properties and neuronal connectivity in a striate and parastriate cortex of contour-deprived cats. J. *Neurophysl.* 39: 613-630.

(120) Singer, W., and Tretter, F. 1976. Unusually large receptive fields in cats with restricted visual experience. *Exp. Brain Res.* 26: 171-184.

(121) Singer, W.; Tretter, F.; and Yinon, U. 1982. Central gating of developmental plasticity in kitten visual cortex. *J. Physl.* 324: 221-237.

(122) Singer, W.; von Grünau, M.; and Rauschecker, J. 1979. Requirements for the disruption of binocularity in the visual cortex of strabismic kittens. *Brain Res.* 171: 536-540.

(123) Sloper, J.J.; Headon, M.P.; and Powell, T.P.S. 1984. Simultaneous hypertrophy of cells related to each eye in the lateral geniculate nucleus of the infant monkey following short-term reverse suture. *Dev. Brain Res.* 15: 295-297.

(124) Stent, G.S. 1973. A physiological mechanism for Hebb's postulate of learning. *Proc. Natl. Acad.* Sci. 70: 997-1001.

(125) Stryker, M.P. 1981. Late segregation of geniculate afferents to the cat's visual cortex after recovery from binocular impulse blockade. *Neurosci. Abstr.* 7: 842.

(126) Stryker, M.P., and Harris, W.A. 1986. Binocular impulse blockade prevents the formation of ocular dominance columns in cat visual cortex. *J. Neurosci.*, in press.

(127) Stryker, M.P.; Sherk, H.; Leventhal, A.G.; and Hirsch, H.V.B. 1978. Physiological consequences for the cat's visual cortex of effectively restricting early visual experience with oriented contours. *J. Neurophysl.* 41: 896-909.

(128) Swindale, N.V. 1982. Absence of ocular dominance patches in dark reared cats. *Nature* 290: 332-333.

(129) Swindale, N.V.; Vital-Durand, F.; and Blakemore, C. 1981. Recovery from monocular deprivation in the monkey. III. Reversal of anatomical effects in the visual cortex. *P. Roy. Soc. Lon. B* 213: 435-450.

(130) Thompson, W.; Kuffler, D.P.; and Jansen, J.K.S. 1979. The effect of prolonged, reversible block of nerve impulses on the elimination of polyneuronal innervation of new-born rat skeletal muscle fibers. *Neuroscience* 4: 271-281.

(131) Tieman, S.B. 1984. Effects of monocular deprivation on geniculocortical synapses in the cat. *J. Comp. Neur.* 222: 166-176.

(132) Tieman, S.B. 1985. The anatomy of geniculocortical connections in monocularly deprived cats. *Cell. Mol. Neurobiol.* 5: 35-45.

(133) Tieman, S.B., and Tumosa, N. 1983. ^{14}C 2-deoxyglucose demonstration of the organization of ocular dominance in areas 17 and 18 of the normal cat. *Brain Res.* 267: 35-46.

(134) Trotter, Y.; Gary-Bobo, E.; and Buisseret, P. 1981. Recovery of orientation selectivity in kitten primary visual cortex is slowed down by bilaterial section of ophthalmic trigeminal nerves. *Dev. Brain Res.* 1: 450-454.

(135) Udin, S. 1983. Abnormal visual input leads to development of abnormal axon trajectories in frogs. *Nature* 301: 336-338.

(136) Udin, S. 1985. The role of visual experience in the formation of binocular projections in frogs. *Cell. Mol. Neurobiol.* 5: 85-102.

(137) Valverde, F. 1971. Rate and extent of recovery from dark rearing in the visual cortex of the mouse. *Brain Res.* 33: 1-11.

(138) Vrensen, G.; and Cardozo, J.N. 1981. Changes in size and shape of synaptic connections after visual training: an ultrastructural approach of synaptic plasticity. *Brain Res.* 218: 79-97.

(139) Wiesel, T.N., and Hubel, D.H. 1965. Comparison of the effects of unilateral and bilateral eye closure on cortical unit responses in kittens. *J. Neurophysl.* 28: 1029-1040.

(140) Wiesel, T.N., and Hubel, D.H. 1965. Extent of recovery from the effects of visual deprivation in kittens. *J. Neurophysl.* 28: 1060-1072.

(141) Wiesel, T.N., and Hubel, D.H. 1974. Ordered arrangement of orientation columns in monkeys lacking visual experience. *J. Comp. Neurol.* 158: 307-318.

(142) Wigström, H., and Gustafsson, B. 1985. On long-lasting potentiation in the hippocampus: a proposed mechanism for its dependence on coincident pre- and postsynaptic activity. *Acta Physl. Scand.* 123: 519-522.

(143) Winfield, D.A. 1983. The postnatal development of synapses in the different laminae of the visual cortex in the normal kitten and in kittens with eyelid suture. *Dev. Brain Res.* 9: 155-169.

(144) Woody, C.D. 1984. The electrical excitability of nerve cells as an index of learned behavior. In *Primary Neural Substrates of Learning and Behavioral Change*, eds. D.L. Alkon and J. Farley, pp. 101-127. New York: Cambridge University Press.

(145) Woody, C.D.; Alkon, D.L.; and Hay, B. 1984. Depolarization-induced effects of Ca2+-calmodulin-dependent protein kinase injection, *in vivo*, in single neurons of cat motor cortex. *Brain Res.* 321: 192-197.

The Neural and Molecular Bases of Learning,
eds. J.-P. Changeux and M. Konishi, pp. 337–358.
John Wiley & Sons Limited.

Dynamic Neocortical Processes and the Origins of Higher Brain Functions

M.M. Merzenich

Dept. of Otolaryngology and Physiology
University of California
San Francisco, CA 94143, USA

INTRODUCTION

The principal objective of this report is to summarize evidence for general, lifelong, self-organizing neocortical processes. The nature and rules of these processes will be outlined, insofar as they are known. Some additional hypotheses based upon these and other relevant experimental findings will be outlined. Some implications of these findings for models of the origins of higher brain functions will be briefly reviewed.

It should be noted from the outset that this general model cannot be fully developed in this abbreviated review. Considerations of the operations of this machinery in the intermediate domain of time (i.e., outline of a specific model for the origins of "complex learning") and of temporally regulated horizontal interactions between functional groups are not considered here, although they constitute crucial facets of this model. Operations and regulation on the affective side of cognitive processes are considered only in passing. Evidence from the behavioral literature consistent with or challenging this general model is not reviewed herein. These topics shall be the subject of later reviews. Some additional conclusions and hypotheses have been described in other reports (24, 25, 27).

CONCLUSIONS AND HYPOTHESES; SUMMARY OF EVIDENCE

Modifiability of Cortical Maps

There are dynamic processes by which the details of somatosensory cortical representations are established, maintained, and altered *by use*.

Cortical "maps" reflect their input histories and change in representational detail continuously, throughout life. Somatosensory cortical representations in adult monkeys undergo a topographic remodeling after peripheral nerve transection (29, 30), amputation of digits (32), syndactyly (1), differential behavioral use of restricted skin surfaces (see Fig. 1, (18, 19)), or restricted cortical lesions (20). Remodelling of skin surface representations in somatosensory cortical fields following peripheral nerve transections, amputations, or in "normal" somatosensory fields over time have also been described in the cat (13, 21), rat (48), flying fox (3), and raccoon (22, 39). These representational changes are ongoing throughout the life of an adult monkey (18). The self-organizing processes, manifested by map remodeling generated by use, appear to account for most of the striking idiosyncratic variation in cortical map detail recorded in a series of normal adult monkeys (25, 31).

Use-dependent Reorganization of Cortical Maps

The capacity for use-dependent alteration of the representational detail of cortical fields is limited by the afferent repertoires ultimately delivered to any given cortical location. Map remodeling by use results from selective changes in input effectiveness and not from changes in the spreads or locations of input afferent arbors. A distance limit for cortical map reorganization has been recorded in all studies in which large peripheral lesions have been introduced. Movements of representational loci across the somatosensory koniocortex (area 3b) in different individual adult owl monkeys were never greater than about 500-1000 microns ((32) and unpublished studies). In behaving animals, locations of representation of heavily stimulated fingertips across the functionally defined area 3b-area 3a border shifted up to about one millimeter, but not further (18). In these animals, and in animals in which the radial side of the hand was deprived of all inputs (Ochs, Merzenich, Allard, and Jenkins, unpublished studies), shifts of the hand-face border of about 300-600 microns –but no farther– were commonly recorded with area 3b.

This "distance limit" for map changes and specific topographical features of the reorganization, in which inputs not overtly represented in a cortical sector nonetheless emerge in reorganization (29, 30) are consistent with the reorganization arising from alterations in synaptic effectiveness of in-place terminal arbors. This point of view is also supported by studies in which receptive fields in somatosensory cortex have been enlarged within a few minutes after bicuculine administration (15) or by the peripheral electrical stimulation of large myelinated afferents in a cutaneous nerve (40). The zone of 2-deoxyglucose labeling

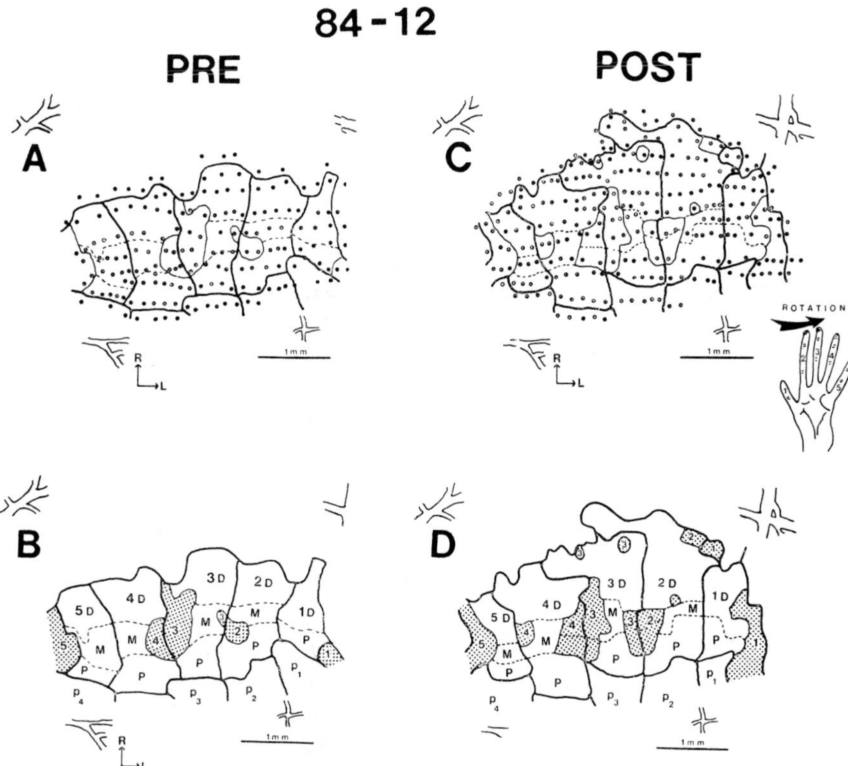

FIG. 1 – Alteration of the details of a cortical map in an adult owl monkey, by use. A map of the representation of the digital surfaces in cortical area 3b is illustrated in B. The penetration grid from which the map was derived is shown in A. Dots represent microelectrode penetration sites. In each penetration receptive fields were defined for neurons within the middle cortical layers. The map in D was derived in the same monkey 84 days later. During the interim the animal was engaged in a behavior that resulted in heavy (1-2 hour/day) differential stimulation of the extreme tips of digits 2, 3, and sometimes 4. The area 3b representation of the hand was completely remodeled over this period, with neurons at nearly every cortical site acquiring a "new" overt receptive field. The heavily stimulated surfaces expanded severalfold in representational extent. The extents of other representational territories were altered little over this period. On the other hand, most representational locations were substantially different. These results are typical of those in a series of map remodeling-by-use experiments (18). Note the highly significant but distance-limited shifts along the area 3b-3a and hand-face borders. Such shifts are recorded, in the same directions, in all of these experiments.

of neocortical fields with skin stimulation is far greater than the zone overtly representing those skin surfaces (17). Cortical receptive fields defined by peripheral electrical stimulation are larger than those derived by peripheral tactile stimulation. There is clear evidence that inputs from surrounding skin fields evoke EPSPs in neurons that are not normally overtly driven by them (52, 53). Finally, the horizontal extents of afferent input arbors defined anatomically (23, 38) or by antidromic electrical stimulation mapping (P. Snow, R. Nudo, W. Jenkins, and W. Rivers, unpublished results) spread, at least usually, more widely across the somatosensory cortical zones than can be accounted for by the functional map of the skin surface in the projection zones of these afferents. All of these studies manifest a repertoire of potentially highly effective driving inputs in the somatosensory cortical fields under study that is far larger than the limited input subset normally effective for driving cortical neurons with natural stimuli.

Input Coincidence Temporal Relationship

The temporal relationship of input activity underlies the establishment of cortical receptive fields and the details of representational topographies. It is clear from map-remodeling experiments that the details of cortical maps and the highly variable extents and shapes of cortical receptive fields are not simple anatomical constructs. How, then, are cortical receptive fields and topographic details generated and maintained? Two test experiments have now demonstrated that the establishment and maintenance of local map order is controlled by the temporal structure of inputs. In the simplest of these studies, the details of cortical maps were defined several months after fusing the glabrous and hairy skin of two adjacent digits with minimal disturbance of their innervation (see Fig. 2, (1,4)). This resulted in a breakdown of the normal discontinuity in the cortical representation of adjacent digits. Following syndactyly, neurons at many locations derived receptive field components that extended across the two digits. In a typical experiment, such 2-digit receptive fields might be seen in 30, 40, or 50 penetrations, while they might normally be encountered along the border between two digits only rarely. At the end of these acute experiments the digits were again surgically separated; now the two field components were clearly evident on the two separated fingers all along their mutual border – again, something rarely recorded normally. Thus, we conclude that the representational discontinuity (nonoverlap of receptive fields) of adjacent digits is a *functional* concept attributable to the fact that the separate digits have largely independent temporal stimulation histories. When temporally independent stimulation of the two digits is disallowed in the syndactyl condition, the cortical representational discontinuity between the two digits disappears.

In a variation of this study we have studied receptive field structure and cortical map order after interdigital transfers of islands of skin with their vascular supply and innervation maintained intact, again in adult monkeys (Clark, Allard, Merzenich, and Jenkins, unpublished observations). Receptive fields, on or bordering the transferred island, commonly incorporate large areal components from skin surfaces both within and outside the boundaries of the island. This dramatic reselection of effective inputs of previously far-separated skin locations into new receptive fields must be a consequence of the new temporal structure of inputs in the island-transfer as compared with the normal case.

A more complex demonstration that the temporal structures of inputs underly receptive field definition and map order is derived from studies of reorganization following peripheral nerve transection and regeneration (36, 49). In such experiments there is a pseudorandom reinnervation effected in nerve regeneration. If anatomical convergences and divergences of inputs in the projection from the skin to the cortex strictly determined receptive fields, then one would predict that with this shuffling of cutaneous inputs into the somatosensory projection system that cortical receptive fields would be greatly enlarged and cortical maps would lose their topographic detail. In fact, quite the opposite is seen. In time, small receptive fields again emerge; and, everywhere within the cortical map, an overlap of receptive fields with those at adjacent cortical sites is re-established (49). Both of these changes can only be accounted for by the operation of coincidence-based, input-selective processes operating on the shuffled inputs now delivered into the central somatosensory system.

One curious aspect of these experiments is an emergence of multiple receptive fields at many sites in the reorganized cortical zone (36, 49). Another is the retention of receptive fields from the ulnar or radial nerve distributions, which often continue to drive neurons along with new receptive field(s) from the reinnervated median nerve distribution (49). In these experimental cases, anomalous multiple receptive fields had minimal distances from each other; they were never recorded on the same functional skin surfaces. Again, there is no plausible anatomical origin of these phenomena; we believe that this invariable separation of small receptive field components can only arise from timing-based, self-organizing processes in the central nervous system. We have interpreted the persistence of multiple receptive fields to be due to the fact that separated functional skin surfaces (e.g., a distal segment of a finger and a pad on the palm) have, again, largely independent temporal stimulation histories. By this argument, this system generates a small receptive field at multiple sites because it has only a limited temporal basis for eliminating other, distant receptive fields. This is an important demonstration that different cortical inputs operating in different temporal domains have a capacity to generate largely independent cortical representations within the same cortical zone.

The Hypercolumn Rule

This "rule" can be stated in three ways: a) at all stages the percentage overlap of receptive fields is roughly maintained as a constant function of cortical distance; b) as the cortical territory representing a given skin surface (representational magnification) grows or contracts over time, that skin surface is represented in correspondingly finer or coarser grain (i.e., by correspondingly smaller or larger receptive fields); c) alterations in receptive fields and alterations in the represented skin location at any given cortical site are actively related, at all stages, with changes in representational detail at surrounding cortical locations.

At any given stage in the life of an adult primate there is a general maintenance of a percentage receptive field overlap (or hypercolumn) rule in somatosensory cortical fields 3b and 1 (46). By this rule, the percentage of receptive field overlap normally changes as a roughly constant function of distance across the neocortical plate, irregardless of the receptive field sizes representing different skin surfaces. This percentage overlap relationship is at least roughly maintained through

---

FIG. 2 – Some features of map remodeling after surgical syndactyly. In this monkey the dorsal and glabrous surfaces of digits 3 and 4 were fused surgically for a period of 64 days prior to derivation of this map (A). Great care was taken to preserve normal innervation of the skin in creating the syndactyly. In all of the penetration sites marked by large dots, receptive fields extended across the surfaces of both digits. A representative sequence of these double-digit receptive fields, derived from a vertical row of penetrations marked by the arrow in A, is shown in B. Such fields are infrequently recorded in a normal monkey (see borders of digits 4 and 5, and 3 and 2, for comparison). At the end of this experiment the digits were surgically separated and the cortical zone again mapped. Cortical receptive fields retained field components on the two adjacent digits. These results are representative of all obtained in this series (1). They are one of several experimental demonstrations that the temporal correlations of inputs underly establishment of cortical receptive fields and map topography.

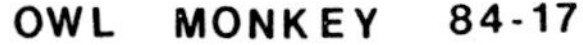
CORTICAL MAP OF SYNDACTYLY HAND

OWL MONKEY 84-17

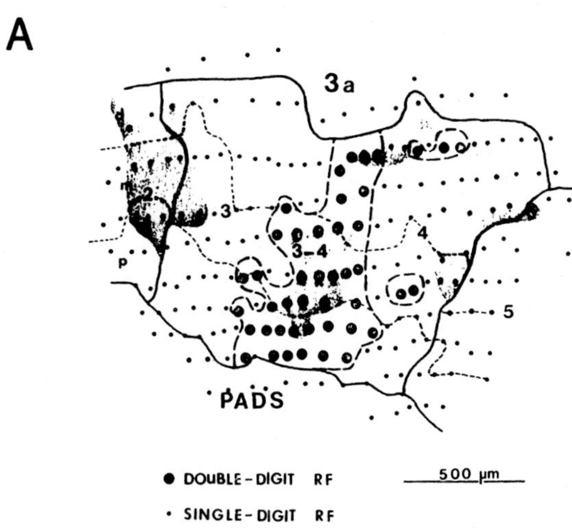
A
3a
3
3-4
4
5
p
PADS
● DOUBLE-DIGIT RF
• SINGLE-DIGIT RF
500 µm

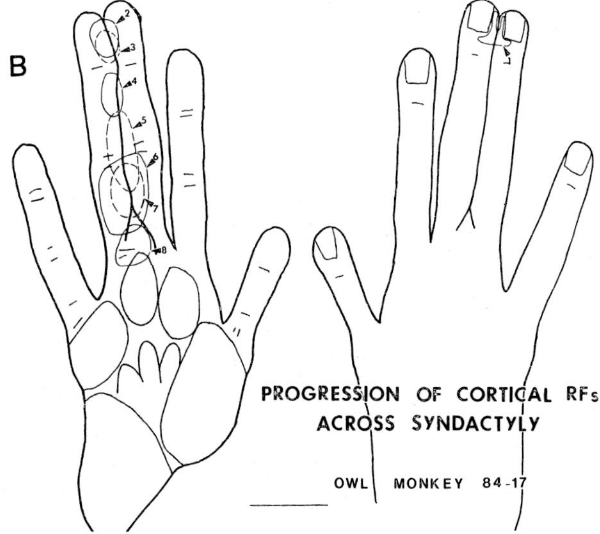
B
2
3
4
5
6
7
8
PROGRESSION OF CORTICAL RFs ACROSS SYNDACTYLY
OWL MONKEY 84-17

map readjustments recorded after *all* of the peripheral lesion, central lesion, and differential use experiments outlined above. That is, as representational magnification changes with the expansion or contraction of the cortical representation of different skin surfaces, there is a roughly proportional, inverse change in average receptive field size (18, 20, 30, 32). This indicates that the receptive field generated at any given cortical location is defined, in part, by interactions across a roughly constant cortical integration distance.

It should be noted that there are a number of specific recorded exceptions to this "rule." In all of these special cases, in which receptive field sizes are inordinately large or small with respect to representational magnification or in which map discontinuities are recorded, effective input selection based on the temporal structure of inputs would appear to supercede a strict enforcement of the percentage-overlap vs. distance rule.

Self-organizing Neural Units

The self-organizing neural unit is a group of cooperating neurons several tens of microns in extent. Neurons within a group collectively derive effective inputs from an ordinarily far more extensive anatomically delivered input repertoire; group members share the "selected" receptive field. Neuron memberships for neuronal groups are subject to continual change; neuronal groups are not only anatomical units, they are functional structures as well. The functionally defined columnar organization of the neocortex (34) is one of its most striking and consistent features. In general, at any given cortical location the "static" response characteristics of neurons in the foreground are shared by neurons in the background, and commonly these static features of the responses of neurons (e.g., their receptive fields) vary little across significant vertical and horizontal electrode penetration distances. Neocortical physiological studies have long suggested that groups of neurons of significant horizontal extent cooperatively generate and maintain cortical receptive fields.

We have sought to further investigate whether the dynamically alterable receptive fields of somatosensory cortical fields are derived and represented cell-by-cell within the neocortex or by cooperating groups of neurons with significant horizontal extents. Results of these studies are, to this point, preliminary. In the first study, the horizontal extents of the peculiar multiple receptive fields recorded after nerve transection and repair were determined (Merzenich, Wall, Sur, and Kaas, unpublished experiments). Each oddly located receptive field was recorded over a horizontal extent of a few tens of microns up to a few hundred microns. As a rule, *every* driven neuron, over the region for which cutaneous driving was evident, was driven from the same oddly located skin field. Transitions were relatively sharp; over a distance of 10, 20, or 30 microns, new fields rose from the recording background and previously recorded fields dropped into the background.

In a second series of experiments, receptive fields were recorded in a series of closely spaced vertical penetrations introduced into the zone of representation of the arm in cortical area 3b. Cortical receptive fields are relatively large in the zone of representation of the arm; the territory of representation of this skin region in neocortical fields is relatively small. We reasoned that if receptive fields changed in a stepwise manner across the neorcortex, then peripheral receptive field territories should vary significantly across those steps, and they should be clearly demonstrable. That was, in fact, the case. Receptive fields changed little for neurons recorded over distances of a few tens of microns up to more than a hundred microns; over a narrow transition distance an overlapping but unequivocally different receptive field emerged. This second receptive field was recorded for neurons over a significant horizontal extent before another receptive field was encountered. Near neuronal group "borders," neurons sometimes (possibly frequently) had composite receptive fields approximately equal to the summed receptive fields of adjacent groups.

Thus, our studies strongly support the concept, stated perhaps most clearly by Mountcastle (34), that the basic functional unit of the cortex is a "minicolumn" of cooperatively linked neurons that is usually several tens of microns across. However, in extension of his arguments, studies also indicate that: a) these small cooperating neuronal groups are functional, not anatomical entities; b) these functional minicolumns continually change neuronal memberships and thereby effectively *move* within the horizontal dimension of the neocortical plate; and c) by changes in neuronal memberships the size of neuronal groups are subject to substantial change.

We have defined, by tactile stimulation, the size of functional mini-columns in an attempt to change neuronal group memberships. Over a period of minutes to hours, receptive fields of studied neurons changed in a stepwise manner, from that characteristic for one minicolumn to that common for neurons within another (Merzenich *et al.*, unpublished experiments). Generated under digital plaster casts (in which large skin surfaces are believed to be more or less synchronously excited whenever the cast is struck), we have also produced greatly enlarged neuronal groups. Using electrical stimulation (delivering an all-synchronous input), we have apparently generated a peripheral cutaneous nerve in some animals for a period of several hours (40).

Accumulated Neural Record in Neocortex

There is an accumulated neural record of input histories within neocortical fields. This storage of information is not fully displayed (indeed, is largely unrepresented) by the pattern of overt action potential responses of cortical neurons. It is clear that inputs over broad cortical zones, including those not overtly driven by them, must produce an accumulated record, as some of those cortical zones will be responsive to those inputs at later times as the cortical representation is altered by use (29, 30, 32). Zarzecki and colleagues have demonstrated that inputs from a skin area broader than that over which they are overtly driven commonly generate EPSPs in cortical neurons (52, 53). These non-driving, as well as overtly driving, inputs must be capable of generating stored, long-term changes.

Behavioral State and Context

The effectiveness of inputs for producing stored and accumulated changes are modulated as a function of behavioral state and context. We have recorded great changes in cortical maps as a function of use in normal monkeys performing a task requiring their dedicated attention and have seen only limited or negative changes in representation in skin surface representations in monkeys performing a similar task while, for the most part, attending to other enterprises (18). This offers preliminary evidence that the alteration of cortical maps by use is modulated by the behavioral state or behavioral context of the applied stimuli. In general, it would be very surprising if this were not the case.

Map changes paralleling those recorded in somatosensory studies have now been described in auditory cortical fields in adult cats. There, shifts of auditory neuron-tuning curves are seen with classical conditioning, with responses in auditory cortex rapidly modified by a tonal stimulus paired with a corneal stimulus (7-9, 50). Changes in tuning curves paralleled conditioning functions. With extinction, auditory tuning curves of cortical neurons shifted back in the direction of their pre-training form.

Thus, in this second sensory system, substantial alteration of neuronal receptive fields was recorded for neurons in each of three studied cortical fields after a relatively small number of stimulus presentations in this highly charged behavioral context. In contrast, neuronal receptive fields were altered little if at all by equivalent schedules of stimulation in the nonreinforced condition. This constitutes a clear demonstration, then, of the modulation of cortical map alteration by behavioral state.

Dynamic Processes in the Neocortex

There can be little doubt that the self-organizing processes operationally manifested in the somatosensory koniocortical field are distributed widely across the neocortex. Moreover, there is growing evidence that similar input-selection or input-filtering processes are in operation at other nervous system levels as well. A review of this literature is beyond the scope of this brief report. To cite several examples from the somatosensory, auditory, and visual systems the following cases are mentioned.

Dynamic alterations of cortical maps, like those recorded in somatosensory area 3b in monkeys, have also been described in somatosensory cortical area 1 (18, 29, 30, 49). There, changes are larger in scale and distance limits appear to be greater. In adults individual maps vary more in area 1 than in area 3b (25, 31), consistent with its apparent modifiability of representational detail. Normal map details or the changes in cortical area 1 driven by differential skin use usually differ widely in any individual animal from the changes recorded in cortical area 3b.

Very substantial individual differences in the details of representation of skin surfaces have been recorded in area 2, the SII fields, and area 5 (37, 41). Again, such marked representational variability indicates that their representational detail is established by use.

The demonstration of tuning curve shifts in response to tonal stimuli, used as the unconditioned stimulus in a classical conditioning behavioral paradigm (7-9, 50) constitutes an apparent auditory system representational plasticity paralleling that recorded in the somatosensory cortex. Again, with repetition of a tonal stimulus in a behavioral context, relatively rapid alterations in auditory cortical receptive fields were recorded. Such changes have been recorded in their most dramatic form in two convergently and divergently connected cortical zones in the cat (a tonotopically organized field "V" and a non-tonotopically organized field AII), but receptive-field changes with stimulus repetition have also been recorded in the koniocortical field, AI.

In tonotopically organized auditory cortical fields the following general observations can be made. a) There are highly divergent and convergent anatomical projections within all binaural columns of the same class in the isofrequency dimensions of these fields (26, 33). b) This nearly all-to-all projection anatomy across all binaural columns of the same class in the isofrequency dimension has been shown physiologically, by a demonstration that there is a remarkably high probability of correlated neuron discharge for pairs of roughly-same-best frequency neurons studied in the thalamus and cortex, or at two different cortical locations (6, 42). c) There are manifest, highly specific responses of neurons at any given location across the isofrequency representational dimension. d) Especially in the isofrequency dimension, cortical maps vary substantially in the representation of neuronal response characteristics as a function of cortical field location. Taken together, these observations indicate that the neocortical machinery in auditory cortical fields must be operating, site by site, to effect an overt response to only a limited set of a very large repertoire of inputs, as in the somatosensory case (27).

In an especially important series of experiments in the auditory cortex, Suga and colleagues have defined a series of orderly representations of a number of different echo-location cues in adult moustache bats (44). For maps derived in different animals, significant variability in representational detail was recorded. While cortical maps were highly ordered there was no clear evidence of equivalent parameter-mapping in the auditory thalamus. Anatomical projections from the thalamus to these cortical zones appeared to be highly divergent and convergent. These very precise, derived maps appear to obey representational rules like those recorded in the somatosensory cortex. Response specificity is described as applying to small columns or groups of cortical neurons.

Taken together, the above observations indicate that somatosensory and auditory representations arise, in general, from intrinsic neocortical input-selection processes paralleling those recorded in somatosensory cortical fields.

Numerous examples and arguments can be drawn from studies of visual, motor, speech recognition, posterior parietal, and chemoreceptive cortical zones. *In general*, neocortical fields have key cytoarchitectural commonalities. *In general*, afferent inputs spread over wider zones than those sectors over which they overtly drive neocortical neurons to discharge. *Commonly*, isorepresentational thalamic axes make a further contribution to this neocortical input spread. *In general*, there is no simple neuroanatomical accounting that can explain neural response specificity or neighborhood response relationships within most studied cortical areas. The more complex the input integration required to account for response specificity and cortical representational order, the greater the requirement for self-organization based on input-coincidence machinery. *In general,* static neuron response characteristics in the neocortex are shared by neighbors, consistent with the conclusion that neuronal responses are defined and refined by groups of cooperating neurons. *In general,* presumptive machinery controlling modulation of input effectivenesses as a function of behavioral state distributes its outputs widely across the neocortex. There is evidence for low frequency oscillatory input in many cortical zones, and REM spikes activate cortical input lines (see below).

Effects of Input Spatial and Temporal Distribution

Field specific sources and distributions of inputs insure production, by use, of field-specific representational constructs. At any moment in the life of any individual, each of these use-driven constructs will be idiosyncratic in representational detail. One major enterprise of the past century of neuroscience research has been the identification, on anatomical then physiological grounds, of functional neocortical "representations" or "areas." In the owl monkey, macaque monkeys, cat, and man (the best studied species with highly developed neocortex) a number of cortical representational fields have been defined in each sensory, motor, and associational sphere (28). These fields are at least usually cytoarchitecturally distinguishable from their neighbors. They are marked by field-specific thalamic and cortical inputs and by field-specific extrinsic projections. When examined, field-specific neuronal response properties are noted. In many instances field-specific behavioral deficits are generated by lesions limited to them. Extrapolating from macaques and by consideration of classical cytoarchitecture and the subsequent refinement of delineable cytoarchitectonic divisions in animal studies, there must be 50-100 representational neocortical zones in humans.

We hypothesize that all of these zones share the same basic, self-organizing neocortical machinery. The details of the representational constructs that they generate from their inputs will be individually dependent upon input sources, upon the spreads of inputs, and upon the temporal relationship between input channels. In some (perhaps most) cortical fields, input effectiveness will be modulated or gated by corticocortical inputs (see below). All fields would be subject to a modulation of input effectiveness as a function of behavioral context or state, but the strength of this modulation, field by field, may be found to be nonuniform. Given field-specific differences in the sources and anatomical spreads of inputs and in input gating in modulation of information storage, each cortical zone will generate an adaptive field-specific representational construct. Apparently at the same time, in the instances in which temporally organizable inputs are delivered in a common form to different cortical zones, similar constructs would be necessarily generated. Thus, for example, some form of detailed "retinotopy," "somatotopy," or "tonotopy" would be conserved in many different cortical fields; where selection for movement or movement direction can arise by input correlations, they will arise, unavoidably, and so forth. That is not to say that these particular maps constitute the primary use-derived product of these cortical zones; input selection can be expected for manifold aspects of delivered inputs.

The capacity for alteration of cortical maps by use should be most limited in koniocortical fields as alterability should be limited by the extents of spreads of convergent inputs. The representation of the skin surface is idiosyncratic, in detail, in the somatosensory koniocortex (25, 31). Correspondingly greater use-derived representational differences should be recorded in more divergently and convergently connected zones.

The Role of Corticocortical Projections

Corticocortical projections are believed to play several different roles in these self-organizing fields. Nelson has shown (35) that inputs from the motor cortex can gate responsivity to tactile stimuli in cortical area 1, but not 3b. The use-generated representations of area 1 are strikingly different from area 3b. This is presumably because inputs derived during active body movements are not allowed to enter the competition matrix during those movements.

We suspect that such input gating is common. Evidence for suppression of neural responses during eye movements has been recorded in several cortical fields (16). In at least the koniocortical auditory field in monkeys neural responses are profoundly suppressed during head and body movements (2). Of course other corticocortical inputs (e.g., the projection from area 17 to field MT) appear to directly enter the input selection machinery.

Intrinsic Mechanisms for Stabilizing Dynamic Neuronal Groups

We hypothesize that there are at least stabilizing mechanisms operating to maintain a functional homeostasis of the neocortical self-organizing machinery. Low frequency oscillations in neuronal discharges are recorded in auditory and somatosensory cortical fields in periods of drowsiness and under certain anesthetic conditions. Discharge oscillation frequencies vary across the horizontal dimensions of auditory and somatosensory cortical fields (43, 45), at any cortical site (i.e., within any given neuronal group) discharge oscillations are in phase (Merzenich and Schreiner, unpublished observations). We hypothesize that a series of low frequency oscillators underly (or at least manifest) neuronal group segregation, that their outputs wax during periods of low input, and that their operation (among other possible romes) effectively stabilizes neuronal group structures and the alterations generated by the preceding active period.

In this self-organizing process an episode of widely distributed synchronous input could be expected to attentuate some of the accumulated consequences of an earlier period of normal input. Effects antagonistic to input selection have been recorded after an all-synchronous input delivered over broad cortical regions, generated by electrical stimulation of peripheral cutaneous nerves (40). We regard these studies as a possible crude simulation of the consequences of episodes of REM sleep. The widely distributed, synchronous spikes delivered across the input latches of the cortex in REM sleep could act to erase weakly recorded changes occurring during periods of waking. This should contribute to the homeostatic maintenance of stable use-selected neuronal groups.

These general processes constitute the basis, on the afferent side, of the ontogeny, maintenance, and adjustment of complex behaviors and cognition. There is a wealth of behavioral evidence that indicates that this general process could account for many aspects of the ontogeny of complex behaviors. As noted at the outset, a fuller consideration of the operation of this machine over the intermediate domain of time and of the effective control of information storage is required for an understanding of the origins of complex learning. These considerations are a subject of ongoing studies and will be reviewed later.

These self-organizing processes constitute a continuation of processes also operating in development. Postnatal developmental processes must play a major and essential role in regulating this self-organization through the course of the ontogenetic development of higher brain functions.

These self-organizing processes operating throughout life are undoubtedly linked and are a possible simple extension of developmental processes that result in the connectional maturation of the forebrain. Other features of system maturation can be expected to have a powerful influence on the establishment of the details of cortical representations and, hence, on the ontogeny of complex behaviors. In this input-coincident machinery, a progressive myelinization would have powerful consequences for establishment of stable input-selected constructs. Myelination sequences (12, 51) could underly cognitive developmental sequences. Such sequencing is requisite in this class of machine as consolidation and stabilization of input repertoires must precede their convergence to "higher" levels. The extended durations of REM sleep episodes would presumably also act to attenuate the effectiveness of inputs in earlier stages of child development.

RELATION TO SOME EXTANT MODELS

Experimental neurobiologists and theoreticians have long sought understanding of elemental, general neurphysiological processes that might account for the development of complex behaviors. A premise of this meeting was that the origins of complex behaviors can be understood on a cellular level. Others have sought understanding of these issues at the level of the general operations of major cortical or subcortical subdivisions, or within the framework of widely inter-connected networks of neurons. This review has outlined some features of a general model of self-organizing processes in the neocortex at an *intermediate* level of organization.

Our search for an understanding of neural mechanisms underlying complex behaviors has been slowed by several self-imposed impediments. First, the primary operating models of experimental neurophysiologists are largely taken from visual system studies which have led to a generation of models of a rigid and unalterable anatomical machine, with responses of neuronal elements fixed in an early, postnatal critical period of life. Second, the nervous system has been studied for the most part through a snapshot approach, in which its functions are considered at a given time slice in the life of an animal or man. This approach has not often been studied in operation. As a consequence, behavioral and cognitive development (as compared with anatomical development and its simple physiological manifestations) has been little studied. Third, when the nervous system is studied in behaviorally trained animals, study has usually begun after the behavioral training is completed (i.e., just when, in terms of understanding the origins of behaviors, the machinery in operation is no longer very interesting). Fourth, the artificial divisions of behaviors and cognitive abilities and distinctions in psychology have been carried into the nervous system, with experimental neurophysiologists often considering these accomplishments (and therefore underlying neural processes) as locationally fragmented. Finally, studies of higher behaviors have been largely cast on a single-cell level in animals and on a macroscopic field level in man. Neither is appropriate for understanding the bases and rules of operation of the cooperating neural groups that control cortical self-organization.

From a wealth of description from psychophysics, cognitive studies, and neuropsychology we have an increasingly clear understanding of what this machinery must accomplish. A wide body of behavioral evidence has long indicated that the correlations of inputs must underly origins of complex behaviors. Many physiologists and theoreticians have considered specific or general physiological processes by which neurons of the neocortex might record or select from information repertoires delivered to it, on the basis of the coincidence among others (see 5, 10, 11, 14, 47). These present studies should be regarded as an empirical extension of the pioneering efforts in these areas. Of these models, the neuronal group selection theory of Edelman ((10, 11), see also (47) and Dudai *et al.*, this volume) has been, in detail, most consistent with our own findings. To this time, a number of Edelman's predictions for neocortical organization have been tested in our experiments; most have been confirmed.

We believe that our studies constitute a further basis of specification of some of the structural features and operational requirements of a general model of neocortical function. If this general model is correct then it should begin to have predictive value for experiments directed toward understanding the origins of higher functions of the brain, the origins of its illnesses, and recovery from injury. A number of these specific predictions are now being tested in our ongoing research.

Acknowledgements. This work was supported by NIH Grant NS-10414, by the Coleman Fund, and by HRI. The author acknowledges the crucial contributions of his colleagues in the many experiments described in this abbreviated review. W. Jenkins and T. Allard provided technical assistance and criticism in the preparation of this manuscript.

REFERENCES

(1) Allard, T.T.; Clark, S.A.; Jenkins, W.M.; and Merzenich, M.M. 1985. Syndactyly results in the emergence of double-digit receptive fields in somatosensory cortex in adult owl monkeys. *Soc. Neurosc. Abstr.* 11(2): 965.

(2) Brugge, J.F., and Merzenich, M.M. 1973. Responses of neurons in auditory cortex of the macaque monkey to monaural and binaural stimuli. *J. Neurophysl.* 36: 1138-1158

(3) Calford, D., and Pettigrew, J. 1985.

(4) Clark, S.A.; Allard, T.T.; Jenkins, W.M.; and Merzenich, M.M. 1985. Syndactyly results in the emergence of double digit receptive fields in somatosensory cortex in adult owl monkeys. *Science*, submitted.

(5) Creutzfeldt, O. 1976. The brain as a functional entity. In *Progress in Brain Research. Perspectives in Brain Research*, vol. 45. Amsterdam: Elsevier.

(6) Creutzfeldt, O.D.; Hellweg, F.-C.; and Schreiner, C. 1980. Thalamocortical transformation of responses to complex auditory stimuli. *Exp. Brain Res.* 39: 87-104.

(7) Diamond, D. 1985. Physiological Plasticity of Single Neurons in Auditory Cortex of the Cat During Learning. Thesis, Univ. of California, Irvine, CA.

(8) Diamond, D. 1985. The expression of learning-induced plasticity of single neurons in auditory cortex is context-dependent. *Neurosci. Abstr.* 11: 834.

(9) Diamond, D.M., and Weinberger, N.M. 1984. Physiological plasticity of single neurons in auditory cortex of the cat during acquisition of the pupillary conditioning response: II. Secondary field AII. *Behav. Neurosci.* 98: 189-210.

(10) Edelman, G.M. 1978. Group selection and phasic reentrant signaling: a theory of higher brain function. In *The Mindful Brain*. Cambridge: MIT Press.

(11) Edelman, G.M., and Finkel, L.H. 1985. Neuronal group selection in the cerebral cortex. In *Dynamic Aspects of Neocortical Function*. New York: J. Wiley & Sons.

(12) Flechzig, P. 1920. Anatomie des menschlichen Gehirns und Rückenmarke auf myelogenetischer Grundlage. Leipzig: Georg Thieme.

(13) Franck, J.L. 1980. Functional reorganization of cat somatic sensory-motor cortex (SmI) after selective dorsal root rhizotomies. *Brain Res.* 186: 458-462.

(14) Hebb, D.O. 1949. Organization of Behavior: New York: J. Wiley & Sons.

(15) Hicks, T.P.; Landry, P.; Metherate, R.; and Dykes, R.W. 1985. Functional properties of neurons mediated by GABA in cat somatosensory cortex under barbiturate and urethan anesthesia.

In *Development, Organization and Processing in Somatosensory Pathways*. Alan R. Liss, Inc.

(16) Judge, S.J.; Wurtz, R.H.; and Richmond, R.H. 1980. Vision during saccadic eye movements. I. Visual interactions in striate cortex. *J. Neurophysl.* 43: 1133-1155.

(17) Juliano, S.L., and Whitsel, B.L. 1985. Metabolic labeling associated with index finger stimulation in monkey SI: between animal variability. *Brain Res.* 342: 242-251.

(18) Jenkins, W.M.; Merzenich, M.M.; Allard, T.T.; and Ochs, M.T. 1986. Behaviorally induced changes in the hand representation in somatosensory cortex of adult owl monkeys. *J. Neurosc.*, submitted.

(19) Jenkins, W.M.; Merzenich, M.M.; and Ochs, M.T. 1984. Behaviorally controlled differential use of restricted hand surfaces induce changes in the cortical representation of the hand in Area 3b of adult owl monkeys. *Soc. Neurosc. Abstr.*

(20) Jenkins, W.M.; Merzenich, M.M.; Zook, J.M.; Fowler, B.C.; and Stryker, M.P. 1982. The area 3b representation of the hand in owl monkeys reorganizes after induction of restricted cortical lesions. *Soc. Neurosc. Abstr.* 8

(21) Kalaska, J., and Pomeranz, B. 1979. Chronic paw deafferentation causes an age-dependent appearance of novel responses from forearm in "paw cortex" of kittens and adult cats. *J. Neurophysl.* 42: 618-633.

(22) Kelahan, A.M., and Doetsch, G.S. 1984. Time-dependent changes in the functional organization of somatosensory cerebral cortex following digit amputation in adult racoons. *Somatosens. Res.* 2: 49-81.

(23) Landry, P., and Deschenes, M. 1981. Intracortical arborizations and receptive fields of identified ventrobasal thalamocortical afferents to the primary somatic sensory cortex in the cat. *J. Comp. Neur.* 199: 345-371.

(24) Merzenich, M.M. 1986. Development and maintenance of cortical somatosensory representations: functional "maps" and neuroanatomical repertoires. In *Touch*, eds. K. Barnard, and T.B. Brazelton. New York: International University Press, in press.

(25) Merzenich, M.M. 1985. Sources of intraspecies and interspecies cortical map variability in mammals: conclusions and hypothesis. In *Comparative Neurobiology: Modes of Communication in the Nervous System*, pp. 138-157. New York: John Wiley & Sons.

(26) Merzenich, M.M.; Colwell, S.A.; and Andersen, R.A. 1982. Thalamocortical and corticothalamic connections in the auditory

system of cat. In *Cortical Sensory Organization*, vol. 3: Multiple Auditory Areas, ed. C.N. Woolsey. Clifton, N.J.: Humana Press.

(27) Merzenich, M.M.; Jenkins, W.M.; and Middlebrooks, J.C. 1984. Observations and hypotheses on special organizational features of the central auditory nervous system. In *Dynamic Aspects of Neocortical Function*, pp. 397-424. New York: John Wiley & Sons.

(28) Merzenich, M.M., and Kaas, J.H. 1980. Principles of organization of sensory-perceptual systems in mammals. *Prog. Psychb.* 9: 1-42.

(29) Merzenich, M.M.; Kaas, J.H.; Wall, J.T.; Nelson, R.J.; Sur, M.; and Felleman, D.J. 1983. Topographic reorganization of somatosensory cortical areas 3b and 1 in adult monkeys following restricted deafferentation. *Neuroscience* 8: 3-55.

(30) Merzenich, M.M., Kaas, J.H.; Wall, J.T.; Sur, M.; Nelson, R.J.; and Felleman, D.J. 1983. Progression of change following median nerve section in the cortical representation of the hand in areas 3b and 1 in adult owl and squirrel monkeys. *Neuroscience* 10: 639-665.

(31) Merzenich, M.M.; Nelson, R.J.; Kaas, J.H.; Stryker, M.P.; Zook, J.M.; Cynader, M.S.; and Schoppmann, A. 1986. Variability in hand surface representations in areas 3b and 1 in adult Owl and Squirrel monkeys. *J. Comp. Neur.*, in press.

(32) Merzenich, M.M.; Nelson, R.J.; Stryker, M.P.; Cynader, M.S.; Schoppman, A.; and Zook, J.M. 1984. Somatosensory cortical map changes following digit amputation in adult monkeys. *J. Comp. Neur.* 224: 591-605.

(33) Middlebrooks, J.C., and Zook, J.M. 1983. Intrinsic organization of the cat's medial geniculate body identified by projections to binaural response-specific bands in the primary auditory cortex. *J. Comp. Neur.* 3: 203-224.

(34) Mountcastle, V.B. 1978. The Mindful Brain, eds. G.M. Edelman and V.B. Mountcastle. Cambridge: MIT Press.

(35) Nelson, R.J. 1984. Sensorimotor cortex responses to vibrotactile stimuli during initiation and execution of hand movement. In *Hand Function and the Neocortex*, eds. A. Goodman and I. Darian-Smith, Berlin: Springer-Verlag.

(36) Paul, R.L.; Goodman, H.; and Merzenich, M.M. 1972. Alterations in mechanoreceptor input to Brodmann's areas 1 and 3 of the postcentral hand area of *Macaca mulatta* after nerve section and regeneration. *Brain Res.* 39: 1-19

(37) Pons, T.P. 1984. The Representation of the Body and Anatomical Connections of Physiologically Defined Regions in Area 2 of the

Macaque Monkey (*Macaca mulatta*). Thesis, Vanderbilt University, Nashville, TN.

(38) Pons, T.P.; Sur, M.; and Kaas, J.H. 1982. Axonal arborizations in area 3b of somatosensory cortex in the owl monkey, *Aotus trivirgatus*. *Anat. Rec.* 202: 151A.

(39) Rasmusson, D. 1982. Reorganization of raccoon somatosensory cortex following removal of the fifth digit. *J. Comp. Neur.* 205: 313-326.

(40) Recanzone, G., and Merzenich, M.M. 1986. Modification of somatosensory cortical fields and representational topographies by electrical stimulation of peripheral cutaneous nerves. *Brain Res.*, submitted.

(41) Robinson, C.J., and Burton, H. 1980. Somatotopic organization in a second somatosensory area of *Macaca fascicularis*. *J. Comp. Neur.* 190: 43-68.

(42) Schreiner, C.E., and Langer, G. 1986. Coding of temporal patterns in the central auditory nervous system. In *Auditory Function*, eds. G. Edelman, S. Hassler, and E. Gall. New York: J. Wiley & Sons, in press.

(43) Schreiner, C.E.; Langner, G.; and Urbas, J.V. 1986. Coding of temporal patterns in the central auditory nervous system. In *Functions of the Auditory System*, eds. G.M. Edelman, E. Gall, and M.W. Cowan. New York: J. Wiley & Sons, in press.

(44) Suga, N. 1985. The extent to which biosonar information is represented in the bat auditory cortex. In *Dynamic Aspects of Neocortical Function*, eds. G. Edelman, E. Gall, and M. Cowan. New York: J. Wiley & Sons.

(45) Sur, M. 1979. Some Principles of Organization of Somatosensory Cortex in Primates. Thesis, Vanderbilt University, Nashville, TN.

(46) Sur, M.; Merzenich, M.M.; and Kaas, J.H. 1980. Magnification, receptive field area and "hypercolumn" size in Areas 3b and 2 of somatosensory cortex in owl monkeys. *J. Comp. Neur.* 44: 295-311.

(47) von der Malsburg, C. 1973. Self organization of orientation sensitive cells in striate cortex. *Kybernetik* 14: 85-100.

(48) Wall, J.T. 1984. Cutaneous responsiveness in primary somatosensory (SI) hindpaw cortex before and after partial hindpaw deafferentation in adult rats. *J. Neurosc.* 4: 1499-1515.

(49) Wall, J.T.; Kaas, J.H.; Sur, M.; Nelson, R.J.; Felleman, D.J.; and Merzenich, M.M. 1986. Functional reorganization in somatosensory cortical areas 3b and 1 of adult monkeys after median nerve repair. *J. Comp. Neur.*, in press.

(50) Weinberger, N.M., and Diamond, D.M. 1986. Dynamic modulation of the auditory system by associative learning. In *Auditory Function*, eds. G. Edelman, S. Hassler, and E. Gall. New York.: J. Wiley & Sons, in press.

(51) Yakolev, P.I., and LeCours, A.R. 1967. The myelogenetic cycles of regional maturation of the brain. In *Regional Developments of the Brain in Early Life*, ed. A. Minkowski. Oxford: Blackwell Sci. Publ.

(52) Zarzecki, P., Blum, P.S.; Bakker, D.A.; and Herman, D. 1983. Convergence of sensory inputs upon projection neurons of somatosensory cortex: vestibular, neck, head, and forelimb inputs. *Exp. Brain Res.* 50: 408-414.

(53) Zarzecki, P., and Wiggin, D.M. 1982. Convergence of sensory inputs upon projection neurons of somatosensory cortex. *Exp. Brain Res.* 48: 28-42.

The Neural and Molecular Bases of Learning,
eds. J.-P. Changeux and M. Konishi, pp. 359–374.
John Wiley & Sons Limited.

Formation of Ectopic Neuromuscular Junctions: Role of Activity and Other Factors

T. Lømo

Institute of Neurophysiology
0162 Oslo 1, Norway

Abstract. Formation of new neuromuscular junctions can be obtained in adult animals by transplanting a nerve to the junction free (ectopic) portion of a skeletal muscle and then sectioning the original nerve to the muscle 2-3 weeks later to make the muscle receptive to innervation. However, the capacity to form such ectopic junctions differs among nerves and muscles. Thus, in the adult rat a transplanted foreign nerve forms numerous ectopic junctions with the soleus muscle but not with the extensor digitorum longus muscle. Furthermore, while foreign axons readily form ectopic junctions with the soleus muscle, soleus axons only very rarely do so after transplantation to the same ectopic region of the soleus muscle.

The formation of ectopic junctions between the fibular nerve and the soleus muscle of adult rats has been extensively studied because it is easy to obtain and manipulate experimentally, and because it recapitulates major events in normal neuromuscular junction formation (e.g., extensive initial polyneuronal innervation followed by elimination, clustering and stabilization of acetylcholine receptors, and appearance of acetylcholinesterase, postjunctional folds and ionic channels with short open times). Through manipulations such as blockage of nerve impulse activity by tetrodotoxin, sectioning of the fibular nerve at different stages of junction formation, and electrical stimulation of the muscle, evidence has been obtained that evoked muscle activity plays a major role in neuromuscular synapse formation. Thus, evoked muscle activity is shown to be important for 1) the elimination of many of the junctions made initially; 2) the maturation and growth to a specified size of the junctions that survive, including the appearance of junctional acetylcholinesterase and probably junctional ionic channels with short open times and postjunctional folds; 3) the number and distribution of junctions on single muscle fibers; and 4) the refractoriness to further innervation in normally innervated muscles.

INTRODUCTION

To understand the development and functional organization of the nervous system it is necessary to know the mechanisms by which synapses are formed and then maintained at appropriate sites in appropriate numbers on target cells. Some insights into these mechanisms can be obtained by studying the neuromuscular junctions that form in adult animals between a transplanted nerve and the nonsynaptic portions of denervated skeletal muscle fibers. Such ectopic junctions became particularly attractive to study when Fex and Thesleff in 1967 (13) showed that these junctions would form quickly and nearly synchronously if the transplanted nerve was left on the muscle for about two weeks before the muscle was made receptive by denervation. The present overview is concerned primarily with ectopic synapse formation in the adult rat soleus muscle. The reasons for this are that in mammals the soleus is more receptive to ectopic synapse formation than many other muscles and has therefore been most extensively studied; that experimental manipulations are relatively easy to perform; and, finally, that the ectopic synapses formed in this preparation appear to recapitulate essential aspects of normal neuromuscular junction formation and may therefore have useful lessons to teach us about neuromuscular junction formation in particular and about synaptogenesis in general. Especially, the preparation has provided information about the role of impulse activity in synapse formation.

DEVELOPMENT OF ECTOPIC NEUROMUSCULAR JUNCTIONS

The fibular nerve is transplanted to the proximal part of the soleus muscle and the soleus is denervated two to three weeks later, usually by cutting or crushing the tibial nerve (14). One to two days after denervation extrajunctional acetylcholine receptors (AChRs) appear along the entire length of the muscle fibers, and 2 1/2 - 3 days after denervation numerous, irregularly distributed AChR clusters and ACh-sensitive "hot spots" appear underneath the fibular nerve ingrowth, which may extend for several mm along the muscle fibers (23, 25, 44). At about three days spontaneous m.e.p.ps and fibular nerve-evoked e.p.ps can be recorded near the AChR clusters (24, 25, 36). Up to about five days after cutting the tibial nerve the innervation is immature. The clustered AChRs have the same short half-lives in the membrane (24 hr, 30) and long mean channel open times (4 ms, 4) as extrajunctional AChRs, presumably because the clusters result, at least in part, from movement of extrajunctional AChRs to the sites of nerve contact. There are no postjunctional folds (18) and no AChE activity (26, 44). The nerve-evoked e.p.ps have low quantal contents and each muscle fiber may be innervated by several fibular axons (6, 20, 23). The efficiency of transmission, however, is relatively high, and already three days after cutting the tibial nerve stimulation of the fibular nerve may elicit action potentials and contractions in the muscle (24, 44). This high efficiency is probably due to a combination of high AChR density, lack of AChE activity, long ionic channel open time, and multiple innervation.

From about five days to three weeks after cutting the tibial nerve some of the ectopic junctions acquire mature, adult characteristics while other junctions disappear. Metabolically stable junctional AChRs (half-life six to ten days) appear at five to six days (30), histochemically detectable AChE and antigens specific for synaptic basal lamina at six to eight days (26, 44), and postjunctional folds and ionic channels with short mean open times (1 ms) within two to three weeks (5, 18). During this period the AChR clusters, which initially were numerous and irregularly distributed often for several mm along individual muscle fibers, condense into one or a few separate clusters (or collections of smaller closely adjacent clusters) (23, 44). At the same time the number of axonal inputs per muscle fiber declines (6, 20, 25). In some cases the axon terminals withdraw from postjunctional specializations that then persist as "empty sites" (20). In other cases no signs of the early innervation remain.

In one study of rat soleus muscles with a transplanted nerve the AChR distribution was examined by autoradiography three weeks or more after the soleus axons were cut ((23) and unpublished observations). Of the 211 fibers studied 41%, 32%, 23%, 3% and 1% contained respectively 1, 2, 3, 4, and 5 separate clusters (or collections of smaller closely adjacent clusters). The length of the fiber segments containing the clusters increased with the number of clusters per fiber. Thus the sum of the lengths of the clusters and the intercluster segments was, on the average, 1.6, 3.4, 4.5, and 7.5 mm for fibers containing respectively 2, 3, 4, and 5 clusters. The average length of the mature clusters was 111 μm. This suggested that at least 1 mm length of muscle fiber is needed to support permanently a neuromuscular junction, or, expressed differently, that refractoriness to synapse formation develops in the segments of the muscle fiber that lie nearest to a maturing neuromuscular junction. Several observations support this conclusion. First, mature ectopic junctions virtually never form closer than about

1 mm to the original endplates (6, 20, 23). Second, in fibers containing more than one ectopic input, the inputs tend to appear either very close together or more than 1 mm apart (23). Third, when two foreign nerves are transplanted to the same region of the soleus, the closely adjacent junctions formed initially are preferentially eliminated (19). The refractory zones are not absolute, however, since adjacent AChRs clusters and AChE plaques may occur also at late times (20).

RELATION TO NORMAL NEUROMUSCULAR JUNCTION FORMATION

Ectopic junction formation in the adult resembles normal junction formation in the embryo in many respects. Also, in the embryo the sequence of events is: clustering of nonjunctional AChRs at sites of nerve contact, AChR stabilization and appearance of junctional specific basal lamina, and, finally, appearance of postjunctional folds and channels with short open times together with a reduction in the number of axonal inputs (6, 11, 30, 33). One difference is that ectopically innervated adult fibers often have more than one permanent junction and more than one permanent axonal input. This difference, however, which may merely be due to the larger size of the muscle fibers and the larger size of the nerve entry zones in the adult, is not absolute since two or more separate endplates may also be found on normal twitch fibers, at least in lower vertebrates, and since extensive polyinnervation has recently been described in normal adult rat lumbrical muscles (38). Other differences are that effective transmission in the embryo may appear before (and not after) AChR clustering and junctional AChE activity at the time or shortly after (and not three to four days after) AChR clustering (11). These differences, however, may be more quantitative than qualitative and may arise partly because cellular processes may be faster in the embryo. Thus, many essential aspects of normal synapse formation appear to be recapitulated in the adult fibular nerve – soleus muscle preparation. It seems useful, therefore, to try to manipulate this system to reveal some of the mechanisms underlying synapse formation.

EXPERIMENTAL MANIPULATIONS

Effects of Evoked Muscle Activity on Receptivity to Innervation and Early Synapse Formation

This has been studied by chronic stimulation of the soleus muscle via implanted electrodes. When denervation and stimulation of the soleus start at the same time a previously transplanted nerve fails to form ectopic neuromuscular junctions (17, 24), probably because stimulation blocks the synthesis of extrajunctional AChRs (12). However, factors other than absence of AChRs may also prevent synapse formation. For example, in the denervated extensor digitorum longus (edl) or in the regions nearest the original endplates of denervated soleus muscles, no ectopic junction formation occurs despite a high sensitivity to ACh (6, 23, 37). Thus, receptivity to innervation may be regulated not only by suppression of AChR synthesis by evoked muscle activity but also by other mechanisms, possibly involving the expression of neural cell adhesion molecules (N-CAM) or other surface molecules (34).

After denervation the original soleus neuromuscular junctions retain a high sensitivity to ACh and can be reinnervated despite chronic direct stimulation of the muscle (14). Such resistance of junctional AChRs to activity can be demonstrated at the earliest stages of synapse formation. Thus, stimulation does not prevent ectopic junction formation when it starts two days after denervation of the soleus muscle (24), i.e., after extrajunctional AChRs appear but before they cluster underneath the fibular nerve. That clustering and synapse formation can occur after the onset of stimulation is probably due to the fact that AChRs (and presumably other properties required for synapse formation) continue to accumulate extrajunctionally for some time despite stimulation because the effects of activity on these membrane properties are delayed by about one day (28). This indicates that AChR clustering is intrinsically resistant to the effects of activity. In other experiments it has been shown that AChR clusters, and an apparatus for effective impulse transmission, develop also when impulse conduction in the nerve is blocked (7, 17). Thus, the first step in ectopic synapse formation is that muscle fibers become receptive to innervation by processes which, at least in some muscles, are elicited by muscle inactivity. Then, nearby appropriate axons may rapidly make functional contact by processes which are activity independent. Finally, by mechanisms which depend strongly on evoked muscle activity (see below), some of the contacts made initially develop into mature adult junctions, while others regress.

Effects of Evoked Muscle Activity on the Development and Distribution of Postjunctional Specializations

This has been studied by cutting the fibular nerve when the ectopic junctions are still very immature (three to five days after cutting the tibial nerve) and then examining the fate of the denervated junctions in the absence or presence of direct stimulation of the muscle. After denervation alone the postjunctional sites fail to develop normally. The ectopic AChR clusters and ACh sensitive "hot spots" remain multiple and irregularly distributed ((23, 25) and unpublished observations), the AChE activity stays low (26), and the AChRs retain their short half-lives (30). The denervated AChR clusters also increase somewhat in size and become more diffuse (30), just as the clusters at denervated neonatal junctions do (35).

Two lines of evidence indicate that this failure of maturation is primarily due to lack of evoked muscle activity. First, when denervation of the ectopic junctions is combined with direct stimulation of the muscle, then the postjunctional sites continue to develop in many respects as if they had been still innervated. After two to three weeks of stimulation only one or a few separate clusters (or collections of smaller closely adjacent clusters), remain (23), and these have virtually the same ACh sensitivity (25), histochemical AChE activity (26), short channel open times (4), average length (107 μm), and distribution along the fibers (23) as the innervated clusters after a comparable time. The effects of stimulation on AChR stabilization and postjunctional folds have not yet been studied, but postjunctional folds appear at denervated ectopic junctions if the muscle is reinnervated (and activated) at the original endplates by the soleus nerve (4) suggesting that activity may be responsible. However, for both postjunctional folds and channel conversion it has not yet been shown that these properties will fail to appear in the absence of evoked muscle activity. Second, when fibular nerve impulse conduction is blocked, but the nerve left otherwise intact, the ectopic junctions, which readily form in the absence of activity, then fail to acquire high AChE activity (7) and a normal distribution of AChR clusters (unpublished observations).

The Nerve Leaves Persistent "Traces" on the Muscle

This has been demonstrated by cutting the fibular nerve at an early stage of ectopic synapse formation and starting stimulation two weeks later. Despite the late onset, stimulation still induces ACh-sensitive "hot spots" and AChE plaques at sites of previous nerve contact (25, 26) indicating that the nerve leaves persistent "traces" on the fiber which interact with activity at a later stage to produce further postjunctional development in the absence of the nerve.

Regulation of Motor Unit Size

Following reinnervation of the soleus and edl muscles by a transplanted sural nerve the distributions of relative motor unit sizes become similar in the two muscles. In soleus and edl muscles innervated or reinnervated by their own nerves, however, the distributions are different (37). This suggests that intrinsic differences among motoneurons are responsible for the fact that different motoneurons innervate different numbers of muscle fibers and, hence, support different numbers of neuromuscular junctions. Normally, the maximum number of neuromuscular junctions that a motoneuron can support is not reached, since motor units usually increase in size after partial denervation (40). Therefore, the actual size of a motor unit may reflect the outcome of a competition between motoneurons for "synaptic space" on the muscle fibers.

Evidence that muscle fibers can support only a limited number of mature neuromuscular junctions has been obtained by Taxt (39), who transplanted either the sural nerve, the lateral planter nerve, or both to the mouse soleus muscle. In each type of experiment the whole soleus was reinnervated by all the motor axons (about 20 in each nerve), which formed new junctions partly at the original endplates and partly ectopically. Interestingly, reinnervation by both nerves (40 axons) led to smaller motor units than reinnervation by either nerve alone (20 axons), while the degree of polyinnervation per muscle fiber, the number of muscle fibers, and the relative motor unit sizes were the same. This suggested that when a given number of muscle fibers becomes reinnervated by an excessive number of motoneurons, the motoneurons must compete for limited synaptic space on the muscle fibers and, as a result, must reduce their number of peripheral contacts in proportion to the motor unit sizes they would normally make. Similarly, when more than one axon innervates one synaptic site on a *Xenopus* or a frog muscle fiber, each axon forms a weaker junction than when it innervates the site alone, suggesting that the axons share a restricted synaptic site between them (1, 41). Since direct stimulation of rat soleus muscles containing early denervated ectopic junctions converts the many small, irregularly distributed AChR clusters into fewer and larger clusters of normal size (see above), it seems likely that the processes restricting the available synaptic space reside in the muscle fiber and depend on evoked muscle activity.

Evidence that impulse activity affects the competition between motoneurons comes from experiments in which impulse conducting axons are found to have a competitive advantage over impulse-blocked axons during reinnervation (31). In other experiments (R. Hennig and T. Lømo, unpublished experiments) the tibial nerve was frozen repeatedly over a period of six weeks to delay reinnervation of the soleus which was stimulated for up to three months starting four weeks before the onset of reinnervation. In the presence of stimulation the regenerating axons reinnervated only 80-96% of the fibers (mean 87%, n = 5), whereas in the absence of stimulation they reinnervated all the fibers (97-100%, mean 99%, n = 6, estimated from differences in the ratio of tetanic tensions to nerve stimulation and direct muscle stimulation). Since the number of muscle fibers was the same and the number of motor axons was probably not reduced, it was concluded that the stimulation had reduced the motor unit size. Such a reduction in motor unit size is consistent with the hypothesis that motor unit size is regulated by some factor produced in limited amounts in active muscle fiber ((29), see also Henderson, this volume).

It is also possible, however, that a competitive advantage may be conferred by factors unrelated to impulse activity, as in the experiments by Bixby and Van Essen (3) where fibular nerve axons, after transplantation to the region of normally innervated soleus endplates, displaced either partially or completely some of the soleus nerve terminals. In this case the fibular nerve axons may have been the more "vigorous" because they were regenerating and without peripheral contacts at the onset of competition. From these results it appears that both motoneuronal and muscular properties determine motor unit size through processes involving impulse activity as well as other factors.

Ability to Form Ectopic Synapses Depends on the Type of the Nerve and Muscle

Evidence for this has been obtained by comparing the capacity of the fibular, the soleus, and the sural nerves to form ectopic junctions with the soleus and the edl muscle. In contrast to the fibular nerve (which grows profusely and usually forms numerous ectopic junctions) the soleus nerve, when transplanted to the same region of the soleus muscle, extends very few regenerating axons and forms ectopic junctions only very rarely (27). The sural nerve behaves similarly to the fibular nerve by forming many ectopic junctions with the soleus muscle. However, when the sural nerve is transplanted to the edl, it almost never forms ectopic junctions regardless of where it is placed on the edl but reinnervates the original denervated junctions (37). Thus, motoneurons appear to be intrinsically different in their capacity to extend axons and form ectopic endplates in foreign territories while muscles appear to be inherently different in their ability to accept ectopic reinnervation by competent axons. Such differences could arise through the irreversible differentiation of motoneurons and muscle fibers into different types early in development. Finally, the formation of ectopic junctions depends on the length of time between transplantation of the nerve and denervation of the muscle. If this time is increased for 3-8, 16, and 24 weeks, then the ectopic junctions form after a longer delay and in smaller numbers (36).

"Fast" and "Slow" Neuromuscular Junctions

The neuromuscular junctions in fast and slow muscles show clear differences in many of their properties, including their appearance in the light microscope after staining with methylene blue (43). The ectopic junctions formed by the fibular nerve have a typically "fast" appearance (many round, discrete boutons connected by thin axon branches), whereas the (relatively few) ectopic junctions formed by the soleus nerve have a typically "slow" appearance (relatively thick, elongated, irregular terminal branches with fewer boutons per unit endplate area (27)). To study the effect of impulse pattern on endplate appearance the transplanted fibular nerve was stimulated continuously at 10 Hz (slow pattern) for three months starting when the soleus was denervated by cutting and reflecting the tibial nerve. The stimulation resulted in slower muscles and some signs of a fast to slow transformation of the appearance of the fibular nerve junctions. The transformation was incomplete, however, perhaps because the junctions received both slow (from the stimulation) and fast (from the fibular motoneurons) impulse patterns or because inherent properties of the fast motoneurons prevented it (27). The results suggested that endplate appearance depends in part on the impulse pattern.

In other experiments single soleus muscle fibers were first reinnervated ectopically by the fast fibular nerve and then at the original endplates by the slow soleus nerve. Such dual innervation did not affect the appearance of either of the two types of junctions, which remained "fast" or "slow" even though the isometric twitch contraction time of the fibers became intermediate between those obtained when the fibers were innervated by either nerve alone (27). These results suggested that the fast and slow appearance of neuromuscular junctions are determined locally by the motoneuron regardless of contraction speed or the presence of junctions elsewhere on the fiber. On the other hand, the contractile properties appear to be determined by the integrated influence of all the synaptic inputs to the fiber.

In a third set of experiments the fibular nerve was transplanted to the entry zone of the cut soleus nerve. Now the fast fibular nerve reinnervated primarily the old slow endplates to form endplates which were identical in appearance to normal slow soleus endplates (27). This indicated that traces, possibly in the basal lamina, persist at the denervated slow endplates forcing the fast fibular axons to terminate along these traces, as observed in the frog (22). Whether these junctions develop fast functional properties, despite their slow appearance, is not known.

POSSIBLE MECHANISMS

The results described suggest that when nerve terminals first contact receptive muscle fibers they induce local changes (imprints) in the fibers. The imprints form independently of impulse activity, possibly by trophic substances and/or contact interactions with the nerve, and persist after destruction of the nerve at an early stage. The nature of the imprint is unknown. Recent evidence suggests that motoneurons produce glycoproteins which become bound to the basal lamina in the synaptic cleft (8). Junctional basal lamina also contains components which cause the formation of clusters of AChRs and AChE activity (42). One possibility, therefore, is that such neurally derived substances direct the initial steps in synapse formation and then either modify the basal lamina or become bound to it, so as to constitute a persistent "imprint." The imprint does not itself lead to mature junctions. This requires muscle activity which is normally evoked at the time of nerve contact, or soon after. Thus, muscle activity, by interacting in some unknown way with the imprints laid down by the nerve, becomes responsible for several important events in the synaptogenesis. First, the activity promotes the stabilization and growth of some junctions while eliminating others. Second, it stimulates the appearance of junctional AChE activity (and probably AChR channels with short open times) and postjunctional folds. Third, it suppresses synthesis of AChRs and promotes other changes in extrajunctional regions which result in refractoriness to subsequent additional innervation.

The mechanisms behind the stabilization of some junctions and the elimination of others are not understood. Depending on the position of the fibular nerve, permanent ectopic junctions may form anywhere on a soleus muscle fiber except for about 1 mm next to the original endplate. This suggests that the position of the successful ectopic junction is determined by chance and the elimination of the other junctions by the outcome of competitive processes. One possibility is that motoneurons initially form an excessive number of synapses because they are stimulated to sprout by substances released from the denervated, inactive muscle ((16), see also Henderson, this volume). Because activity appears to suppress this release, the motoneurons must withdraw some of the terminals when the muscle becomes active.

Another possibility is that as one junction grows other adjacent junctions must regress, either because the more successful junction produces an inhibitory factor that spreads into the nearest segments of that fiber or because the more successful junction deprives the nearest segments of some essential factor. One candidate for such a factor is the substance mentioned above, which is produced in larger amounts in denervated muscles than in active muscles. This could explain the tendency of neuromuscular junctions in some systems to be distributed at intervals of about 1 mm or more, as well as the existence of only a single endplate on most normal mammalian fibers. Since embryonic muscle fibers are short (about 300 µm) when they are first contacted by axons (2), the refractory regions established on each side of a successful junction will extend to the ends of the fiber and force other axons to converge on the same site. Later, as the fiber grows, conducted activity will suppress synapse formation along the rest of the fiber. Through all these effects impulse activity becomes instrumental in stabilizing the individual synapse and in regulating the size, number, and distribution of synapses on single muscle fibers.

Although this scheme may be valid for normal neuromuscular junction formation, some discrepancies exist. In the rat embryo, junctional AChE also appears when evoked muscle activity is prevented (15). In *Xenopus laevis* there is evidence that both short ionic channel open times and AChE activity develop at neuromuscular junctions formed in the absence of activity (9, 21). These differences, however, may be more quantitative than qualitative. Thus, junctional AChE activity may be influenced both by muscle activity and activity-independent neural influences and derived from both the muscle and the nerve (10, 26)). Clusters of AChRs, high AChE activity, and short ionic channel open time may also appear at sites that lack nerve terminals. Apparently, the properties of a mature neuromuscular junction may be influenced by both postjunctional impulse activity, activity-independent neural influences, and intrinsic developmental programs but to varying degrees in different preparations and species.

REFERENCES

(1) Angaut-Petit, D., and Mallart, A. 1979. Dual innervation of endplate sites and its consequences for neuromuscular transmission in muscles of adult *Xenopus laaevis*. *J. Physl.* 289: 203-218.

(2) Bennett, M.R., and Pettigrew, A.G. 1974. The formation of synapses in striated muscle during development. *J. Physl.* 241: 515-545.

(3) Bixby, J.L., and Van Essen, D.C. 1979. Competition between foreign and original nerves in adult mammalian skeletal muscle. *Nature* 282: 726-728.

(4) Brenner, H.R.; Meier, T.; and Widmer, B. 1983. Early action of nerve determines motor endplate differentiation in rat muscle. *Nature* 305: 536-537.

(5) Brenner, H.R., and Sakmann, B. 1983. Neurotrophic control of channel properties at neuromuscular synapses of rat muscle. *J. Physl.* 337: 159-171.

(6) Brown, M.C.; Jansen, J.K.S.; and Van Essen, D. 1976. Polyneuronal innervation of skeletal muscle in new-born rats and its elimination during maturation. *J. Physl.* 261: 387-422.

(7) Cangiano, A.; Lømo, T.; Lutzemberger, L.; and Sveen, O. 1980. Effects of chronic nerve conduction block on formation of neuromuscular junctions and junctional AChE in rat. *Acta Physl. Scand.* 109: 253-296.

(8) Caroni, P.; Carlson, S.S.; Schweitzer, E.; and Kelly, R.B. 1985. Presynaptic neurones may contribute a unique glycoprotein to the extracellular matrix at the synapse. *Nature* 314: 441-443.

(9) Cohen, M.W.; Greschner, M.; and Tucci, M. 1984. *In vivo* development of cholinesterase at a neuromuscular junction in the absence of motor activity in *Xenopus laevis*. *J. Physl.* 348: 57-66.

(10) Davey, B.; Younkin, L.H.; and Younkin, S.G. 1979. Neural control of skeletal muscle cholinesterase: a study using organ-cultured rat muscle. *J. Physl.* 289: 501-515.

(11) Dennis, M.J. 1981. Development of the neuromuscular junction: inductive interactions between cells. *Ann. R. Neurosci.* 4: 43-68.

(12) Fambrough, D. 1979. Control of acetylcholine receptors in skeletal muscle. *Phys. Rev.* 59: 165-227.

(13) Fex, S., and Thesleff, S. 1967. The time required for innervation of denervated muscles by nerve implants. *Life Science* 6: 635-639.

(14) Frank, E.; Jansen, J.K.S.; Lømo, T.; and Westgaard, R.H. 1975. The interaction between foreign and original motor nerves innervating the soleus muscle of rats. *J. Physl.* 247: 725-743.

(15) Harris, A.J. 1981. Embryonic growth and innervation of rat skeletal muscles. II. Neural regulation of muscle cholinesterase. *Phil. Trans. R. Soc. Lon. B* 293: 279-286.

(16) Henderson, C.E.; Huchet, M.; and Changeux, J.-P. 1983. Denervation increases a neurite-promoting activity in extracts of skeletal muscles. *Nature* 302: 609-611.

(17) Jansen, J.K.S.; Lømo, T.; Nicolaysen, K.; and Westgaard, R.H. 1973. Hyperinnervation of skeletal muscle fibers. Dependence on muscle activity. *Science* 181: 559-561.

(18) Korneliussen, H., and Sommerschild, H. 1976. Ultrastructure of the new neuromuscular junctions formed during reinnervation of rat soleus muscles by a foreign nerve. *Cell Tis. Res.* 167: 439-452.

(19) Kuffler, D.; Thompson, W.; and Jansen, J.K.S. 1977. The elimination of synapses in multiply-innervated skeletal muscle fibres of the rat: dependence on distance between end-plates. *Brain Res.* 138: 353-358.

(20) Kuffler, D.P.; Thompson, W; and Jansen, J.K.S. 1980. The fate of foreign endplates in cross-innervated rat soleus muscle. *Proc. R. Soc. Lon. B* 208: 189-222.

(21) Kullberg, R.; Owens, J.L.; and Vickers, J. 1985. Development of synaptic currents in immobilized muscle of *Xenopus laevis*. *J. Physl.* 364: 57-68.

(22) Letinsky, M.S.; Fischbeck, K.H.; and McMahan, U.J. 1976. Precision of reinnervation of original postsynaptic sites in frog muscle after nerve crush. *J. Neurocytol.* 5: 691-718.

(23) Lømo, T.; Mirsky, R.; and Pockett, S. 1984. Formation of neuromuscular junctions in adult rats: role of postsynaptic impulse activity. In *Neuromuscular Diseases*, eds. G. Serratrice *et al.*, pp. 393-399. New York: Raven Press.

(24) Lømo. T., and Slater, C.R. 1978. Control of acetylcholine sensitivity and synapse formation by muscle activity. *J. Physl.* 275: 391-402.

(25) Lømo, T., and Slater, C.R. 1980. Acetylcholine sensitivity of developing ectopic nerve-muscle junctions in adult rat soleus muscles. *J. Physl.* 303: 173-189.

(26) Lømo, T., and Slater, C.R. 1980. Control of junctional acetylcholinesterase by neural and muscular influences in the rat. *J. Physl.* 303: 191-202.

(27) Lømo, T., and Waerhaug, O. 1985. Motor endplates in fast and slow muscles of the rat: what determines their differences? *J. Physl. Paris* 80: 290-297.

(28) Lømo, T., and Westgaard, R.H. 1975. Further studies on the control of ACh sensitivity by muscle activity in the rat. *J. Physl.* 252: 603-626.

(29) Purves, D., and Lichtman, J.W. 1980. Elimination of synapses in the developing nervous system. *Science* 210: 153-157.

(30) Reiness, C.G., and Weinberg, C.B. 1981. Metabolic stabilization of acetylcholine receptors at newly formed neuromuscular junctions in rat. *Develop. Biol.* 84: 247-254.

(31) Ribchester, R.R., and Taxt, T. 1983. Motor unit size and synaptic competition in rat lumbrical muscles reinnervated by active and inactive motor axons. *J. Physl.* 344: 89-111.

(32) Rubin, L.; Schuetze, C.; Weill, C.; and Fischbach, G. 1980. Regulation of acetylcholinesterase appearance at the neuromuscular junction *in vitro*. *Nature* 287: 264-267.

(33) Sanes, J.R., and Chiu, A.Y. 1983. The basal lamina of the neuromuscular junction. *Cold S.H. Quant. Biol.* XLVIII: 667-678.

(34) Sanes, J.R., and Covault, J. 1985. Axon guidance during reinnervation of muscle. *Trends Neur.* 8: 523-528.

(35) Slater, C.R. 1982. Neural influence on the postnatal changes in acetylcholine receptor distribution at nerve-muscle junctions in the mouse. *Develop. Biol.* 94: 23-30.

(36) Sommerschild, H. 1981. Formation of ectopic neuromuscular junctions in adult rats. *Acta Physl. Scand.* 111: 151-158.

(37) Taxt, T. 1983. Cross-innervation of fast and slow-twitch muscles by motor axons of the sural nerve in the mouse. *Acta Physl. Scand.* 117: 331-341.

(38) Taxt, T. 1983. Local and systemic effects of tetrodotoxin on the formation and elimination of synapses in reinnervated adult rat muscle. *J. Physl.* 340: 175-194.

(39) Taxt, T. 1983. Motor unit numbers, motor unit sizes and innervation of single muscle fibres in hyperinnervated adult mouse soleus muscle. *Acta Physl. Scand.* 117: 571-580.

(40) Thompson, W., and Jansen, J.K.S. 1977. The extent of sprouting of remaining motor units in partly denervated immature and adult rat soleus muscle. *Neuroscience* 2: 523-535.

(41) Trussel, L.O., and Grinnell, A.D. 1985. The regulation of synaptic strength within motor units of the frog cutaneous pectoris muscle. *J. Neurosci.* 5: 243-254.

(42) Wallace, B.G.; Nitkin, R.M.; Reist, N.E.; Fallon, J.R.; Moayeri, N.N.; and McMahan, U.J. 1985. Aggregates of acetylcholinesterase induced by acetylcholine receptor-aggregating factor. *Nature* 315: 574-577.

(43) Waerhaug, O., and Korneliussen, H. 1974. Morphological types of motor nerve terminals in rat hindlimb muscles possibly

innervating different muscle fibre types. *Z. Anat. Entwickl.-Gesch.* 144: 237-247.

(44) Weinberg, C.B.; Sanes, J.R.; and Hall, Z.W. 1981. Formation of neuromuscular junctions in adult rats: accumulation of acetylcholine receptors, acetylcholinesterase and components of synaptic basal lamina. *Develop. Biol.* 84: 255-266.

The Neural and Molecular Bases of Learning,
eds. J.-P. Changeux and M. Konishi, pp. 375–398.
John Wiley & Sons Limited.

Synapse Turnover in the Central Nervous System

C.W. Cotman, R.G. Gibbs, and M. Nieto-Sampedro

Dept. of Psychobiology
University of California
Irvine, CA 92717, USA

Abstract. Synapse turnover has been documented at many sites throughout the mammalian central nervous system. Synapse loss and replacement can occur as an adaptation to altered environments and is associated with normal aging. Numerous animal studies have also shown that synaptogenesis will occur in response to injury and, in some cases, appears to restore behavior. We have studied the hippocampal formation as a model system for reactive synaptogenesis. Major synaptic rearrangements occur in both denervated and nondenervated regions of the hippocampus following entorhinal lesions. Recently, we observed similar changes in the hippocampus of patients with Alzheimer's disease. We propose that reactive synaptogenesis occurs in the human brain as a means of compensating for ongoing neuronal loss which occurs as a result of aging and/or disease.

INTRODUCTION

Synapse turnover, defined as the loss and replacement of synapses, appears to be an ongoing process in the mammalian brain which can take place as a function of experience and environmental change as well as in response to injury. Although relatively little is known about the relationship between synapse turnover and behavior, it seems logical to assume that the ability of the brain to alter its synaptic circuitry in response to stimuli is somehow related to the adaptive abilities of the nervous system. In this sense synapse turnover is probably involved in ongoing learning and memory processes. Synapse turnover, in the context of reactive synaptogenesis and sprouting, has also been implicated as a mechanism by which the brain may compensate for functions lost due to brain injury. Consequently, a long-term goal of studies on synapse turnover is to understand the mechanisms by which the gain and loss of synapses occurs as well as affects on behavior.

WHEN AND WHERE DOES SYNAPSE TURNOVER OCCUR?

Natural Synapse Turnover

Natural synapse turnover, meaning synapse turnover evoked by nondamaging stimuli and the normal physiological activity of the organism, is known to occur in several regions of the mature nervous system. Synapse turnover has been well documented in the peripheral nervous system including the parasympathetic innervation of the ciliary muscle (42), the innervation of skeletal muscles by motor neurons (2), and at sensory nerve endings (6). Here, however, we will focus exclusively on synapse turnover in the mature central nervous system (CNS).

Perhaps the most remarkable example of stimulus evoked synapse turnover occurs in the hypothalamus and neurohypophysis (23). Cells in the supraoptic nucleus of the hypothalamus project to the posterior lobe of the pituitary where they terminate around fenestrated capillaries and release small peptide hormones. In particular, these cells release vasopressin and oxytocin which have important roles in the regulation of water retention and smooth muscle contractions. In a well-hydrated, nonpregnant and nonlactating rat, neurons in the supraoptic nucleus are separated from each other by glial processes. Similarly, in the pituitary, specialized astrocytes (pituicytes) surround and engulf axon terminals from the supraoptic nucleus effectively separating them from the capillaries. Water deprivation, lactation, or late pregnancy and parturition causes the glial processes and pituicytes to withdraw resulting in (2) the appearance of synaptic contacts between adjacent magnocellular neurons in the supraoptic nucleus and (3) access of the axon endings to the perivascular space in the neurohypophysis (23). These events are soon followed by (2) the initiation of fast continuous firing of supraoptic neurons with occasional high frequency bursts and (3) an increase in the synthesis of peptide hormones and their precursors (23). These events result in increased water retention in the kidneys or a rise in mammary pressure and are totally reversible.

Natural synapse turnover has also been described in the olfactory system (19), vestibular nucleus (38), cerebral cortex, and cerebellum. In the cortex and cerebellum the number of dendritic spines and size of the dendritic tree can be significantly affected by behavioral experience. For example, mice raised for 17 days in an environment where they could exercise and be as active as they like showed a 23% increase in the number of spines on the dendrites of Purkinje cells beyond that of mice housed in cages with only enough space to allow access to food and water (35). Similar results were obtained in young monkeys. Likewise, rats raised in an "enriched" environment showed an increase in dendritic branching in the occipital cortex (45) as well as an increase in the number of synapses per neuron (44) relative to rats raised in an "impoverished" environment. Whether the increase in the number of synapses per neuron is due to additional synapse formation or to the stabilization of existing synapses is, as yet, unclear. Changes in dendritic morphology have also been observed with aging (experience?) in both rodents and humans.

Natural synapse turnover has also been correlated with learning. As one example, Greenough *et al.* (21) trained rats to reach for food with the nonpreferred paw. Normally, apical dendritic branching in layer V pyramidal cells of motor cortex is greater on the side opposite the preferred paw. After 16 days of training branching was greater on the side opposite the trained paw (see also (20) for discussion).

Another case worth noting is the observation by Lipp *et al.* (30) that the rate of two-way avoidance learning in rats and mice is inversely correlated with the size of the intra- and infrapyramidal mossy fiber projection in the hippocampus. In other words, rats which are good learners have a small mossy fiber projection whereas rats which are poor learners have a larger mossy fiber projection. This relationship is maintained following experimental manipulation of the mossy fiber projection by thyroxin treatment. Thus, rat pups obtained from a line of good learners and injected with thyroxin show an increase in mossy fiber projections and a decrease in their rate of learning as adults. While this does not represent natural synapse turnover *per se*, the fact that learning ability is predictable on the basis of mossy fiber anatomy attains special significance in view of age-related increases in mossy fiber terminals in the hippocampus and dentate gyrus of humans (7).

In spite of the need to know more about the effects of experience and aging on synaptic rearrangements, natural synapse turnover has been difficult to study due to the inability to distinguish new from old synapses. As an alternative, synapse turnover has been extensively studied as it occurs in response to brain injury. Such studies are particularly relevant to synaptic changes which occur in response to cell loss associated with normal aging and with certain disease states such as Alzheimer's disease (see below).

Lesion-induced Synapse Turnover

Synapse loss and replacement typically occurs in a target structure after the removal of one or more of its major afferents (see (9-11) for reviews). For example, the number of synapses in the outer two thirds of the molecular layer of the dentate gyrus is decreased by 85% two days after the removal of its inputs from entorhinal cortex but begins to rise again within an additional two days. Similarly, kainic acid lesions of CA3 and CA4 pyramidal cells in the hippocampus produce a selective, though temporary, loss of synapses in stratum radiatum and stratum oriens. In the former case, synapses in the dentate molecular layer are replaced by sprouting fibers originating in the contralateral entorhinal cortex, the septum, and hippocampal subfield CA4 whereas synapses in stratum radiatum and stratum oriens are replaced by sprouts from residual commissural and associational CA4 fibers (see Figs. 1 and 2).

Injury can also induce synapse turnover in areas outside of the denervated zones. For example, following an entorhinal lesion 20% of the synapses in the inner third of the dentate molecular layer are lost within four days, and then return by ten days, even though most of the synapses in this area originate from cells in area CA4 of the

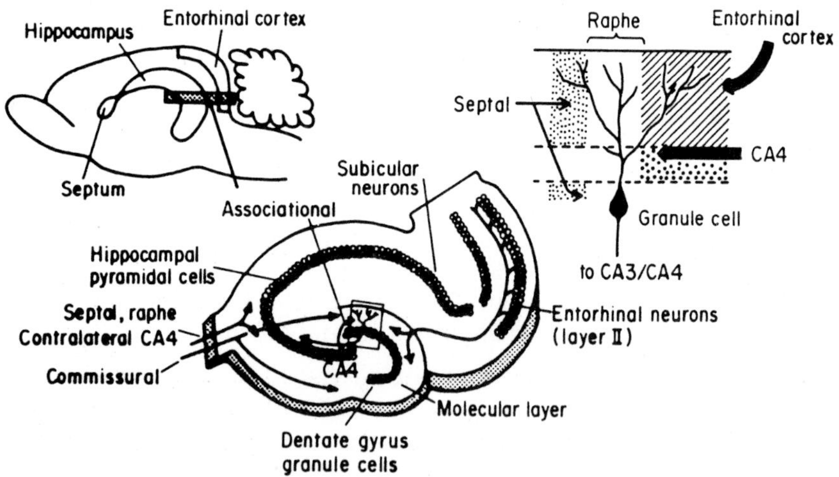

FIG. 1 – Normal distribution of extrinsic afferents projecting onto dentate granule cells. Center: cross-section taken through the hippocampus and dentate gyrus as depicted in upper left. Upper right: representation of the normal distribution of afferent fibers which innervate the dentate granule cells.

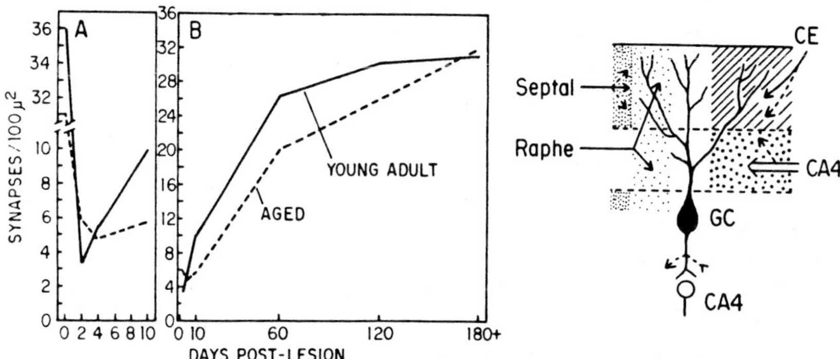

FIG. 2 – Left: time course of synapse replacement in the dentate gyrus following an entorhinal lesion in young and aged rats. Right: diagram depicting the sprouting of remaining afferents in the dentate following an entorhinal lesion (broken arrows represent sprouting; solid arrows represent the normal projection).

hippocampus (11). It should be noted that there are no observable degenerating synapses in the inner third of the molecular layer suggesting that the turnover observed is the result of synaptic disconnection and reconnection. Similar changes are observed in the contralateral hippocampus, although at a much slower rate.

Entorhinal lesions also induce synaptic changes in the CA4/Hilus of the dentate (25). Forty percent of the synaptic contacts in the ipsilateral hilus are lost within four days after an entorhinal lesion and are gradually replaced over a period of six months. In contrast, the density of mossy fiber terminals in the hilus does not decrease, but increases 125% over the same six month period. In the contralateral hilus there is no change in the density of normal synaptic contacts. However, the density of mossy fiber terminals increases approximately 150%, analogous to the increase observed ipsilateral to the lesion. These findings demonstrate that pronounced transneuronal events may occur after major insults to the adult CNS and suggest that, aside from restoring synaptic input to the denervated region, reactive synaptogenesis may serve to restore the functional integrity of complex circuit loops.

WHAT RULES GOVERN SYNAPSE REPLACEMENT?

Overview on Reactive Synaptogenesis

Several rules appear to govern the reinnervation of a target structure in the mature CNS. First, reinnervation completely restores the synaptic complement in the denervated zone. This has been demonstrated in the dentate molecular layer following entorhinal lesions (9, 11), in hippocampal subfield CA1 following lesions of CA3 (9, 11), and in the lateral septum following transection of the fimbria (36). These findings probably reflect a more general tendency to maintain the average area of contact on postsynaptic densities (PSDs) within the denervated area. Hilman and co-workers (24) have shown that as parallel fiber inputs to the cerebellum are lost the remaining parallel fiber synapses rapidly increase in size, the net effect being that the total contact area of PSDs on each Purkinje cell is maintained even though the total number of synapses declines. It is probable that similar changes in synapse size also occur in other areas of the brain in response to natural and injury-induced synapse loss.

Second, an afferent will reinnervate a denervated zone only if its terminal field overlaps with that of the damaged input. This is illustrated in the example above where entorhinal terminals are replaced by commissural, temporo-dentate, and septal fibers. In contrast, retino-thalamic fibers, which have highly exclusive terminal fields, do not reinnervate adjacent portions of the lateral geniculate following enucleation (22). Similarly, neurons in the medial superior olivary nucleus receive nonoverlapping inputs from the ipsilateral and contralateral anteroventral cochlear nucleus which innervate their medial and lateral dendrites respectively. Selective removal of one of these inputs does not induce sprouting of the other (46). Again, this rule only applies to the mature CNS – in the developing CNS, anomolous pathways can be induced by injury (1).

Third, in the event that a terminal field receives more than one type of afferent, there is an hierarchy in the ability of each afferent to reinnervate synaptic territory vacated as the result of destruction of one of the other inputs. This hierarchy reflects competition between different fiber populations for available synaptic space. This is best illustrated in the hippocampus where the pattern of septal cholinergic innervation in the dentate molecular layer is determined by the distribution of commissural and associational (C/A) fibers (8). In the molecular layer, C/A fibers synapse along the proximal 1/3 of the granule cell dendrites while septal cholinergic and entorhinal fibers terminate predominantly along the outer 2/3 of the dendritic field. After an entorhinal lesion the septal cholinergic fibers sprout to help replace the entorhinal input; however, at the same time the C/A terminal field expands causing cholinergic terminals to move to more distal areas of the dendrites. Conversely, when the C/A fibers are removed, septal cholinergic fibers proceed to occupy the entire width of the molecular layer, including that portion previously occupied by the C/A fibers. However, the nature of the competition is such that nearly all C/A fibers must be removed before any cholinergic fibers will sprout into the denervated area. If the lesion is incomplete cholinergic fibers will continue to be excluded and residual CA4 fibers will sprout and reinnervate the denervated zone. A similar mechanism appears to operate during development to produce the pattern of cholinergic innervation observed in the adult.

Implications for Synapse Turnover Derived from Transplant Studies

Much has been learned about reinnervation of a target structure from studies of CNS transplants. Reinnervation by transplants differs from sprouting in that new fibers enter a target region and travel relatively long distances (several millimeters) whereas sprouting occurs locally. Transplants of CNS tissues have been shown to selectively innervate appropriate targets in the host brain and to restore function in both young and aged rats. Transplanted tissues are highly selective in the areas they innervate. For example, septal transplants placed into either a fimbrial cavity or an entorhinal cavity, or injected into the hippocampus directly, accurately reproduce the normal pattern of cholinergic innervation in both the hippocampus and entorhinal cortex following removal of their native cholinergic inputs (4, 28). Similarly, transplants of entorhinal cortex selectively reinnervate appropriate regions of the host hippocampus and amygdala while essentially ignoring other denervated regions to which the entorhinal cortex does not normally project (18) (see Fig. 3).

The distribution of transplant fibers in a target structure appears to be correlated with their transmitter type. For example, transplants of dopaminergic, noradrenergic, serotoninergic, and cholinergic tissues differentially innervate the host in patterns characteristic of the normal innervation by each transmitter type (5) (see Fig. 3). In addition, cholinergic striatal (29) or habenular tissues produces the same pattern of innervation in the host hippocampus as produced by septal transplants, even though these cells normally do not innervate the hippocampus. However, unlike septal transplants which nearly always successfully reinnervate the host hippocampus, habenular transplants were successful in only 35% of the cases examined (unpublished observations). Habenular transplants had a high rate of survival and were

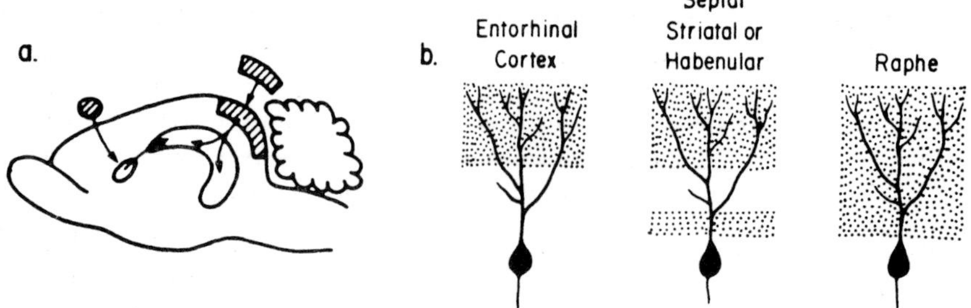

FIG. 3 – a) Diagram depicting the transplantation of embryonic CNS tissues into either the septal or retrohippocampal regions. b) Patterns of innervation produced by transplants of different tissues within the host dentate gyrus.

shown to contain ChAT-positive cells, but in many cases no innervation was observed. Therefore, although the pattern of innervation appears to be determined by transmitter type, differences in the propensity for different tissues to innervate a given target structure suggest that some mechanism of target selection is at work, possibly related to differences in competition between transplant fibers and other afferents within a terminal field (see below).

Selective competition between host and transplant fibers have been demonstrated in several systems. As previously mentioned, septal transplants will restore the normal pattern of cholinergic innervation in the host hippocampus provided the native septal cholinergic innervation has been removed. If, however, the native projection is left intact, innervation by the transplant is significantly impaired even when massive deafferentation of the target region is produced by the removal of other inputs (5, 29). This demonstrates a competitive interaction between homologous transplant and host fibers. Similarly, entorhinal transplants fail to innervate the host hippocampus while the native entorhinal inputs are intact even after denervation of the target by septal lesions (Gibbs and Cotman, submitted). Some innervation is observed following transection of the fimbria, probably in response to the removal of contralateral entorhinal inputs.

In short, it would appear that not only are the number of synapses in the target region fully restored but the number and distribution of synapses formed by different afferents is highly regulated as well. Since, after an entorhinal lesion, synaptic rearrangements occur not only in the denervated region, but in nondenervated, interconnected regions of both the ipsilateral and contralateral hippocampus as well, it seems likely that the rearrangements observed do more than restore synapse numbers in the denervated target, they restore specific types of interactions between the two hippocampi as well (see above). This kind of transynaptic response should have significant effects on brain function following synapse loss due to injury or normal aging.

Another important issue which has emerged from studies of CNS transplants is whether synaptic rearrangements can be reversed once they have occurred. The significance of transplants in relation to behavioral recovery is derived from the fact that axons in the CNS do not regenerate after being damaged as do axons in the PNS (although significant progress is being made in this area). Consequently, transplants have been viewed as a way of replacing projections which have been lost due to injury, disease, or aging. However, in most cases transplant fibers do not reach their targets until well after local synaptic rearrangements have begun to occur. For example, by the time the majority of entorhinal transplant fibers reach the host hippocampus, septal sprouting, sprouting of contralateral entorhinal inputs, and expansion of the C/A fiber terminal field has already occurred. In most cases (>95%) there is no indication that any of these changes have been reversed by the transplant, even as long as nine months post-implantation. Consequently, it may be that the brain's initial response to injury precludes the possibility of completely restoring the normal synaptic composition of a terminal field, whether through implants or through the regeneration of the native projection. Nevertheless, complete restoration of normal circuitry is often unnecessary for functional recovery to be produced (see below).

WHAT HAPPENS DURING SYNAPSE TURNOVER?

By definition the process of synapse turnover requires that synapses become disconnected (or degenerate) and that new connections be formed. Most of our knowledge of the mechanism of synapse turnover is derived from anatomical studies in which synaptic rearrangements have been observed at the light and electron microscopic levels. Success with this approach has been limited, however, for the reasons that a) during natural synapse turnover, only a small population of synapses are being replaced at any given time, and b) there is as yet no way to distinguish new from old connections or to identify the stage of synapse turnover in which a synapse is engaged. Consequently, the molecular mechanisms responsible for synapse turnover are largely unknown. However, enough morphological evidence has accumulated to make some inferences as to the events which occur during synapse removal and replacement.

Synapse Disconnection

At least two mechanisms of synapse disconnection occur in the adult: disconnection due to degeneration of the synaptic ending and disconnection due to the interposition of a glial cell or process between pre- and postsynaptic elements (see above). Morphological intermediates indicative of degeneration have been found but are typically rare (see (11) for discussion). In cases where synapse turnover is induced in nondenervated areas the only probably intermediates observed at the electron microscopic level are large perforated postsynaptic densities (34). This may represent a mechanism by which existing synapses increase in size and then break apart, forming new synaptic contacts in the absence of degeneration.

Synapse Formation

Synapse formation is almost always preceded by some form of process outgrowth (axon regeneration, sprouting, etc.). Factors in normal and injured brain which promote cell survival and neurite outgrowth have been described (3, 33, 41). Recently, we found a neurite-stimulating activity that increases in response to injury with a time course of induction that parallels reactive sprouting (32) (Fig. 4).

Neurite-promoting activity was tested using primary cultures of ciliary ganglion neurons freed of non-neuronal cells and plated at low density to avoid indirect interfering effects. Neurons could be kept alive either by supplying them with survival factors that lacked neurite-promoting activity or by increasing the K^+ concentration of the culture medium. Cells maintained in this way assumed a rounded morphology which persisted for long periods of time. Subsequently, neurite-promoting activity could be assayed by monitoring neurite formation after the addition of brain extract to the ciliary neuron cultures.

Bilateral entorhinal lesions were performed in adult rats. At various times post-lesion the animals were sacrificed and extracts prepared from the deafferented hippocampi and from the cortex surrounding the wound. These extracts were found to contain neurite-promoting activity beyond that present in uninjured brain beginning at 5 days post-lesion and reaching a maximum at 10-15 days post-lesion (Fig. 4). This time course parallels the commissural sprouting and slightly precedes the reactive synaptogenesis which occurs in the hippocampus following

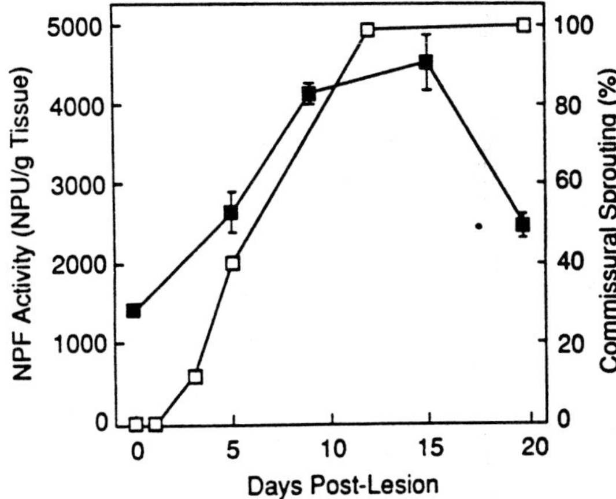

FIG. 4 – Diagram shows the time course for the appearance of NPF activity in the hippocampus following a unilateral entorhinal lesion along with the time course for the sprouting of commissural entorhinal fibers.

entorhinal lesions, suggesting that this activity has a physiological role. Similarly, one might predict that like factors are released in response to cell loss associated with minor vascular injury, aging, stroke, or major trauma in an effort to maintain the circuitry and normal synaptic abundance in affected areas.

After process growth has occurred, new synaptic junctions must be formed. Junctions may form *de novo* in which case they probably use the same mechanisms which operate during development. Some sprouts, however, may reoccupy vacated postsynaptic sites which remain after terminal debris is removed. There is considerable evidence that both mechanisms are operative following lesion induced turnover in denervated areas of the brain. In contrast, detailed studies of lesion induced synaptogenesis in nondenervated zones suggests that synaptic junctions may be involved in a cycle of growth and breakdown. In this model the junction matures and becomes larger until it becomes so large that it literally splits into smaller junctions which can then either degenerate or grow again into one or more mature synapses (34).

Concomitant with synapse formation is the redistribution of receptors in the target area. For example, following entorhinal lesions, the kainic acid-type glutamate receptors redistribute themselves in parallel with the expansion of the commissural and associational fiber terminal field in the hippocampus and dentate gyrus (17).

Clearly, while there is considerable evidence documenting the existence and functional importance of synapse turnover, considerably less is known about the molecular events which occur during synapse loss and replacement. What the field needs is to develop molecular probes specific to different stages of synapse turnover. The development of synapse-specific antibodies which specifically recognize developing synapses might ultimately provide the tools necessary for a more complete study of the mechanism of synapse replacement.

ARE ANIMAL MODELS OF SYNAPSE TURNOVER RELEVANT TO THE HUMAN BRAIN?

Several lines of evidence suggest that the synaptic rearrangements observed in animals can and do occur in the human brain. In humans, mossy fiber terminals are abundant in the inner molecule layer of the dentate gyrus of aged subjects but are virtually absent in young individuals (7). This proliferation may be the result of natural growth or may be induced by the loss of pyramidal neurons as the result of aging. In rodents the destruction of mossy fiber targets induces the same type of growth (10).

A more recently discovered example involves changes in hippocampal circuitry in patients with Alzheimer's disease (17). Brains from Alzheimer's patients show a selective loss of cells in layer II of entorhinal cortex. These cells normally give rise to the perforant path which constitutes the major cortical excitatory input to the hippocampus. In rodents, entorhinal lesions produce a series of synaptic rearrangements in the hippocampus including expansion of the commissural and assocational fiber terminal field and sprouting of septal cholinergic fibers in the molecular layer of the dentate (see above). We have recently observed that similar changes occur in the hippocampus of Alzheimer's patients, thereby exemplifying the relevance of animal models to studies of synaptic rearrangements which occur in association with pathology and aging in humans.

IS SYNAPSE TURNOVER FUNCTIONALLY RELEVANT?

Functional Recovery with CNS Transplants

Studies of CNS transplants demonstrate that, at least in some cases, functional recovery does not require the precise reestablishment of point-to-point circuitries. Labbe *et al.* (27) have shown that cortical transplants can increase the rate of recovery of reinforced alternation following lesions of frontal cortex prior to the establishment of tranplant-host connections. In this case, transplants may be facilitating the functional recovery of partially damaged circuits in the host or the induction of alternate circuits capable of supporting the behavior.

As another example, transplants of dopaminergic tissues into the CNS of adult rats have been shown to ameliorate sensorimotor asymmetries produced by unilateral destruction of the nigro-striatal pathway (12, 14) and to reduce the severity of motor deficits associated with aging (16). Transplanted cells of both central and peripheral origin have been successful in correcting behavioral deficits with the greatest recovery observed when cells are placed directly into the denervated striatum; transplants placed into the region of the substantia nigra have no effect. Consequently, the transplanted cells do not receive their normal inputs and do not recreate the normal circuitry of the nigrostriatal pathway. Rather, functional recovery is related to the ability of the transplants to increase dopaminergic activity within the denervated striatum. Similarly, septal transplants placed into the host hippocampus have been shown to improve spatial memory abilities in animals in which the native cholinergic input to the hippocampus has been removed (13) and in aged animals with spatial memory deficits (15). Analogous to the dopaminergic transplants, the ability of septal transplants to restore function is contingent upon their ability to provide cholinergic innervation to the denervated areas of the host. Clearly these transplants are not reconstituting damaged circuits but most likely restore function by altering levels of cellular excitability and spontaneous activity within the denervated zones.

In other cases the reestablishment of specific circuitries appears to be necessary for functional recovery to be achieved. For example, transplants of entorhinal cortex were shown to reinnervate appropriate regions of the host hippocampus following removal of the native entorhinal inputs (18). However, these transplants did not induce the recovery of spontaneous or reinforced alternation in a T-maze or improve the animals' performance in an 8-arm radial maze following bilateral entorhinal lesions (unpublished observations). All animals were tested repeatedly for eight months following the lesion surgery without any sign of improved performance, demonstrating the magnitude and the stability of the deficit. As with the cholinergic and dopaminergic transplants mentioned above, entorhinal transplants failed to receive many of the inputs which normally project to entorhinal cortex. Although this did not impair the ability of septal and nigral implants to restore behavior, it may account for the lack of recovery observed with entorhinal transplants.

Correlations between Synapse Turnover and Behavior

Examples of natural synapse turnover and its correlation with behavior have already been discussed (see above). The functionality of fibers which sprout in response to surgical manipulation has also been demonstrated in the CNS. Perhaps the best example comes from the work of Tsukahara and co-workers (43) and their studies of synaptic plasticity in the red nucleus. The red nucleus (RN) receives inputs from ipsilateral cerebral cortex (via the cerebral peduncle) and contralateral cerebellum (from the nucleus interpositus). Axons from the RN project to spinal cord. Cortical inputs synapse upon the distal dendrites of RN cells whereas cerebellar inputs synapse upon somatic regions of the cells. Correspondingly, electrical stimulation of the cortical inputs produces a characteristic slow-rising, dendritic EPSP whereas stimulation of the cerebellar inputs produces a fast-rising EPSP. These two responses are easily distinguished and predictable based upon the location of the afferent terminals relative to the cell body. In the adult, destruction of the cerebellar input causes the cortical input to sprout and form new synapses onto proximal regions of the dendrites. Within ten days after destroying the cerebellar inputs the rise-time of cortically evoked EPSPs in the RN is significantly reduced. The prediction that cortical fibers had indeed formed new synapses closer to the cell body has been confirmed by combining lesion studies with electron microscopic examination of HRP-filled cells in the RN.

Tsukahara and co-workers have also shown that synaptic rearrangements in the RN can be induced in the absence of direct lesions, either in response to cross innervation of flexor and extensor nerves of the forelimb or as the result of classical conditioning. Two to six months after cross innervation of forelimb nerves, the rise time of cortically evoked EPSPs in the RN is signficantly reduced. This effect is almost exclusively restricted to cells innervating the upper regions of the spinal cord where the motor neurons contributing to the affected nerves are located. A similar effect is produced in response to the classical conditioning of elbow flexion in response to electrical stimulation of the contralateral cerebral peduncle. In this study, cortical outflow was restricted mainly to the cortico-rubral fibers by lesioning cortico-fugal fibers below the level of the RN. This eliminated the contribution of pyramidal tract fibers as well as the cortico-pontocerebellar and other cortico-bulbar fibers in this reflex. Initially, stimulation of the cerebral peduncle elicited no forearm movement. After seven days of pairing stimulation of the cerebral peduncle with electrical stimulation of the forearm, forearm flexion could be elicited by stimulation of the cerebral peduncle alone. Analysis of cortically evoked EPSPs in the RN revealed that a new fast-rising EPSP had emerged which was superimposed onto the slow-rising EPSP normally observed. These data suggest that cortical fibers innervating the distal dendrites of RN cells sprouted additional terminals which formed synapses along regions of the dendrites more proximal to the cell bodies during the acquisition of the learned response.

Lesion-induced synaptic plasticity has been correlated with functional recovery in other areas of the CNS as well. As previously mentioned, the entorhinal cortex provides excitatory input to both the ipsilateral and contralateral hippocampus and dentate gyrus. While the ipsilateral projection is massive, the contralateral projection is comparatively minor. Unilateral ablation of the entorhinal cortex produces a temporary deficit in the performance of both spontaneous and reinforced alternation in a T-maze, followed by recovery over a period of 10-14 days (31, 37). In contrast, these deficits are permanent following a bilateral entorhinal lesion (40).

Following unilateral entorhinal ablation, the fibers which constitute the commissural entorhinal projection sprout within the denervated zones and form new synapses with granule cell dendrites (39). Correspondingly, the amplitude of extracellular field potentials evoked in the dentate by electrical stimulation of the contralateral entorhinal inputs increases by as much as 200% over a period of ten days following the lesion. Finally, the time course of this increase in synaptic efficacy parallels the time course of recovery of spontaneous and reinforced alternation in the T-maze, following which destruction of the contralateral entorhinal cortex results in the permanent reinstatement of the deficits. These data strongly suggest that sprouting of the commissural entorhinal input is responsible for the behavioral recovery observed. Behavioral recovery has also been correlated with sprouting of peripheral noradrenergic fibers in the hippocampus following kainic acid lesions of areas CA3 and CA4 (26).

Synapse turnover may have its most obvious and immediate functional significance as a compensatory mechanism in aging and disease-related neuronal loss within defined neuronal populations. In the previous section we illustrated that in Alzheimer's disease the loss of entorhinal neurons seems to be accompanied by the sprouting of fibers from residual neurons. This may restore input to an otherwise progressively denervated neuron, thereby stabilizing it and protecting it from overall loss of trophic influences.

It should be noted that in no case does sprouting "recreate" the missing afferent system in an anatomical sense. Even the sprouting of contralateral entorhinal fibers following a unilateral entorhinal lesion does not recreate the missing entorhinal input – the sprouted system is neither topographically organized nor is it as massive as the ipsilateral entorhinal input. Furthermore, other synaptic rearrangements also occur in the hippocampus following entorhinal lesions (see above). Therefore, the notion that sprouting can restore function following injury further suggests that functional recovery does not always require the precise reestablishment of point-to-point circuitries but may involve reestablishing specific patterns of activity within compromised neural loops or the fine tuning and amplification of remaining inputs. Thus, with regards to the reestablishment of neural circuits, it seems necessary to consider each case separately. As an example, possible functional consequences of the changes in connectivity which occur following unilateral vs. bilateral entorhinal lesions are considered below.

Unilateral Injury

After unilateral loss of entorhinal neurons, contralateral neurons sprout new fibers and increase their synaptic drive onto dentate granule cells on the opposite side. As noted above, this enhances the restoration of alternation behavior and perhaps other behaviors as well. In systems with multiple positive feedback, the growth of such inputs may enhance the functional amplification of otherwise weak signals. Lesions cause network assymmetries in the circuitry related to the damage. Compensation for this may be achieved by synapse turnover in nondenervated zones. After unilateral entorhinal ablation, synapse loss in the contralateral hippocampus appears to reduce synapse number to approximately the values on the injured side. Synapses then reappear at a rate such that, at all times postlesion, the repopulation of both sides occurs to a similar extent. Thus, this loss and gain over time may serve to rebalance the network and stabilize information processing in a coordinated fashion.

Following bilateral injury to the entorhinal cortex, as in the case of Alzheimer's disease, the minor loss of entorhinal neurons in early stages is probably compensated for by axon sprouting by residual neurons. That is, the sprouting of remaining entrorhinal fibers may serve to maintain synaptic drive with fewer neurons present. As the injury progresses, other heterologous afferents such as CA4 fibers, mossy fibers, and cholinergic septal fibers also sprout, possibly increasing their correlational coefficient with respect to remaining entorhinal fibers. Additional cholinergic input appears to be beneficial with regard to hippocampal function as demonstrated by the effects of transplanting cholinergic tissues into the hippocampus of aged rodents (15). Additional cholinergic input may likewise be beneficial during the course of Alzheimer's disease considering that the disease also results in some cholinergic cell loss (Fig. 5).

CA4 fiber sprouting in the hippocampus provides another example of a possible beneficial reaction. CA4 fibers comprise one of several feedback loops which are part of many reverberating loops within the limbic system. After the loss of entorhinal input, the growth of these fibers may act to enhance and build up signals which otherwise would be too weak. For example, a train of impulses activating entorhinal neurons

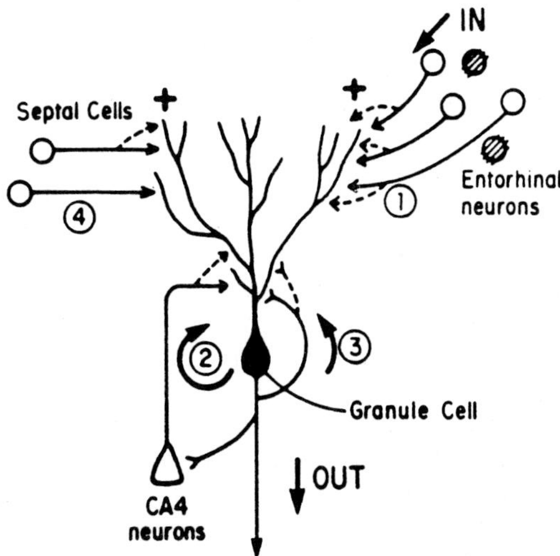

FIG. 5 – Diagram of compensatory sprouting which may serve to maintain the level of excitatory input onto granule cells during the gradual loss of entorhinal neurons in patients with Alzheimer's disease. Cases 1-4 each provide additional excitatory input to the granule cell dendrites thereby compensating for the loss of entorhinal cells: 1) sprouting of remaining entorhinal neurons; 2) sprouting of commissural and associational fibers; 3) sprouting of mossy fiber terminals feeding back onto granule cell dendrites; 4) sprouting of septal fibers.

stimulates dentate granule cells which, in turn, excite CA4 cells whose collaterals feed back onto the dentate granule cells in a positive feedback system. This enhances granule cell firing. In addition, granule cells appear to sprout within their own dendritic field to further compensate for entorhinal cell loss by establishing yet another positive feedback mechanism. The hippocampus is particularly vulnerable to neuronal loss. The fact that it is also highly plastic suggests that the synapse turnover observed is one of many mechanisms by which it compensates for its own losses and injuries

CONCLUSIONS

At this time we must conclude that there is too little data to evaluate the role of synapse turnover in learning. Certainly, prolonged training can induce morphological changes in dendritic trees which, presumably, reflect synaptic changes. However, whether these changes reflect learning *per se* or merely an increase in the activity of certain pathways is still unknown. Clearly, the process is sufficiently subtle so that it requires refined multilevel analysis on a case by case basis. From such detailed analyses it may ultimately be possible to derive an overall conclusion as to the role of synapse turnover in normal learning and memory processes. At the present time, however, evidence keeps accumulating that the process is part of an adaptive response of the brain to different challenges that come its way, including those associated with normal learning.

REFERENCES

(1) Angaut, P.; Alvardo-Mallart, R.M.; and Sotelo, C. 1985. Compensatory climbing fiber innervation after unilateral pendunculotomy in the newborn rat: origin and topographic organization. *J. Comp. Neur.* 236: 161-178.

(2) Barker, D., and Ip, M.C. 1966. Sprouting and degeneration of mammalian motor axons in normal and deafferented skeletal muscle. *P. Roy. Soc. Lon. B* 163: 538-556.

(3) Berg, D.K. 1984. New neuronal growth factors. *Ann. R. Neurosci.* 7: 149-170.

(4) Bjorklund, A., and Stenevi, U. 1977. Reformation of severed septohippocampal cholinergic pathway in the adult rat by transplanted septal neurons. *Cell Tis. Res.* 185: 289-302.

(5) Bjorklund, A., and Stenevi, U. 1979. Regeneration of monoaminergic and cholinergic neurons in the mammalian central nervous system. *Physiol. Rev.* 59: 62-100.

(6) Burgess, P.R.; English, K.B.; Horch, K.W.; and Stensaas, L.J. 1974. Patterning in the regeneration of type I cutaneous receptors. *J. Physl. Lon.* 236: 57-87.

(7) Cassell, M.D., and Brown, M.W. 1984. The distribution of Timm's stain in the nonsulphide-perfused human hippocampal formation. *J. Comp. Neur.* 222: 461.

(8) Cotman, C.W.; Lewis, E.R.; and Hand, D. 1981. The critical afferent theory: a mechanism to account for septohippocampal development and plasticity. In *Lesion-Induced Neuronal Plasticity in Sensorimotor Systems*, eds. H. Flohr and W. Precht, pp. 13-27. Heidelberg: Springer.

(9) Cotman, C.W., and Nieto-Sampedro, M. 1982. Brain function, synapse renewal, and plasticity. *Ann. R. Psychol.* 33: 371-401.

(10) Cotman, C.W., and Nieto-Sampedro, M. 1984. Cell biology of synaptic plasticity. *Science* 225: 1287-1294.

(11) Cotman, C.W.; Nieto-Sampedro, M.; and Harris, E.W. 1981. Synapse replacement in the nervous system of adult vertebrates. *Physiol. Rev.* 61: 684-784.

(12) Dunnett, S.B.; Bjorklund, A.; Schmidt, R.H.; Stenevi, U.; and Iversen, S.D. 1984. Intracerebral Grafting of Neuronal Cell Suspensions, IV: Behavioral recovery in rats with unilateral 6-OH lesions following implantation of nigral cell suspensions in different brain sites. *Acta Physl. Scand. Supp.* 522: 29-37.

(13) Dunnett, S.B.; Low, W.C.; Iversen, S.D.; Stenevi, U.; and Bjorklund, A. 1982. Septal transplants restore maze learning in rats with fornix-fimbria lesions. *Brain Res.* 251: 335-348.

(14) Freed, W.J. 1983. Functional brain tissue transplantation: reversal of lesion-induced rotation by intraventricular substantia nigra and adrenal medulla grafts, with a note on intracranial retinal grafts. *Biol. Psychiatr.* 18(11): 1205-1267.

(15) Gage, F.H.; Bjorklund, A.; Stenevi, U.; Dunnett, S.B.; and Kelly, P.A.T. 1984. Intrahippocampal septal grafts ameliorate learning impairments in aged rats. *Science* 225: 533-535.

(16) Gage, F.H.; Dunnett, S.B.; Stenevi, U.; and Bjorklund, A. 1983. Aged rats: recovery of motor impairments by intrastriatal nigral grafts. *Science* 221: 966-969.

(17) Geddes, J.; Monaghan, D.T.; Cotman, C.W.; Kim Lott, I.; and Chui, H. 1985. Plasticity of hippocampal circuitry in Alzheimer's disease. *Science* 230: 1179-1181.

(18) Gibbs, R.B.; Harris, E.W.; and Cotman, C.W. 1985. Replacement of damaged cortical projections with transplants of entorhinal cortex. *J. Comp. Neur.* 26: 47-65.

(19) Graziadei, P.P.C., and Graziadei, G.A.M. 1979. Neurogenesis and neuron regeneration in the olfactory system of mammals. I. Morphological aspects of differentiation and structural organization of the olfactory sensory neurons. *J. Neurocytol.* 8: 1-17.

(20) Greenough, W.T., and Chang, F.-L.F. 1985. Synaptic structural correlates of information storage in mammalian nervous systems. In *Synaptic Plasticity*, ed. C.W. Cotman, chap. 12. New York: Guilford Press.

(21) Greenough, W.T.; Larson, J.R.; and Withers, G.S. 1985. Effects of unilateral and bilateral training in a reaching task on dendritic branching of neurons in the rat motor-sensory forelimb cortex. *Behav. Neural Biol.* 44: 301-314.

(22) Guillery, R.W. 1977. Experiments to determine whether the retino geniculate axons can form translaminar collateral sprouts in the dorsal lateral geniculate of the cat. *J. Comp. Neur.* 146: 407-419.

(23) Hatton, G.I. 1985. Reversible synapse formation and modulation of cellular relationships in the adult hypothalamus under physiological conditions. In *Synaptic Plasticity*, ed. C.W. Cotman, chap. 13. New York: Guilford Press.

(24) Hillman, D.E., and Chen, S. 1985. Plasticity in the size of pre- and postsynaptic membrane specializations. In *Synaptic Plasticity*, ed. C.W. Cotman, chap. 3. New York: Guilford Press.

(25) Hoff, S.F. 1986. Lesion-induced transneuronal plasticity in the adult rat hippocampus. *Neuroscience*, in press.

(26) Kesslak, J.P., and Gage, F.H. 1986. Recovery of spatial alternation deficits following selective hippocampal destruction using kainic acid. *Behav. Neurosci.*, in press.

(27) Labbe, R.; Firl, A., Jr.; Mufson, E.J.; and Stein, D.G. 1983. Fetal brain transplants: reduction of cognitive deficits in rats with frontal cortex lesions. *Science* 221: 470-472.

(28) Lewis, E.R., and Cotman, C.W. 1980. Mechanisms of septal lamination in the developing hippocampus revealed by outgrowth of fibers from septal implants I. Positional and temporal factors. *Brain Res.* 196: 307-330.

(29) Lewis, E.R., and Cotman, C.W. 1982. Mechanisms of septal lamination in the developing hippocampus revealed by outgrowth of fibers from septal implants. III. Competitive interactions. *Brain Res.* 233: 29-44.

(30) Lipp, H.-P.; Schwegler, H.; and Driscoll, P. 1984. Postnatal modification of hippocampal circuitry alters avoidance learning in adult rats. *Science* 225: 80-82.

(31) Loesche, J., and Steward, O. 1977. Behavioral correlates of denervation and reinnervation of the hippocampal formation of the rat: recovery of alternation performance following unilateral entorhinal cortex lesions. *Brain Res. Bull.* 2: 31-39.

(32) Needels, D.L.; Nieto-Sampedro, M.; and Cotman, C.W. 1986. Induction of a novel neurite-promoting activity in rat brain following injury. *Neuroscience*, in press.

(33) Nieto-Sampedro, M., and Cotman, C.W. 1985. Growth factor induction and temporal order in CNS repair. In *Synaptic Plasticity and Remodeling*, ed. C.W. Cotman, chap. 14. New York: Guilford Press.

(34) Nieto-Sampedro, M.; Hoff, S.F.; and Cotman, C.W. 1982. Perforated postsynaptic densities: probable intermediates in synapse turnover. *Proc. Natl. Acad. Sci.* 79(18): 5718-5722.

(35) Pysh, J.J., and Weiss, G.M. 1979. Exercise during development induces an increase in Purkinje cell dendritic tree size. *Science* 206: 230-232.

(36) Raisman, G., and Field, P.M. 1973. A quantitative investigation of the development of collateral reinnervation after partial deafferentation of the septal nuclei. *Brain Res.* 50: 241-264.

(37) Scheff, S.W., and Cotman, C.W. 1977. Recovery of spontaneous alternation following lesions of the entorhinal cortex in adult rats: possible correlation to axon sprouting. *Behav. Biol.* 21: 286-293.

(38) Sotelo, C., and Palay, S.L. 1971. Altered axons and axon terminals in the lateral vestibular nucleus of the rat. Possible example of axon remodeling. *Lab. Inv.* 25: 653-671.

(39) Steward, O.; Cotman, C.W.; and Lynch, G. 1976. A quantitative autoradiographic and electrophysiological study of the reinnervation of the dentate gyrus by the contralateral entorhinal cortex following ipsilateral entorhinal lesions. *Brain Res.* 114: 181-200.

(40) Steward, O.; Loesche, J.; and Horton, W.C. 1976. Behavioral correlates of denervation and reinnervation of the hippocampal formation of the rat: open field activity and cue utilization following biolateral entorhinal cortex lesions. *Brain Res. Bull.* 2: 41-48.

(41) Thoenen, H., and Edgar, D. 1985. Neurotrophic factors. *Science* 229: 238-242.

(42) Townes-Anderson, E., and Raviola, G. 1978. Degeneration and regeneration of autonomic nerve endings in the anterior part of rhesus monkey ciliary muscle. *J. Neurocytol.* 7: 583-600.

(43) Tsukahara, N. 1985. Synaptic plasticity in the red nucleus and its possible behavioral correlates. In *Synaptic Plasticity*, ed. C.W. Cotman, chap. 7. New York: Guilford Press.

(44) Turner, A.M., and Greenough, W.T. 1983. Synapses per neuron and synaptic dimensions in occipital cortex of rats reared in complex, social or isolation housing. *Acta Stereologica Suppl.* 2: 239-244.

(45) Uylings, H.B.M.; Kuypers, K.; Diamond, M.C.; and Eltman, W.A.M. 1978. Effects of differential environments on plasticity of dendrites of cortical pyramidal neurons in adult rats. *Exp. Neurol.* 62: 658-677.

(46) White, E.L., and Nolan, F.D. 1974. Absence of reinnervation in the chinchilla medial superior olive. *Anat. Rec.* 178: 486.

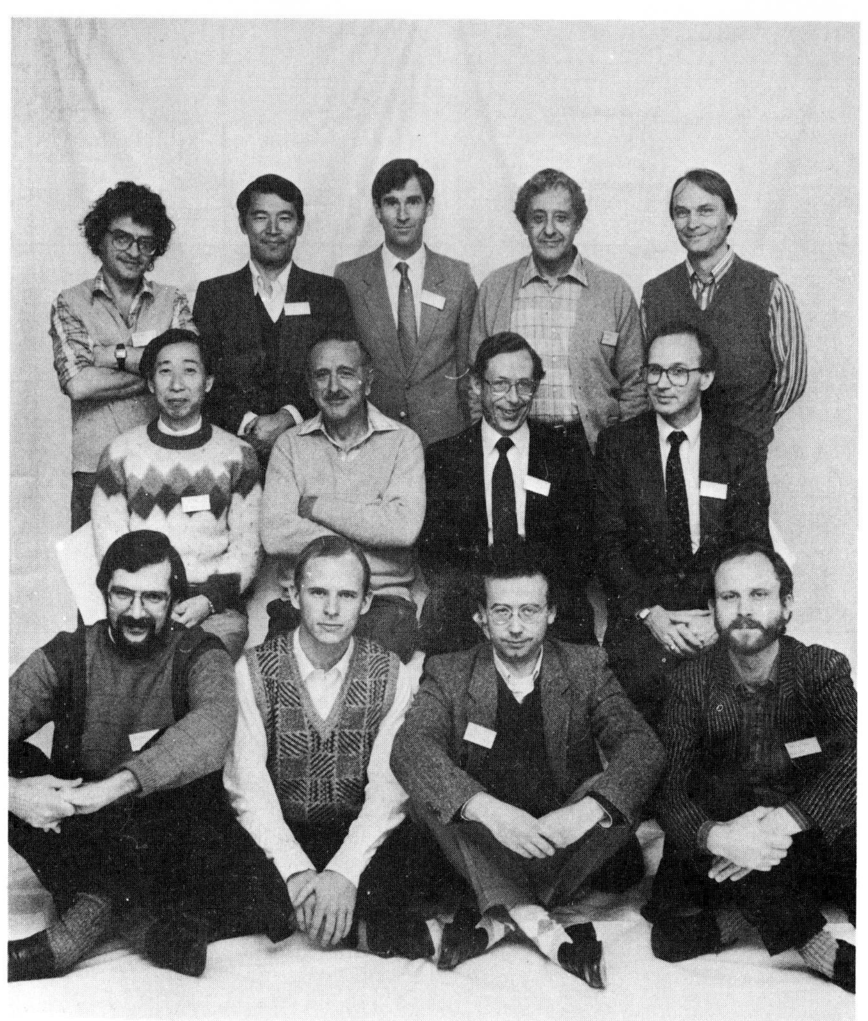

Back row, left to right:
Yadin Dudai, Mark Konishi, Edmund Rolls, Mort Mishkin, Randolf Menzel

Middle row, left to right:
Shun-ichi Amari, Joaquin Fuster, Graham Goddard, Christoph von der Malsburg

Bottom row, left to right:
Herbert Schwegler, Stanislas Dehaene, Elie Bienenstock, Christain Müller

The Neural and Molecular Bases of Learning,
eds. J.-P. Changeux and M. Konishi, pp. 399–410.
John Wiley & Sons Limited.

On Neuronal Assemblies and Memories
Group Report

Y. Dudai, Rapporteur

S.I. Amari	R. Menzel
E. Bienenstock	M. Mishkin
S. Dehaene	C.M. Müller
J. Fuster	E.T. Rolls
G.V. Goddard	H.H. Schwegler
M. Konishi	C. von der Malsburg

INTRODUCTION

Most memories are expected to involve the cooperation of many neurons. In discussing the memory one has therefore to address the structure and properties of functionally related sets of neurons. Understanding the operations of such sets may require theoretical and experimental tools in addition to those which are required for the study of more simple levels of neuronal organization. For our purpose we heuristically and generally define neuronal assemblies as *sets of coactive neurons*. Psychophysiological considerations lead to the assumption that coactivation should occur within a temporal window in the millisecond to second range. However, the temporal constraints on coactivation may vary according to the type and function of the assembly. Complementary definitions of assemblies will follow (see also von der Malsburg, this volume, and (17, 20, 22, 41)).

Neuronal assemblies may differ in the number of neurons, in their architecture and localization, and in their function. Different assemblies may share components. It is not unlikely that even relatively simple behavioral modifications in invertebrates involve activity-dependent modulations of neuronal assemblies, even though major sites of plasticity can be reduced in such cases to single synaptic or cellular loci (reviewed in (43); Menzel and Bicker, this volume).

Nevertheless, when considering assemblies, it is assumed that multiple, dispersed sites of plasticity exist and that plasticity could not be completely reduced to identified cellular components, i.e., no discrete identifiable loci within the network could account for the plastic change in the output of the entire network or for most of it. This does not necessarily imply that the assembly has emergent properties that could not be explained by summation of individual properties of its neuronal components; it just implies that the complexity of the system requires taking into account the concomitant properties of many neuronal components at a time.

Various mathematical representations have been suggested for assemblies. These models are therefore based on the concept of ensemble encoding. Several such models have been reviewed (see (1, 2, 11, 20-22, 24-26, 32, 41, 44, 46) and von der Malsburg, this volume). An important class of models exploits analogies with large systems of interacting particles, as studied in statistical mechanics (21, 22, 32, 44, 46). In these models the set of synaptic strengths between neurons, which determine the properties of the assembly, is generally represented by a matrix of real numbers, hence the term matrix models (see Rolls, this volume). The models place constraints on the structure and function of the assemblies, and hence on the brain, on the mode of interaction of its units, and on the resulting system properties. These constraints and properties, and the rationale underlying them, are discussed in detail in the above-mentioned references.

NEURONAL CODING AND REPRESENTATIONS

For studies of assemblies in general, and learning and memory in particular, it is crucial to elucidate how events and their relationship are encoded. Several principles of the neuronal coding operations, which are involved in the function of assemblies, often emerge from studies of central processing in sensory systems. The main characteristics are:

1. Different stimulus qualities may be kept separate and processed in parallel (e.g., in the owl's auditory system (28), in the electroreceptor system of electric fish (19), or in the visual system of mammals (45).

2. The code may be transformed from spike temporal- or rate-code into place code (e.g., in the owl's auditory system the transformation involves delay lines and coincidence detection and yields resolution of ca. 150 μs in the interaural convergence site). The place code usually involves topographical representation (29).

3. There is hierarchical sequence of data processing (e.g., resulting in fine tuning up to ca. 10 μs in the above-mentioned owl system).

4. There may be convergence as well as divergence or segregation of place codes for different stimulus parameters.

The sensory space is thus transformed into an internal representational map. In other words, a single neuron in the map could be regarded as standing for a representational atom. Assemblies could thus be defined as *sets of neurons necessary to achieve a certain internal representation.* Events, then, would be represented by combinations of atoms, i.e., by the coactivation of the appropriate neurons. Representation of complex events would necessitate hierarchies formed by combination of assemblies. This might necessitate some mechanism to keep the superimposed assemblies from fusing into one assembly. Such mechanisms may involve, for example, the segregation of separate, prewired loosely coupled subsystems or the usage of time tags. In the latter case the postulated hierarchical organization would be a dynamic reorganization process occurring on a fast time scle (von der Malsburg, this volume, and (9, 46)).

So far the assembly could be described as being passively formed by sensory information, although the machinery involved in the formation of the neuronal code is a result of an active phylogenetic and ontogenetic process (see below). However, assemblies could also be regarded as having active properties in their self-interaction and in interaction with other assemblies. The dynamic interaction between neuronal assemblies may suffice to explain self-evaluation of performance by sets of assemblies, making it unnecessary to assume the presence of a homunculus that reads the information. The internal state of the brain would then be regarded solely as *the sum of the functional interactions between the neuronal assemblies in the brain at a given time.* This raises again the question of the temporal constraints on the coactivation of members of the assembly and the time-sharing strategy between assemblies which might be used by the brain. The cross talk between assemblies does not exclude the possibility that some assemblies function as evaluators of other assemblies which communicate with them.

HOW ARE ASSEMBLIES GENERATED AND MODIFIED?

One could consider the question from two points of view: history and mechanism. The organism's brain is not a *tabula rasa* (see also, in this context, (42) and references therein). It is therefore very likely that some assemblies, or predispositions of assemblies, are built into the brain by genetic instructions as a consequence of phylogenesis. These *a priori* patterns impose constraints on the ontogenesis of assemblies, i.e., on development and learning. Two major organizational mechanisms may be considered for ontogenesis: instruction and selection ((4, 5, 11, 17, 42, 44), and von der Malsburg, this volume). The latter mechanism is postulated to operate on fluctuating spontaneous activity according to Darwinian rules, probably involving the temporary existence of pre-assemblies and hence pre-representations (e.g., (18)), and potentially yielding an almost infinite number of phenotypic variations in internal representations. The selection may operate on the local level (e.g., via Hebb synapses, activity-induced synaptic stabilization, and elimination processes (4, 5, 17), as well as on the global level (e.g., via bias towards cooperative activity within assemblies).

It might be worthwhile to suggest a heuristic unifying selection/evaluation principle that operates from the local to the global level and could account for developmental ontogenesis and for learning (i.e., for association of internal representations as well as for association of the latter with external stimuli and for the internal association of external stimuli between themselves). Loops that contain external elements (i.e., sensory input) are thus treated here in the same way as loops that contain only internal elements. Such a universal principle may have evolved during phylogenesis and accomodate for usage in more complex nervous systems and tasks. This might be the Darwinian selection principle itself, reinforcing cooperative patterns of activity, which, as a result, self-reproduce. Such a picture thus depicts the brain as a set of assemblies in which neurons respond both to signals from other assemblies and from sensory input channels, and their activity is modified in accord by obeying a single unifying rule of reinforcement.

WHAT IS THE RELATIONSHIP BETWEEN NEURONAL ASSEMBLIES AND MEMORIES?

To understand this an understanding of perception must first be obtained, e.g., how can our representational system combine perceptual primitives with relationships, and how can it perform very rapidly tasks such as completion and perceptual generalization across transforms of size, position, and rotation. Mathematical models can not yet provide satisfactory algorithms for the latter, and electrophysiological data are still lacking. It is likely that these perceptual problems are solved before representations of objects are stored. As for the memory of the representation, one may suggest that neuronal activity due to cross-correlational or auto-correlational associations, emerging from alterations in sensory input or in internal states, modifies the connectivity and thus the representation of information. Physiological and molecular mechanisms revealed by studies of learning in reduced or simple neuronal systems (e.g., activity-dependent modulation of transmitter release or alterations in postsynaptic receptors or ionic channels (5, 43)) may underlie the persistent alterations in information transfer in the appropriate loci in the modulated assembly. On the other hand, additional molecular and cellular mechanisms (e.g., on a very fast time scale), not revealed in simple networks, should not be excluded (e.g., see (8)).

Retrieval would then be the reactivation of an earlier assembly. The reactivated assembly is a memory (but see below). Descriptions of assemblies that incorporate notions such as parallel processing or matrix operations predict that in some circumstances activation of a sufficient part of the assembly should yield the full internal representation (completion property), and destruction of part of the assembly should leave memory largely intact (graceful degradation property) ((25, 26, 41); and Rolls, this volume).

But what is the stored memory? A representational memory should require operation of several assemblies that differ in their hierarchical status (see also above). Should we consider as the memory the entire meta-assembly system involved in generating the representation? In such a case memory is the assembly engram. Alternatively, it is possible that the memory is only those fragments of a preexisting assembly that are modified – either strengthened or weakened – due to the association. If this is the case then memory of a given representation is smaller than the assembly that yields the representation or the assembly active at the time of experience.

One can contrast representational (or cognitive or declarative) memory, in which what is stored and retrieved is a representation of a stimulus or response, with another type of memory (7, 37-39) which is procedural and also includes, in its primitive forms, the memory of modified reflexes in reduced preparations or simple organisms (43). In the latter case, a substantial part of the information may be stored at few discrete loci, e.g., synapses in the network. What is stored is the altered probability for a stimulus-evoked response and retrieval is actually the readout of the information in the reflex.

Declarative and procedural memories (see below with regard to their nomenclature) can clearly be distinguished in man and probably also in other mammals (7, 37-40). Global amnesia (e.g., due to Korsakoff's syndrome) abolishes declarative memory but not procedural memory. The former is affected by various lesions in the limbic system, especially the hippocampus, amygdala, and mammilary bodies. The latter probably requires the participation of the basal ganglia and cerebellum. Anatomical and functional models for the operations of both memory systems have been described (13, 37).

It is, however, evident that most cognitive memories are not stored in the subcortical areas that are required for their acquisition and probably also for their retrieval (areas that play a crucial role in reward mechanisms, too). Rather, lesion experiments, stimulation, single-unit recordings, and clinical data all seem to point to *sites of storage* in association areas of the cerebral cortex (7, 12-14, 23, 33, 37-40). There is a differentiation in postulated storage locations; memories for items in a particular modality are probably located in areas close to the corresponding cortical primary sensory areas. Thus visual memories may be located in the inferior-temporal cortex, auditory memories in the superior-temporal, somatic memories in the posterior-parietal, and olfactory and gustatory memories in the orbital-prefrontal areas. Cross-modality memories are presumably stored at temporo-parietal and dorsolateral prefrontal areas. In addition, integration of events that are temporally separate and behaviorally contingent takes place with the participation of dorsolateral prefrontal cortex. In the latter, subsidiary circuits seem to exist that deal specifically with such temporally related events. For temporal integration, the prefrontal cortex probably works in conjunction with other cortical assocation areas, limbic structures, and the cerebellum.

There is two-way communication between acquisition, storage, and retrieval systems and reciprocal activation of limbic and cortical areas in these processes. The former may act as multiselector switches of the latter.

It is not yet clear whether the molecular and cellular mechanisms that underlie cognitive memory differ from those that underlie procedural memory, or whether it is only the topology and algorithms that differ between the two types of memory. It is also not yet clear at what stage in the phylogenetic scale cognitive memory emerges. The molecular and cellular research on memory in animals done to date has been performed mostly on models of procedural memory. Reevaluation of current definitions of memory types, and clearer definitions (and/or redefinitions) based on updated experimental data and notions, may provide common conceptual denominators for the analysis of memory systems at various levels of the phylogenetic scale, and may also facilitate the identification of memory systems which involve the operation and modification of assemblies in animals. Such systems might offer great advantages from an experimental point of view.

EXPERIMENTAL APPROACHES

Indeed, one should consider experimental approaches to the study of neuronal assemblies. Such experimental approaches are not easy to design and execute because of the extreme complexity of the nervous system at this level of organization and the lack of some crucial experimental (and analytical) tools. Nevertheless, some approaches utilizing different experimental attitudes and techniques, and tackling the problems on different levels of complexity, could be suggested.

1. One could attempt to *reduce the complexity* of the problem as much as possible without losing crucial complex characteristics of assemblies (i.e., without reducing the system onto the level of a prewired rigid network or a single cell and synapse analysis). In this context, relatively simple nervous systems (e.g., in invertebrates), which have proven very valuable in investigating lower levels of neuronal complexity, may be of help (see Menzel and Bicker, this volume, and (43)). Since organization of nervous systems in assemblies should have evolved on a phylogenetic time scale, it is reasonable to assume that at least some (rudimentary?) properties of assemblies could be revealed in relatively simple organisms. One could consider as candidates, for example, the neuronal systems that modulate body posture in the lobster (in which case the postulated assembly is modulated by an aminergic signal (31)) or the system that controls the locust escape behavior (3). Especially rewarding might be attempts to identify in invertebrates cognitive types of learning, e.g., in bees (15, 36). In other words, the interdisciplinary usage in relatively simple invertebrates of concepts and techniques borrowed from studies of assemblies and representational memory in vertebrates might yield some insight into problems which are more difficult to analyze in a mammalian brain.

2. *Behavioral analysis*, especially in an ethological context (e.g., (35) and references therein), *combined with electrophysiology and neuroanatomy*, could shed more light on the tasks that assemblies are encountered with and on how they perform these tasks. Such an analysis could assist in the identification of topography of assemblies and their ontogenesis. Bird song may provide an example for such an integrated experimental approach (27, 34). In this case, unique neuronal assembly(ies) become(s)

gradually established for a specific function. The diversity of sounds produced by different individuals of the same species, and during song development within an individual, suggests that the brain song control system can produce many output patterns. It is likely that the same set of neurons produces all the patterns by their combinatorial assemblage (see, in this respect, (5)). The final selection of a particular pattern depends on many factors including innate perceptual bias and motor constraints, early auditory experience, and vocal-auditory interactions. This process takes place gradually, involves stabilization of connections and interactions between specific neurons, and leads to the stage where a particular song becomes crystallized (27, 34).

3. Some information regarding assemblies could be gathered by the use of existing *neurophysiological and neuroanatomical* techniques in the *mammalian brain*. Among these one could consider the combined psychophysical and neuroanatomical analysis of pathological lesions in man, with a special emphasis on their effect on complex cognitive tasks (7, 12, 30, 33, 38, 39); mapping of detailed anatomical connections within the brain (e.g., determination of probabilities of connections between specific types of cells, convergence of pathways); analysis of response modifiability (e.g., determination of signals coming on adjacent pathways, temporal specificity properties in identified central neurons); analysis of responses of identified cells to discrete stimuli when these stimuli are part of a structure of a larger sensory stimulus, contrasted with the response to the same stimuli when presented in a nonrelated way; and recordings from association cortex areas in behaving animals in associative paradigms, in which neuroelectrical responses to discrete stimuli are analyzed as a function of discrete changes in the physical characteristics of the stimulus and the behavioral response to it.

4. It is, however, apparent that *novel techniques* are crucial for further research of assemblies. Activity-dependent stains with high spatial and temporal resolution, which allow the simultaneous scanning of activity at real time over large brain regions, preferably in behaving animals, are a prime example (6, 16). Affinity-tagging (e.g., by quick-reacting, highly permeable affinity labels) of macromolecules, which are crucial for memory processes and specific for it, are another example. Identification of specific gene products that are crucial for the proper operation of biological learning and memory mechanisms may prove valuable in generating such affinity tags (10, 43).

5. The construction of *functional models* ((11, 20-22, 24-26, 32, 46) and von der Malsburg, this volume) and their tests, e.g., by computer

simulation, is an additional approach. Specific predictions of such models may then be tested by the use of the techniques mentioned above. Such predictions may permit assessment of the model without necessarily evoking the need to elucidate·the entire structure and function of an assembly.

REFERENCES

(1) Amari, S.I. 1983. Field theory of self-organizing neural nets. *IEEE SMC* 13: 741-748.

(2) Anderson, J.A. 1972. A simple neural network generating an interactive memory. *Math. Biosci.* 14: 197-220.

(3) Bicker, G., and Pearson, K.G. 1983. Initiation of flight by an identified wind sensitive neuron (TCG) in the locust. *J. Exp. Biol. 104*: 289-293.

(4) Changeux, J.-P., and Danchin, A. 1976. Selective stabilisation of developing synapses as a mechanism for the specification of neuronal networks. *Nature* 264: 705-712.

(5) Changeux, J.-P.; Heidemann, T.; and Patte, P. 1984. Learning by selection. In *The Biology of Learning*, eds. P. Marler and H.S. Terrace, pp. 115-133. Dahlem Konferenzen. Berlin, Heidelberg, New York, Tokyo: Springer-Verlag.

(6) Cohen, L.B.; Salzberg, B.M.; and Grinvald, A. 1978. Optical methods for monitoring neuron activity. *Ann. R. Neurosci.* 1: 171-182.

(7) Cohen, N.J., and Squire, L.R. 1980. Preserved learning and retention of patterrn analyzing skill in amnesia: dissociation of knowing how and knowing that. *Science* 210: 207-209.

(8) Crick, F. 1982. Do dendritic spines twitch? *Trends Neur.* 5: 44-46.

(9) Crick, F. 1984. Function of the thalamic reticular complex: the searchlight hypothesis. *Proc. Natl. Acad. Sci.* 81: 4585-4590.

(10) Dudai, Y. 1985. Genes, enzymes, and learning in *Drosophila. Trends Neur.* 8: 18-21.

(11) Edelman, G., and Mountcastle, V.B. 1978. The Mindful Brain. Cambridge, MIT Press.

(12) Fuster, J.M. 1980. The Prefrontal Cortex. New York: Raven Press.

(13) Fuster, J.M. 1984. The cortical substrate of memory. In *Neuropsychology of Memory*, eds. L.R. Squire and N. Butters, pp. 25-31. New York: Guilford Press.

(14) Fuster, J.M. 1985. The prefrontal cortex, mediator of cross-temporal contingencies. *Human Neurobiol.* 4: 169-179.

(15) Gould, J.L. 1984. Natural history of honey bee learning. In *The Biology of Learning*, eds. P. Marler and H.S. Terrace, pp. 149-180, Dahlem Konferenzen. Berlin, Heidelberg, New York, Tokyo: Springer Verlag.

(16) Grinvald, A.; Manker, A.; and Segal, M. 1982. Visualization of the spread of electrical activity in rat hippocampal slices by voltage-sensitive optical probes. *J. Physl.* 333: 269-291.

(17) Hebb, D.O. 1949. The Organization of Behavior. A Neuropsychological Theory. New York: Wiley.

(18) Heidmann, A.; Heidmann, T.M.; and Changeux, J.-P. 1984. Stabilisation sélective de représentations neuronales par resonance entre "préreprésentations" spontanées du réseau cérébral et "percepts" évoqués par interaction avec le monde extérieur. *C.R. Acad. S. III* 299: 839-844.

(19) Heiligenberg, W. 1984. The electric sense of weakly electric fish. *Ann. R. Physl.* 46: 561-583.

(20) Hinton, G.E., and Anderson, J.A., eds. 1981. Parallel Models of Associative Memory. Hillsdale, NJ: Erlbaum.

(21) Hinton, G.E.; Sejnowski, T.J.; and Ackley, D.H. 1984. Boltzmann machines: constraint satisfaction networks that learn. Technical report CMU CS-84-119, Dept. Computer Sci. Pittsburgh, PA: Carnegie Mellon University.

(22) Hopfield, J.J. 1982. Neural networks and physical systems with emergent collective properties. *Proc. Natl. Acad. Sci.* 79: 2554-2558.

(23) Hyvarinen, J. 1982. Posterior parietal lobe of the primate brain. *Physiol. Rev.* 62: 1060-1129.

(24) Kohonen, T. 1977. Associative Memory: A System-theoretical Approach. Berlin, Heidelberg, New York, Tokyo: Springer-Verlag.

(25) Kohonen, T. 1984. Self-organization and Associative Memory. Berlin, Heidelberg, New York, Tokyo: Springer-Verlag.

(26) Kohonen, T.; Oja, E.; and Lehtio, P. 1981. Storage and processing of information in distributed associative memory systems. In *Parallel Models of Associative Memory*, eds. G.E. Hinton and J.A. Anderson, pp. 105-143. Hillsdale, NJ: Erlbaum.

(27) Konishi, M. 1985. Birdsong: from behavior to neuron. *Ann. R. Neurosci.* 8: 125-170.

(28) Konishi, M. 1985. How auditory space is encoded in the owl's brain. In *Comparative Neurobiology, Modes of Communication in the Nervous System*, eds. M.J. Cohen and F. Strumwasser, pp. 335-349. New York: J. Wiley.

(29) Konishi, M. 1986. Centrally synthesized maps of sensory space. *Trends Neur.*, in press.

(30) Kosslyn, S.M.; Holtzman, J.D.; Farah, M.J.; and Gazzaniga, M.S. 1985. A computational analysis of mental image generation: evidence from functional dissociations in split brain patients. *J. Exp. Psy. G.* 114: 311-341.

(31) Kravitz, E.A.; Beltz, B.S.; Glusman, S.; Goy, M.F.; Harris-Warrick, R.M.; Johnston, M.F.; Livingstone, M.S.; Schwartz, T.L.; and Siwicki, K.K. 1983. Neurohormones and lobsters: biochemistry to behavior. *Trends Neur.* 6: 345-349.

(32) Little, W.A. 1974. The existence of persistent states in the brain. *Math. Biosci.* 19: 101-120.

(33) Luria, A.R. 1966. Higher Cortical Function in Man. London: Tavistock Publications.

(34) Marler, P. 1984. Song learning: innate species differences in the learning process. In *The Biology of Learning*, eds. P. Marler and H.S. Terrace, pp. 289-309. Dahlem Konferenzen. Berlin, Heidelberg, New York, Tokyo: Springer-Verlag.

(35) Marler, P., and Terrace, H.S., eds. 1984. The Biology of Learning. Dahlem Konferenzen. Berlin, Heidelberg, New York, Tokyo: Springer-Verlag.

(36) Menzel, R. 1983. Neurobiology of learning and memory: the honey bee as a model system. *Naturwissen.* 70: 504-511.

(37) Mishkin, M. 1982. A memory system in the monkey. *Phil. Trans. R. Soc. Lon. B* 298: 85-95.

(38) Mishkin, M.; Malamut, B.; and Bachevalier, J. 1984. Memories and habits: two neural systems. In *Neurobiology of Learning and Memory*, eds. G. Lynch, J.L. McGaugh, and N.M. Weinberger, pp. 65-77. New York: Guilford Press.

(39) Mishkin, M., and Petri, H.L. 1984. Memories and habits: some implications for the analysis of learning and retention. In *Neuropsychology of Memory*, eds. L.R. Squire and N. Butters, pp. 287-296. New York: The Guilford Press.

(40) Murray, E.A., and Mishkin, M. 1985. Amygdalectomy impairs cross modal association in monkeys. *Science* 228: 604-606.

(41) Palm, G. 1982. Neural Assemblies. Berlin, Heidelberg, New York, Tokyo: Springer-Verlag.

(42) Piatelli-Palmarini, M., ed. 1980. Language and Learning: The Debate Between Jean Piaget and Noam Chomsky. Cambridge, MA: Harvard University Press.

(43) Quinn, W.G. 1984. Work in invertebrates on the mechanisms underlying learning. In *The Biology of Learning*, eds. P. Marler and H.S. Terrace, pp. 197-246. Dahlem Konferenzen. Berlin, Heidelberg, New York, Tokyo: Springer-Verlag.

(44) Toulouse, G.; Dehaene, S.; and Changeux, J.-P. 1986. A spin glass model of learning by selection. *Proc. Natl. Acad. Sci.*, in press.

(45) Van Essen, D.C. 1985. Functional organization of primate visual cortex. In *Cerebral Cortex*, eds. A. Peters and E.D. Jones, vol. 3. New York: Plenum Press.

(46) von der Malsburg, C., and Bienenstock, E. 1986. Statistical coding and short-term synaptic plasticity: a scheme for knowledge representation in the brain. In *Disordered Systems and Biological Organization*, eds. E. Bienenstock, F. Fogelman, and G. Weisbuch, pp. 247-272. Berlin, Heidelberg, New York, Tokyo: Springer-Verlag.

The Neural and Molecular Bases of Learning,
eds. J.-P. Changeux and M. Konishi, pp. 411–432.
John Wiley & Sons Limited.

Synaptic Plasticity as Basis of Brain Organization

C. von der Malsburg

Abt. Neurobiologie
Max-Planck-Institut für Biophysikalische Chemie
3400 Göttingen, F.R. Germany

Abstract. Synaptic plasticity may be regarded as the basis of brain organization. We have two sources of knowledge: physiological experiments on simple model systems and considerations flowing from functional requirements. This investigation tries to exploit the second source. The vital task of the nervous system is appropriate response to external situations. This requires a mapping of external situations into inner states which preserves the relevant metric of the environment. This in turn requires an appropriate configuration space of inner states of "symbols." According to classical theories the state of the brain is aptly described by noting the set of cells – the "assembly" – active within a psychological moment. This view is criticized here. States which have the same global distribution of features would be confused with each other. Attempts to repair the situation, with the help of an unnatural representation by cardinal units and restrictions on nervous connectivity, lead to an unrealistically narrow configuration space. The difficulties can, however, be solved with the help of a more differentiated interpretation of physiology, in which temporal correlations between cellular signals play the role of relational variables, and with a new hypothetical physiological function, synaptic modulation, according to which synaptic weights undergo temporary changes under the control of the temproal fine-structure in cellular signals. According to this new interpretation the nervous system can rely on the "natural representation" of an internal pattern by its own elements. Synaptic plasticity as a basis for memory is transformed into a two-step process in which rapid modulations play the role of short-term memory and are transferred into long-term changes under the control of central signals.

WHAT IS THE PHYSICAL BASIS OF MIND?

The Greeks reduced the multiplicity of materials to a conceptually simple basis: a small number of atomic types and their chemical combination. Such conceptual unification has yet to be attained for the phenomena of mind. One of the important functions of our mind is the construction of models or "symbols" for external objects and situations. What will be discussed here is the structure of the symbols of mind and the processes by which they develop.

Regulative Principles

The discussion may gain in focus by contrast and analogy to the symbols of human communication. The following principles are formulated from this point of view.

Hierarchical structure. The symbols of communication are hierarchically composed of subsymbols. For instance, a book is composed of chapters, paragraphs, sentences, phrases, and words. Such hierarchical structure must also be required of the symbols of mind.

Full Representation. The symbols of communication are mere, parsimonious tokens for the images they are to evoke in the reader's mind. In contrast, symbols of the mind have to fully represent all aspects of our imaginations.

Physical closure. Each written symbol of communication is represented by a dedicated piece of matter, e.g., a drop of ink on virgin paper. Symbols of the mind have to coexist within the same physical system. New symbols should not require new pieces of hardware.

A basis for organization. The symbols of communication are passive products. In contrast, symbols of the mind have to serve as the basis for active organization.

THE CELL-ASSEMBLY FRAMEWORK

The fundamental tenets of the cell-assembly framework have been stated in the works of Hebb (9) and Hayek (8), but most of them are much older. Since then this framework has been developed into a full-fledged dynamical theory by, for example, more precise definitions of synaptic plasticity, the introduction of stabilizing inhibition, and the development of appropriate mathematical tools. The classical theories of the Perceptron (7, 14, 15) and Associative Memory (5, 10, 12, 18, 25) have been formulated entirely within the cell-assembly framework. These two theories are to be regarded as central paradigms from which many of our present-day concepts of brain function derive their specific meaning. The concept of hierarchies of pattern-representing cells, which has been so fruitfully exploited in cortical neurophysiology, is most explicitly crystallized in the perceptron. Associative memory with its beautiful properties of distributed storage of information, graceful degradation, and pattern completion (described by Rolls, this volume) will surely survive as a milestone on the way to functional theories of the brain.

Semantics

Physical states of the brain are to be regarded as symbols for objects, situations, etc. What is the structure of these symbols and in what way do they refer to their subject?

Semantic atoms. The complete symbol characterizing the present state of my mind can be decomposed into smallest units, *semantic atoms* (the term "atom" is commonly used in logic and linguistics to designate indivisible constituent elements). Each atom can be interpreted as an elementary symbol with its own meaning. Typical subjects for atoms are "a blue line of orientation a and stereo depth r at position x of retina," or "there is a face." Semantic atoms are represented in the brain by physical units (nerve cells or disjunctive groups of nerve cells). Atoms can be in an active or inactive state.

Combination by coactivation. The complete symbol characterizing the present state of my mind has been composed by the coactivation of a number of semantic atoms. The symbolic meaning of the composite symbol is additively composed of the elementary meanings of the constituent atoms. The sets of coactive units are often called assemblies, a term introduced by Hebb.

Organization

How are the symbols of mind organized, i.e., how do they come into existence? This organization proceeds in steps which are discussed in reverse chronological order.

Assembly dynamics. Units, or atoms, are activated or inactivated by excitatory and inhibitory interactions. These are channeled by slowly changing physical connections (see below). There are two sources of influences on a unit: external and internal to the brain. The external influences are controlled by stimuli to the sense organs. The internal influences are controlled by the activity of other units. The symbols of mind are quasi-stationary assemblies stabilized by the input and exchange of excitation and inhibition.

Ontogenesis. (The term ontogenesis is taken here in the special sense of referring to that part of structural genesis of our mind and brain which is shaped by our mental history. Those structural aspects which are under more direct control of the genes, and consequently of evolution, are counted under the section on *Phylogenesis*.) The internal connectivity patterns necessary to stabilize assemblies are created by synaptic plasticity. If an assembly is to be "written" into the system, connections between its active units are strengthened (Hebb plasticity). An assembly thus "stored" can later be recovered from partial input. This function is called associative memory.

Phylogenesis. In order for the system to work in the way described it has to be placed in an appropriate initial state with respect both to the basic machinery and to the initial connectivity. This initial state is realized with the help of information stored in the genes.

Two Remarks

An accurate and complete statement of the assembly theory is impossible. As is the case with most fundamental conceptual frameworks, their basic tenets are implicit in all detailed work yet are subconscious and sometimes inconsistent. The account given here of the classical framework, therefore, is necessarily an idealization.

In the ensuing discussion the assembly framework is taken as a comprehensive system for the brain as far as it is concerned with the symbolic representation of the world (internal and external), although this claim of comprehensiveness is rarely made by anybody.

CRITIQUE OF THE ASSEMBLY FRAMEWORK

If I ask you to pass me that book over there – and you do so – you demonstrate a number of abilities of your brain: language interpretation, pattern recognition and visual scene analysis, planning of action, visuo-motor coordination, and motor pattern generation. For decades attempts have been made to understand and model those abilities and others within the assembly framework, all without much success. Maybe the problem is still simply that of finding the right initial connectivity diagrams or the right set of trigger features to make the system work. Maybe, on the other hand - as is assumed here - there is a deeper reason for this failure and the assembly framework itself is to be blamed. Although my discussion seems to be philosophical in nature, the thrust of it is directed at the solution of technical problems. To put it in computer language, without appropriate data structures one cannot write appropriate algorithms. This section raises a number of objections to the assembly framework. The next chapter proposes solutions to the issues raised.

Semantics

The assembly has no structure. The mental symbol in the classical framework – the assembly – is a set of coactive units. As such it has no internal structure. (I should mention here that the lack of syntactical structure in the assembly has been criticized before by Legéndy (13)). Put the other way around, if two symbols (two sets of units) are made coactive, all information on the partition of units among the original symbols is lost. The classical symbol thus violates regulative principles. One cannot avoid coactivating symbols, e.g., those referring to parts of a scene to be described. In such cases the features and modifiers which appertain to the simultaneously represented objects begin to float and form illusory conjunctions, i.e., they trigger consequences which should be reserved for objects combining the features differently. This problem may be called the superposition catastrophe of the classical framework (see Fig.1).

There are various ways in which one may attempt to avoid this difficulty. The most widespread of them consists in a severe restriction of the network to those connections which draw the right consequences. One important scheme is as follows (see Fig.2): keep the part-assemblies in physically distinct subsystems within the brain (e.g., different parts of a topologically organized visual area) – no confusion is possible so far; let the pattern within a subsystem be classified by a set of specialized units ("cardinal cells"); let the subsystem speak to the rest of the brain exclusively with the help of those "labeled lines." The symbols within the subsystems can interact with each other on a higher level without confusion because all detail is invisible on that higher level. To

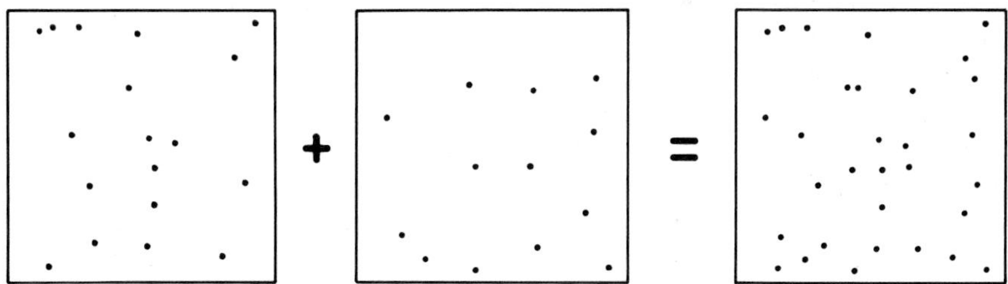

FIG. 1 – Superposition catastrophe. The box symbolizes some part of the brain and is imagined to be filled with neurons. Each dot represents an active cell. On the left, there are two different subassemblies. On the right, the two subassemblies are superposed by coactivation. Information on the partition of the superposition into subassemblies is lost. The rest of the brain can only react to the whole assembly, not to the original subassemblies. False conjunctions of features will therefore lead to erroneous reactions.

illustrate, if the linguistic part of the brain received a full list of the visual features seen at present, it would infer illusory patterns from false conjunctions of features. The presence of patterns has to be evaluated on a level, near to retina, where the relative positions of features are still known and must be sent in encoded form to the linguistic part. Knowledge of the features is useless if it is not complemented with knowledge about their grouping into patterns. Therefore, visual features are to be hidden from the rest of the brain.

This solution creates more difficulties than it solves. Cutting the network into subsystems severely restricts flexibility. It puts a heavy burden on phylogenesis (if it is not possible to derive the subsystem

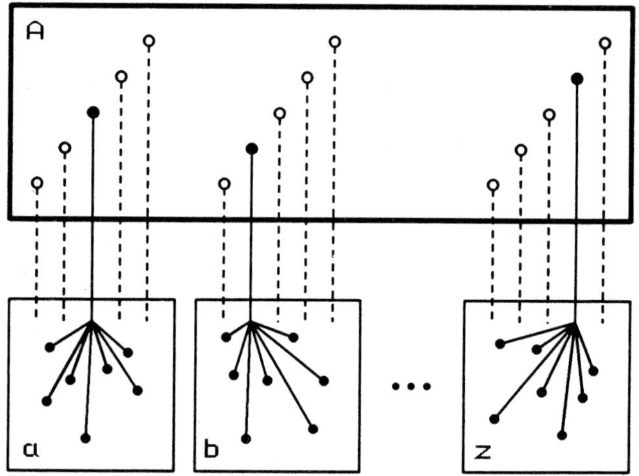

FIG. 2 – Avoidance of the superposition catastrophe in the assembly framework. Assemblies are enclosed in subsystems, represented here as boxes A and a,b,...,z. Active units are represented by filled circles, inactive units (in A) by open circles. Patterns within the lower boxes are represented, within A, by cardinal cells (labeled lines). Boundaries of subsystems are not crossed by connections, except for the ones shown. Specifically, output from the lower boxes is provided exclusively by cardinal cells. The associative connections necessary to store and stabilize assemblies are restricted to within subsystems. The hierarchy can be continued above and below. Patterns in different subsystems can be superposed without confusion since no unit is sensitive to coactivity of units in different subsystems.

structure from a process of ontogenetic organization). Putting patterns (e.g., visual patterns) into subsystems is a difficult problem itself (visual patterns may overlap on the retina!). The scheme presupposes the existence of dedicated units to represent high-level patterns (e.g., "grandmother"). New patterns require new units (thus violating the regulative principle of physical closure). Awful administrative problems are involved in deciding when to represent a new pattern and in finding virgin units to represent them. All variable detail describing the patterns within the subsystems (e.g., "grandmother has a good-humored smile on her face and wears a blue hat") are stripped off on the way to higher levels, thus violating the principle of full representation. In summary, the scheme only works in very restricted environments and with rigid patterns for which the machine has been specifically designed.

Another solution to the superposition catastrophe problem involves selective attention (6, 11, 20). The total symbol which is relevant to the actual situation is not simultaneously active. At a given moment activity is restricted by a central-command system (directing a "searchlight") to a smaller subsymbol. Conjunctions are only permitted between units which are coactivated in one "fixation" of the searchlight. In this scheme a history of consecutive fixations can express a symbol which is hierarchically structured into subsymbols, thus solving the problem in principle. Remaining problems with this scheme are the generation of appropriate activations (the special case of the activation of compact areas in visual space has been worked out in (6, 17)) and with the generation and the evaluation of this history. Evaluation necessitates a temporal storage medium which can be sensitive to the whole history, i.e., to a comprehensive symbol.

No assignment of meaning to connections. The assembly framework assigns meaning to units. This assignment is possible on the basis of the special contexts in the external and internal environment of the brain in which the units are active. Connections are laid down by synaptic plasticity in response to coincident unit activity. Thus, in comparison to units, connections are tied to much more specific contexts. Accordingly, specific meaning could be assigned to connections. However, classical theory does not do so. The reason for this is that individual connections are not expressed in the symbols (assemblies) and connections are not dynamical variables (they cannot be activated and inactivated like units). This point will be discussed further below.

ASSEMBLY DYNAMICS

Some readers may be inclined to shrug off semantics as an epiphenomenon, insignificant for the dynamics of the brain. However, the points of criticism raised in the last section materialize in terms of dynamics. The important point is that situations which are represented by indistinguishable states cannot be expected to lead to distinguishable consequences in the brain.

Interference by irrelevant connections. The point of dynamics in the assembly framework is to coactivate units which are part of the same context. This process is plagued by the presence of connections which have been formed, and which make sense exclusively, in presently irrelevant contexts.

In the associative memory scheme of the classical framework this problem is solved statistically. A unit which should be on in a given assembly receives many excitatory connections from within the assembly, whereas a unit which should be off receives only a few connections from those other units in the assembly with which it happens to be co-member in another assembly. This system works well as long as the assemblies stored in the memory have little overlap with each other. If, however, assemblies have large subsets in common they start to create strong shadows, partly activating other, overlapping assemblies. Now, overlap between mental symbols is the rule rather than the exception. Traditionally, one avoids the difficulty by introducing more units. If there are several units for each elementary symbol different copies can be dedicated (together with their connections) to different assemblies. Thus, a given assembly gets rid of irrelevant connections by avoiding the activation of the units that comman them.

This "solution" necessarily has an unwanted side effect. The overlap between mental symbols is an important basis for vital generalizations. When I consider a particular scene I absorb knowledge about the objects involved by modifying the interactions within and between the corresponding mental symbols. I want to be able to have this knowledge at my disposal in other situations if they partly involve the same objects or aspects. This, however, is possible only through physical overlap between mental symbols. Avoiding this overlap destroys the basis for generalization.

What is needed is a system in which presently irrelevant connections can be switched off, precisely as the presently irrelevant units can be switched off. This would make connections the subject of "meta-interactions." Such a system is discussed later in the section on *NATURAL REPRESENTATION*.

Overlay of functions. This paragraph treats a special aspect of the preceding section. Neural modelers usually take the liberty of concentrating at any one time on one function of the nervous system, correspondingly dedicating their hypothetical neural hardware to that function. This is an understandable habit but it hides the fact that all functions of which our mind is capable have to somehow coexist in the same brain. An obvious solution to the problem is the juxtaposition of dedicated hardware. As far as the functions have been already known to phylogeny, this is a viable solution. However, many functions are learned during ontogeny and they naturally involve symbols which are partly identical. Functions are defined by appropriate systems of interconnections. While the system is performing one function, connections subserving other functions are highly disturbing. Ontogeny may be able to slowly separate the important functions physically from each other (e.g., by developing connections mediated y specialized units which are gated by excitation and inhibition). However, this will not always be possible (due to anatomical constraints), it will take time (during which an overlay of functions has to be borne), and it may not be desirable (since new functions have to partly use old functions). Again, it would be nice if there was a way to temporarily inactivate all connections subserving functions which presently are not relevant.

Ontogenesis

Ontogenesis speaks of the formation of memory. For this discussion it is advantageous to distinguish two types of memory: *historical* and *structural memory*. A similar distinction is made by many neurologists although they refer to it by a variety of names. Historical memory allows us to store specific high-level knowledge, such as "Paris is the capital of France," and to recall specific events of our personal biography complete with detail: circumstances and persons involved, thoughts we had at the time, and so on. Structural memory stores structures and knowledge in a way independent of specific contexts. The two types of memory serve different important purposes. They seem to be implemented by different structures or mechanisms in our brain (it has been shown that patients with amnesia, in whom the ability to lay down historical memory traces is destroyed, may still have structural memory (4)).

In the assembly framework, memory is implemented by Hebb's rule of synaptic plasticity. It connects units which are coactive in a mental state. Let me first discuss structural memory. Certain coactivity relationships in the scene represented by the actual mental symbol are essential, others are accidental. The internal structure of objects is much more stable and consequently more significant than, for instance, their spatial relationships, which vary frequently. (This difference in significance of relationships in an observed scene is a direct reflection of the difference in strength of physical interactions within and among the objects making up the scene.) It is usually useless to couple two units which correspond to features which are part of different objects. Such connections, created by the indiscriminate stickiness of Hebb's rule, would soon clutter up the whole brain with unspecific connections.

In assembly theory there are two solutions to this problem. The first relies on the fact that physically nonexistent connections cannot be plastically strengthened. It therefore suffices to restrict the physical network to such connections as can be expected to correspond to significant relations resorting, for instance, to division into subsystems as discussed in the section entitled *The assembly has no structure* and in Fig. 2. This solution is to be rejected with the same arguments used in that section. The second solution permits all associations between the units active in a mental symbol but puts connections under the constraint of competion (e.g., by limiting the total strength of connections going into or coming out of a unit). After sufficient statistics have been gathered, the strengths of connections will reflect the frequency with which they have been strengthened and thus will reflect the significance of interactions. This solution takes prohibitive amounts of time. In reality we often have to base vital decisions on inspection of a single scene. Somehow synaptic plasticity must be conditioned by a significance of relations which can be deduced directly from the structure of a scene. Such a system will be discussed below.

Historical memory seems to require the coupling of all units which happen to be united in the mental symbol to be memorized so that an indiscriminate stickiness is required here. However, historical memory apparently cannot store just any conceivable situation – it seems to be good only for situations which are "legal" according to our structural memory (1). It may therefore be useful to discriminate a "strong force," which constitutes structural memory, from a "weak force" responsible for historical memory. The weak force becomes perceptible only if the mental symbol comes sufficiently close to one of the historical memory traces, in which case a large number of individually weak connections coherently add up to perceptible influences. Under ordinary circumstances the weak force is nothing but an unimportant random perturbation. In any case the existence of historical memory cannot distract from the conclusion that structural memory cannot consist in an indiscriminate stickiness, as is implied in the c assical framework.

Phylogenesis

Throughout centuries one of the great themes about the brain has been the balance between nature and nurture, between phylogeny and the more fluid types of organization, ontogeny and the spontaneous organization of thought. The genetically determined brain is certainly not a *tabula rasa*. On the other hand, it is to be regarded a weakness of most classical theories that for every function there is a specialized connectivity pattern invoked, and that whenever it is difficult to explain it by ontogenetic mechanisms, one invokes genetic determination, i.e., one makes phylogeny responsible for it. This "phylogenetic loophole" is favored by an important scientific idea, the algorithmic scheme (sometimes referred to by the adjective computational). It proceeds in four sequential steps: a) identification of a problem, b) formulation of an algorithm, c) implementation (in a computer or in the form of a nervous network), and d) execution of the algorithm. If the scheme is applied to specific functions in the b ain, it is only too tempting for the modeler to restrict his explicit presentation to steps c) and d) and to assign steps a) and b) to phylogeny. However, with a problem presenting itself to an individual for the first time in evolution, all four steps have to be performed by ontogeny and assembly dynamics in his brain and the role of phylogeny must be restricted to providing a "meta-algorithm": the physical framework for the whole scheme which includes the formulation of the problem and the "invention" of an appropriate "algorithm" (22)! In other terms, we must not only understand how the brain performs certain specific functions but also how the brain finds them! If it is necessary to invoke specific connectivity structures (cardinal cells, division into subsystems, gated pathways) we also have to specify the process of ontogenetic organization for it. Only structures of a general type can be put off to phylogeny.

Violation of the Regulative Principles

Assemblies as symbols of the mind violate all of the regulative principles stated earlier.

(Hierarchical structure.) The only subsymbols of an assembly are individual atoms. All information represented by the activity of an assembly can be stated by giving a list of active units (the order in the list having no significance). The absence of any intermediate levels in this "hierarchical structure" is most drastically illustrated by the loss in grouping information when several subassemblies are coactive (superposition catastrophe, see Fig. 1). Several stages of hierarchical structure are only possible if the multi-unit detail of one level is encoded by units (cardinal cells) on the next level, a solution which, in turn, can only be bought at the price of cutting the network into subsystems (see above).

Some authors have pointed out that there may be a system of hierarchical relations between different assemblies. (This is particularly the case in models of the spin-glass type (19).) Such structure is, however, not expressed in a given state, and there are no provisions within the assembly framework for forming appropriate hierarchies of assemblies and for storing and retrieving them.

(Full representation.) To avoid false conjunctions all specification of intermediate objects in terms of sets of units must be hidden from the view of consecutive stages of processing. Objects are represented by cardinal units, i.e., by mere tokens. In communicating, parsimony forces us to abbreviate complicated structures and convey them by symbolic tokens. In the brain, however, the full structure of the objects represented should be made available to all subsystems without being deformed and mutilated by the prejudice of a narrow and rigid coding scheme.

(Physical closure.) It is remarkable how flexible the brain is in dealing with new phenomena and problems. Apparently our mind can build up new symbols and new functional structures. If, as seems to be necessary within the assembly framework, patterns and interactions are represented by dedicated units, new units must continuously be actuated. Whereas with communiction, where each new letter is a new piece of paper and a new drop of ink, this creates no harm, it cannot be tolerated for the brain. There is now way in which new units could inherit structure from the sets of units they are to represent and from other patterns with which those sets overlap - all their connections must be specified from scratch. Moreoever, there are terrible administrative problems with the actuation of new units. When is it time to create a new unit: when a new pattern appears for the first time? If not, how does one keep track of multiple occurrences before having a unit dedicated? How does one select a candidate unit which happens to have appropriate anatomical connections and which is not yet dedicated? When will one liberate units standing for ephemeral patterns? All of these problems could be avoided if patterns were represented by those units of which they are composed.

(**A basis for organization!**) The assembly framework starts with a very simple principle of organization, synaptic plasticity. Certain steps of organization have been successfully described on that basis, among them the formation of feature-representing cells and the formation of interconnection patterns to store and stabilize assemblies. However, the assembly as a symbol of the mind forces one to assume operations and interconnection patterns which are so peculiar that it is difficult to imagine the form of their ontogenetic organization, to say the least.

For all these reasons the classical assembly theory does not deserve the status of a comprehensive framework for a theory of brain function; it cannot be accepted as a description of the physical basis of mind.

NATURAL REPRESENTATION

My criticism of the assembly framework raised above would be incomprehensible if it was not complemented by some constructive response. I therefore present here a concise description of a different theoretical framework which has been described in more detail elsewhere (3, 21-24).

The physical world is hierarchically structured into objects, their arrangements, and their parts. There is no need for an object to be represented by a new type of cardinal unit. A coherent object is simply formed by cohesively binding its constituent elements (crystallites, molecules, atoms, elementary particles). The interaction between objects is not mediated by representatives. In fact, it takes place as a direct interaction between the constituents. Correspondingly one could think of a symbol system in which a pattern formed by a set of elementary symbols is represented collectively by just those elementary symbols! Let me call this a *natural representation*. High-level symbols in such a system are large structured sets of elementary symbols; interactions between high-level symbols result from the combination of interactions between "atoms." In order for such a system to work one has to introduce degrees of freedom and interactions which allow the atoms to bind to each other in a flexible way. Both the physical world and the systems of visual communication use spatial degrees of freedom to bind elements and form aggregates. If in the brain atoms are to be identified with nerve cells, spatial degrees of freedom cannot be used since nerve cells are immobile.

Temporal Correlations

Time is divided into two scales: a *psychological time scale* (some tenths of a second), which is characteristic of mental processes, and a *fast time scale* (some thousandths of a second). Mean unit activity evolves on the psychological time scale but the activity fluctuates around this mean on the fast temporal scale. Units bind to each other by correlating their activity fluctuations. A set of units can be bound into a block by synchronizing their fast activity fluctuations. Several such blocks can coexist if their activity is desynchronized relative to each other: this is the solution to the superposition catastrophe. (Legéndy has already mentioned temporal relations as a solution to the syntax problem (13).)

Fluctuations are the expression of an intrinsic instability of units. Correlations naturally arise in sets of units which receive excitation from a common origin or which are synaptically coupled. (Processing of correlations in nervous networks has been discussed before by Sejnowski (16).) The useless and trivial state of global correlation is suppressed by an inhibitory system.

As we know, correlations have important consequences for the activation of nerve cells: neurons are coincidence detectors! If two units are desynchronized with each other they cannot cooperate to excite a third unit. If they are synchronized, they can.

Dynamical Connections

Modulating connections. Correlations are shaped by connections. If correlations are to represent variable bindings, connection strengths must vary. This function is called synaptic modulation. Correlation between two units increases the strength of an excitatory connection between them up to a maximum strength which is characteristic of the connection. (The set of maximum strengths for all connections defines the "permanent" network.) Anticorrelation between two units decreases the strength of an excitatory connection between them down to the value zero. These changes take place on the psychological time scale. If there are no signals in the two units the connection slowly relaxes, within times characteristic of short-term memory, to a resting state in which it conducts with a constant fraction of its maximum strength. (A different system for reducing the physical network to a sparse "skeleton" has been described by Sejnowski (16).)

Meta-interactions. Connections interact with themselves and with each other. A connection self-reinforces: the existence of an excitatory connection leads to correlation, which in turn strengthens the connection. Connections cooperate: connections between the same source and the same target help each other to synchronize the source with the target and consequently help each other to grow if they do not differ too much in length (number of intermediary units). Connections compete with each other as far as they run against the boundary condition of excluded global synchrony. Thus there exists a system of meta-interactions, to which was alluded in the section *Interference by irrelevant connections*.

Logogenesis
Assembly theory has to work with very restricted permanent connectivity patterns in order to avoid confusion (e.g., patterns are allowed to converse with each other only through their cardinal units). These restricted connectivity patterns have to be formed during ontogenesis or even during phylogenesis. With natural representation, highly specific connection patterns are formed on the fast psychological timescale. Two constraints contribute to the specificity of those connection patterns: the structure of the permanent network and the rules of the pattern formation process described in the previous section. In the context of the present paper the term "logogenesis" will be used for this fast process to emphasize its similarity with the processes of phylogenesis and ontogenesis. All three are evolution processes involving natural selection from a large repertoire created by random fluctuations. The criterion for selection during logogenesis is described next.

Connection patterns are distinguished by sparsity of activated connections (due to the competition between connections) and optimal cooperation between the surviving connections. Simulation studies (3, 23, 24) suggest that connection patterns have topological structure, i.e., they can be decomposed into many "neighborhoods" of directly coupled units which are sometimes coupled by long indirect pathways. (In a random graph any two units have fairly direct connections.)

Projections between patterns. Topological connection patterns can be combined, by sparse projections, to form larger topological connection patterns. Thus, rich hierarchies of symbols can be formed. An important, special case is constituted by homeomorphic projections in which two connection patterns of equal inner structure are joined together by a neighborhood-preserving projection of connections between corresponding units, thus forming a larger connection pattern. Homeomorphic projections between patterns replace the association of representative units in assembly theory.

Restrictions imposed by permanent connectivity. Connection pattern formation is a highly spontaneous process. This process is influenced by the memory inherent in the structure of the permanent network which systematically favors certain connection patterns. In an extreme case the permanent network among a given set of units has itself the structure of a connection pattern. In a less radical extreme case, corresponding to the classical associative memory, the permanent network is a superposition of connection patterns. In order to represent particular situations connectivity dynamics then has to reduce the superposition and recover one of the stored patterns. Unit-wise overlap between the stored patterns does not lead to confusion. In the extreme case several connection patterns coexist on an identical support of units and can still be selectively activated (this process has been simulated (23)). In general, permanent connectivity just imposes certain "grammatical" rules on the form of possible connection patterns, leaving great freedom to the patterns formed.

The evaluation of correlations. What are the dynamical consequences of the correlation structure of the signals emitted by a given set a of units? Suppose the set of units has permanent sparse projections to a number of other sets of units. Set a can excite activity in one of the other sets only if the correlation pattern on a fits the structure of connections in that other set, because only then can the individual signals sent by a cooperate with the help of inner connections in the other set. In addition, the signals coming from a select that connection pattern on the other set of units which fits the connection pattern in a. Different correlation structures in a thus establish "resonance" with (and arouse activity in) different sets of units.

Ontogenesis

Plasticity increases the "permanent" strength of those connections which are strongly activated. (In addition, it is probably necessary to require that new connections be formed between cellular processes over small distances for cells which are stronlgy correlated.) A compensating process must decrease connections (and finally break them) under appropriate conditions.

This type of plasticity is far from being an indiscriminate stickiness because two units are permanently connected only after having been bound to each other in a connection pattern. In other words, a new connection is stored only if stabilized and validated by existing indirect connections: already in a single situation it can be decided by logogeny whether a particular connection fits the context. In comparison to the assembly framework, slow ontogeny has to carry a much lower organizational burden.

Semantics

Atoms plus relations. A sentence cannot be described by an unstructured sum of the symbolic meanings of its letters (or even of its words). The order of the elements establishes relations. These relations are as much carriers of meaning as the elements. (Any long message has a standard distribution of letter frequencies so that information is contained *exclusively* in the system of neighborhood relationships!) Natural representation, i.e., the representation of a pattern by its elements, is possible only if relations of the elements within the pattern are represented as well. In the system discussed here for the brain, the general type of relationship can be interpreted as common membership in synchronously firing subsets (where the subsets firing at different times can overlap). If the whole pattern is the visual description of a scene, and units represent local visual features, relations bind those features to each other which apply to the same object, to the same part of an object, or to a local neighborhood, in increasing order of correlation strength. (If the individual feature units are not specific as to retinal position, the patterns of activity and relations among the units are then position-invariant representatives of visual patterns (24).) If the whole pattern is a linguistic structure, units may represent phonemes or morphemes and grammatical roles, and relations bind the phonemes or morphemes into higher units, attach grammatical roles to them, and assemble those elements into phrases and sentences. Any mental symbol can be further specified by attaching modifying symbols to it. This attachment has to be made precise by specifying to which part of the symbol each modifier applies. The mental symbols which constitute our thoughts are huge systems of cross-referenced active units, all having vague meaning by themselves, creating precision only in their structured ensemble.

Symbols to whom? The symbols of communication are sent by one individual and received by others. Who is the recipient of mental symbols? Let us leave aside the behaviorist answer according to which the only recipient would be the motor output, i.e., those subsysymbols which form in the motor modality of the brain. Instead we have to ask, who is the subject of perception and how is the unity of perception established in the brain? It is an ineradicable misconception that the unity of perception has to be established in a separate center which, in addition, is often imagined as being of structureless unity itself. This mental archetype leads to infinite regress and absurdity. Instead, the unity of mind has to be seen as an organic equilibrium among a great multitude of elements. The mental symbols both send and receive at the same time. Signals sent by one subsymbol are deciphered by other subsymbols and the sending symbol can in turn only establish itself, momentarily, if it responds to the messages and questions sent by others. In the state of unity each subsymbol encodes in its own terms the situation described by the others. This unity is not reached by *leaving out* detail but by *uniting* all detail with the help of relations.

CONSEQUENCES REGARDING THE FORM OF SYNAPTIC PLASTICITY

What is the upshot of all of this for synaptic plasticity? Let us imagine that we were able to induce tissue cultures of the relevant types of neurons to form isolated pairs of cells with a direct synaptic link. Let us imagine further that we were able to contact both cells with intracellular electrodes so that we could record from them, influence their membrane potential, or apply specific drugs to their interior. We then could measure the postsynaptic conductance change induced in one of the cells by a spike triggered in the other cell, thereby measuring the weight of the synaptic connection. What changes in this weight could we expect to happen in response to which signals in the two neurons?

Global Control

The whole purpose of synaptic plasticity is growth of those connection patterns which are successful. Success can be measured on two levels, on a global and on a local one. The global level concerns the teleonomic value of recent action for the animal. It can be evaluated by central structures, and plastic changes can be gated accordingly. Such gating systems appear to be implemented with the help of central nuclei and extensive fiber systems which are able to distribute appropriate transmitters to specific sites, to large regions, or to the entire brain (2).

Local Control

Such global decisions are necessary to impart specific, biologically useful directions to the development of the brain. However, it is not possible to optimize billions of variables with the help of global signals. There must be a local criterion of success which can be evaluated in many places simultaneously. The general type of success criterion for synaptic configurations is the degree of cooperativity, or consistency, between different connections (where causal interactions in the external world may be counted as a special kind of connection). Synapses are consistent with each other if there is synergy between the effects relayed by their signals, i.e., if they exert the same type of influence (excitatory or inhibitory) on the same target (e.g., the same postsynaptic cell) at the same time. Hebb plasticity and synaptic modulation, as proposed here, are specific realizations of this local control scheme.

This general scheme leaves open a number of questions: What is the temporal resolution with which coincidences are measured? What is the necessary coincidence order, i.e., how many fibers must be coactive? What is the postsynaptic integration unit: an entire neuron, an entire dendrite, or a dendritic patch? What is the nature of the signal by which one synapse learns of the synergy with others, e.g., postsynaptic membrane potential, the concentration of Ca^{2+} or of another second messenger in the postsynaptic medium (or even some signal exchanged on the presynaptic side)? What is the time course with which plastic changes become effective in a synapse? Finally, what is the nature and form of the mechanism by which the instability inherent in synaptic plasticity is finally checked: conservation of total presynaptic weight (for which integration unit?), homeostasy of mean postsynaptic activity?

Experimental Predictions

Ultimate answers to these questions must come from experiments. Such experiments should be conducted under conditions in which all relevant signals can be controlled, i.e., in a culture dish or perhaps in a tissue slice. It may be useful to list some predictions which flow from the considerations presented in this paper:

Synaptic plasticity is (at least) at two-step process. Rapid synaptic changes which become effective in fractions of a second are transferred into permanent changes, probably under control of central gating signals.

The rapid changes (synaptic modulation) increase or decrease PSP size by considerable factors. Coincidences increase PSP size, anticoincidences decrease it.

Coincidences are measured with a high temporal resolution. This is measured in milliseconds or in tens of milliseconds (rather than the hundreds of milliseconds suggested by the assembly concept).

Coincidences must be of high order. High order may mean five or eight action potentials which must arrive simultaneously at the same target. Low order (especially binary) coincidences are drowned in noise. There may be complicated trade-offs between coincidence time, coincidence order, and size of the integrative unit.

Acknowledgement. I would like to thank E. Bienenstock, G. Toulouse, J.-P. Changeux, and S.-I. Amari for important and very helpful remarks on an earlier version of this paper. A large part of this material is already contained in the article "Am I thinking assemblies?" by the same author, which appeared in "Brain Theory," eds. G. Palm and A. Aertsen (1986), pp. 161-176. Permission by Springer-Verlag, Heidelberg.

REFERENCES

(1) Bartlett, F.C. 1932. Remembering. Cambridge: Cambridge University Press.

(2) Bear, M.F., and Singer, W. 1986. Acetylcholine, noradrenaline and the extrathalamic modulation of visual cortical plasticity. *Nature*, in press.

(3) Bienenstock, E. 1986. Dynamics of central nervous system. *Proceedings of the Workshop on Dynamics of Macrosystems*, IIASA Laxenburg, Sept. 1984, eds. J.P. Aubin and K. Sigmund. Berlin, Heidelberg, New York, Toyko: Springer-Verlag, in press.

(4) Cohen, N.J., and Squire, L.R. 1980. Preserved learning and retention of pattern analyzing skill in amnesia: dissociation of knowing how and knowing that. *Science* 210: 207-209.

(5) Cooper, L.N. 1973. A possible organization of animal memory and learning. In *Collective Properties of Physical Systems*, Proceedings of the Twenty-Fourth Nobel Symposium, eds. B. Lundqvist and S. Lundqvist, pp. 252-264. New York: Academic Press.

(6) Crick, F. 1984. Function of the thalamic reticular complex: the searchlight hypothesis. *Proc. Natl. Acad. Sci.* 81: 4568-4590.

(7) Fukushima, K., and Miyake, S. 1982. Neocognitron: a new algorithm for pattern recognition tolerant of deformations and shifts in position. *Patt. Recog.* 15: 455-469.

(8) Hayek, F.A. 1952. The Sensory Order. An Inquiry into the Foundations of Theoretical Psychology. Chicago: University of Chicago Press.

(9) Hebb, D.O. 1949. The Organization of Behaviour. A Neuropsychological Theory. New York: Wiley.

(10) Hopfield, J.J. 1982. Neural networks and physical systems with emergent collective computational abilities. *Proc. Natl. Acad. Sci.* 79: 2554-2558.

(11) Julesz, B. 1981. Textons, the elements of texture perception, and their interactions. *Nature* 290: 91-97.

(12) Kohonen, T. 1977. Associative Memory. Berlin, Heidelberg, New York, Tokyo: Springer-Verlag.

(13) Legéndy, C.R. 1970. The brain and its information trapping device. In *Progress in Cybernetics*, ed. J. Rose, vol. 1, pp. 309-338. New York: Gordon and Breach.

(14) Marko, H., and Giebel, H. 1970. Recognition of handwritten characters with a system of homogeneous layers. *Nachrichtentec. Z. Heft* 9: 455-459.

(15) Rosenblatt, F. 1961. Principles of Neurodynamics: Perceptrons and the Theory of Brain Mechanism. Washington: Spartan Books.

(16) Sejnowski, T.J. 1981. Skeleton filters in the brain. In *Parallel Models of Associative Memory*, eds. G.E. Hinton and J.A. Anderson, pp. 189-212. Hillsdale, NJ: Lawrence Erlbaum.

(17) Sejowski, T.J., and Hinton, G.E. 1985. Separating figure from ground with a Boltzmann machine. In *Vision, Brain and Cooperative Computation*, eds. M.A. Arbib and A.R. Hanson, Cambridge: MIT Press.

(18) Steinbuch, K. 1961. Die Lernmatrix. *Kybernetik* 1: 36-45.

(19) Toulouse, G.; Dehaene, S.; and Changeux, J.-P. 1986. A spin glass model of learning by selection. *Proc. Natl. Acad. Sci.*, submitted.

(20) Treisman, A., and Gelade, G. 1980. A feature integration theory of attention. *Cog. Psych.* 12: 97-136.

(21) von der Malsburg, C. 1981. The correlation theory of brain function. *Internal Report 81-2*, Dept. Neurobiol., Max-Planck-Institute for Biophysical Chemistry, P.O. Box 2841, Göttingen, F.R. Germany.

(22) von der Malsburg, C. 1985. Algorithms, brain and organization. In *Dynamical Systems and Cellular Automata*, eds. J. Demongeot, E. Golès and M. Tchuente, pp. 235-246. London: Academic Press.

(23) von der Malsburg, C. 1985. Nervous structures with dynamical links. Berichte Bunsenges. *Phys. Chem.* 89: 703-710.

(24) von der Malsburg, C., and Bienenstock, E. 1986. Statistical coding and short-term synaptic plasticity: a scheme for knowledge representation in the brain. In *Disordered Systems and Biological Organization. Proceedings*. Les Houches, Feb. 1985, eds. E. Bienenstock, F. Fogelman, and G. Weisbuch, pp. 249-272. Berlin, Heidelberg, New York, Toyko: Springer-Verlag.

(25) Willshaw, D.J. 1972. A simple network capable of inductive generalization. *P. Roy. Soc. Lon. B* 182: 233-247.

The Neural and Molecular Bases of Learning,
eds. J.-P. Changeux and M. Konishi, pp. 433–472.
John Wiley & Sons Limited.

Plasticity in Neuronal Circuits and Assemblies of Invertebrates

R. Menzel and G. Bicker

Institut für Tierphysiologie, Neurobiologie
Freie Universität Berlin
1000 Berlin (West) 33

Abstract. Invertebrate neuronal circuits are composed of identifiable neurons which interact to process sensory information and generate motor programs. Electrical signalling in neuronal circuits depends on the history of previous use and on concomitant activity in extrinsic neuronal pathways. Changes in synaptic transmission intrinsic to circuits account for behavioral phenomena such as habituation. Modification of synaptic transmission by extrinsic pathways uses different mechanisms ranging from presynaptic inhibition of a specific synapse to the release of neuromodulatory substances which modify a whole array of cells depending on receptor specificity for the modulator. At various levels of the nervous system, neuromodulators coordinate and integrate components of motor programs into meaningful behavior. In some instances release of neuromodulatory substances can even trigger whole behavioral sequences. Animals which have to process, learn, and memorize a wealth of complex stimuli use assemblies composed of neuronal circuits. Information processing in neuronal assemblies is poorly understood but is probably an extension of the principles operating in neuronal circuits. Invertebrates may offer advantageous preparations to study assemblies because neural activity in assemblies is integrated by accessible identified neurons which convey the output to segmental ganglia or to neuropils of the brain.

INTRODUCTION

All animals have to adapt to changing environmental and internal conditions. Thus the properties of behavioral plasticity should be shared by nervous systems all the way from lower invertebrates to the higher evolved invertebrate and vertebrate phyla. Adaptive changes occur at all levels of neuronal complexity and it is a topic of current research whether adaptations on molecular, cellular, and circuit levels are homologous in animal species phylogenetically as distant as worms and mammals. Many invertebrates provide less complex nervous systems and technically accessible neurons, a fact which allows assignation of adaptive behaviors to synaptic changes within a neuronal circuit of known connectivity. Our review will first illustrate how changes in transmission of known synapses affect flexibility in those behaviors, which at first glance are often thought to represent rather stereotyped routines. We then will move on to look into the neural basis of changes of more complex behavior. Insects, in particular, display a rich behavioral repertoire including complex sensory processing and motor control, a variety of forms of learning, lifelong memory, and behavior which suggests "mental images."

Variable and complex behavior requires nervous systems which combine circuits into (large) communities of circuits. Since the combination of circuits into functional neural communities is a dynamic process depending on stimulus combinations, behavioral status of the whole animal, epigenetic programming, and individual history, we might call the set of all participating cells a neural assembly. Hebb (39) envisaged cell assemblies in the brain as dynamic combinations of well-defined local circuits which "can act briefly as a closed system" and "constitute the simplest instance of a representative process (image or idea)." Neither the single synapse, the single neuron, nor the local circuit are considered to be relevant units in terms of behavioral (and cognitive) structure but rather the flexible compound of many circuits into "assemblies." Plasticity of the nervous system, though based on molecular and cellular switches, is thus thought to be represented in the flexibility of cell assemblies.

We shall use the term "neural assembly" in a somewhat broader sense than Hebb, defining assemblies as coactive cells which are put together by learning and which essentially represent the "engram" or a stored representation of past experience. We would like to include the "epigenetic engram" and view the neural assembly as a group of cells which join together at a certain time to serve a particular behavior. In accordance with our colleagues, who study the large vertebrate brains, we expect to find self-organizing and self-instructing properties from the assembly which lead to the preference of certain activity stages. In extreme cases there may be very few activity stages (e.g., in small ganglia), but the large amount of behavioral patterns of highly evolved arthropods, such as the social insects, suggests many activity stages of assemblies and their combinations. The concept of neural assembly has been productive in contrast to Lashley's (73) view of brain function because it opened the experimental approach to the cellular elements. However, very little is known about the properties of these assemblies. Here again the work with invertebrates might be particularly promising because the small number of neurons favors an economy of the nervous system to an extent that even single neurons or small sets of neurons control complete behavioral (and sensory integrative) subroutines and the behavioral repertoire is strongly controlled by innate, hard-wired circuits. Plasticity of synapses and circuits appears, therefore, as a particular property on the backbone of stereotyped and rigid wiring. We will discuss examples of innate, hard-wired circuits capable of changing synaptic transmission by intrinsic as well as neuromodulatory extrinsic mechansisms and, finally, we will describe some associative learning phenomena in circuits and assemblies. Three invertebrate favorites for a molecular approach to learning, *Aplysia*, *Hermissenda*, and *Drosophila*, have already been extensively reviewed and will be referenced in a somewhat different context.

NONASSOCIATIVE PLASTICITY

Plasticity in the Crayfish's Tail Flip

Activity in single interneurons can initiate complete behavioral acts in several invertebrate species. The earliest and probably most extreme example of this rather straightforward organization of motor control was discovered in 1938 by Wiersma in the crayfish nervous system (127). A single electrical shock applied to one of the four giant fibers of the ventral nerve chord triggers a complete escape response which consists of appropriate positioning of various body appendages and a fast flexion and extension of the abdomen, the tail flip. The description of other neurons that could elicit rhythmic beating of the swimmerets introduced the term "command neuron" into the literature (128). Crayfish evade noxious stimuli in at least three different types of escape responses (72, 132) which partly involve different but overlapping circuits. The responses that Wiersma studied are mediated by the medial and lateral giant command fibers. Visual or sudden tactile stimuli delivered to the frontal part of the animal cause firing of the medial giants which command a flexion that moves the animal backwards away form the stimulus. Caudally applied tactile stimuli can initiate an action potential in the two lateral giant fibers resulting in a tail flip that pitches the animal up and forward. All repetitive sequences of tail flips during centrally patterned swimming episodes that follow the initial flip are mediated by nongiant circuits.

The neural pathways of the nongiant circuitry are almost unknown but the organization of the giant-mediated circuits is well established (see Fig. 1). In fact, the lateral giant-mediated escape response represents, in neural terms, the best understood escape behavior in the animal kingdom. We will now focus on the inital giant-mediated tail flip which is the first unit of a behavior sequence that comprises the whole escape response (131). Abdominal tactile afferents (TA) connect to the lateral giants either directly or via a group of 60 sensory interneurons (SI). The excitatory monosynaptic pathway from the primary sensory afferents is rather weak, whereas the sensory interneurons provide the major path of excitation to the lateral giant fibers. The excitation is conveyed via electrical synapses to the two lateral giants which function as a single unit because they are electrically coupled. The lateral giants have divergent connections to a giant motor neuron (MoG), via a driver neuron (SG), and to a group of fast flexor motor neurons (FF) which in turn exite phasic flexor muscles (110).

The lateral giant command neuron is embedded between the convergent sensory and divergent motor pathways. It decides whether a tail flip will occur and it organizes the exact movement during the flip. The *decision process* is a simple *threshold mechanism* for eliciting a single-action potential in the lateral giant fiber while the performance of the flip is shaped by means of the connections to driver and motor neurons in the abdominal segments. Repeated stimulation leads to habituation of giant as well as nongiant-mediated escape behavior. Up to ten elicitations of the lateral giant-mediated tail flip cause a reflex failure in most animals (69). Recovery is slow and requires more than eight hours to reach a 60% level. In an isolated abdomen preparation, repetitive stimulation of the afferents causes a decrease of the compound EPSP in the lateral giant whereas prolonged stimulation of the command neuron is always accompanied by a tail flip (66). The work of Zucker (136, 137) established that depression in synaptic transmission between tactile afferents and sensory interneurons can account for the habituation. The tactile sensory neurons do not adapt to repeated stimuli but the decrease of the EPSP in the lateral giants is paralleled by a decline in the chemically mediated EPSP in the presynaptic sensory interneurons. No change in the membrane properties of neurons postsynaptic to the site of habituation could be found, and Zucker (137) suggested that repeated stimulation of the sensory neuron to

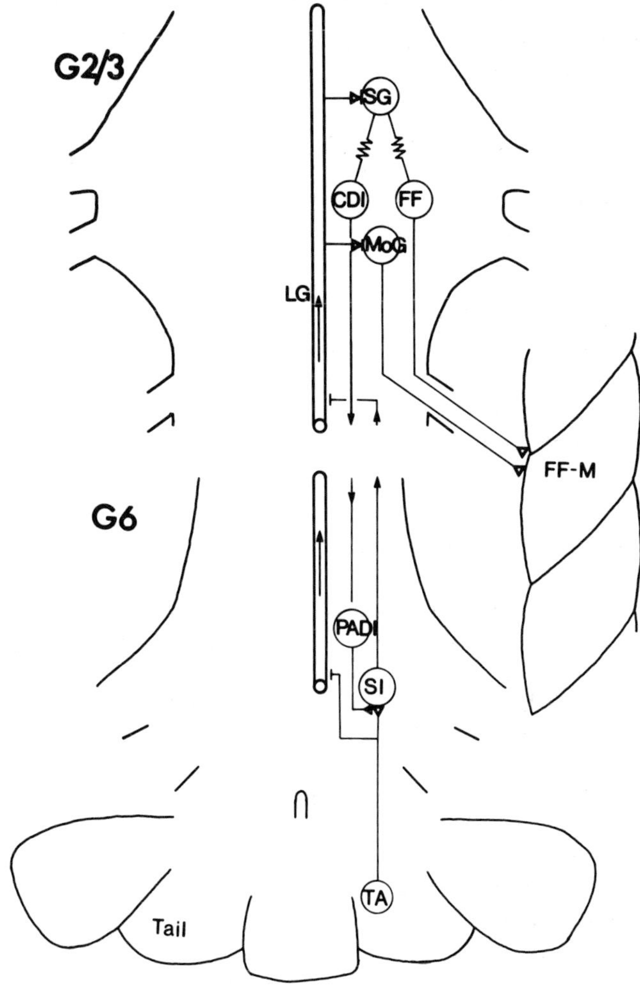

FIG. 1 – Some pathways of the lateral giant-mediated tail flip circuitry of the crayfish (see text for references). G 2/3, G 6: abdominal ganglion 2 or 3 and 6; LG: lateral giant interneuron; SG: driver neuron; CDI: corollary discharge interneurons; MoG: giant motor neuron; FF: fast flexor motor neurons; FF-M: fast flexor muscles; PADI: primary afferents depolarizing interneurons; SI: sensory interneurons; TA: tactile afferents; ⊣ : electrical synapse; →| : rectifying electrical synapse; ▲ : inhibitory synapses; △ : excitatory synapses.

interneuron synapse causes a decrease in the number of transmitter quanta released by each action potential. The locus for this homosynaptic depression which underlies the habituation is thus thought to be presynaptic. A similar result has been obtained for the gill withdrawal reflex in *Aplysia*. The short-term habituation of this graded reflex, as was shown by quantal analysis (12), is accompanied by a decrease in the number of transmitter quanta released by the sensory neurons onto motor neurons.

Thus, the graded gill withdrawal reflex and an all-or-none fixed act, the tail flip, share a common locus and mechanism for habituation. Escape behavior underlies strong selection pressure and it is not unreasonable to assume that mechanisms discovered in the crayfish's tail flip are applicable to other animals as well. A giant interneuron system between abdominal ganglion and thoracic ganglia mediates escape to wind puffs applied to the cerci of the cockroach (11, 59, 111). Repeated cercal stimulation leads again to depression at the chemical synapse between sensory and giant neurons.

The ability to ignore repetitive noxious stimuli helps the crayfish avoid energy-consuming escape maneuvers. The actual performance of swimming or other tail movements could cause a dangerous self-produced habituation of the tail flip response because the tactile afferents are massively stimulated during these movements. However, the synapse between sensory afferents and interneurons (see Fig. 1) is protected from habituation during tail movements by presynaptic inhibition (61, 68) which is effected by a population of PADI (62). A piece of control circuitry is set aside to modulate plasticity inherent in a neural pathway (67). Every tail flip is accompanied by a corollary discharge in this control circuitry (CDI, corollary discharge interneurons) which protects the escape response from self-induced habituation. This is accomplished, without any changes in the excitability of the escape pathways as a whole, by means of strategic presynaptic inhibition of the first labile synapse in the pathway.

Mechanisms of Locust Jump

Most behavioral responses to the same stimulus are variable depending on a manifold of internal and external factors which influence the behavior of an animal. This section will treat the question of how information about certain novel, visual stimuli is channeled to a particular motor pattern, the jump circuitry of the locust, and will outline some neuronal mechanisms which render jumping behavior labile. This information processing task involves the dioptric apparatus of the compound eyes, three optic ganglia, descending neurons in the ventral nerve chord as the connection between brain and thoracic ganglia, and some circuitry in the metathoracic ganglion. Thus, the locust will serve as an example of how, at various well-defined stages in the nervous system, synaptic transmission is influenced according to the needs of the animal and how several mechanisms are responsible for synaptic plasticity. The locust possesses a pair of large interneurons that can be readily recorded from within the ventral nerve chord. This descending contralateral movement detector (DCMD) responds to the movement of small objects in the visual field of the contralateral eye. The integrative properties of the DCMD and its presynaptic circuitry have been subject to a number of reviews (99, 112). Here we will mainly focus on the plastic properties of the circuitry.

The DCMD receives its visual input via chemical transmission from the lobula giant movement detector (LGMD; see Fig. 2) (109). The dendrites of the LGMD arborize in a fan-like manner across the third optic ganglion and the axon projects within the protocerebrum onto dendrites of the DCMD. The DCMD neuron functions mainly as relay between head and thorax because spikes in the LGMD are usually followed by DCMD spikes in a one-to-one relationship. The axon of the DCMD crosses in the brain to the contralateral side and conducts the spike down the ventral nerve chord to its main output targets in the metathoracic ganglion. The dendritic subfields of the LGMD integrate retinotopic as well as nonretinotopic output channels of the optic ganglia. The LGMD serves as an excellent example of how an identified neuron integrates neural activity concerning a certain aspect of visual stimulation. Thousands of afferent retinotopic on and off units are thought to converge onto the field A of the LGMD that form excitator chemical synapses which are subject to habituation (97, 98). The afferents are protected by a lateral inhibitory network (LI) from responding to stationary large field stimuli. Additional feed-forward inhibition (FFI) mediated by nonhabituating pathways in a nonretinotopic fashion blanks transient large-field stimuli. Thus the system is sensitive to small, novel stimuli moving within the whole visual field of one eye. When stimuli are repeatedly applied to the same area of the eye the movement detection system habituates. Habituation is localized because a shift of the stimulus over as little as one interommatidial distance causes recovery. This indicates that the decremental process lies in the periphery prior to the convergence of the retinotopic input onto the LGMD. Electric stimulation experiments in the second optic chiasma revealed that decrementing EPSPs in the fan dendrite of the LGMD can account for the habituation. No conductance or spike threshold changes were recorded in the LGMD. Thus it is likely that a process in the synaptic terminals of the excitatory afferents to the LGMD is responsible for the site-specific response decrement in the movement detection system. Various stimulus modalities can arouse locusts and dishabituate the movement detection system. Dishabituation is not site-specific, affects the whole visual field, and is likely to operate presynaptically to the LGMD because no accompanying electrophysiological events can be recorded in the dendrite during dishabituation.

How does the locust solve the problem of protecting the sensory system from habituation due to its own movements? Repeated small field movements rapidly habituate the movement detection system whereas large field movements do not depress the responsiveness to small field stimuli. This property of the movement detection system is largely due to lateral inhibition which prevents the response to large field stimuli. The distal-positioned lateral inhibitory network protects the labile synapses which connect to the LGMD from habituation (97). A novel function besides contrast enhancement or preference for small field stimuli is thus ascribed to lateral inhibition. An additional mechansism that prevents the locust from confusing self-generated with external movements operates during rapid head movements. Voluntary or optokinetically induced saccades cause inhibition of the DCMD response (134). A command to turn the head is sufficient to cause the inhibition. Experiments performed on animals with cut neck muscles showed that the inhibition can not be explained by proprioceptive feedback but that a corollary discharge mechanism has to be assumed. Once electrical impulses have struggled through the jungle of lateral inhibitory connections, labile synapses, and FFI in the movement detection system, they are then transmitted via a strong chemical synapse between LGMD and DCMD (see Fig. 2). Early work (10) suggested that the DCMD is in some way involved in the escape jump of the locust because it connects weakly to the already defined FETi in the metathoracic ganglion which excites the extensor tibiae muscles of the hind legs. These muscles are exclusively used in jumps and kicks. Before we describe the jumping circuitry we will briefly describe the motor program for the jump (42-44).

In the initial cocking phase both hind leg tibiae are rapidly flexed and locked in parallel aginst the femur. During the co-contraction phase the antagonistic flexors and extensors counteract each other which results

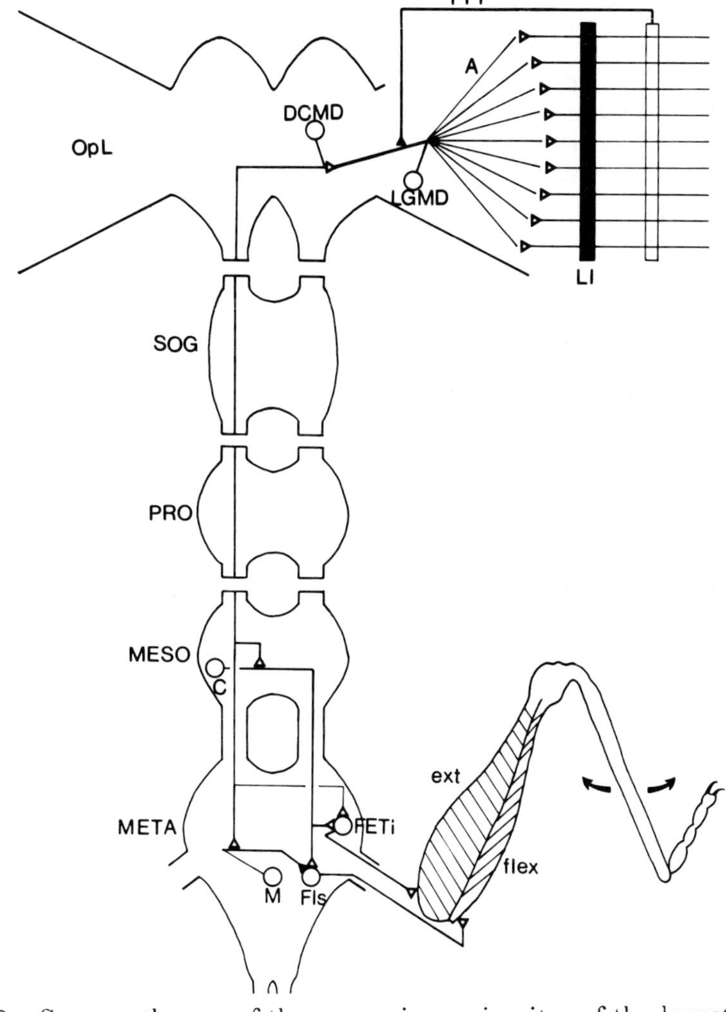

FIG. 2 – Some pathways of the escape jump circuitry of the locust (see text for references). LGMD: lobula giant movement detector with dentritic subfield A; DCMD: descending contralateral movement detector; FFI: neurons mediating feed-forward inhibition; LI: lateral inhibitory network; C: coactivating interneuron to FETi (fast extensor tibiae motoneurons) and FLs (flexor tibiae motoneurons); M: multimodal interneuron; OpL: optic lobe; SOG: subesophageal ganglion, PRO, MESO, META: pro-, meso-, and metathoracic ganglion; △ : excitatory synapses; ▲ : inhibitatory synapses.

in a flexed position of the tibia. The purpose of co-contraction is to store elastic energy in cuticle spring deformation by a slow isometric contraction of extensor and flexor muscles in the femur which counteract each other (4). The jump is finally released by a sudden inhibition of flexor activity which allows rapid contraction of the extensors and the release of stored elastic energy. The extension of both hind tibiae pitches the locust into the air. The jump and defensive kick of the hind legs share a motor program with the same three essential phases (104). This enables probing of the jumping circuitry with intracellular electrodes while the locust preparation actually tries to defend itself with kicks. An interneuron (103) was discovered in the meso- and metathoracic ganglion which can simultaneously coactivate the FETi and Fls by means of strong excitatatory monosynaptic connections. This C-neuron is perfectly suited for producing the cocking phase. It receives large EPSPs from DCMD and is also excited by hissing sounds and tactile stimulation of the abdomen, all stimuli which lead to cocking in aroused animals. The amplitude of the EPSP that C produced in FETi depends on the position of the tibia, being largest when the tibia is already in close apposition to the femur. A simultaneous activation of the antagonistic muscles in extended hind legs would lead, due to mechanical reasons, to tibial extension rather than the required tibial flexion.

After a phasic signal from the C-neurons has coactivated the antagonistic muscles, the co-contraction phase is maintained by positive feedback pathways from mechanorecptors in the leg, which re-excite flexor and extensor motoneurons, and excitatory pathways from extensor to flexor motoneurons. Since peripheral circuits are sufficient to maintain co-contraction, central pathways can now focus their attention on the final trigger phase. An important interneuron of this circuitry is the multimodal M-neuron (see Fig. 2) whose branches are mainly confined within the metathoracic ganglion. Excitatory input from visual, auditory, tactile, and proprioceptive sensory systems are integrated by M which links in a disynaptic pathway DCMD with hind leg flexor motoneurons (101). M receives a strong monosynaptic EPSP from DCMD and in turn inhibits the hind leg flexor motoneurons. During the triggering phase of a defensive kick a high frequency burst appears in M (122) which precedes the sudden inhibition of flexor activity. Thus, M is possibly the last neural element to take part in the decision whether the locust will jump. Several mechanisms ensure that M does not inhibit the flexors inadvertently. The high threshold for spike initiation lies between 12 to 15 mV above resting potential which prevents weak sensory input from activating M when the animal is not prepared to jump. The strong excitatory pathway from DCMD to M underlies a presynaptic inhibition mechanism which is probably due to an increased chloride conductance produced by depolarization of the presynaptic terminals (100). This leads to a reduction in amplitude of DCMD spikes and eventually to nonlinear summation of EPSPs in M.

A final feature of the whole circuit was discovered by Heitler (41). Similar to the suppression that DCMD undergoes during saccadic head movement (134), it is also suppressed during defensive kicks in restrained animals. Whether the suppression also occurs during the jumping motor program involving both hind legs is unknown. If this is the case one becomes skeptical as to whether DCMD can actually trigger the flexor inhibition during the last phase of the jump. Several possibilities have been discussed (41), one of which explains suppression as serving a sensory filtering function. Since DCMD performs a dual role, initial excitation of C and the excitation of M, the production of the cocking response should have a lower threshold. Thus the suppression may raise the threshold for the activation of M and prevent weak stimuli from triggering the jump.

Once the locust is in the air things run smoothly. Already during tibial extension a central program triggers a set of neurons that initiate the central oscillation which is responsible for the wingbeat (102, 130). The pattern of activity across these neurons may determine the direction of the initial flight trajectory. A second peripheral mechanism, driven by the windstream on the head, backs the central mechanism (5) during take off. Finally, reesponsibility is handed over to the autopilot in the cockpit. It consists of a population of descending interneurons which are sensitive to the position of the horizon and the wind direction (108). These interneurons which project from the brain to the thoracic ganglia serve as course deviation detectors. A gating process in the thoracic ganglia translates their deviation signals into correctional steering commands (107). It is evident that the story we have told does not account for all aspects of variability in the described circuits. The role of M during co-contraction is presently being reinvestigated (Pearson, personal communication), and DCMD may be facultatively turned off whenever the locust "thinks" it is appropriate (113). Thus the nervous system may generate time windows for the responsiveness of its decision neurons, a mechanism that makes it difficult for the experimenter who works with a more or less restrained preparation.

Labile Behavior in Crayfish and Locust Allows some Conclusions

Decisions to perform rapid escape behavior are based on activity in single identifiable cells. These decision elements integrate convergent sensory input and channel the resulting signals to appropriate motor circuits. Simple threshold mechanisms in these identifiable cells explain the decision process. The decision elements monitor proprioceptive input which raises or lowers the firing threshold. Proprioceptive gating processes partly account for the lability of behavior. A simple form of plasticity, habituation, is explained by depression of synaptic transmission. Actual movements of the animal may stimulate sensory pathways which in turn are protected by various inhibitory mechanisms from self-induced habituation. These inhibitory mechanisms most likely operate at the presynaptic side. It is difficult to envisage a nonassociative cell biological mechanism that changes the sensitivity to input from cell A but not to its neighboring synaptic input from cell B in the dendritic field of a follower cell receiving input from many intermingled synapses. In other words, the postsynaptic terminals of a cell do not "know" whether they receive synaptic input from cell A or B, and a differential modulation of synaptic strength on the postsynaptic side is, therefore, hard to accomplish. It is far easier to install some circuitry that can differentiate between the presynaptic terminals of A and B. The presynaptic A terminal may express a receptor molecule that renders A, but not B, sensitive to the action of the transmitter of the modulatory pathway. Under conditions where the transmitter action remains fairly localized, the transmission of A to one follower cell may be modulated whereas the transmission to an other follower cell in a different area of the nervous system remains unaffected even though all presynaptic terminals of A may express the receptor.

Action of Neuromodulators on Neuronal Circuits

Even the most stereotyped rhythmic behaviors have to be adapted to environmental changes. The probability of occurrence, the repetition rate of the motor pattern, the phase relationship between the motor components, and the fine tuning of the strength of muscle contractions have to be optimized to different environmental conditions. We have pointed out in the few examples described above that plasticity is intrinsic even in anatomically hard-wired circuits that mediate reflex behavior. We will now discuss some examples where particular extrinsic cells modulate already functioning neuronal circuits. These cells release substances which alter the transmission across conventional synapses.

Probably the most completely understood circuit producing a rhythmic output is the central pattern generator (CPG) in the stomatogastric ganglion of decapod crustaceans which produces alternating dilations and constrictions of the muscles of the pyloric and gastric system (82, 117, 118). Fourteen neurons whose synaptic interaction are completely established comprise the CPG for the pyloric rhythm and about the same number of cells for that of the gastric mill. The pyloric rhythm is active even in an isolated stomatogastric ganglion since one of the cells (the anterior buster cell, AB) is an endogenous pacemaker (90,91). However, it remains to be explained how neurons projecting from the CNS initiate, modulate, and turn off the oscillations. For example, a single cholinergic neuron, the anterior pyloric modulator cell (AMP) projecting from the esophageal ganglion to the stomatogastric ganglion, induces long-lasting depolarization in several identified neurons of the circuit (79). By this action both the oscillation is started (start-stop function) and driven to higher or lower frequencies (modulatory function). The neuropeptides proctolin and FMRFamide activate the quiescent pyloric and gastric rhythm (80). Several other transmitters, including dopamine and serotonin, enhance bursting in the pacemaker cells and thus change the overall frequency of the pyloric rhythm. A phase shift between the cellular components of the circuit appears in the presence of dopamine or proctolin and this is thought to result from a modulation of the synaptic strength among the neurons of the CPG. We may learn from this example that even a small circuit has the intrinsic capacity to generate a variety of neural outputs and that modulatory neurons projecting from outside the circuit onto strategic points specifically change certain components of the output pattern. In essence, the extrinsic modulatory neurons, like the AMP-neuron, convert the rigid machinery of a CPG into a flexible network with rudimentary properties of a cell assembly. The neurons join together to produce different output patterns at different times and these changes are adaptive with respect to the needs of the animal. Thus, the circuitry including the modulatory neurons have self-organizing and self-instructive properties which express the epigenetic rules for the dynamics of the network.

Several other examples of extrinsic modulatory neurons, which exemplify more complex adaptive changes in well-defined circuits, are known in the invertebrate nervous system. For example, the metacerebral cell (MCC) of *Aplysia*, which is homologous to the MCC of many other gastropods, increases the frequency of the feeding rhythm and rouses biting behavior by releasing serotonin (5-HT) in the CNS and the periphery (71). The MCC interacts with neuronal circuits and muscles controlling feeding on many levels of the nervous system. Thus, food arousal is regulated by activity-dependent 5-HT release from a single cell. Another example for neuromodulation of rhythmic motor outputs is furnished by the leech whose segmental ventral ganglia contain "neuronal analogs" of the MCC, the serotonergic Retzius cell. The central swimming oscillator of the leech is stimulated by 5-HT circulating in the blood (129). Pharmacological lesions of the Retzius and other serotonergic cells abolish feeding and swimming behavior (35, 74), which is later restored by application of 5-HT. Neuromodulatory 5-HT neurons serve to integrate several components of feeding behavior including swimming towards food sources, bite frequency, and blood meal size. In insects, feeding is controlled by octopamine (OA). Honeybees (87-89) and flies (77) respond more strongly to water and sucrose solution and imbibe much more when injected with OA or agonists. OA injected into the brain in small doses (10 nl, 10^{-6} M) is much more effective than injections into the hemolymph. We shall see below that OA sensitizes several other reflex behaviors in insects such as (walking, flying, and jumping and that the neurons responsible for this action are known. It appears that some octopaminergic neurons of the brain modulate feeding whereas those of the thoracic ganglia modulate the other behaviors.

Antagonistic behavior is frequently controlled by two different modulators. In the lobster, for example, injection of OA and 5-HT into the hemolymph causes two opposing static postures: tonic extension of all extremities under OA and tonic flexion under 5-HT (38,75). The two postures resemble behavioral components during an aggressive and submissive stance, respectively. Since both amines act synergistically in the periphery as neurohormones by enhancing the motor response of several muscles, their antagonistic action must result from a modulation of circuits within the CNS which control postural flexion and extension. If the amines are supplied to the motoneurons in the ganglia of the ventral chord the flexor muscles contract in response to 5-HT and relax in response to OA, whereas opposite patterns were found for extensor muscles. A corresponding antagonism of the two amines was found for the excitatory motoneurons and the inhibitory motoneurons which innervate the same muscle (70). It was concluded that OA enhances the readout of a central motor pattern which causes extension (contraction of extensors, relaxation of flexors) while 5-HT leads to the readout of a pattern for flexion. The 5-HT neurons in the lobster CNS have been localized by immunohistochemistry (3), whereas less is known about the neuroanatomy of the OA neurons. Most of the ca. 100 5-HT neurons have their somata in central ganglia with at least one serotonergic cell body in each ganglion of the ventral chord. Each neuron in the thoracic region arborizes both in the CNS and in a peripheral nerve plexus along the second root. The peripheral nerve plexus is a neurohemoral organ which supplies the hemolymph with 5-HT and OA. Thus, the amine produced by such a neuron acts as a neurohormone in the periphery and as a transmitter or modulator centrally. It is reasonable to assume that these 5-HT and OA neurons release their substances simultaneously in the periphery and in the CNS when excited. The peripheral action of both amines is to prime the muscles for stronger and faster action independent of their recent histoy and is nonselective for a motor pattern, whereas their central action is decisive for the motor pattern to be executed.

5-HT and OA have also opposite modulatory effects upon EPSPs in the lateral giants of crayfish (34). When OA is perfused through the arterial system the EPSP is enhanced, wherease 5-HT depresses the EPSP. Indirect evidence suggests that the monamines act on the synapse between tactile afferents and the sensory interneurons. It is well known that the threshold for a tail flip is raised in crayfish which are restrained or feeding. Glanzman and Krasne (34) suggest that 5-HT might mediate these supprssive effect whereas OA mediates a possible sensitization of the escape response.

The network properties of neuromodulation are, under those circumstances, understandable where particularly well-defined neurons release the modulators. The ventral nerve chord of insects, for example, contains OA in a particular set of well-described neurons, the dorsal unpaired median (DUM) neurons of bilateral symmetry. DUM cells have been investigated mainly in locusts and cockroaches (24, 49, 51, 55, 105). Most of the locust DUM cells are interneurons whose processes are confined to their ganglion of origin (36), whereas a minimum of nine cells send their bifurcating axons peripherally out of the metathoracic ganglion (126) into the musculature. The physiology of one particular DUM neuron, the DUMETi which innervates the extensor tibiae muscle of the hind leg, has been extensively studied. When DUMETi is stimulated intracellularly or when OA (10^{-6} M) is locally supplied to the muscle, it suppresses intrinsic rhythmicity of the muscle and potentiates neuromuscular transmission (25, 56, 96). Thus, the peripheral action of the modulatory neuron is to favor rapid movement and to remove catch tension from the muscle. The muscle's responses will then be more closely matched to its pattern of neuronal input (22, 23). In the CNS, OA released by an excited DUM cell or by local injection of OA into the regions of its output branches potentiates synaptic transmission between motoneurons, between sensory to motor neurons, interneurons, and motor neurons, and dishabituates synapses projecting onto fast excitatory motoneurons (e.g., FETi) (120, 121).

The integration process with respect to a certain behavior is, therefore, the release of a modulator in a particular spatiotemporal pattern into the neuropil. Sombati and Hoyle (121) speculated about a neuropilar compartmentation of micro-behaviors or behavioral components and condensed this view in the catchphrase "orchestration hypothesis of neural function." In their own words ((121), see pp. 503, 504):

> "While general release of the common excitatory modulator OA will increase the probability of occurrence of any behavior, which behavior will in fact appear depends, on the orchestration hypothesis, on which modulatory neurons are most strongly active at the time. On that will depend the locations within the neuropil where the highest concentrations occur at any given time, and therefore which parts of which circuits are most likely to be thrown into (or out of) action."

The DUM neurons which synthesize, transport, and release OA satisfy the needs for raising the general excitatory state or readiness to behave and are according to the orchestration hypothesis, the mediators of specific behaviors. Neuromodulators seem to be important in integration and fine tuning of behavioral components but their role in initiation of behavior is not yet understood. The Ddc mutant of *Drosophila* is deficient in the synthesis of dopamine and serotonin and the per^o mutation reduced OA level to one third of normal, yet flies with temperature-sensitive alleles of these mutants seem to behave normally except in learning (Ddc) and circadian rhythm (per^o) (76). These examples may suggest that modulatory circuits are not vital for the hard-wired routine operations of the nervous system. However, the life of a mutant in a genetics lab is obviously very different from that under natural conditions.

Hoyle's "orchestration hypothesis" is an attempt to integrate modulatory neurons into the concept of hard-wired circuits. We might, therefore, view the function of modulatory neurons as driving the neural assemblies from one to another preferred activity stage. If this view is correct we should find multisensory convergence and activity-dependent plasticity particularly emphasized in the modulatory neurons. Future work will have to address this question.

ASSOCIATIVE PLASTICITY

Associative plasticity is a widespread property of invertebrate nervous systems. It is an interesting, but as yet unsolved, question how small a nervous system capable of associative learning can be. There is no firm evidence for associative learning in unicellular organisms such as protozoans or "brainless" multicellular organisms such as the coelenterates, whereas nonassociative plasticity is found in both phyla (85). Fused neural networks appear first in the lower worms (*Plathelminthes*), and there is no doubt that these animals learn in a true sense. We have concentrated our discussion of the higher invertebrates (molluscs and arthropods). Since we addressed our attention to the network properties we have not considered the extensive work on the cellular basis of learning in molluscs. For these aspects, see the reviews by Alkon and Carew (both this volume).

Food Avoidance Conditioning in Gastropod Molluscs

Pleurobranchaea californica, a gastropod mollusc of the Pacific Ocean, preys on sea anemones at the bottom of the sea. Food is recognized by anterior chemosensory body appendages, (the oral veil with the tentacles) and the rhinophores, grasped in a bite strike by the proboscis, and is swallowed in rhythmic feeding movements by the muscular buccal mass (16). The feeding rhythm is generated by a central oscillator system in the cerebropleural ganglion (brain) and in the buccal ganglion, which innervates the buccal mass. Many interneurons and connections of the feeding circuitry are mapped but the detailed mechanisms of why this system oscillates are not known (17, 32). Inspired by traditional command neuron philosophy, Davis, Mpitsos, Gillette and their colleagues (14-18, 33, 94) looked for plasticity in key elements of this circuitry. *Pleurobranchaea* learns to reject and withdraw from food that has been previously paired with an electric stimulus. The paradigm is associative with memory staying stable for days to weeks (18, 94), and differential conditioning to different food substances can be shown. After conditioning has occurred Davis and Gillette (14) found changes in the response of the paracerebral neurons (PCNs), which they recorded in the living animal. The PCNs are a group of ca. 8 cells in each hemiganglion and constitute an essential element of the feeding oscillator. The importance of these interneurons is demonstrated by the facts that they become phasically depolarized and hyperpolarized during the feeding rhythm; depolarization of a certain PCN type (the phasic PCNs, PCp) elicits feeding in the living animal, and they are capable of resetting the feeding rhythm in the isolated nervous system (22).

Food stimuli applied to the chemosensory body appendages depolarize the PCNs. However, the PCNs of conditioned animals receive a barrage of inhibitory postsynaptic potentials (IPSPs) and EPSPs. The change occuring in the feeding circuitry is due to associative learning because control animals which receive food and shock unpaired do not show the change from excitation to inhibition (15). The change, however, can not only be caused by learning, because the PCNs of food-satiated animals become hyperpolarized, as well, when food contacts their sensory organs. Food avoidance and food satiation join into a common neural pathway which provides a nice example of a neural correlation of a motivational state. As the next step towards a cellular analysis of learning, Kovac *et al.* (64) tackled the question of whether isolated nervous systems feel hungry. They removed the nervous system with attached chemosensory organs from naive, conditioned, satiated, and control animals with unpaired food and shock application. Fortunately, the memory trace survives the operation. PCNs in conditioned animals receive a barrage of IPSPs when food is applied to the chemosensory structures. In addition, an excitatory polysynaptic pathway leading from identified feeding interneurons to the PCNs is reduced in its efficacy in conditioned nervous systems. In contrast to the results obtained in whole animal preparations, PCNs from satiated animals show excitatory responses towards food stimulation. The deprivation from the sensory input of the gut obviously stimulates a healthy appetite in the isolated nervous system of a previously satiated animal.

Bath and iontophoretic application of cholinergic agents provides evidence that the PCNs carry acetylcholine receptors on their somata (93) and can, therefore, be depolarized by acetylcholine (ACh). Conditioning reduces the ACh sensitivity of the PCNs. It is now possible to explain the decreased excitability of the PCNs in conditioned animals. It appears that desensitization of an ACh receptor may be part of a mechanism for learning in a mollusc. This conclusion is supported by the finding that the garden slug *Limax* shows longer memory retention in a similar paradigm if fed on a choline enriched diet, which increases ACh levels (114). In a rhythm-generating circuit which is almost certainly organized in loops, it is difficult to talk in terms of which neuron is pre- or postsynaptic to another. But in contrast to the *Aplysia* model, where an associative amplification of cAMP level causes a reduction in a potassium conductance on the *presynaptic* side of a modifiable synapse, the decreased ACh sensit iity of the PCNs implies a mechanism acting on the *postsynaptic* side of a connection.

The increased inhibition of the PCNs during conditioning is yet unaccounted for but an inhibitory pathway, presynaptic to the PCNs, has already been described (77). The conditioning procedure seems to distribute inhibition onto other neurons of the feeding circuitry. Thus *re-routing* of inhibitory pathways may be a feature of learning in a paradigm that changes appetitive into avoidance behavior. Even in relatively simple nervous systems a cellular mechanism of learning may require changes at multiple sites within the circuitry. However, a fair amount of circuit chasing in a gastropod nervous system could keep track of a distributed memory trace which is so easily lost in the vertebrate brain.

Similar to *Pleurobranchaea*, *Limax* decreases its appetite towards food paired with unpleasant chemostimulation (31, 115). The underlying learning psychology of this paradigm is nicely worked out (114) and a reduced preparation displaying the feeding motor program as well as learning is available. The properties of food avoidance learning in *Limax* have recently been modelled in a simulation program (32, see Fig. 3). Although only few of the network assumptions are actually supported by neurophysiological results, the model is interesting because it poses questions which are amenable at the cellular level with current technology. Taste receptors (1) provide an autocorrelation matrix (II) with a profile of parallel inputs, which are though to be categorized partially be preexisting (genetically defined) synaptic connections and modifiable synapses. The result is a stable activity pattern for each set of input (see Rolls, this volume, for the properties of an autocorrelation matrix). The outputs of the matrix (S1-S4) are all connected to the trigger neurons of the conditionable behaviors. A Hebb-like synapse was chosen to account for associative plasticity but this is not essential for the model; a presynaptic activity-dependent facilitation as proposed for associative learning in *Aplysia* (see Carew, this volume) would have the same function. Most importantly, the two antagonistic "behaviors" are mutually exclusive by a strong inhibitory connection .

Now one can see what synaptic modifications are required when an initially attractive food (A) is paired with an aversive stimulus (Q).

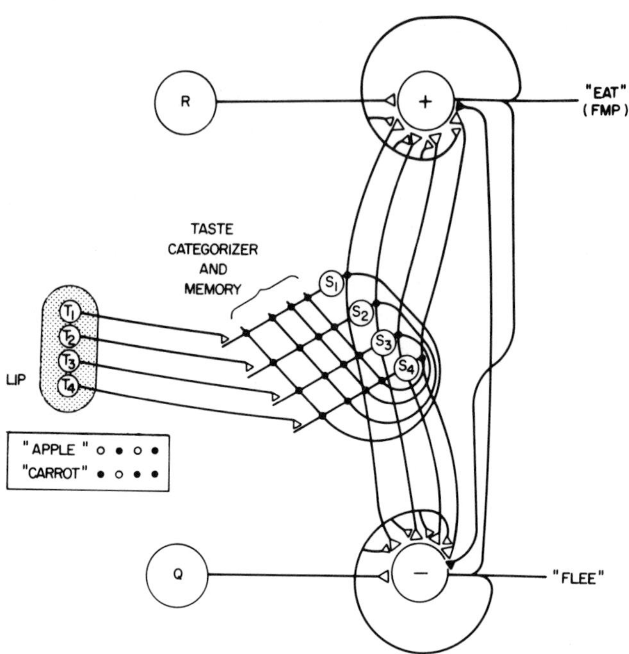

FIG. 3 – A diagram of the components of the *Limax* simulation program (from (32)). T1-T4: taste receptors in the lip (coding for "apple" or "carrot" taste with different patterns of excitation); S1-S4: outputs of taste categorizer matrix and sensory memory matrix; R: "reward" cell driving the + cell, which produces the feeding motor program (FMP); Q: punishment cell ("quinine") driving the - cell, which produces the "flee" motor program; △ : excitatory synapses; ▲ : inhibitory synapses.

Initially the categorized internal representation of A in the matrix I drives the + cell, which turns off the – cell even though there is weak excitatory input from S1-S4. Pairing with Q in the correct temporal order enhances the excitatory input to the – cell to a level that it switches off the + cell. This model predicts the following properties of the network which can be tested: a) the sensory autocorrelation matrix is separate from the memory storing synapses; b) the representations of the taste stimuli are connected to all "behaviors," which can be conditioned – this alpha-conditioning design is in contrast to the establishment of new connections during learning; c) learning does not change the preexisting reflex connections (in our example, the synaptic connections between S1-S4 with the + cell); and d) memories for aversively and appetitively conditioned tastes ar represented at different locations.

Operant Conditioning of Leg Posture in Insects

True operant conditioning with the perspective of a cellular analysis is still very rare in neurobiology and thus demands particular attention. The studies on the so-called "Horridge paradigm" are of additional interest because Hoyle (52) has tentatively advanced the opinion that at least some cellular correlates of this associative motor learning are independent of any synaptic plasticity and relate to a change of potassium ion conductance in certain identified motoneurons. Although synaptic plasticity is generally considered to be the most likely mechanism of the neural basis of learning, it can not be ruled out on *a priori* grounds that other cellular mechanisms, even nonneural phenomena (e.g, in glia elements), are involved in learning. It is thus worthwhile to look more closely into the evidence indicating a modulation of spike initiation in the output neuron. Furthermore, motor learning in a set of identified neurons should help to elucidate the contributions from the periphery and central nervous system to associative learning. Since so much is known about transmission and modulation in the motor system of decapod crustaceans (see above), it is unfortunate that very little effort has been invested so far in the analysis of associative motor learning of crustaceans although it unquestionably exists in the ghost crab *Ocypode* and the crayfish (50, 123).

Locusts and cockroaches keep a hind leg at a certain position if a deviation from that position is followed by an electrical stimulation of its tarsus (2, 20, 45, 52). Yoked animal controls reveal the operant nature of conditioning. About 2/3 of the animals learn. The speed of learning depends on the unconditioned stimulus (UCS) and mode of conditioning (increase in spike frequency: up-learning, or decrease in spike activity: down-learning). Sensory feedback about the position of the leg is not necessary but proprioceptive reflexes are known to change during the course of training (135). Isolated ganglion-nerve-muscle preparations are successfully trained in a similar way (48). The aversive electric shock can be replaced in a whole animal preparation by a loud, disturbing high frequency sound which stimulates the animal both through airborne sound and vibration (each stimulus component presented separately does not serve as an UCS or by a reward (fresh grass fed to the animal) (52, 125). Animals placed in a cold room learn quickly to heat themselves to a comfortable temperature (28). Avoidance of noise and shock is learned within 1-2 hours, but appetitive learning is slower.

The cellular analysis of a particular motoneuron, the anterior adductor (AAdc), is simplified by the fact that the postural changes it controls are shifts in muscle tone which result from an altered mean frequency of discharge in this tonic neuron (47, 54, 125, 133). AAdc discharges regularly under high Mg^{2+}, low Ca^{2+} conditions and thus spontaneous firing seems to be independent of inputs from chemical synapses. When the motoneuron has been conditioned to a higher discharge rate in Ringer, five out of eight preparations gave a more than 50% higher rate also at high Mg^{2+}, low Ca^{2+} conditions. It was concluded that the major change induced by operant conditioning resides in the motoneuron and not in synaptic input. This conclusion is supported by the finding that the input resistance of the AAdc motoneuron decreases parallel to the increase in spontaneous firing rate. The change in membrane resistance might be due to an increase in potassium flux (52). Training might, therefore, change the membrane potential at a strategic point of the neuron, the locus of spike initiation. Since synaptic potentials are hardly seen in the soma recordings the conclusions rest exclusively on the questionable assumpmtion that the high Mg^{2+}, low Ca^{2+} treatment totally eliminates synaptic input under the available experimental conditions. Furthermore, Hoyle and Field (57) succeeded in conditioning leg posture in the primitive orthopteran, the New Zealand weta. This insect has a muscle catch mechanism to lock the hind legs upwards in a defense response. Leg positioning, therefore, does not require ongoing activity in the respective motoneurons but only a burst of activity in the octopaminergic, neuromodulatory neuron DUMETi preceding a short burst in the slow extensor tibia neuron (SETi). And indeed, the authors did not find any spontaneous activity in SETi, the motoneuron homologous to that in the locust. The positive outcome of their training experiments in the weta indicates a learning mechanism which does not need the pacemaker properties of the motoneurons but rather a synaptic interaction between SETi, DUMETi, and the common inhibitor neuron. We conclude that Hoyle's interpretation of a nonsynaptic process in the operant conditioning of a motor neuron is not conclusive and that a synaptic mechanism seems more likely.

The importance of synaptic plasticity in the circuit driving the motoneuron is stressed by the finding that the leg uses at least three different motor patterns to adjust the femur-tibia joint to a conditioned position, depending on how much the joint has to be bent (29). So far only SETi or AAdc have been recorded intracellularly during conditioning, but all other motoneurons involved in adjusting this joint are individually known (8, 9) and an analysis of their interaction should be possible. Also, many premotor interneurons and sensory neurons in the metathoracic ganglion are known, which control the movement of the hind legs (8, 26, 119). Since instrumental conditioning alters the connection between the chordotonal input and the motor output (135), interneurons are intimately involved in the modulation of the circuit for leg posture.

All evidence indicates plastic changes in many neurons of a circuit, even in such a simple learning task as leg posture in insects. At the molecular level Kerkut *et al.* (61, 62) observed that many biochemical processes change in the thoracic ganglion when a leg is conditioned. Using the classical procedure of conditioning (up-learning, a mild electroshock to the tarsi as UCS), they found effects of associative learning on the following processes:

a) RNA synthesis: inhibition of RNA synthesis by actinomycin D, acridine orange, congo red, and chloramphenicol reduces learning in a dose- and time-dependent fashion.

b) Protein synthesis: inhibition of protein synthesis inhibits learning in a similar way. Uridine and leucine incorporation is higher in the experimental animals than in the control (untreated) and yoked animals.

c) ACh: activity of acetylcholinesterase (AChE) decreases during acquisition. Retention is correlated with the level of AChE activity. Physostigmine and prostigmine injected into the ganglion enhance learning in a dose-dependent way; it is thought that these drugs acts as anticholinesterases.

d) GABA: glutamate decarboxylase may have a reduced activity and thus produce less γ-aminobutyric acid (GABA) in the trained ganglia.

A new protein of low molecular weight appears during conditioning, although it is not yet firmly established how much of the changes accounts for shock stimulation alone and how much is specific for the associative process. These results demonstrate measurable effects which should be followed up with today's better techniques and the knowledge we have about the sensory, motor, and interneurons in the thoracic ganglia. It is assumed, but not yet critically tested, that adaptive changes at the level of translation and transcription are responsible for long-lasting changes whereas immediate associative learning is independent of these processes. Conditioning with the heat stimulus (see above) provides a method of fast learning and thus could be used to separate short- and long-term retention effects. Finally, the contribution of individual cells in the circuit can be tested by blocking RNA and protein synthesis in specific cells through intracellular injection of the inhibitors or even by killing specific cells. The leg-lift preparation offers ample opportunities to study the cellular and molecular events involved in instrumental learning since the behavioral paradigm is firmly established and conditioning is possible within a few minutes under conditions suitable for intracellular recordings from identified cells.

Learning with the Insect Brain

The richness of learned behavior in insects depends on the complex neuronal machinery of the brain which is composed of several hundred thousands of neurons (e.g., in the honeybee 950,000). The fruitfly *Drosophila melanogaster* and the honeybee *Apis mellifera* are the two species which have been most successfully used in learning studies: *Drosophila* because single gene mutations effecting learning can be studied with behavioral, genetic, and biochemical methods (106); *Apis* because learning exists in many forms and long-term memory is a very important component in its life cycle (30, 37, 84, 85). The behavioral analysis of learning, particularly in the honeybee, has revealed many phenomena reminiscent of those known from learning studies in vertebrates (84).

The genetic and biochemical aspects of learning mutants of *Drosophila* have been reviewed recently (19, 106). Six mutations are known, meanwhile, which are deficient in olfactory learning and/or memory. The metabolic abnormalities are known for four mutations. They are thought to affect different steps in a molecular cascade from a monoamine-activated adenylate cyclase to a protein kinase which might be involved in the phosphorylation of an ion channel. These mutations support the notion that a molecular mechanism similar to that underlying nonassociative and associative plasticity in *Aplysia* plays an essential part in olfactory learning of *Drosophila*. Additional neurotransmitter pathways may also be involved, e.g., other biogenic amines and ACh (19, 27).

In our context those mutants which affect the neuroarchitecture of the brain are of particular interest. Heisenberg *et al.* (40) describe two mutants of the mushroom bodies (m.b.) (see Fig. 4) which are very poor in olfactory learning but have no defects in motor performance, courtship behavior, olfaction (as far as spontaneous odor preference is concerned), visual learning (83), and learning of a particular visuomotor coordination. Aversive olfactor conditioning is more strongly impaired than appetitive olfactory learning. The authors concluded that the structural misarrangements and losses in the m.b. neuropil are the primary causes for the deficits in learning. These results are in agreement with studies on honeybees aimed at elucidating the localization of transfer from short-term to long-term memory (21, 86). Consolidation into long-term memory can be interrupted by cooling the whole bee shortly (<2 min) after a one-trial learning or by localized cooling of the m.b.s. The time course of interference by cooling is the same in both cases, whereas cooling of the antennal lobes (the primary olfactory projection area) has only a very transient effect, and cooling of other brain parts does not interfere with memory consolidation at all. We have concluded from these studies that the m.b. neuropil is intimately involved in the establishment of a long-term memory trace. It is thus tempting to search for particular features of the m.b. which might be obligatory for the establishment of LTM.

The m.b.s are formed by bundles of densely packed parallel projecting fibers called Kenyon cells (K-cells: 340,000 in the bee, 2,500 in *Drosophila*) (see Fig. 4). K-cell processes of the bee receive sensory input in the dorsal cup-like neuropil structure (calyx) mainly from olfactory relay neurons (of the antenno-glomerularis tract), but also from other sensory systems (visual, mechanosensory, chemosensory from the mouth parts)(92). The projection fibers of the K-cells travel down the pedunculus and branch half of their length into two output regions: the α-lobe (frontal) and the β-lobe. Arborizations of extrinsic output neurons of the m.b. form layers oriented perpendicularly to the K-cell projections, particularly in the α-lobe. Fig. 4 shows, for example, one of the many α-lobe extrinsic fiber bundles, the P.C.T.

The overall neuroanatomical organization of the m.b. is surprisingly similar to that of the cerebellum (116), where hundred thousands of parallel fibers synapse onto the perpendicularly oriented planes formed by the dendrites of Purkinje cells. Inhibitory connections via Golgi, stellate, and basket cells help to shape the discharge pattern within cerebellar circuits. Similarly, the P.C.T. mentioned above is thought to function as an inhibitory loop between output and input areas in the m.b. because it exhibits GABA immunoreactivity (6). It is well established that the cerebellum is involved in motor learning and

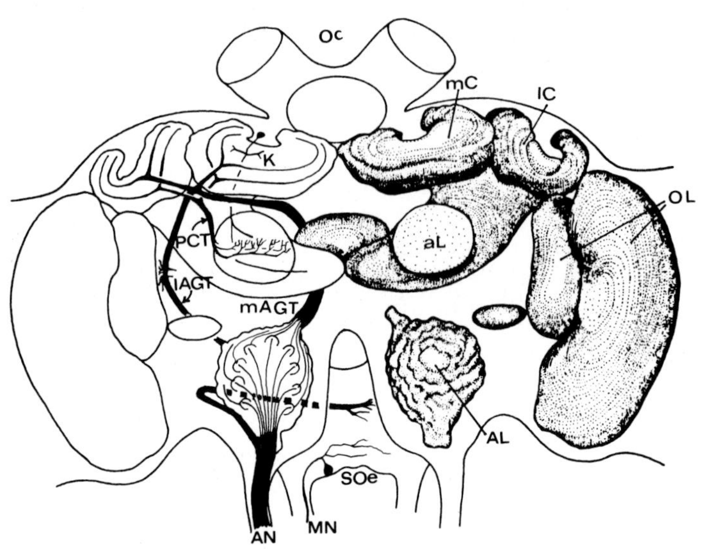

FIG. 4 – The brain of the honeybee. mC and lC: median and lateral calyx of the m.b.; aL: alpha lobe of the m.b.; K: Kenyon cells, the intrinsic neurons of the m.b.; mAGT and lAGT: median and lateral antenno-glomerularis tract; PCT: protocerebro-calycal tract; Oc: ocelli; AL: antennal lobe; SOe: subesophageal ganglion; AN: antennal nerve; MN: motoneuron to muscles moving the proboscis (tongue); OL: optic lobes.

particular models of this function have been proposed ((1, 81), see also Ito, this volume). The conjunction of climbing fiber input with ongoing parallel fiber activity is thought to modify the efficacy of the parallel fiber synapses onto Purkinje cells. Ito and his colleagues (60) demonstrated long-term synaptic depression, by conjunctive parallel and climbing fiber activity, and provided evidence that an adaptive change in gain control of the vestibulo-ocular reflex is mediated by a side path of this reflex through the flocculus of the cerebellum. It appears from many studies (46, 58) that the m.b., similar to the cerebellum, coordinates motor patterns by exerting inhibition on motor command pathways (see (40) for further discussion). Furthermore, the m.b.s are located in parallel rather than serial pathways, as is the cerebellum. Olfactory reflexes in *Drosophila* and bees, for example, do not depend on functioning m.b.s because additional sensory pathways bypass the m.b.s. Thus, the anatomical division of olfactory pathways may reflect an underlaying functional separation. It is tempting to speculate that the memory trace in the m.b.s is not located in the main line of sensory-motor control but in a parallel pathway and operates on motor subroutines through selective gain control as the Ito hypothesis suggests for the cerebellum.

Pharmacological experiments provide evidence for the selective involvement of some neurotransmitters in associative learning of insects and the role of the m.b.s. Injections of drugs into the bee brain, which interfere with aminergic transmission during or after one-trial appetitive olfactory conditioning, reveal that: a) dopamine (DA) is specifically involved in the retrieval of stored information but not in the sensory or motor aspects of the reflex and not in the storage process; b) OA modulates the sensory-motor components by enhancing the motor response and sensitizing the chemosensory input but does not interfere with the storage and retrieval processes; and c) norepinephrine (NE) and amphetamine are the only substances affecting the storage process (the bee brain contains no epinephrine (88)). DA appears in large quantities in the layers of the α-lobe and may thus be a transmitter of m.b. extrinsic fibers. NE is detected only in very small quantities in the bee brain. Interestingly, young be s (<3 days after emergence) do not contain NE in their brains and are unable to learn. Local injections of NE (10^{-8} M) or amphetamine (10^{-8} M) in small quantities (10 nl) into each α-lobe shortly before conditioning enhances the probability of conditioned responding at a time when their immediate effect has faded away.

CONCLUSIONS

Individually identified neurons located in relatively small nervous systems render the cellular and molecular analysis of neuronal plasticity possible and allow the examination of the contribution of single cells to the adaptive plasticity in neuronal circuits and assemblies. We encounter two principles in the examples described above. *Intrinsic plasticity* attentuates or potentiates transmission of signals through certain, modifiable synapses by the activity of the circuit itself. The result is, therefore, habituation by repeated stimulation, spontaneous recovery from habituation with time, and recruitment of new synapses by excess of stimulation (this developmental plasticity has not been discussed in detail here but is well documented in invertebrates, e.g. (95, 124)). The cellular mechanisms of intrinsic plasticity are likely to be found at the presynaptic terminal. There is evidence that not all synapses of a circuit are modifiable. Synapses with constant gain guarantee the automatic functioning of circuits and leave adaptive modification to certain strategically located plastic synapses. It is not known, however, in which cellular and molecular aspects these synapses differ.

Extrinsic plasticity is a mechanism of circuits to adapt their internal properties as a result of additional, modificatory input (67). Single modulatory neurons have been identified in various invertebrate nervous systems. They may act simultaneously in the periphery and in the CNS or are confined to the CNS. Little is known regarding in which respect modulatory neurons or circuits differ from sensory integration and motor output neurons or circuits and how they receive sensory input. Particularly, it is unknown whether modulatory circuits are specially designed to respond to temporally contingent stimuli, to certain stimulus combinations, or to combinations of stimuli and motor patterns. All modulatory neurons in invertebrates studied so far synthesize biogenic amines (5-HT, OA, NE) or neuropeptides. Aminergic modulators are indeed the magic substances which transpose local circuits into "dynamic combinations of circuits."

Another common property of modulatory neurons is their wide arborization throughout large parts of a ganglion by which each cell reaches many neuropilar compartments. It is an attractive idea to interpret the packages of neuropil, which are served by an axonal arborization of a modulatory neuron, as a functional unit in the sense that all synapses in this compartment may be modulated simultaneously by one neuron. The "orchestration hypothesis" advanced by Hoyle (121) adds an important feature to the cellular connectivity pattern of circuits. It appears that not only the network of interconnected neurons but also the brickwork of densely packed synapses from many neurons are the functional elements of the nervous system. Methods other than single cell recordings are needed to test this idea.

Associative learning appears as an extension of extrinsic plasticity, but so far too little is known about the contribution of modulatory neurons to the establishment of the memory trace. Neurons acting as general facilitator for many circuits may transmit the UCS to circuits dedicated specifically to learning, probably via monoaminergic neurotransmission, which is thought to be involved in learning in *Aplysia*, *Hermissenda*, *Drosophila*, and *Apis*. Recently, cholinergic transmission has been implied in visual learning of *Drosophila* (27), retention of taste conditioning in *Limax*, and food avoidance conditioning in *Pleurobranchea*. Whether ACh just happens to be a transmitter needed for the transmission of CS and UCS or whether it is linked to the memory trace remains to be seen.

Learning at the circuit level appears as a selection of a particular pattern of synapses by extrinsic pathways. It is unlikely, however, that a simple switching of existing pathways is the only mechanism of neuronal plasticity in invertebrates. Preliminary observations suggest that in invertebrates, as well, enriched and deprived environments alter considerably the structural features of the neurons (e.g., (44, 124)). We believe that it is only for technical reasons that the appearance of novel synapses and novel network properties during learning have not yet been described. The enormous learning capacity of highly evolved invertebrates and the large possibilities of their behavior exclude simple α-conditioning as a general strategy of learning in higher invertebrates. Instead, properties of information processing in neuronal assemblies, only slightly different from those in large brains, may determine the rules of learning. As in vertebrates, the information processing capabilities in these neuronal ssemblies are poorly understood.

Neuronal plasticity, including associative plasticity, seems to be interwoven with stereotyped neuronal processing. Nevertheless, associative learning processes which include the brain reside in structures which, like the mushroom bodies, are not in the main line of the sensory-motor pathways but in a parallel pathway. We compared the neuronal assembly of the m.b. with the cerebellum and, indeed, the structural and functional analogies are amazing. This analogy tells us that the architecture of assemblies might be similar in brains which differ profoundly in their phylogenetic origin. It is, therefore, not astonishing that learning and memory in higher invertebrates resembles surprisingly many features of their vertebrate colleagues.

Acknowledgements. We are grateful to our colleagues for helpful comments and Frau Cwienczek for typing the manuscript.

REFERENCES

(1) Albus, J.S. 1971. A theory of cerebellar function. *Math. Biosci.* 10: 26-61.

(2) Alloway, M. 1972. Learning and memory in insects. *Ann. Rev. Entom.* 17: 43-56.

(3) Beltz, B.S., and Kravitz, E.A. 1983. Mapping of serotonin-like immunoreactivity in the lobster nervous system. *J. Neurosci.* 3: 585-602.

(4) Bennet-Clarke, H.C. 1975. The energetics of the jump of the locust *Schistocerca gregaria*. J. *Exp. Biol.* 63: 53-83.

(5) Bicker, G., and Pearson, K.C. 1983. Initiation of flight by an identified wind sensitive neurone (TCG) in the locust. *J. Exp. Biol.* 104: 289-293.

(6) Bicker, G.; Schäfer, S.; and Kingan, T.G. 1985. Mushroom body feedback interneurones in the honeybee show GABA-like immunoreactivity. *Brain Res.* 360: 394-397.

(7) Breen, C.A., and Atwood, H.L. 1983. Octopamine – a neurohormone with presynaptic activity-dependent effects at crayfish neuromuscular junction. *Nature* 303: 716-718.

(8) Burrows, M. 1980. The control of sets of motoneurones by local interneurones in the locust. *J. Physl.* 298: 213-233.

(9) Burrows, M. 1983. Local interneurons and the control of movement in insects. In *Neuroethology and Behavioral Physiology*, eds. F. Huber and H. Markl, pp. 26-41. Berlin, Heidelberg, New York, Tokyo: Springer-Verlag.

(10) Burrows, M., and Rowell, C.H.F. 1973. Connections between descending visual interneurons and metathoracic motoneurons in the locust. *J. Comp. Physl.* 85: 221-234.

(11) Callec, J.J.; Guillet, J.C.; Pichon, Y.; and Boistel, J. 1971. Further studies on synaptic transmission in insects. II. Relation between sensory information and its synaptic integration at the level of a single giant axon in the cockroach. *J. Exp. Biol.* 55: 123-149.

(12) Castelluci, V., and Kandel, E.R. 1974. A quantal analysis of the synaptic depression underlying habituation of the gill-withdrawal reflex in *Aplysia*. *Proc. Natl. Acad. Sci.* 71: 5004-5008.

(13) Changeux, J.-P.; Heidmann, T.; and Patte, P. 1984. Learning by selection. In *The Biology of Learning*, eds. P. Marler and H.S. Terrace, pp. 115-133. Dahlem Konferenzen. Berlin, Heidelberg, New York, Tokyo: Springer-Verlag.

(14) Davis, W.J., and Gillette, R. 1978. Neural correlate of behavioral plasticity in command neurons of *Pleurobranchaea*. *Science* 199: 801-804.

(15) Davis, W.J.; Gillette, R.; Kovac, M.P.; Croll, R.P.; and Matera, E.M. 1983. Organization of synaptic inputs to paracerebral feeding command interneurons of *Pleurobranchaea californica*. III. Modifications induced by experience. *J. Neurophysl.* 49: 1557-1571.

(16) Davis, W.J., and Mpitsos, G.J. 1971. Behavioral choice and habituation in the marine mollusc *Pleurobranchaea californica*

MacFarland (Gastropoda, Opisthobranchia). *Z. Vergl. Physl.* 75: 207-232.

(17) Davis, W.J.; Siegler, M.V.S.; and Mpitsos, G.J. 1973. Distributed neuronal oscillators and efference copy in the feeding system of *Pleurobranchaea. J. Neurophysl.* 36: 258-274.

(18) Davis, W.J.; Villet, J.; Lee, D.; Rigler, M.; Gillette, R.; and Prince, E. 1980. Selective and differential avoidance learning in the feeding and withdrawal behavior of *Pleurobranchaea. J. Comp. Physl.* 138: 157-165.

(19) Dudai, Y. 1985. Genes, enzymes and learning in *Drosophila. TINS* 8: 18-21.

(20) Eisenstein, E.M. 1972. Learning and memory in isolated insect ganglia. *Adv. Insect* 9: 111-181.

(21) Erber, J.; Masuhr, Th.; and Menzel, R. 1980. Localization of short-term memory in the brain of the bee, *Apis mellifera. Physl. Entom.* 5: 343-358.

(22) Evans, P.D. 1980. Biogenic amines in the insect nervous system. *Adv. Insect* 15: 317-473.

(23) Evans, P.D. 1982. Properties of modulatory octopamine receptors in the locust. In *Neuropharmacology of Insects.* Ciba Foundation Symposium 88, pp. 48-69. London: Pitman.

(24) Evans, P.D., and O'Shea, M. 1978. The identification of an octopaminergic neurone and the modulations of a myogenic rhythm in the locust. *J. Exp. Biol.* 73: 235-260.

(25) Evans, P.D., and Siegler, M.V.S. 1982. Octopamine mediated relaxation of maintained and catch tension in locust skeletal muscle. *J. Physl.* 324: 93-112.

(26) Field, L.H., and Burrows, M. 1982. Reflex effects of the femoral chordotonal organ upon leg motor neurones of the locust. *J. Exp. Biol.* 101: 265-285.

(27) Folkers, E., and Spatz, H.-Ch. 1984. Visual learning performance of *Drosophila melanogaster* is altered by neuropharmaca affecting phosphodiesterase activity and acetylcholine transmission. *J. Insect Physl.* 30: 957-965.

(28) Forman, R.R. 1983. Leg position learning by an insect. I. A heat avoidance learning paradigm. *J. Neurobiol.* 15: 127-140.

(29) Forman, R.R., and Zill, S.N. 1984. Leg position learning by an insect. II. Motor strategies underlying learned leg extension. *J. Neurobiol.* 15: 221-237.

(30) v. Frisch, K. 1967. The Dance Language and Orientation of Bees. Cambridge: University Press.

(31) Gelperin, A. 1975. Rapid food aversion learning by a terrestrial mollusc. *Science* 185: 567-570.

(32) Gelperin, A.; Hopfield, J.J.; and Tank, D.W. 1985. The logic of Limax learning. In Model Neural Network and Behavior, ed. A.I. Selverston. New York: Plenum Publishing Corporation.

(33) Gillette, R.; Kovac, M.P.; and Davis, W.J. 1982. Control of feeding motor output by paracerebral neurons in the brain of *Pleurobranchaea californica*. *J. Neurophysl.* 47: 885-908.

(34) Glanzman, D.L., and Krasne, F.B. 1983. Serotonin and octopamine have opposite modulatory effects on the crayfish's lateral giant escape reaction. *J. Neurosci.* 3: 2263-2269.

(35) Glover, J.C., and Kramer, A.P. 1982. Sertonin analogue selectively ablates identified neurons in the leech embryo. *Science* 216: 317-319.

(36) Goodman, C.S.; Pearson, K.G.; and Spitzer, N.C. 1980. Electrical excitability: a spectrum of properties in the progeny of a single embryonic neuroblast. *Proc. Nat. Acad. Sci.* 77: 1676-1680.

(37) Gould, J.L. 1984. Natural history of honeybee learning. In *The Biology of Learning*, eds. P. Marler and H.S. Terrace, pp. 149-180. Dahlem Konferenzen. Berlin, Heidelberg, New York, Tokyo: Springer-Verlag.

(38) Harris-Warrick, R.M., and Kravitz, E.A. 1984. Cellular mechanisms for modulation of posture by octopamine and serotonin in the lobster. *J. Neurosci.* 4: 1976-1993.

(39) Hebb, D.O. 1949. The Organization of Behavior. New York: Wiley.

(40) Heisenberg, M.; Borst, A.; Wagner, S.; and Byers, D. 1985. Drosophila mushroom body mutants are deficient in olfactory learning. *J. Neurogenetics* 2: 1-30.

(41) Heitler, W.J. 1983. Suppression of a locust visual interneuron (DCMD) during defensive kicking. *J. Exp. Biol.* 104: 203-215.

(42) Heitler, W.J., and Burrows, M. 1977. The locust jump. I. The motor programme. *J. Exp. Biol.* 66: 203-219.

(43) Heitler, W.J., and Burrows, M. 1977. The locust jump. II. Neural circuits of the motor programme. *J. Exp. Biol.* 66: 221-241.

(44) Hertel, H. 1983. Change of synapse frequency in certain photoreceptors of the honeybee after chromatic deprivation. *J. Comp. Physl.* 151: 477-482.

(45) Horridge, G.A. 1962. Learning leg position by the ventral nerve cord in headless insects. *P. Roy. Soc. Lon.* B 157: 35-52.

(46) Howse, P.E. 1974. Design and function in the insect brain. In *Experimental Analysis of Insect Behavior*, ed. L.B. Brown, pp. 180-194. Berlin, Heidelberg, New York, Tokyo: Springer-Verlag.

(47) Hoyle, G. 1965. Neurophysiological studies on learning in headless insects. In *The Physiology of the Insect Central Nervous System*, eds. J.E. Treherne and J.W.L. Blament, pp. 203-232. New York, London: Academic Press.

(48) Hoyle, G. 1966. An isolated insect ganglion-nerve-muscle preparation. *J. Exp. Biol.* 44: 413-427.

(49) Hoyle, G. 1975. Evidence that insect dorsal unpaired median (DUM) neurones are octopaminergic. *J. Exp. Biol.* 193: 425-431.

(50) Hoyle, G. 1976. Learning of leg position by the ghost crab, *Ocypode certophthalma*. *Behav. Biol.* 18: 147-163.

(51) Hoyle, G. 1978. Intrinsic rhythm and basic tonus in insect skeletal muscle. *J. Exp. Biol.* 73: 173-203.

(52) Hoyle, G. 1979. Mechanisms of simple motor learning. *TINS* 2: 153-155.

(53) Hoyle, G. 1980. Learning, using natural reinforcement, in insect preparations that permit cellular neuronal analysis. *J. Neurobiol.* 11: 323-354.

(54) Hoyle, G. 1982. The role of pacemaker activity in learning. In *Cellular Pacemakers*, ed. D.O. Carpenter, pp. 142-161. New York, London: Academic Press.

(55) Hoyle, D., and Dagan, D. 1978. Physiological characteristics and reflex activation of DUM (octopaminergic) neurons of locus metathoracic ganglion. *J. Neurobiol.* 9: 59-79.

(56) Hoyle, G.; Dagan, D.; Moberly, B.; and Colquhoun, W. 1974. Dorsal unpaired median insect neurons make neurosecretory endings on skeletal muscle. *J. Exp. Zool.* 187: 159-165.

(57) Hoyle, G., and Field, L.H. 1983. Defense posture and leg-position learning in a primitive insect utilize catchlike tension. *J. Neurobiol.* 14: 285-298.

(58) Huber, F. 1960. Untersuchungen über die Funktion des Zentralnervensystems und insbesondere des Gehirns bei der Fortbewegung und Lauterzeugung der Grillen. *Z. Vergl. Physl.* 44: 60-132.

(59) Hue, B., and Callec, J. 1983. Presynaptic inhibition in the cercal-afferent giant interneurone synapses of the cockroach, *Periplaneta americana L.* *J. Insect Physl.* 29: 741-748.

(60) Ito, M. 1984. The Cerebellum and Neural Contral. New York: Raven Press.

(61) Kennedy, D.; Calabrese, R.L.; and Wine, J.J. 1974. Presynaptic inhibition: primary afferent depolarization in crayfish neurons. *Science* 185: 451-454.

(62) Kerkut, G.A.; Emson, P.C.; and Beesley, P.W. 1972. Effect of leg-raising learning on protein synthesis and AChE activity in the cockroach CNS. *Comp. Biochem.* 41 (3B): 635-645.

(63) Kerkut, G.A.; Oliver, G.W.O.; Rick, J.T.; and Walker, R.J. 1970. The effects of drugs on learning in a simple preparation. *Comp. Gen. Pharmac.* 1: 437-483.

(64) Kirk, M.D. 1985. Presynaptic inhibiton in the crayfish CNS: pathways and synaptic mechanisms. *J. Neurophysl.* 54: 1305-1325.

(65) Kovac, M.P.; Davis, W.J.; Matera, M.E.; Morielli, A.; and Croll, R.P. 1985. Learning: neural analysis in the isolated brain of a previously trained mollusc, *Pleurobranchaea californica. Brain Res.* 331: 275-284.

(66) Krasne, F.B. 1969. Excitation and habituation of the crayfish escape reflex: the depolarising response in lateral giant fibres of the isolated abdomen. *J. Exp. Biol.* 50: 29-46.

(67) Krasne, F.B. 1978. Extrinsic control of intrinsic neuronal plasticity: a hypothesis from work on simple systems. *Brain Res.* 140: 197-216.

(68) Krasne, F.B., and Bryan, M.S. 1973. Habituation: regulation through presynaptic inhibition. *Science* 182: 590-592.

(69) Krasne, F.B., and Woodsmall, K.S. 1969. Waning of the crayfish escape response as a result of repeated stimulation. *Anim. Behav.* 17: 416-424.

(70) Kravitz, E.A.; Beltz, B.S.; Glusman, S.; Goy, M.F.; Harris-Warrick, R.M.; Johnston, M.F.; Livingstone, M.S.; Schwarz, T.L.; and Siwicki, K.K. 1983. Neurohormones and lobsters: biochemistry to behavior. *TINS* 6: 345-349.

(71) Kupfermann, I., and Weiss, K.R. 1981. The role of serotonin in arousal of feeding behavior of Aplysia. In *Serotonin Neurotransmission and Behavior*, eds. D.L. Jacobs and A. Gelperin. Cambridge, MA, London: MIT Press.

(72) Larimer, J.L.; Eggleston, A.C.; Masukawa, L.M.; and Kennedy, D. 1971. The different connections and motor outputs of lateral and medial giant fibres in the crayfish. *J. Exp. Biol.* 54: 391-402.

(73) Lashley, K.S. 1950. In search of the engram. *Soc. Exp. Biol. Symp.* 4: 454-482.

(74) Lent, C.M., and Dickinson, M.H. 1984. Serotonin integrates the feeding behavior of the medicinal leech. *J. Comp. Physl.* A 154: 457-471.

(75) Livingstone, M.S.; Harris-Warrick, R.M.; and Kravitz, E.A. 1980. Serotonin and octopamine produce opposite postures in lobster. *Science* (NY) 208: 76-79.

(76) Livingstone, M.S., and Tempel, B.L. 1983. Genetic dissection of monamine transmitter synthesis in *Drosophila. Nature* 303: 67.

(77) London, J.A., and Gilette. 1984. Functional roles and circuitry in an inhibitory pathway to feeding command neurons in *Pleurobranchaea. J. Exp. Biol.* 113: 423-446.

(78) Long, T.F., and Murdock, L.L. 1983. Stimulation of blowfly feeding behavior by octopaminergic drugs. *Proc. Natl. Acad. Sci.* 80: 4159-4163.

(79) Marder, E. 1984. Mechanisms underlying neurotransmitter modulation of a neuronal circuit. *TINS* 7: 48-53.

(80) Marder, E., and Hooper, S.L. 1984. Neurotransmitter modulation of the stomatogastric ganglion of decapod crustraceans. In *Model Neural Networks and Behavior*, ed. A.A. Selverston. New York, London: Plenum.

(81) Marr, D.A. 1969. A theory of cerebellar cortex. *J. Physl. Lon.* 202: 437-470.

(82) Maynard, D.M. 1972. Simpler networks. *Ann. NY Acad.* 193: 59-72.

(83) Menne, D., and Spatz, H.-Ch. 1977. Colour vision in *Drosophila melanogaster. J. Comp. Physl.* 114: 302-312.

(84) Menzel, R. 1983. Neurobiology of learning and memory: the honey bee as a model system. *Naturwiss.* 70: 504-511.

(85) Menzel, R. *et al.* 1984. Biology of invertebrate learning. In *The Biology of Learning*, eds. P. Marler and H.S. Terrace, pp. 249-270. Dahlem Konferenzen. Berlin, Heidelberg, New York, Tokyo: Springer-Verlag.

(86) Menzel, R.; Erber, J.; and Masuhr, Th. 1974. Learning and memory in the honeybee. In Experimental Analysis of Insect Behavior, ed. Barton-Browne, pp. 195-217. Berlin, Heidelberg, New York: Springer-Verlag.

(87) Mercer, A.R., and Menzel, R. 1982. The effect of biogenic amines on conditioned and unconditioned responses to olfactory stimuli in the honeybee, *Apis mellifera. J. Comp. Physl.* 145: 363-368.

(88) Mercer, A.R.; Mobbs, P.G.; Davenport, A.P.; and Evans, P.D. 1983. Biogenic amines in the brain of the honeybee, *Apis mellifera*. *Cell Tis. Res.* 234: 655-677.

(89) Michelsen, B., and Menzel, R. 1984. The effects of catecholamines on odour learning in honeybees. Verh. Deut. G. Zool. 77: 232. Stuttgart: G. Fischer Verlag.

(90) Miller, J.P., and Selverston, A.J. 1982. Mechanisms underlying pattern generation in lobster stomatogastric ganglion as determined by selective inactivation of identified neurons. II. Oscillatory properties of pyloric neurons. *J. Neurophysl.* 48: 1378-1391.

(91) Miller, J.P., and Selverston, A.J. 1982. Mechanisms underlying pattern generation in lobster stomatogastric ganglion as determined by selective inactivation of identified neurons. IV. Network properties of pyloric system. *J. Neurophysl.* 48: 1416-1432.

(92) Mobbs, P.G. 1982. The brain of the honeybee *Apis mellifera*. I. The connections and spatial organization of the mushroom bodies. *Phil. Trans. R. Soc. Lon.* B 298: 309-354.

(93) Morielli, A.D.; Matera, E.M.; Kovac, M.P.; Shrum, R.G.; McCormack, K.J.; and Davis, W.J. 1986. Cholinergic suppression: a postsynaptic mechanism of long-term associative learning. *Proc. Nat. Acad. Sci.* 83: 4556-4560.

(94) Mpitsos, G.J.; Collins, S.D.; and McClellan, A.D. 1978. Learning: a model system for physiological studies. *Science* 199: 497-506.

(95) Murphey, R.K., and Matsumoto, S.G. 1976. Experience modifies the plastic properties of identified neurons. *Science* 191: 564-566.

(96) O'Shea, M., and Evans, P.D. 1979. Potentiation of neuromuscular transmission by octopaminergic neuron in the locust. *J. Exp. Biol.* 79: 169-190.

(97) O'Shea, M., and Rowell, C.H.F. 1975. Protection from habituation by lateral inhibition. *Nature* 254: 53-55.

(98) O'Shea, M., and Rowell, C.H.F. 1976. The neuronal basis of a sensory analyser, the acridid movement detector system. II. Response decrement, convergence, the nature of the excitatory efferents of the LGMD. *J. Exp. Biol.* 65: 289-308.

(99) O'Shea, M., and Rowell, C.H.F. 1977. Complex neural integration and identified interneurons in the locust brain. In *Identified Neurons and Behavior of Arthropods*, ed. G. Hoyle. New York and London: Plenum Press.

(100) Pearson, K.G., and Goodman, C.S. 1981. Presynaptic inhibition of transmission from identified interneurons in locust central nervous system. *J. Neurophysl.* 45: 501-515.

(101) Pearson, K.G.; Heitler, W.J.; and Steeves, J.D. 1980. Triggering of locust jump by multimodal inhibitory interneurons. *J. Neurophysl.* 43: 257-278.

(102) Pearson, K.G.; Reye, D.N.; Parsons, D.W.; and Bicker, G. 1985. Flight initiating interneurons in the locust. *J. Neurophysl.* 53: 910-925.

(103) Pearson, K.G., and Robertson, R.M. 1981. Interneurons coactivating hind leg flexor and extensor motoneurons in the locust. *J. Comp. Physl.* 144: 391-400.

(104) Pflüger, H.-J., and Burrows, M. 1978. Locust use the same basic motor pattern in swimming as in jumping and kicking. *J. Exp. Biol.* 75: 95-100.

(105) Platnikova, S.J. 1969. Effectory neurons with several axons in the ventral nerve cord of the Asian grasshopper, *Locusta migratoria*. *J. Evol. Biochem. Physl.* 5: 276-278.

(106) Quinn, W.G. 1984. Work in invertebrates on the mechanisms underlying learning. In *The Biology of Learning*, eds. P. Marler and H.S. Terrace, pp. 197-246. Dahlem Konferenzen. Berlin, Heidelberg, New York, Tokyo: Springer-Verlag.

(107) Reichert, H., and Rowell, C.H.F. 1985. Integration of nonphaselocked exteroceptive information in the control of rhythmic flight in the locust. *J. Neurophysl.* 53: 1201-1217.

(108) Reichert, H.; Rowell, C.H.F.; and Griss, C. 1985. Course correction circuitry translates feature detection into behavioral action in locusts. *Nature* 315: 142-144.

(109) Rind, F.C. 1984. A chemical synapse between two motion detecting neurons in the locust brain. *J. Exp. Biol.* 110: 143-167.

(110) Roberts, A.; Krasne, F.B.; Hagiwara, G.; Wine, J.J.; and Kramer, A.P. 1982. Segmental giant: evidence for a driver neuron interposed between command and motor neurons in the crayfish escape system. *J. Neurophysl.* 47: 761-781.

(111) Roeder, K.D. 1948. Organization of the ascending giant fiber system in the cockroach *Periplaneta americana*. *J. Exp. Zool.* 108: 243-261.

(112) Rowell, C.H.F. 1976. Small system neurophysiology and the study of plasticity. In *Neural Mechanisms of Learning and Memory*, eds. M.R. Rosenzweig and E.L. Bennett. Cambridge, MA, London: MIT Press.

(113) Rowell, C.H.F., and O'Shea, M. 1980. Modulation of transmission at an electrical synapse in the locust movement detector mechanism system. *J. Comp. Physl.* 137: 233-241.

(114) Sahley, C.L.; Barry, S.R.; and Gelperin, A. 1986. Dietary choline augments associative memory function in *Limax maximus*. *J.Neurobiol.* 17: 113-120.

(115) Sahley, C.L.; Rudy, J.W.; and Gelperin, A. 1983. Associative learning in a mollusc: a comparative analysis. In *Primary Neural Substrates of Learning and Behavioral Change*, eds. D. Alkon and J. Farley. Cambridge, MA.: University Press.

(116) Schürmann, F.W. 1974. Bemerkungen zur Funktion der corpora pedunculata im Gehirn der Insekten aus morphologischer Sicht. *Exp. Brain Res.* 19: 406-432.

(117) Selverston, A.I.; King, D.G.; Russel, D.F.; and Miller, J.P. 1976. The stomatogastric nervous system: structure and function of a small neural network. *Prog. Neurobiol.* 7: 215-290.

(118) Selverston, A.I., and Miller, J.P. 1980. Mechanisms underlying pattern generation in lobster stomatogastric ganglia as determined by selective indication of identified neurons. I. Pyloric system. *J. Neurophysl.* 44: 1102-1121.

(119) Siegler, M.V.S. 1981. Postural changes alter synaptic interactions between nonspiking interneurons and motor neurons in the locust. *J. Neurophysl.* 46: 310-323.

(120) Sombati, S., and Hoyle, G. 1984. Central nervous sensitization and dishabituation of reflex action in an insect by the neuromodulator octapamine. *J. Neurobiol.* 15: 455-480.

(121) Sombati, S., and Hoyle, G. 1984. Generation of specific behaviors in a locust by local release into neuropil of the natural neuromodulator octopamine. *J. Neurobiol.* 15: 481-506.

(122) Steeves, J.D., and Pearson, K.G. 1982. Proprioceptive gating of inhibitory pathways to hind leg flexor motoneurons in the locust. *J. Comp. Physl.* 146: 507-515.

(123) Strafstrom, C.E., and Gerstein, G.L. 1977. A paradigm for position learning in the crayfish claw. *Brain Res.* 134: 185-190.

(124) Technau, G., and Heisenberg, M. 1982. Neural reorganization during metamorphosis of the corpora pedunculata in *Drosophila melanogaster*. *Nature* 295: 405-407.

(125) Tosney, T., and Hoyle, G. 1977. Computer-controlled learning in a simple system. *P. Roy. Soc. Lon.* B 195: 365-393.

(126) Watson, A.H.D. 1984. The dorsal unpaired median neurons of the locust metathoracic ganglion: neuronal structure and diversity, and synapse distribution. *J. Neurocyt.* 13: 303-327.

(127) Wiersma, C.A.G. 1938. Function of giant fibres of the central nervous system of the crayfish. *Proc. Soc. Exp. M.* 38: 661-662.

(128) Wiersma, C.A.G., and Ikeda, K. 1964. Interneurons commanding swimmeret movements in the crayfish, *Procamborus clarkii* (Girard). *Comp. Biochem. Physl.* 12: 509-525.

(129) Willard, A.L. 1981. Effects of serotonin on the generation of the motor program for swimming by the medicinal leech. *J. Neurosci.* 1: 936-944.

(130) Wilson, D.M. 1961. The central control of flight in a locust. *J. Exp. Biol.* 38: 471-490.

(131) Wine, J.J. 1984. The structural basis of an innate behavioral pattern. *J. Exp. Biol.* 112: 283-319.

(132) Wine, J.J., and Krasne, F.B. 1972. The organization of escape behavior in the crayfish. J. *Exp. Biol.* 56: 1-18.

(133) Woollacott, M., and Hoyle, G. 1977. Neural events underlying learning in insects: changes in pacemaker. *P. Roy. Soc. Lon. B* 195: 395-415.

(134) Zaretzky, M., and Rowell, C.H.F. 1979. Saccadic suppression by corollary discharge in the locust. *Nature* 280: 583-585.

(135) Zill, S.N., and Forman, R.R. 1983. Proprioceptive reflexes change when an insect assumes an active, learned posture. *J. Exp. Biol.* 107: 385-390.

(136) Zucker, R.S. 1972. Crayfish escape behavior and central synapses. I. Neural circuits exciting lateral giant fiber. *J. Neurophysl.* 35: 599-620.

(137) Zucker, R.S. 1972. Crayfish escape behavior and central synapses. II. Physiological mechanism underlying behavioral habituation. *J. Neurophysl.* 35: 638-651.

The Neural and Molecular Bases of Learning,
eds. J.-P. Changeux and M. Konishi, pp. 473–502.
John Wiley & Sons Limited.

Activity-dependence of Network Properties

R.F. Thompson

Dept. of Psychology
Stanford University
Stanford, CA 94305, USA

INTRODUCTION

Perhaps the greatest scientific challenge of our time is to understand the functioning of nervous systems and how their operation governs the behavior of organisms. Of particular interest are the ways in which nervous systems acquire, store, integrate, and utilize information about experienced events and the ways such information interacts with more genetically determined behavioral capacities and tendencies to determine the behaviors that organisms exhibit. In this overview – written, I trust, in the spirit of what Dr. Tsukahara would have done – the focus is on networks, structures, and systems in the mammalian brain where behavioral learning and training procedures result in altered neuronal activity and where there is at least suggestive evidence for the occurrence of neuronal plasticity.

A BRIEF HISTORY

The belief that learning results from changes in the structural and functional properties of neurons and their interconnections has its basis in the work of Cajal who first demonstrated that nervous systems are made up of discrete units, i.e., neurons (21). Given the framework of the "neuron doctrine," early neuroscientists such as Lugaro (81), Tanzi (133), and Cajal (21) proposed that learning might be due to changes in cell to cell interactions. Indeed, they suggested that the processes of growth and development of the embryonic nervous system might in fact continue on a more subtile scale into adulthood and serve as the basic processes underlying learning and memory. Since then the growth in knowledge about the architecture, neurophysiology, and neurohumoral properties of nervous systems has been staggering, especially in the past twenty-five years with the emergence of the discipline of neuroscience. Yet in spite of this deluge of facts our understanding of the mechanisms of learning and memory remains rudimentary. The advances of the past quarter of a century have brought the field to a point to where we can now *begin* to identify neural mechanisms that may be responsible for learning and memory. As might be expected, given such a complex problem, the most striking progress has been made in the analysis of simpler forms of learning in vertebrates and in organisms having relatively simple nervous systems – certain invertebrates.

The history of views of brain substrates of learning and memory is directly related to the history of psychology. Psychology is somewhat unique among fields in that it started on a particular day in 1879, when Wilhelm Wundt founded the first psychology laboratory in Leipzig. He developed the method of introspection which involves analyzing one's experiences and sensations into their essential elements. Wundt's approach was particularly successful in the analysis of sensations and told us what types of skin receptors ought to exist almost 100 years ago.

Wundt's laboratory was visited by many Americans. Among them was William James (64), who established the young field of psychology in the U.S. with his classic text, *Principles of Psychology*, published in 1890. James was strongly influenced in his thinking by the British associationists (e.g., Locke and Hume) who believed that we learn associations by contiguity of experiences. James illustrated how the brain might build on reflexes to learn by association.

Meanwhile, Darwinism was at its peak in England and led to the study of animal behavior and the animal mind. The method of introspection was used in which a naturalist would put himself in the place of the animal and introspect about how the animal felt and thought about the situation. This method was founded on the idea that the mind evolved by small changes, just as did the body. By putting themselves into human mazes, naturalists learned much about how rats learned mazes. It was found that humans and rats learn comparable mazes at about the same rate and in much the same way.

Edward Thorndike, an undergraduate at Wesleyan in the early 1890s, read James' text, became excited about the new field of psychology, and entered graduate school at Harvard to study with James. He was fascinated by the study of animal intelligence and began independent experiments with chicks in his apartment. His landlady threw him out but James took Thorndike, and his chicks, into his own basement. To survive financially Thorndike (140) had to later accept a fellowship at Columbia, where he did his classic work on cats in puzzle boxes (1898). The cats learned to find a food reward by trial and error. These experiments, using objective measures of animal learning, led Thorndike to state the law of effect: the probability of a given behavior increases if it is associated with reward and decreases if associated with punishment.

Meanwhile, parallel developments were occurring in Russia. The eminent physiologist Sechenov published a paper (1863) entitled "Who must investigate the problems of psychology?" (see (15)). His answer was that physiologists should investigate psychology by studying reflexes. His view and his books were condemned by the Czarist censor committee and a court action was started against him but was later dropped. His writings exerted a profound influence on two young physiologists, Pavlov and Bechterev. Pavlov acknowledges major intellectual debts to Sechenov and also to Thorndike, whose objective measurements of animal behavior impressed him greatly.

When Pavlov discovered the conditioned salivary response he immediately realized that this "psychic reflex" provided a method for studying higher mental processes in animals. His impact on the West was gradual and much more in terms of the vast body of data his laboratory collected on conditioned reflexes and his basic approach of using conditioned reflexes to study learning as opposed to his theory of cortical function. Pavlov did not at first take the neuron doctrine seriously and spoke of waves of excitation and inhibition spreading across the cortex to account for learning. An early study in his laboratory by Zeliony, in 1911, seemed to show that the neocortex was essential for conditioned responses and this became the accepted dogma, held more rigidly by some of his students than by Pavlov himself (111). This later proved not to be the case (17, 113).

Bechterev also investigated conditioned reflexes using skeletal muscle responses such as leg flexion (see (15)). Initially his work had a greater impact on the West than did Pavlov's. This influence, similar to Thorndike's, was to show the value of objective methods to study learning and brain function in animals.

At this time in the West students of animal behavior were still required to interpret results in terms of the experience of the animal. In 1903 at the University of Chicago, John B. Watson completed his PhD under Angell, a psychologist, and Donaldson, a neurologist, and stayed on to complete a paper in 1907 investigating the sensations and experiences the rat used to solve the problem of the maze. In 1908 he accepted a professorship at Johns Hopkins and began increasingly to rebel against interpretations of behavior in terms of consciousness. In 1913 he published an important paper entitled "Psychology as a behaviorist views it" that founded behaviorism and ultimately led to the disappearance of the introspectionist school (148).

Watson emphasized that to understand behavior, all that was necessary was to measure the stimuli that went in and the responses that came out. Consciousness or awareness was an unnecessary construct. For Watson, all behavior could be explained in terms of learning. Given twelve babies, he claimed he could make any one an artist or a baker by training them. His view of learning was similar to that of Bechterev, Pavlov, and Thorndike, involving conditioned reflexes and trial-and-error learning. Unlike Pavlov and Bechterev, Watson ignored biology and placed all emphasis on a switchboard association notion of learning, similar to the theory of James and the much earlier view of Descartes.

Watson established behaviorism at about the same time that logical positivism came to the fore in the philosphy of science: all science is measurements, and theories are simply ways of relating sets of measurements. For the more advanced sciences, such as physics, this could be done by equations. In order for psychology to be a science it had to begin with the establishment of measurable relationships between stimuli and responses.

At least four major theories of learning developed as a result of Watson's ideas: 1) the systematic and mechanistic system of C. Hull emphasized drive reduction as the mechanism of reinforcement; 2) Guthrie's notion of elemental stimulus-response associations (50); 3) Skinner's development of the effect of schedules of reward and punishment on operant behaviors; and, 4) Tolman's emphasis on the cognitive nature of animal behavior. All these approaches were behavioristic and not concerned directly with biological mechanisms. In the 1940s and 1950s these were the dominant theories of learning. The majority of workers did not follow any one theory but were more empirical in approach. As a result of these theories and the research they stimulated, much was discovered about learning in animals.

The modern field concerned with the biological substrates of learning and memory was begun in the United States by Karl Lashley, then a graduate student working with Watson:

> "In 1914, I think, Watson called attention of his seminar to the French edition of Bechterev [on conditioned reflexes], and that winter the seminar was devoted to translation and discussion of the book. In the spring I served as a sort of unpaid assistant and we constructed apparatus and planned experiments together. We simply attempted to repeat Bechterev's experiments. We worked with withdrawal reflexes, knee jerk, pupillary reflexes... Our whole program was then disrupted by the move to the lab in Meyer's clinic. There were no adequate animal quarters there. Watson started work with the infants as the next best material available. I tagged along for awhile, but disliked the babies and found me a rat lab in another building. We accumulated a considerable amount of experimental material on the conditioned reflex which has never been published. Watson saw it as a basis for a systematic psychology and was not greatly concerned with the nature of the reaction itself. I got interested in the physiology of the reaction and the attempt to trace conditioned reflex paths through the nervous system started my program of cerebral work." (Letter of May 14, 1935, K.S. Lashley to E.R. Hilgard, reproduced with the kind permission of E.R. Hilgard).

One has the feeling that then, as well as throughout his life, Lashley wanted to believe in localization of the memory trace but his own results kept confounding his belief (76). Lashley began his empirical search for the memory trace at Johns Hopkins University in a collaborative study with Sheppard Franz, who worked at St. Elizabeth's Hospital in Washington, D.C. Lashley and Franz (77) presented a very balanced and modern treatment of the issues of the localization of memory.

Lashley continued to pursue localization of the memory trace in the cerebral cortex, culminating in his classic 1929 monograph (75). There he stated the extreme cortical localization view, the switchboard theory, and then proceeded to demolish it with experimental data. He concluded that memory traces were stored in the cerebral cortex but were not localized. He did not consider, in any detail, the alternative possibility he and Franz raised earlier, that memory traces for certain forms of learning might be localized subcortically. Nevertheless, Lashley continued in search of the cortical engram and in 1950 drew his oft-quoted conclusion:

> "This series of experiments has yielded a good bit of information about what and where the memory trace is not. It has discovered nothing directly of the real nature of the engram. I sometimes feel, in reviewing the evidence on the localization of the memory trace, that the necessary conclusion is that learning just is not possible. It is difficult to conceive of a mechanism which can satisfy the conditions set for it. Nevertheless, in spite of such evidence against it, learning does sometimes occur" (see pp. 477-478 (76)).

Lashley moved from the University of Chicago to Harvard in 1937 and became Director of the Yerkes Laboratory in Orange Park Florida in 1942. He disliked Cambridge and travelled there only once a year to give two weeks of seminars in order to keep his chair. At Orange Park, as at Chicago earlier, he had many of the people with him who became leaders in the fields of brain and behavior: Beach, Hebb, Schneirla, Leeper, Krechevsky-Krech, Griffin, Chow, Nissen, Riesen, Sperry, Pribram, Evarts, and many others. A major goal at Orange Park was to define the functions of primate association cortex. Much of our initial understanding of the behavioral roles of association cortex came from this work. Learning was the primary method used to define the various behavioral functions of association areas, as in complex sensory discriminations. However, Lashley remained pessimistic about ever understanding brain substrates of learning and memory as such.

Lashley's 1929 monograph brought the developing field concerned with brain substrates of memory almost to a halt. The switchboard theory seemed to be wrong, but what were the alternatives? One alternative was field theory. The Gestalt psychologists, Wertheimer, Koffka, and Köhler, developed the notion that perceptions and memories exist as electric fields in the brain. Köhler did a number of animal studies of recording DC potentials from the cortex, with inconclusive results. Lashley and Sperry followed up these notions by implanting conducting and insultating sheets in the cortex and found no effect on learning or memory.

In 1949 Lashley's former student, Donald Hebb, published a theory of brain function and learning that he hoped would rescue the field (54). It had a considerable impact and indeed revitalized the field. Basically it was a modified switchboard theory. A given memory was represented by a set of neurons that had developed increased functional connections. The memories were not thought to be localized to one place but rather to be "distributed." A given memory was represented by a network, or cell assembly, in the cortex and the same neuron could participate in more than one memory. Hebb was deliberately vague about the network of neurons but quite specific about the synaptic mechanisms involved, which has come to be termed the Hebb synapse. He stated that a synaptic connection to a given neuron is strengthened when the synapse is activated in temporal conjunction with the occurrence of an action potential in the postsynaptic neuron. Hebb's synaptic theory was perhaps less important than the fact that he developed a connectionistic view that could work.

Electrical stimulation of the brain as a tool for localization of the memory trace was first used systematically in a now classic series of studies from the laboratory of W. Horsley Gantt at Johns Hopkins (Gantt trained with Pavlov). Gantt, Loucks, Brogden, and others working in Gantt's laboratory attempted to define "the relation of conditioned reflex function to anatomic pathways" using electrical stimulation to elicit the conditioned behavioral response. Brogden and Gantt (16) completed an extremely important series of experiments using electrical stimulation of the cerebellum as the UCS (1942). In brief, they found that a variety of movements elicited by cerebellar stimulation could be conditioned to a tone or a light. Responses as diverse as forelimb flexion and discrete closure of the ipsilateral eyelid conditioned easily.

DEFINITIONS AND ISSUES

Lasting changes in behavior resulting from prior experience can be characterized as the result of learning, memory, and retrieval processes. Most psychologists would agree that there are several forms or categories of learning but would be less likely to agree on the properties that uniquely distinguish them. At this point it is useful to keep the basic definition of learning broad. Thus, bacteria show a kind of memory, their behavior can change as a result of experience (e.g., with certain molecules), and this change can persist after the experience. This example does not fit neatly into any of the common categories of learning but it may well serve as an important model (4, 71).

It has been useful to distinguish two basic categories of learning: nonassociative and associative. Nonassociative learning is said to result from experience with one type of event (e.g., habituation – a decrease in response to repeated stimulation and sensitization – a increase in response following (usually strong) stimulation). Associative learning, resulting from the conjunction of two or more events, is commonly categorized as Pavlovian (or classical) and instrumental conditioning.

In classical conditioning two stimuli are presented with the conditioned stimulus (CS) onset preceding the UCS onset in time. The key defining feature is that the CS and UCS always occur regardless of what the organism does. The UCS typically elicits some type of reflex response. Many psychologists would add that the UCS has a "reinforcement" value, either negative as in shock or positive as in food. Typically the CS does not elicit the response that is elicited by the UCS before training but comes to elicit a (usually) similar response as a result of temporally paired or contingent (but not uncontingent) presentations of CS and UCS. In instrumental learning, presentation of the UCS is made contingent upon the behavior of the organism, as in pressing a lever to obtain food or flexing a limb to avoid shock. At the most basic level, associative learning concerns learning about the causal relationships between events occurring in the organism's environment. From the point of view of neurobiological analysis Pavlovian conditioning has several advantages over instrumental learning, the most important being that the effects of experimental manipulations on learning rather than performance can be more easily evaluated, but both exhibit similar basic properties of associative learning.

The problem of localizing the neuronal substrates of learning and memory has been the greatest barrier to progress and remains fundamental to all work on the biological basis of learning and memory, particularly in the mammalian nervous system, as stressed by Lashley and by Hebb. In order to analyze the biophysical mechanisms that form memory traces it is, obviously, necessary to localize the memory traces, particularly essential memory traces (traces essential, i.e., necessary and sufficient, for the learning and memory of behavioral responses), and this in turn requires identification of the essential memory trace circuits. In the mammalian brain, identification of essential memory trace circuits for associative learning is only now being achieved.

IDENTIFICATION OF ESSENTIAL MEMORY TRACE CIRCUITS IN THE MAMMALIAN BRAIN

Recent evidence strongly supports the view that memory trace circuits, and by inference memory traces, are localized rather than widely distributed in the mammalian brain. But within localized cellular regions the trace(s) can still be distributed among the neural elements or ensembles. Although controversies still exist the weight of evidence argues against memory traces being localized to sensory relay nuclei, motor nuclei, or reflex pathways. The structures currently thought to be most involved in memory trace formation are the cerebellum, hippocampus, amygdala, and the cerebral cortex.

Red Nucleus

A major efferent target of the cerebellar hemisphere, via the superior cerebellar peduncle, is the contralateral red nucleus. It is also a major ipsilateral target of descending fibers from the motor cortex (corticorubral fibers). In turn it gives rise to descending fibers to brain stem and spinal cord (rubrospinal path) which cross and descend contralateral to the cells of origin in the red nucleus. In a most interesting study Smith (127) reported that large unilateral lesions in the red nucleus and vicinity markedly impaired a classically conditioned flexion response of the forelimb contralateral to, but not ipsilateral to, the lesion in cats. (He did not report what effect the lesion had on the reflex response.)

Tsukahara (142, 143) developed an ingenious simplified preparation based on this paradigm. A stimulating electrode serving as the CS is implanted in the cerebral peduncle and the peduncle lesioned caudal to the corticorubral fibers. The UCS is the shock to the contralateral forepaw. The CS pulse train is adjusted to produce a weak flexion response of the forelimb and then the CS and UCS are paired in training. Animals learn the leg-flexion response to peduncle stimulation in several days of training. The shortest latency forelimb EMG response to peduncle stimulation is 8 ms and the latency range is 8 to 34 ms. Excitability and threshold of the system is measured in terms of the behavioral limb flexion to peduncle stimulation. Over the course of training this excitability measure (termed "performance") increases markedly but excitability of the behavioral response to interpositus stimulation does not. Tsukahara argues that since the two pathways are presumably the same from red nucleus to forelimb, the excitability increase is at the synaptic junctions of peduncle fibers on the red nucleus. Recordings from red nucleus neurons show that their probability of response to the CS increases significantly after training. In other work, Tsukahara and associates have shown that lesion-induced sprouting of corticorubral synapses occurs in both neonatal and adult animals and that the newly formed synapses are physiologically effective (142, 143, 144). The corticorubral system is capable of considerable plasticity.

In the case of learning of discrete, adaptive CRs with peripheral stimuli in the normal intact mammal, the red nucleus appears to be efferent from the memory trace (see below). Earlier literature indicates that carnivores can learn a discrete leg-flexion-response following complete neodecortication (see above and (17, 113)). Consequently, although the corticorubral tract may normally be involved in leg-flexion conditioning in the intact animal it is not essential. Cerebellar lesions, on the other hand, do permanently abolish the discrete leg-flexion conditioned response (32). This of course does not rule out plasticity developing in the red nucleus. Indeed, Tsukahara's simplified preparation provides an elegant and important model system for analysis of mechanisms of training-induced neuronal plasticity.

Cerebellum

Ito has developed a most important experimental model of induced neuronal plasticity using plasticity of the vestibulo-ocular reflex (VOR) and applied the general Marr-Albus cerebellar model of motor learning (see e.g. (59, 61, 62)). Plasticity of the VOR was recently reviewed in depth by Miles and Lisberger (95) and Ito (61). In brief, gain control can be altered by using lenses or by moving the visual field and head. The VOR shows a long-lasting adaptation to changed gain. This adaption appears to be neuronal and not simply due to a learned strategy (95). Ablation of the flocculus (60) or of the vestibular cerebellum including the flocculus (117) abolishes VOR adaptation. Miles and Lisberger developed a case against VOR plasticity occurring in the cerebellum in the primate, based primarily on the properties on neuronal unit responses in the flocculus, and suggested instead that it occurs in the brain stem (95). They interpreted the flocculus lesion effect as afferent or modulatory, i.e., the flocculus is important in the induction of VOR plasticity in brain stem neurons (see (95)).

Recent evidence from Ito's laboratory supports his view that plasticity can in fact be established in the flocculus of the rabbit (62). In brief, using the high decerebrate rabbit, responses of identified Purkinje cells were recorded in response to single-pulse stimulation of vestibular nerve (2/s). They showed a short-latency excitatory response. Similar excitation was shown by putative basket cells. Conjunctive stimulation of vestibular nerve (20/s) and inferior olive (4/s) for 25 s (and only conjunctive stimulation) depressed the subsequent excitatory Purkinje cell response to single-pulse stimulation of vestibular nerve for periods as long as a hour (see also (35)). Similarly, iontophoretic application of glutamate (the putative parallel fiber neurotransmitter) (122) in conjunction with 4/s olivary stimulation depressed the subsequent glutamate sensitivity on the Purkinje cells for a period of an hour. Ito thus developed a model of the process where cellular plasticity can develop in the cerebellar cortex. He suggested two possible cellular mechanisms, both of which involve decreased sensitivity of chemical (glutamate?) receptors on Purkinje cells (62). Under different conditions of paired stimulation of mossy fibers and climbing fibers in the intact-behaving rabbit, normal behavioral learned responses (eyelid closure, head turn) can be established (132).

Recent evidence, based primarily on eyelid conditioning as a model system (48, 138), overwhelmingly favors an essential role for the cerebellum in both learning and memory of discrete, adaptive behavioral responses learned to deal with aversive events, thus supporting the general spirit of earlier theories of the role of the cerebellum in motor learning (e.g., 2, 34, 58, 85). Utilizing lesions, electrophysiological recordings, electrical microstimulation, microinfusion of drugs, and anatomical methods a region of the cerebellum ipsilateral to the trained eye (lateral interpositus nucleus) has been shown to be essential for the learning and memory of the conditioned eyelid response but not for the reflex response (23, 78, 88, 90, 91, 139). These effects are ipsilateral in that unilateral cerebellar lesions do not impair learning of responses on the contralateral side of the body. Additional work suggests that this effect holds across CS modalities, skeletal response systems, species, and with instrumental ontingencies (32, 112, 151). Electrophysiological analysis reveals several localized regions of cerebellar cortex and the lateral interpositus nucleus, where neurons (including identified Purkinje cells) develop patterned changes in discharge frequency that precede and predict ("model") the occurrence and form of the learned behavioral response within trials (31, 36, 91).

The essential efferent CR pathway appears to consist of fibers exiting from the interpositus nucleus ipsilateral to the trained side of the body in the superior cerebellar peduncle, crossing to relay in the contralateral magnocellular division of the red nucleus, and crossing back to descend in the rubral pathway to act ultimately on motor neurons (22, 51, 82, 87, 90, 119). Recent lesion and microstimulation evidence argues that the essential UCS-reinforcing pathway, the necessary and sufficient pathway conveying information about the UCS to the cerebellar memory trace circuit, consists of climbing fibers from the dorsal accessory olive projecting via the inferior cerebellar peduncle. Thus, lesions of the appropriate region prevent acquisition and produce normal extinction of the behavioral CR with continued paired training in already trained animals (89), and electrical microstimulation of this same region elicits behavioral responses and serves as an effective UCS for normal learning of behavioral CRs (86). Lesions of the middle cerebellar peduncle, conveying afferents from many sources to the cerebellum as mossy fibers, prevent acquisition and immediately abolish retention of the eyelid CR suggesting that this may be the essential CS pathway (129). Indeed, electrical microstimulation of the mossy fiber system can serve as a very effective CS producing rapid learning when paired with, for example, a corneal airpuff UCS. Finally, appropriate conjoint stimulation of mossy fibers as a CS and climbing fibers as a UCS in the intact behaving animal yields normal behavioral learned responses (132). All of these results taken together build an increasingly strong case for localization of the essential memory traces to the cerebellum. Assuming this to be the case the exact location(s) of the essential memory trace(s) within the cerebellum have not yet been determined (90, 91, 150, 152), but multiple sites are perhaps most consistent with the organization of somatosensory projections to cerebellum (66, 126)

Hypothalamus and Amygdala - Learned Cardiovascular Responses and "Fear"

A relatively consistent picture is emerging from studies on cardiovascular conditioning in three vertebrates. The paradigm is classical conditioning in which a several second auditory or visual CS terminates with an electric shock UCS to some portion of the head or body. In the baboon, small, discrete bilateral lesions of the perifornical region of the hypothalamus abolish the entire learned cardiovascular response complex (heart rate increase, blood pressure increase, etc.) completely, permanently, and selectively (128). The lesion has no effect on reflex cardiovascular responses, on cardiovascular responses associated with exercise, or on a behavioral measure of conditioned "fear" - conditioned suppression of lever pressing. (It is not yet clear whether the critical lesion here is to neuron cell bodies or fibers of passage.) Utilizing lesions, electrical stimulation, neural unit recording, microinfusion of drugs, and anatomical methods much of the essential circuitry for cardiovascular conditioning has been identified in the pigeon (24, 25) and rabbit (41, 65, 123). The essential efferent pathway includes portions of the amygdala, hypothalamus, and descending pathways to brain stem and spinal cord. In the rabbit the lateral subthalamic region appears to be a critical portion of the efferent pathway from the amygdala. Some neurons in the amygdala (rabbit) show increases during the development of the heart rate CR that correlate with the magnitude of the CR (65). In the pigeon, with a visual

CS, any one of three visual pathways can support conditioning, and training-induced modification of neural unit activity occurs at, but not afferent to, central thalamic optic relays. Although it is not yet known where the memory traces are located the amygdala is a possibility; generally it seems more involved in conditioned emotional responses ("fear") (67).

Davis and colleagues have utilized conditioned potentiation of the acoustic startle response in the rat as a model of conditioned emotional state ("fear"). Having earlier defined the acoustic startle reflex pathway (ventral cochlear nucleus to nuclei of lateral lemniscus to nucleus reticularis pontis caudalis to spinal interneurons to motor neurons (26)), they determined that the potentiating effect of a light, previously paired with shock, on the startle response appears to act on the startle circuit at the ventral nucleus of the lateral leminiscus (141). Essential components of the potentiation circuit include the geniculo-cortical visual system and the amygdala (57), as in the cardiovascular learning circuit for a visual CS in the pigeon.

Hippocampus

There exists an extensive literature involving lesion, stimulation, and recording studies of the hippocampus in learning and memory. Olds and co-workers began a pioneering and extensive analysis of cellular responses during a conditioned food retrieval task that involved both classical and instrumental learning (107, 125).

The activity of neurons was usually multiple unit, recorded during paired and unpaired presentations of conditioned stimuli where compared. Localization of primary sites of neural change was a central issue in these studies, and Olds *et al.* (107) reasoned that, during paired conditioning, cells responding with the shortest latencies after CS onset represent such sites. Such cells could not reflect phasic responses of other afferent cells. However, Olds *et al.* recognized the possibility that "short latency sites" may still be reflecting changes in tonic activity from afferent projections. In a wide sample of brain areas Olds *et al.* showed that the hippocampus, specifically the CA3 field, exhibited among the shortest latency responses after CS presentation. Segal and Olds (125) continued analysis of the hippocampal system and reported, in terms of changes in cell activity across trials, that the dentate gyrus was the first component of the hippocampus to reveal significant increases above spontaneous firing rates. Later in training, CA3 and then CA1 cell regions exhibited discriminative responding in accordance with the principle circuit of the hippocampus.

The effect of hippocampal ablation was not specifically tested on the paradigm used by Olds, but all other evidence suggests that an intact hippocampus is not required for learning such a task (33, 56, 68, 106). Discrimination reversal is one type of learning which is consistently impaired by damage to the hippocampal system (7, 56), and Disterhoft and Segal (30) examined the activity of hippocampal pyramidal and granule cells during two-tone discrimination and reversal of food retrieval behavior. They showed that hipppocampal cells exhibited differentially enhanced discharges to the CS+ after differential behavioral responding had stabilized. Interestingly, within subsequent reversal session, hippocampal neurons maintained elevated rates of response to the previous CS+ (the new CS-) and changed (increased) response rates only to the new CS+ (the previous CS-). Thus, hippocampal activity was more closely related to changing behavioral responsiveness than to the positively reinforced stimulus and did not orrelate well with changing behavioral responsiveness to the nonreinforced CS.

Berger and Thompson (9, 10) used classical conditioning of the rabbit nictitating membrane eyelid response to study the activity of hippocampus and other limbic system neurons during classical conditioning (see also (5, 13)). Initial studies showed that neurons recorded from the pyramidal cell region of the hippocampus increased the frequency of discharge very early during the course of training and preceded onset of conditioned behavioral responding by a considerable number of trials. Extinction of the behavioral response is associated with a decrease in the frequency of firing hippocampal neurons. Within conditioning trials hippocampal cells exhibit a distinctive pattern of firing that correlates highly with amplitude of the conditioned behavioral response (6). In this sense the firing of hippocampal neurons produces a "temporal model" of the learned behavior (137). Berry and associates (12) used an appetitive classical conitioning task, conditioned jaw movements to sweetened water in water-deprived rabbits, and showed that unit activity in the CA1 pyramidal region shows contingency-dependent responses that develop in the first 5-10 trials and form a predictive temporal model of the behavioral conditioned response, which is a rhythmic 7-9 Hz jaw movement, thus extending the hippocampal "temporal model" phenomenon to appetitive learning.

Single unit analyses of physiologically identified cell groups in eyelid conditioning have shown that pyramidal neurons are the hippocampal cell type modified during conditioning and that other cell types exhibit different response patterns (8, 11). Additional studies have demonstrated that hippocampal cellular plasticity also occurs with these characteristics in other species besides the rabbit (110), with the use of at least two different sensory modalities as the CS, and when response systems other than the nictitating membrane are conditioned (136). Although the hippocampus is not essential for the basic learned behavioral response, several lines of evidence indicate that long-lasting neuronal plasticity coding this hippocampal "memory trace" develops within the hippocampus. Thus, there is a persisting increase in the perforant path-granule cell synapse excitability analogous to that seen with long-term potentiation (LTP) (149). In addition, there is a learning-specific, persistent increase in glutam te receptor binding in hippocampal membranes following training (84). Finally, Disterhoft, Coulter, and Alkon (29) reported a persistent decrease in afterhyperpolarization in pyramidal neurons studied in the hippocampal explant in trained vs control animals, thought due to a decrease in Ca^{2+} activated outward K^+ conductance.

In an appetitive instrumental learning task in the rat, Deadwyler and associates (27, 28) have shown that two-tone, CS-evoked dentate field potentials of differing waveform and latency develop differentially over training, discrimination, and reversal. Both the shorter latency response and differential behavioral response are impaired by damage to entorhinal cortex. Lesions of the hippocampus (and septal nuclei) have also been shown to impair severely learning of spatial tasks in the rat (see (106)), but so have frontal cortical lesions (69). Consistent with the hippocampal lesion effect are electrophysiological data demonstrating strong correlations between increased firing of certain hippocampal neurons and location of an animal in space (97, 104, 105, 109). This evidence has been interpreted within the framework of "spatial memory" (106), but Olton *et al.* (108) have developed an alternative interpretation in terms of "working memory." It is not clear whether the spatial correlates of hippocampal neurons develop as a result of learning. In fact, available evidence indicates that spatial correlates of hippocampal cells are present at an animal's first exposure to a new environment and are not modified by time or experience in that environment (55, 72). Furthermore, the same unit will respond in a particular place in a maze and in half of a lever press box (72). Thus, although demonstrations of spatially related unit correlates are quite striking their relation to specific sensory information and to associative learning is uncertain. The syndrome of HM (human amnesia resulting from bilateral temporal lobe damage) has proved very difficult to replicate in animals. Indeed, it was only in 1978 that Mishkin (101) showed that a similar deficit in memory function (recent visual memory – delayed nonmatching to sample) can be produced in monkeys subjected to bilateral ablation of both the hippocampus and amygdala. The deficit that follows bilateral ablation of either structure alone is much less pronounced (see following section on *Temporal lobes*). But Squire and Zola-Morgan (130) have recently shown that lesions of the hippocampus alone can also yield this deficit, so the role of the amygdala is not clear.

To state some oversimplified conclusions the hippocampus appears to play some kind of role in the storage and/or retrieval of memories but is not itself the essential site of long-term memory storage in animals or humans. In many cases the role the hippocampus plays is modulatory in nature. Manipulations of it can influence performance in learning and memory tasks but it is not itself an essential part of the memory trace circuits. Possible exceptions to this last generalization are the important role the hippocampus appears to play in certain spatial memory tasks in the rat and in recent visual memory performance in the monkey, not to mention its apparently critical role in certain aspects of human memory.

Cerebral Cortex

Frontal lobes. The most prominent, consistent, and general behavioral deficit following frontal lobe lesions is seen in the delayed-response problem (37, 63, 80, 98, 114, 115, 135) as an inability to remember, even for very short durations, under which cup a reward is placed if a screen is lowered during the delay. The first demonstration of double dissociation (a criterion proposed by Teuber, (134)) was made between the functions of the frontal and temporal cortices (53). Lesions of the frontal cortex resulted in a deficit delayed response but not visual discrimination tasks, whereas lesions of the temporal lobe had the opposite results. The effective frontal locus for delayed response is a few millimeters in the middle of the principle sulcus (19, 20).

The deficit can be seen as memorial or attentional (or both); these interpretations are given full consideration in a detailed review by Fuster (38). Distractions interfere with memory storage and such effects may account in part for the delayed response deficit. Animals with frontal lesions can have very good memories if not distracted (53, 83, 92, 94). The pause in delayed response testing (e.g., (63)) and in delayed alternation testing (120, 121, 131) may cause performance deficits in part through distractions and massed testing, which enhance perseverative tendencies (93, 116). The deficits caused by frontal lobe lesions on conditioned inhibition (18, 70, 80) and discrimination reversal (see (147)) may share a similar problem of interpretation.

Recent studies have added significantly to our understanding of the frontal lobes. Modern anatomical studies demonstrate afferent (47) and efferent connections (124) between the frontal and parietal cortices as well as columnar organization within the frontal cortex (44). Similarly, functional differences between the orbital (e.g., object discrimination) and dorsolateral (e.g., delayed response) prefrontal cortices have been described (1, 42, 43, 45, 46, 52, 96, 99, 145, 146).

Unit activity in the frontal cortex has been measured extensively in behaving animals since it was first described for monkeys trained on delayed response (14, 40) or delayed alternation (74). Several basic firing patterns have been described (39). Most cells react to stimulus presentation. Many cells react to the stimulus if it has meaning due to previous experience (i.e., learning, context?). Some cells react to the rewarding stimulus. Some display sustained cell discharge during the delay period that appears to be related to performance of the task and may be involved in temporal integration. A particularly interesting type of cell seems to be related to sensory-motor integration (73). It appears, then, that the types of cell activities found in the frontal cortex support the notion that the frontal cortex is involved in determining situational context and appropriate goal-directed behaviors and perhaps in the retention process itself.

Temporal lobes. In general, bilateral lesions of the inferotemporal area do not abolish the ability of monkeys to discriminate between real objects but do abolish their ability to discriminate visual forms (i.e., two-dimensional pictures of forms). The essential circuit for this latter discrimination includes the striate, peristriate, and inferotemporal areas (100). Monkeys were trained to discriminate between pictures of a cross and square. Serial lesions were performed to make lesions of the unilateral inferotemporal cortex and contralateral occipital cortex. Relearning between operations and re-relearning after the two surgeries yielded good retention. However, when the splenium of the corpus callosum was subsequently cut, thus preventing visual processing between the intact striate-peristriate cortex on one side with the contralateral peristriate-inferotemporal cortex, the animals lost the ability to discriminate the visual patterns. This result supports the idea that cortical processing is serial.

Mishkin (102) recently demonstrated an interaction between inferotemporal cortex and the amygdala-hippocampus in an analogous crossed-lesion experiment for recent visual memory. The test used was delayed nonmatching-to-sample with increasing delays and increasing lists of stimuli. Monkeys with crossed inferotemporal cortex and amygdala-hippocampal lesions and with resection of the anterior commissure performed nearly as poorly on visual recognition as did monkeys given bilateral amygdala-hippocampal lesions (103). Mishkin (102) proposes that short-term visual memories may be stored within the inferotemporal cortex by actions of the amygdala-hippopcampus complex, but the actual locus of storage is, of course, not yet known (see above section on *Hippocampus*).

Consistent with these observations are the recent findings from Rolls' laboratory (3). They found that 26 of 421 neurons sampled in the inferotemporal cortex of monkey showed activity that appeared related to memorial function in a delayed matching-to-sample task. Specifically, they responded to a familiar stimulus if it was presented after having been presented as a novel stimulus, but only if no other stimuli intervened. Thus, such neurons respond only "in relation to relatively short-term memory aspects of these tasks so that the longer term aspects of the memory required for this type of recognition appear to be processed in structures beyond the ITC."

CONCLUSION

In so far as candidate sites for memory storage in the mammalian brain are concerned, current evidence is strongest for the cerebellum as the storage site for the learning of discrete, adaptive skeletal muscle responses, and plasticity of the vestibulo-ocular reflex. The red nucleus is capable of experience-induced neuronal plasticity but such plasticity does not appear to be essential for normal behavioral learning of discrete, adaptive responses. Similarly learning-induced plasticity develops in the hippocampus in a range of paradigms but the hippocampus itself does not appear to be the site of long-term storage. The amygdala is critically involved in learned cardiovascular responses and in "conditioned fear" but it is not yet known whether the essential memory traces are in fact stored there. In the cerebral cortex, perhaps the most suggestive evidence comes from studies of the sulcus principalis in the frontal lobe, which appears to be critically involved in, and might even be a locus for, short-term memory, at least in the delayed response paradigm. In general, other clear evidence regarding memory storage in the cerebral cortex is surprisingly sparse (but see recent work from Rolls' laboratory (118)). The human clinical literature would certainly seem to suggest that memories for language are stored in the cerebral cortex.

Acknowledgements. Supported in part by grants from the National Science Foundation (BNS-8106648), the Office of Naval Research (N00014-83-K-0238), the McKnight Foundation and the Sloan Foundation.

REFERENCES

(1) Akert, K.; Orth, O.S.; Harlow, H.F.; and Schiltz, K.A. 1960. Learned behavior of rhesus monkeys following neonatal prefrontal lobotomy. *Science* 132: 1944-1945.

(2) Albus, J.S. 1971. A theory of cerebellar function. *Math. Biosci.* 10: 25-61.

(3) Baylis, G.C., and Rolls, E.T. 1983. Responses of neurons in the inferior temporal visual cortex in long and short term memory tasks. *Soc. Neurosc. Abstr.* 9: 21.

(4) Berg, H.C. 1975. Bacterial behavior. *Nature* 254: 389.

(5) Berger, T.W.; Berry, S.D.; and Thompson, R.F., 1986. Role of the hippocampus in classical conditioning of the aversive and appetitive behavior. In *The Hippocampus*, eds. R.L. Isaacson and K.H. Pribram, vol. II and IV. New York: Plenum Press, in press.

(6) Berger, T.W.; Clark, G.A.; and Thompson, R.F. 1980. Learning-dependent neuronal responses recorded from limbic system brain structures during classical conditioning. *Physl. Psych.* 8(2): 155-167.

(7) Berger, T.W.; and Orr, W.B. 1982. In *Conditioning: Representation of Involved Neural Functions*, ed. C.D. Woody, pp. 1-12. New York: Plenum.

(8) Berger, T.W.; Rinaldi, P.; Weisz, D.J.; and Thompson, R.F. 1983. Single unit analysis of different hippocampal cell types during classical conditioning of the rabbit nictitating membrane response. *J. Neurophysl.* 50(5): 1197-1219.

(9) Berger, T.W., and Thompson, R.F. 1978. Identification of pyramidal cells as the critical elements in hippocampal neuronal plasticity during learning. *Proc. Natl. Acad. Sci.* 75: 1572-1576.

(10) Berger, T.W., and Thompson, R.F. 1978. Neuronal plasticity in the limbic system during classical conditioning of the rabbit

nictitating membrane response. I. The hippocampus. *Brain Res.* 145: 323-346.

(11) Berger, T.W., and Thompson, R.F. 1978. Neuronal plasticity in the limbic system during classical conditioning of the rabbit nictitating membrane response. II. Septum and mamillary bodies. *Brain Res.* 156: 293-314.

(12) Berry, S.D., and Oliver, C.G. 1983. Hippocampal activity during appetitive classical conditioning in rabbits. *Soc. Neurosc. Abstr.* 9: 645.

(13) Berry, S.D., and Thompson, R.F. 1978. Prediction of learning rate from the hippocampal EEG. *Science* 200: 1298-1300.

(14) Blake, M.O.; Meyer, D.R.; and Meyer, P.M. 1966. Enforced observation in delayed response learning by frontal monkeys. *J. Comp. Physl. Psych.* 61: 374-379.

(15) Boring, E.G. 1950. A History of Experimental Psychology, 2nd. ed. New York: Appleton-Century-Crofts.

(16) Brogden, W.J., and Gantt, W.H. 1942. Interneural conditioning: cerebellar conditioned reflexes. *Arch. Neurol. Psychiat.* 48: 437-455.

(17) Bromily, R.B. 1948. Conditioned responses in a dog after removal of neocortex. *J. Comp. Physl. Psych.* 41: 102-110.

(18) Brutkowski, S. 1964. Prefrontal cortex and drive inhibition. In *The Frontal Granular Cortex and Behavior*, eds. J.S. Warren and K. Akert. New York: McGraw-Hill.

(19) Butters, N., and Pandya, D. 1969. Retention of delayed-alternation: effect of selective lesions of sulcus principalis. *Science* 165: 1271-1273.

(20) Butters, N.; Pandya, D.; Sanders, K; and Dye, P. Behavioral deficits in monkeys after selective lesions within the middle third of sulcus principalis. *J. Comp. Physl. Psych.* 76: 8-14.

(21) Cajal, S.R. 1894. La fine structure des centres nerveux. *P. Roy. Soc. Lon.* B 55: 444-468.

(22) Chapman, P.F.; Steinmetz, J.E.; and Thompson, R.F. 1985. Classical conditioning of the rabbit eyeblink does not occur with stimulation of the cerebellar nuclei as the unconditioned stimulus. *Neurosci. Abstr.* 11: 835.

(23) Clark, G.A.; McCormick, D.A.; Lavond, D.G.; and Thompson, R.F. 1984. Effects of lesions of cerebellar nuclei on conditioned behavioral and hippocampal neuronal responses. *Brain Res.* 291: 125-136.

(24) Cohen, D.H. 1980. The functional neuroanatomy of a conditioned response. In *Neural Mechanisms of Goal-directed Behavior and Learning*, eds. R.F. Thompson, L.H. Hicks, and V.B. Shvyrkov. New York: Academic Press.

(25) Cohen, D.H. 1982. Central processing time for a conditioned response in a vertebrate model system. In *Conditioning: Representation of Involved Neural Functions*, ed. C.D. Woody, pp. 517-534. New York: Plenum Press.

(26) Davis, M.; Gendelman, D.S.; Tischler, M.D.; and Gendelman, P.M. 1982. A primary acoustic startle circuit: lesion and stimulation studies. *J. Neurosci.* 2: 791-805.

(27) Deadwyler, S.A.; West, M.; and Lynch, G. 1979. Activity of dentate granule cells during learning: differentiation of perforant path input. *Brain Res.* 169: 29-43.

(28) Deadwyler, S.A.; West, M.; and Robinson, J.H. 1981. Entorhinal and septal inputs differentially control sensory-evoked responses in the rat dentate gyrus. *Science* 211: 1181-1183.

(29) Disterhoft, J.F.; Coulter, D.A.; and Alkon, D.L. 1986. Conditioning-specific membrane changes of rabbit hippocampal neurons measured *in vitro*. *Proc. Natl. Acad. Sci.*, in press.

(30) Disterhoft, J.F., and Segal, M. 1978. Neuron activity in rat hippocampus and motor cortex during discrimination reversal. *Brain Res. B*. 3: 583-588.

(31) Donegan, N.H.; Foy, M.R.; and Thompson, R.F. 1985. Neuronal responses of the rabbit cerebellar cortex during performance of the classically conditioned eyelid response. *Neurosci. Abstr.* 11: 835.

(32) Donegan, N.H.; Lowry, R.W.; and Thompson, R.F. 1983. Effects of lesioning cerebellar nuclei on coditioned leg-flexion responses. *Neurosci. Abstr.* 9: 331.

(33) Douglas, R.J. 1967. The hippocampus and behavior. *Psychol.* 67: 416-442.

(34) Eccles, J.C. 1977. An instruction-selection theory of learning in the cerebellar cortex. *Brain Res.* 127: 327-352.

(35) Ekerot, C.F., and Kano, M. 1985. Long-term depression of parallel fibre synapses following stimulation of climbing fibres. *Brain Res.* 342: 357-360.

(36) Foy, M.R.; Steinmetz, J.E.; and Thompson, R.F. 1984. Single unit analysis of cerebellum during classically conditioned eyelid response. *Neurosci. Abstr.* 10: 122.

(37) French, G.M., and Harlow, H.F. 1962. Variability of delayed-reaction performance and in normal and brain-damaged rhesus monkeys. *J. Neurophysl.* 25: 585-599.

(38) Fuster, J.M. 1980. The Prefrontal Cortex: Anatomy, Physiology and Neuropsychology of the Frontal Lobes. New York: Raven.

(39) Fuster, J.M. 1984. Behavioral electrophysiology of the prefrontal cortex. *Trends Neur.* 7: 408-414.

(40) Fuster, J.M., and Alexander, G.E. 1971. Neuronal activity related to short-term and memory. *Science* 173: 652-654.

(41) Gallagher, M.; Kapp, B.S.; McNall, C.L.; and Pascoe, J.P. 1981. Opiate effects in the amygdala central nucleus on heart rate conditioning in rabbits. *Pharm. Biochem. Behav.* 14: 497-505.

(42) Goldman, P.S. 1971. Functional development of the prefrontal cortex in early life and the problem of neuronal plasticity. *Exp. Neurol.* 32: 366-387.

(43) Goldman, P.S. 1972. Developmental determinants of cortical plasticity. *Acta Neurobiol. Exp.* 32: 495-511.

(44) Goldman, P.S., and Nauta, W.J.H. 1977. Columnar distribution of cortico-cortical fibers in the frontal association, motor, and limbic cortex of the developing rhesus monkey. *Brain Res.* 122: 393-413.

(45) Goldman, P.S.; Rosvold, H.E.; and Mishkin, M. 1970. Evidence for behavioral impairment following prefrontal lobectomy in the infant monkey. *J. Comp. Physl. Psych.* 70: 454-463.

(46) Goldman, P.S.; Rosvold, H.E.; Mishkin, M. 1970. Selective sparing of function following prefrontal lobectomy in infant monkeys. *Exp. Neurol.* 29: 221-226.

(47) Goldman-Rakic, P.S., and Schwartz, M.L. 1982. Interdigitation of contralateral and ipsilateral columnar projections to frontal association cortex in primates. *Science* 216: 755-757.

(48) Gormezano, I. 1972. Investigations of defense and reward conditioning in the rabbit. In *Classical Conditioning II: Current Research and Theory*, eds. A.H. Black and W.F. Prokasy, pp. 151-181. New York: Appleton-Century-Crofts.

(49) Groves, P.M., and Thompson, R.F. 1970. Habituation: a dual-process theory. *Anal. Rev.* 77: 419-450.

(50) Guthrie, E. 1935. The Psychology of Learning. New York: Harper & Row.

(51) Haley, D.A.; Lavond, D.G.; and Thompson R.F. 1983. Effects of contralateral red nucleaer lesions on retention of the classically conditioned nictitating membrane/eyelid response. *Neurosci. Abstr.* 9: 643.

(52) Harlow, H.F.; Blomquist, A.J.; Thompson, C.I.; Schiltz, K.A.; and Harlow, M.K. 1968. In *The Neuropsychology of Development, ed. R. Isaacson*, pp. 79-120. New York: J.Wiley and Sons.

(53) Harlow, H.F.; Davis, R.T.; Settlage, P.H.; and Meyer, D.R. 1952. Analysis of frontal and posterior association syndromes in brain-damaged monkeys. *J. Comp. Physl. Psych.* 45: 419-429.

(54) Hebb, D.O. 1949. The Organization of Behavior. New York: J. Wiley & Sons.

(55) Hill, A.J. 1978. First occurrence of hippocampal spatial firing in a new environment. *Exp. Neurol.* 62: 282-297.

(56) Hirsh, R. 1974. The hippopcampus and contextual retrieval of information from memory: a theory. *Behav. Biol.* 12: 421-444.

(57) Hitchcock, J.M., and Davis, M. 1986. Lesions of the amygdala, but not of the cerebellum or red nucleus, block conditioned fear as measured with the potentiated startle paradigm. *Behav. Neur.* 100(1): 11-22.

(58) Ito, M. 1968. Neurophysiological aspects of the cerebellar motor control system. *Int. J. Neurol.* 7: 162-176.

(59) Ito, M. 1970. Neurophysiological aspects of the cerebellar motor control system. *Int. J. Neurol.* 7: 162-176.

(60) Ito, M. 1974. The control mechanisms of cerebellar motor system. In *The Neurosciences, Third Study Program*, eds. F.O. Schmitt and R.G. Worden. Boston: MIT Press.

(61) Ito, M. 1982. Cerebellar control of the vestibulo-ocular reflex around the flocculus hypothesis. *Ann. R. Neurosci.* 5: 275-296.

(62) Ito, M. 1984. The Cerebellum and Neural Control. New York: Raven Press.

(63) Jacobsen, C.F. 1936. Studies of cerebral functions in primates. I. The functions of the frontal association areas in monkeys. *Comp. Psychol. Monogr.* 23: 101-112.

(64) James, W. 1890. Principles of Psychology. New York: Holt.

(65) Kapp, B.S.; Gallagher, M.; Applegate, C.D.; and Frysinger, R.C. 1982. The amygdala central nucleus: contributions to conditioned cardiovascular responding during aversive Pavlovian conditioning in the rabbit. In *Conditioning: Representation of Involved Neural Functions*, ed. C.D. Woody, pp. 581-600. New York: Plenum.

(66) Kassel, J.; Shambes, G.M.; and Welker, W. 1984. Fractured cutaneous projections to the granule cell layer of the posterior cerebellar hemmisphere of the domestic cat. *J. Comp. Neur.* 225: 458-468.

(67) Kesner, R.P., and Wilbrun, M.W. 1974. A review of electrical stimulation of the brain in the context of learning and retention. *Behav. Biol.* 10: 259-293.

(68) Kimble, D.P. 1968. Hippocampus and internal inhibition. *Psychol. B.* 70: 285-295.

(69) Kolb, B.; Sutherland, R.J.; and Wishaw, I.Q. 1982. A comparison of the contributions of the frontal and parietal association cortex to spatial localization in rats. *Behav. Neuro.* 97: 13-27.

(70) Konorski, J. 1961. The physiological approach to the problem of recent memory. In *Brain Mechanisms and Learning*, ed. J.F. Delafresnaye. Oxford: Blackwell.

(71) Koshland, D.E. 1980. Bacterial Chemotoxis as a Model Behavioral System. New York: Raven Press.

(72) Kubie, J.L., and Ranck, J.G., Jr. 1982. Tonic and phasic firing of rat hippocampal complex-spike cells in three different situations: context and place. In *Conditioning: Representation of Involved Neural Functions*, ed. C.D. Woody. New York: Plenum Press.

(73) Kubota, K.; Iwamoto, T.; and Suzuki, H. 1974. Visuokinetic activities of primate prefrontal neurons during delayed-response performance. *J. Neurophysl.* 37: 1197-1212.

(74) Kubota, K., and Niki, H. 1971. Prefrontal cortical unit activity and delayed alternation performance in monkeys. *J. Neurophysl.* 34: 337-347.

(75) Lashley, K.S. 1929. Brain Mechanisms and Intelligence. Chicago: University of Chicago Press.

(76) Lashley, K.S. 1950. In search of the engram. In *Symp. Soc. Exp. Biol.*, no. 4: 454-482. New York: Cambridge University Press.

(77) Lashley, K.S., and Franz, S.I. 1917. The effects of cerebral destruction upon habit-formation and retention in the albino rat. *Psychobiology* 71-139.

(78) Lavond, D.G.; Lincoln, J.S.; McCormick, D.A.; and Thompson, R.F. 1984. Effect of bilateral lesions of the dentate interpositus cerebellar nuclei on conditioning of heart-rate and nictitating membrane/eyelid responses in the rabbit. *Brain Res.* 305: 323-330.

(79) Lavond, D.G.; McCormick, D.A.; and Thompson, R.F. 1984. A nonrecoverable learning deficit. *Physl. Psych.* 12(2): 103-110.

(80) Lawicka, W., and Konorski, J. 1959. The physiological mechanism of delayed reations. III. The effects of prefrontal ablations on delayed reactions in dogs. *Acta Biol. Exp.* 19: 221-231.

(81) Lugaro, E. 1899. I recenti progressi dell' anatomia del sistema nervoso in repporto alla psicologia et alla psichiatria. Riv. Patol. nerv. ment., t. IV: fasc. 11-12- (Cited in Cajal, 1911).

(82) Madden, J., IV; Haley, D.A.; Barchas, J.D.; and Thompson, R.F. 1983. Microinfusion of picrotoxin into the caudal red nucleus selectively abolishes the classically conditioned nictitating membrane/eyelid response in the rabbit. *Neurosci. Abstr.* 9: 830.

(83) Malmo, R.B. 1984. Interference factors in delayed response in monkeys after removal of frontal lobes. *J. Neurophysl.* 5: 295-308.

(84) Mamounas, L.A.; Thompson, R.F.; Lynch, D.G.; and Baudry, M. 1984. Classical conditioning of the rabbit eyelid response increases glutamate receptor binding in hippocampal synaptic membranes. *Proc. Natl. Acad. Sci.* 81(8): 2548-2552.

(85) Marr, D. 1969. A theory of cerebellar cortex. *J. Physl. Lon.* 202: 437-470.

(86) Mauk, M.D., and Thompson, R.F. 1984. Classical conditioning using stimulation of the inferior olive as the unconditioned stimulus. *Neurosci. Abstr.* 10: 122.

(87) McCormick, D.A.; Guyer, P.E.; and Thompson, R.F. 1982. Superior cerebellar peduncle lesions selectively abolish the ipsilateral classically conditioned nictitating membrane/eyelid response of the rabbit. *Brain Res.* 244: 347-350.

(88) McCormick, D.A.; Lavond, D.G.; Clark, G.A.; Kettner, R.E.; Rising, C.E.; and Thompson, R.F. 1981. The engram found? Role of the cerebellum in classical conditioning of nictitating membrane and eyelid responses. *B. Psychon. Soc.* 18(3): 103-105.

(89) McCormick, D.A.; Steinmetz, J.E.; and Thompson, R.F. 1985. Lesions of the inferior olivary complex cause extinction of the classically conditioned eyeblink response. *Brain Res.* 359: 120-130.

(90) McCormick, D.A., and Thompson, R.F. 1984. Cerebellum: essential involvement in the classically conditioned eyelid response. *Science* 223: 269-299.

(91) McMcCormick, D.A., and Thompson, R.F. 1984. Neuronal responses of the rabbit cerebellum during acquisition and performance of a classically conditioned nictitating membrane-eyelid response. *J. Neurosci.* 4(11): 2811-2822.

(92) Meyer, D.R. 1972. Some features of the dorsolateral frontal and infero-temporal syndromes in monkeys. *Acta Neurobiol. Exp.* 32: 235-260.

(93) Meyer, D.R.; Hughes, H.C.; Buchholz, D.J.; Dalhouse, A.D.; Enlow, L.J.; and Meyer, P.M. 1976. Effects of successive

unilateral ablations of principalis cortex upon performances of delayed alternation and delayed response by monkeys. *Brain Res.* 108: 397-412.

(94) Meyer, D.R., and Settlage, P.H. 1958. Analysis of simple searching behavior in the frontal monkey. *J. Comp. Physl. Psych.* 51: 408-410.

(95) Miles, F.A., and Lisberger, S.G. 1981. Plasticity in the vestibulo-ocular reflex: a new hypothesis. *Ann. R. Neur.* 4: 273-299.

(96) Miller, E.A.; Goldman, P.S.; and Rosvold, H.E. 1973. Delayed recovery of function following orbital prefrontal lesions in infant monkeys. *Science* 182: 304-306.

(97) Miller, V.M., and Best, P.J. 1980. Spatial correlates of hippocampal unit activity are altered by lesions of the fornix and endorhinal cortex. *Brain Res.* 194: 311-323.

(98) Milner, B. 1972. Disorders of learning and memory after temporal lobe lesions in man. *Clin. Neurosurg.* 19: 421-446.

(99) Mishkin, M. 1964. Perseveration of central sets after frontal lesions in monkeys. In *The Frontal Granular Cortex and Behavior*, eds. J.M. Warren and K. Akert, pp. 219-237. New York: McGraw-Hill.

(100) Mishkin, M. 1966. Visual mechanisms beyond the striate cortex. In *Frontiers in Physiological Psychology*, ed. R.W. Russell, pp, 93-119. New York: Academic Press.

(101) Mishkin, M. 1978. Memory in monkeys severely impaired by combined but not by separate removal of amygdala and hippocampus. *Nature* 273: 297-298.

(102) Mishkin, M. 1982. A memory system in the monkey. *Phil. Trans. Roy. Soc. Lon. B.* 298: 85-95.

(103) Mishkin, M.; Spiegler, B.J.; Saunders, R.C.; and Malamut, B.L. 1982. An animal model of global amnesia. In *Alzheimer's Disease: A Review of Progress*, eds. S. Corkin, K.L. Davies, J.H. Growde, E. Usdin, and R.J. Wurtman. New York: Raven Press.

(104) O'Keefe, J. 1979. Place units in the hippocampus of the freely moving rat. *Exp. Neurol.* 51: 78-109.

(105) O'Keefe, J., and Conway, D.H. 1978. Hippocampal place units in the freely moving rat: why they fire where they fire. *Exp. Brain Res.* 31: 573-590.

(106) O'Keefe, J., and Nadel, L. 1978. The Hippocampus as a Cognitive Map. Oxford: Clarendon Press.

(107) Olds, J.; Disterfhoft, J.F.; Segal, M.; Hornblith, C.L.; and Hirsch, R. 1972. Learning centers of rat brain mapped by measuring

latencies of conditioned unit responses. *J. Neurophysics* 35: 202-219.

(108) Olton, D.S.; Becker, J.T.; and Handelmann, G.E. 1980. Hippocampal function: working memory or cognitive mapping. *Physl. Psych.* 8(2): 239-246.

(109) Olton, D.S.; Branch, M.; and Best, P.J. 1978. Spatial correlates of hippocampal unit activity. *Exp. Neurol.* 58: 387-409.

(110) Patterson, M.M.; Berger, T.W.; and Thompson, R.F. 1979. Neuronal plasticity recorded from cat hippocampus during classical conditioning. *Brain Res.* 163: 339-343.

(111) Pavlov, I.P. 1927. Conditioned Reflexes. Oxford: Oxford University Press.

(112) Polenchar, B.E., and Patterson, M.M. 1984. Cerebellar deep nuclei lesions abolish or impair an instrumental avoidance response in rabbit. *Soc. Neurosc. Abstr.* 10(1): 123.

(113) Poltrew, S.S., and Zeliony, G.P. 1930. Grosshirnrinde und Assoziationsfunction. *Zoologie Biologie* 90: 157-160.

(114) Pribram, K.H.; Krugger, L.; Robinson, F.; and Berman, A.J. 1955. The effects of precentral lesions on the behavior of monkeys. *Yale J. Biol.* 28: 428-443.

(115) Pribram, K.H.; Mishkin, M.; Rosvold, H.E.; and Kaplan, S.J. 1952. Effects on delayed-response performance of lesions of dorsolateral and ventromedial cortex of baboons. *J. Comp. Physl. Psych.* 45: 567-575.

(116) Pribram, K.H., and Tubbs, W.E. 1967. Short-term memory, parsing, and the primate frontal cortex. *Science* 156: 1765-1767.

(117) Robinson, D.A. 1976. Adaptive gain control of vestibulo-ocular reflex by the cerebellum. *J. Neurophysl.* 39: 954-969.

(118) Rolls, E.T. 1984. Neurons in the cortex of the temporal lobe and in the amygdala of the monkey with responses selective for faces. *Human Neurobiol.* 3: 209-222.

(119) Rosenfield, M.E.; Devydaitis, A.; and Moore, J.W. 1985. *Brachium conjunctivum* and rubrobulbar tract: brainstem projections of red nucleus essential for the conditioned nictitating membrane response. *Physl. Behav.* 34: 751-759.

(120) Rosvold, H.E., and Delgado, J.M.R. 1956. The effect on delayed alternation test performance of stimulating or destroying electrically structures within the frontal lobes of the monkey's brain. *J. Comp. Physl. Psych.* 49: 365-372.

(121) Rosvold, H.E.; Mishkin, M.; and Szwarcbart, M.K. 1958. Effects of subcortical lesions in monkeys on visual-discrimination and

single-alternation performance. *J. Comp. Physl. Psych.* 51: 437-444.

(122) Sandoval, M.E., and Cotman, C.W. 1978. Evaluation of glutamate as a neurotransmitter of cerebellar parallel fibers. *Neuroscience* 3: 199-206.

(123) Schneiderman, N.; McCabe, P.M.; Haselton, J.R.; and Ellenberger, H.H. 1986. Neurobiological bases of conditioned bradycardia. In *Classical Conditioning III: Behavioral, Neurophysiological, and Neurochemical Studies in the Rabbit*, eds. I. Gormezano, W.F. Prokasy, and R.F. Thompson. Hillsdale, NJ: Erlbaum, in press.

(124) Schwartz, M.L., and Goldman-Rakic, P.S. 1984. Ipsilateral and contralateral connectivity of the prefrontal association cortex: relation between intraparietal and principal sulcal cortex. *J. Comp. Neur.* 226: 403-420.

(125) Segal, M., and Olds, J. 1972. The behavior of units in the hippocampal circuit of the rat during learning. *J. Neurophysl.* 35: 680-690.

(126) Shambes, G.M.; Gibson, J.M.; and Welker, W. 1978. Fractured somatotopy in granule cell tactile areas of rat cerebellar hemispheres revealed by micromapping. *Brain Behav.* 15: 94-140.

(127) Smith, A.M. 1970. The effects of rubral lesions and stimulation on conditioned forelimb flexion responses in the cat. *Physl. Behav.* 5: 1121-1126.

(128) Smith, O.A.; Astley, C.A.; DeVit, J.L.; Stein, J.M.; and Walsh, K.E. 1980. Functional analysis of hypothalamic control of the cardiovascular responses accompanying emotional behavior. *Fed. Proc.* 39(8): 2487-2494.

(129) Solomon, P.R.; Lewis, J.L.; LoTurco, J.J.; Steinmetz J.E.; and Thompson, R.F. 1986. The role of the middle cerebellar peduncle in acquisition and retention of the rabbits classically conditioned nictitating membrane response. *B. Psychon. Soc.*, in press.

(130) Squire, L.R., and Zola-Morgan, S. 1983. The neurology of memory: the case for correspondence between the findings for man and non-human primate. In *The Physiological Basis of Memory*, 2nd. ed., ed. J.A. Deutsch. New York: Academic Press.

(131) Stamm, J.S. 1964. Retardation and facilitation in learning by stimulation of frontal cortex in monkeys. In *The Frontal Granular Cortex and Behavior*, eds. J.M. Warren and K. Akert, pp. 102-125. New York: McGraw-Hill.

(132) Steinmetz, J.E.; Lavond, D.G.; and Thompson, R.F. 1985. Classical conditioning of the rabbit eyelid response with mossy

fiber stimulation as the conditioned stimulus. *B. Psychon. Soc.* 23(3): 245-248.

(133) Tanzi, E. 1893. I fatti e le induzioni nell'odierna istologia del sistema nervoso. *Riv. sper. Freniat. Med. Leg Alien. ment.* 19: 419-472.

(134) Teuber, H.L. 1955. Physiological psychology. *Ann. R. Psych.* 6: 267-296.

(135) Teuber, H.L. 1964. The riddle of frontal function in man. In *The Frontal Granular Cortex and Behavior*, eds. J.M. Warren and K. Adert, pp. 410-444. New York: McGraw-Hill.

(136) Thompson, R.F.; Berger, T.W.; Berry, S.D.; and Hoehler, F.K. 1980. The search for the engram, II. In *Brain Mechanisms in Behavior*, ed. D. McFaddem. New York: Springer-Verlag.

(137) Thompson, R.F.; Berger, T.W.; Berry, S.D.; Hoehler, F.K.; Kettner, R.S.; and Weisz, D.J. 1980. Hippocampal substrates of classical conditioning. *Physl. Psych.* 8(2): 262-279.

(138) Thompson, R.F.; Berger, T.W.; Cegavske, C.F.; Patterson, M.M.; Roemer, R.A.; Teyler, T.J.; and Young, R.A. 1976. The search for the engram. *Am. Psychol.* 31: 209-227.

(139) Thompson, R.F.; McCormick, D.A.; and Lavond, D.G. 1986. Localization of the essential memory trace system for a basic form of associative learning in the mammalian brain. In *One Hundred Years of Psychological Research in America*, eds. S.H. Hulse and B.F. Green, pp. 125-171. Baltimore, MD: Johns Hopkins University Press.

(140) Thorndike, E.L. 1898. Animal intelligence: an experimental study of the associative processes in animals. *Psychol. Rev. Monogr. Suppl.* 2(8): 1-109.

(141) Tischler, M.D., and Davis, M. 1983. A visual pathway that mediates fear-conditioned enhancement of acoustic startle. *Brain Res.* 276: 55-71.

(142) Tsukahara, N. 1981. Synaptic plasticity in the mammalian central nervous system. *Ann. R. Neur.* 4: 351-379.

(143) Tsukahara, N. 1982. Classical conditioning mediated by the red nucleus in the cat. In *Conditioning: Representation of Involved Neural Functions*, ed. C.D. Woody. New York: Plenum.

(144) Tsukahara, N.; Oda, Y.; and Notsu, T. 1981. Classical conditioning mediated by the red nucleus in the cat. *J. Neurosc.* 1: 72-79.

(145) Tucker, T.J., and Kling, A. 1967. Differential effects of early and late lesions of frontal granular cortex in the monkey. *Brain Res.* 5: 377-389.

(146) Tucker, T.J., and Kling, A. 1969. Perseveration of delayed response following combined lesions of prefrontal and posterior association cortex in infant monkeys. *Exp. Neurol.* 23: 491-502.

(147) Warren, J.M. 1964. The behavior of carnivores and primates with lesions in the prefrontal cortex. In *The Frontal Granular Cortex and Behavior*, eds. J.M. Warren and K. Akert. New York: McGraw-Hill.

(148) Watson, J.B. 1913. Psychology as the behaviorist views it. *Psychol. Rev.* 20: 158-177.

(149) Weisz, D.J.; Clark, G.A.; and Thompson, R.F. 1984. Increased activity of dentate granule cells during nictitating membrane response conditioning in rabbits. *Beh. Brain Res.* 12: 145-154.

(150) Woodruff-Pak, D.S.; Lavond, D.G.; Logan, C.G.; Steinmetz, J.E.; and Thompson, R.F. 1985. The continuing search for a role of the cerebellar cortex in eyelid conditioning. *Neurosci. Abstr.* 11: 333.

(151) Yeo, C.H.; Hardiman, M.J.; and Glickstein, M. 1984. Discrete lesions of the cerebellar cortex abolish the classically conditioned nictitating membrane response of the rabbit. *Beh. Brain Res.* 13: 261-266.

(152) Yeo, C.H.; Hardiman, M.J.; and Glickstein, M. 1985. Classical conditioning of the nictitating membrane response of the rabbit. *Exp. Brain Res.* 60: 87-98.

The Neural and Molecular Bases of Learning,
eds. J.-P. Changeux and M. Konishi, pp. 503–540.
John Wiley & Sons Limited.

Information Representation, Processing, and Storage in the Brain: Analysis at the Single Neuron Level

E.T. Rolls

Dept. of Experimental Psychology
University of Oxford
Oxford OX1 3UD, England

Abstract. The ways in which information is represented, processed, and stored in the nervous system of primates as shown by recording from single neurons are considered.

1) Individual stimuli, objects, or responses (termed events) are coded as the pattern of firing across a population of neurons. That is, ensemble encoding rather than "grandmother cell" encoding is used. Evidence for this from recordings in temporal cortical areas involved in face recognition is presented.

2) In order to clarify how the nervous system would function with such ensemble encoding, and to clarify how single neurons might respond in such a system, a theoretical analysis of information representation and storage in matrix memories formed by neuronal networks is presented. It is shown that such distributed information processing and storage has a number of advantages, including completion of an incomplete pattern, generalization, graceful degradation when the system is damaged or incomplete, and speed. It is also shown that these properties arise only if ensemble coding for information across subpopulations of neurons is used. It is further noted that the tuning of neurons, which is graded differentially to different events rather than being so specific that it occurs only to one event, is advantageous in making many fine discriminations. Also, it is shown that such neuronal networks allow any pattern of firing to be interfaced to any other pattern of firing, providing a basis for information transmission from sensory input through to motor output with no special "homunculus" required.

3) Through the connected stages of a processing system the representation of information becomes more sharply differentiated between events, as shown by the fineness of tuning of single neurons in different stages of the taste system and in temporal lobe visual areas.

One reason that this is necessary is to reduce interference in the transfer of information across and storage of information within matrix memories. Neuronal networks which will perform this categorization, or orthogonalization (decorrelation) of the representations of stimuli or events using learning to achieve the necessary mountain climbing, are described.

4) Evidence that neurons in the amygdala and orbitofrontal cortex of the primate are involved in association memory, for example in cross-modality associations and in stimulus-reinforcement associations, is described. It is shown that sensory information processing occurs through several areas in the primate before it is interfaced with such associational and motivational systems. This is illustrated by taste and visual information processing systems involved in the control of feeding in which modulation by hunger occurs only after several cortical stages of analysis. The theoretical significance of this is that particular stimuli, such as a particular food, can only be represented across a limited ensemble of neurons which is well differentiated from other ensembles representing non-foods or other foods after several stages of analysis; and that this differentiation is necessary so that when motivation acts, or association learning occurs, it does so with sufficient specificity for that particular food or stimulus and not for other stimuli.

5) Evidence that neurons in the hippocampus of the primate are involved in memories for combinations of events, such as where in the environment a particular object was seen or which motor response should be made to a particular stimulus, is described. Evidence on how hippocampal circuitry may be appropriate for detecting such conjunctions or combinations of events which may reach it from different areas of the temporal, parietal, and frontal cortex is described.

6) The storage of information in short-term memories is shown to usually involve short-term changes in synaptic efficacy (e.g., in the inferior temporal visual cortex in delayed matching-to-sample tasks) but in a few cases involves holding a pattern of firing during a delay period (e.g., in the dorsolateral prefrontal cortex in delayed response tasks).

INTRODUCTION

In this paper the ways in which information is represented, processed, and stored in the nervous system of primates will be considered. The evidence will be based on analysis of the activity of single neurons because this is the basic level at which information is transferred over any distance in the nervous system, so that the information being processed must be represented (at least when transferred over any distance) in the firing pattern of single neurons. The examples will be drawn from work on the nonhuman primate to make it as relevant as possible to understanding brain function in man.

Evidence will be presented to show that information is represented over ensembles of neurons. Theoretical analyses, which show how such distributed information processing occurs and which highlight its advantages for brain function, are described first in order to make the understanding of these neuronal operations involved in information processing and the types of response which are obtained from single neurons more precise. After this, the ways in which information is represented across ensembles of neurons will be described. Then the changes in information representation which take place through the sensory systems as information is categorized by cortical processing are described. Also discussed are the ways in which such information is used in different information storage and processing systems in the brain; those involved in association memory and short-term memory will be described.

MODELS OF NEURONAL INFORMATION PROCESSING AND STORAGE

Matrix models of memory (25, 33, 34, 51) provide useful insight into information processing in groups of neurons. They can be used to help understand the types of response found in single neurons in the brain by analyzing how the equivalent of single neurons in a computer simulation of a matrix memory respond. Matrix models can be modified to provide more complex models of information processing in brain regions such as the neocortex and hippocampus (66).

Consider a population of n neurons with vertically oriented dendrites intersected by a set of n horizontally running axons (see Fig. 1). At each intersection of an axon with a dendrite there is a modifiable synpase. (This situation is almost exactly what is found in the cerebellum (see (26)). The unconditioned (unlearned) response is represented by the pattern of firing of the n vertically oriented neurons in Fig. 1. The conditioned stimulus is represented by the pattern of firing of the n horizontal axons. When there is simultaneous activity in a horizontal axon and a vertical neuron, the synapse becomes modified. (This is a very simple learning rule. The modification can consist of a decrease or an increase of synaptic strength.) In such a memory information is thus stored in a correlation matrix formed by the product of a vector of n neurons representing the conditioned stimulus with a vector (perhaps also of n neurons) representing the unconditioned stimulus. Many associations can be stored in the same matrix by adding each product to the previous summed contents of the matrix. This process of storage is illustrated in Fig. 2.

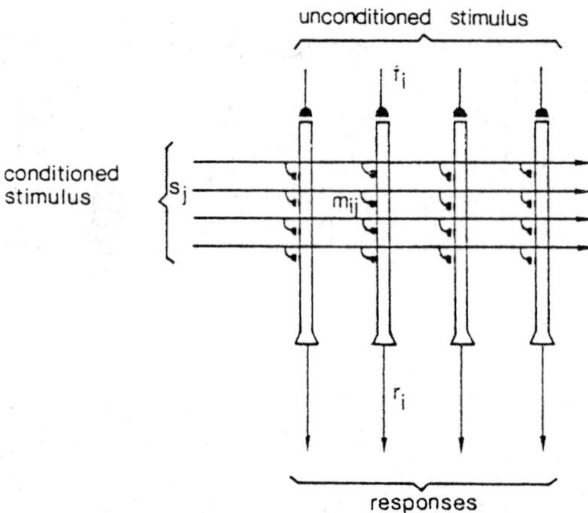

FIG. 1 – Neurons connected to form a matrix memory. The vertical rectangles represent the dendrites of the neurons which respond unconditionally to application of the unconditioned or forcing stimuli (f) to produce the responses (r). The conditioned stimuli (s) are applied to the horizontally running axons, each one of which forms a modifiable synapse with each dendrite it passes (see text).

To recall an association from the matrix memory the conditioned stimulus is applied to the horizontal axons. Each axon activates each dendrite in proportion to how much the particular synapse was modified during learning. The firing of each vertical neuron then represents the sum of effects produced through all its synapses. This is the sum over all conditioned stimulus input axons of the firing on that axon multiplied by the synaptic strength at the synapse at each axon-dendrite intersection in the matrix. An example of how this recall process functions is shown in Fig. 3.

There are many biologically desirable properties of this type of information store, including recall of a complete stimulus from the memory when only a part of a stimulus is shown, generalization to a similar stimulus if a stimulus which has never been seen before is shown (see Fig. 4), and considerable tolerance to partial destruction or absence during development of synapses or neurons in it (i.e., graceful degradation in performance as damage to the memory increases; see Fig. 5). This type of information store also shows some of the other features of biological memory such as interference. This interference can be reduced by thresholding (see Figs. 4 and 5). Anatomical and

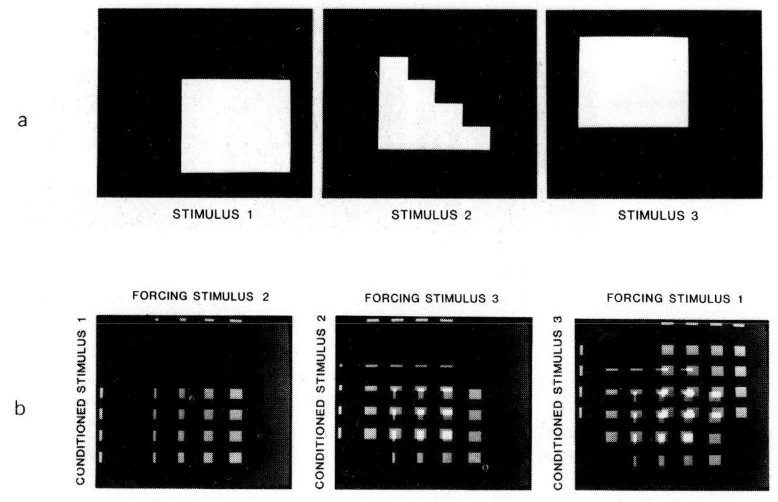

FIG. 2 – Storage of information in a matrix memory. a) The stimuli used consisted of 8 by 8 pixels and were read off by rows to form 64-element vectors applied as stimuli to the matrix memory. b) The matrix memory with three different associations being stored. In A, stimulus 1 is used as the conditioned stimulus and stimulus 2 as the unconditioned or forcing stimulus. The 64 dendrites in the matrix run as 64 vertical columns across which the unconditioned stimulus (represented as a 64-element vector and shown above the matrix) is applied. The 64 horizontal axons run as the rows of the matrix, and to these the conditioned stimulus is applied (represented as a 64-element vector and shown at the left of the matrix). The gray scale values within the matrix are proportional to synaptic strength formed by the conditioning. The gray values of the vectors are proportional to firing rate. B and C show the formation of further associations, which overlap and add to the strength of some synapses in the memory.

physiological evidence is also consistent with the idea that information storage in some parts of the brain uses such a distributed storage system (65, 66). Another useful property of this type of memory is that it is fast, with only one synaptic delay being interposed between application of the input stimulus pattern and appearance of the output pattern.

The types of response shown by single neurons and populations of neurons can be clarified by considering how a single neuron in such a memory might respond using computer simulations. These included 64 neuron (a 64 by 64 storage matrix) and 1024 neuron (a 1024 by 1024

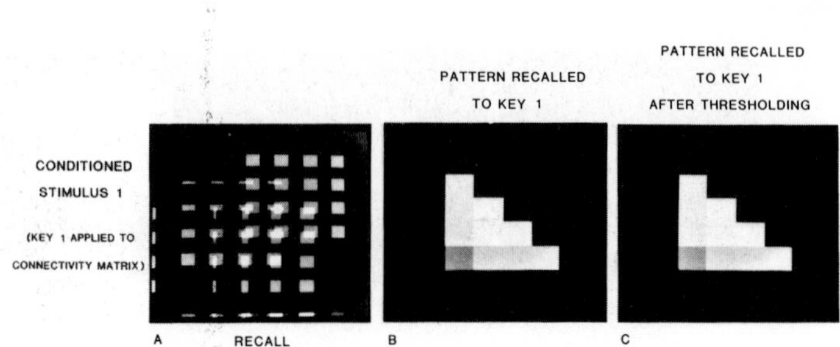

FIG. 3 – The recall of information from a matrix memory. A) Application of conditioned stimulus 1 (shown on the left of the diagram) to the matrix containing three stored associations results in the pattern of firing of the output neurons represented as a vector across the bottom of the diagram (cf. Fig. 1). B) The recalled pattern (i.e., the pattern of firing of the output neurons) represented as an 8 by 8 image (cf. Fig. 2a). C) The recalled pattern after thresholding at half the maximal firing rate (brightness level).

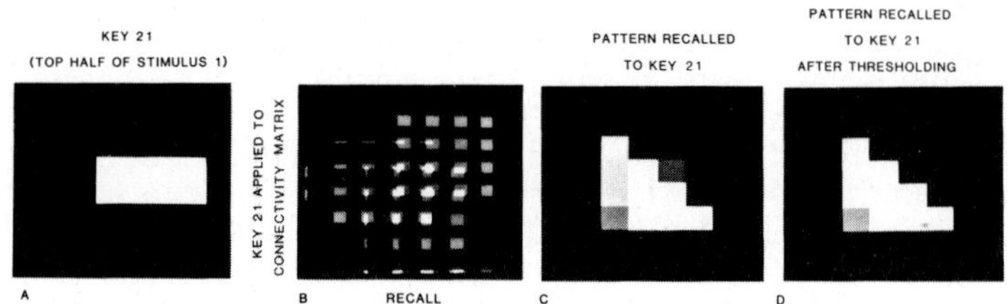

FIG. 4 – Completion and generalization in the recall from a matrix memory. The upper half of stimulus 1 (A) is applied to the connectivity matrix (B) and results in recall of the pattern in (C) shown after thresholding in (D).

storage matrix) linear associative matrix memories. In the 1024 neuron network, lateral inhibition was applied to the input stimulus vectors in order to orthogonalize the stimuli and thus improve the storage capability of the network (see Kohonen *et al.* (34)). It should be remembered that each neuron in the matrix is represented by each vertical dendrite (see Fig. 1). The information stored on such a single neuron i by modification of its synapses is the sum over every stimulus pair of the pattern of the conditioned stimulus multiplied by the firing of that (i'th) neuron to the unconditioned stimulus. Thus the i'th neuron

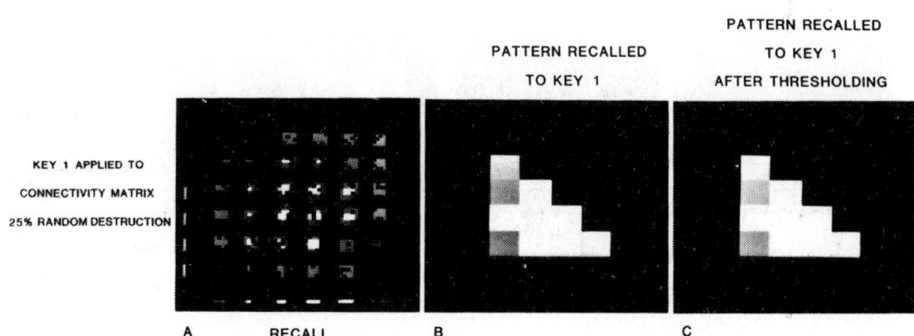

FIG. 5 – Graceful degradation of the performance of a matrix memory when it is damaged. The application of key 1 to the matrix after 25% of the synapses had been removed at random (A) resulted in the recall shown in (B) and after thresholding in (C).

responds best in such a memory to a combination of one to many of the conditioned stimuli. In one extreme condition, if neuron i fires to only one of the unconditioned stimuli, then it responds best to the conditioned stimulus associated with that unconditioned stimulus. In the other extreme condition, if neuron i fires to all the unconditioned stimuli, then it is most responsive to a combination of all the conditioned stimuli. Between these limits, neuron i will respond best to a combination of a subset of the conditioned stimuli, and will respond partly to each of the stimuli in the subset. The results of the simulation show that in some cases the neurons respond best to one of the conditioned stimuli applied to the network, and in other cases to several of the conditioned stimuli applied to the network (see Fig. 6). This is remarkably similar to what is found when recordings are made from single neurons in the cortex in the superior temporal sulcus of the monkey, for in this region each neuron typically responds to only a subset of the stimuli (which in this case are faces) which are effective for activating the different neurons in this region (see below and (4, 58)).

This type of information storage in neuronal networks also has implications for the representation of information in the brain. In order to derive the benefits of information storage in a matrix memory noted above (such as completion, generalization, and graceful degradation) it is essential that each individual object in the environment (such as a particular grandmother) be represented by the firing pattern of an ensemble of neurons. (This pattern of firing is termed an "event.") This is because completion, generalization, and graceful degradation rely on some of the neurons which represented the original object or event being

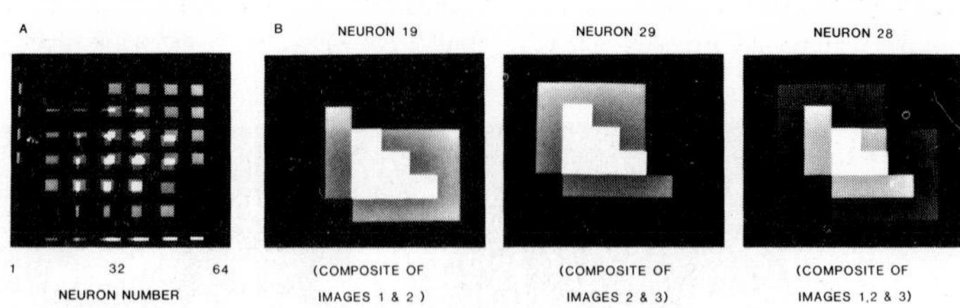

FIG. 6 – Response properties of single neurons in a matrix memory. A) The association matrix containing 3 associations. The 64 "neurons" in the matrix are 64 vertical columns, each of which has synapses modified on it which represent the patterns of none, one, or several of the conditioned stimuli. Examples of the information stored on single neurons are shown in B.

activated by the incomplete event, by the similar event, or after some of the synapses or neurons in the network have been destroyed. On the other hand, each event must not be represented over a very large population of neurons which overlaps almost completely with the population activated by a different event; if this were the case then the matrix memory would display great interference and would be a very inefficient memory storage or interfacing system. These two arguments lead to the conclusion that in a matrix memory system each event must be represented across an ensemble of neurons but that the ensemble must be of limited size. In such an ensemble, in which information represented could individuate an event (e.g., the face of a particular person), it would be expected that each neuron would be tuned to differentiate quite sharply between the different members of the set of individual stimuli represented in that matrix but would typically respond to more than one member of the set of stimuli. That is, neurons which responded only to one object or event (e.g., grandmother Smith) would not be useful in a matrix memory system. This theoretical analysis thus explains the utility of the type of information representation across the neurons in the cortex in the superior temporal sulcus of the monkey, where it is found that each neuron typically responds to a limited subset of the stimuli (which in this case are faces) which are effective for activating the different neurons in this region (see above).

Another advantage of such ensemble encoding is that if neurons are not tuned to only one stimulus, but instead each stimulus activates differentially its own set of graded filters, then fine, continuous discriminations between the members of that set are enhanced.

Potentially more discriminations are possible than with the one neuron-one stimulus type of encoding (for further discussion see Erickson (17, 18)).

Another problem which is clarified by this theoretical analysis is sensory to motor or input-output processing in the brain. The analysis shows that such neuronal nets effectively enable an input vector of n elements (represented by the firing of the conditioned stimulus axons in Fig. 1) to be connected to an output vector of (for example) n elements (represented by the firing of the unconditioned stimulus neurons in Fig. 1) in such a way that any particular pattern of firing in the input vector or population of neurons can produce any particular pattern in the output vector or population of neurons. An ensemble of neurons in this analysis is the pattern of firing in a subset of the neurons in a vector. (The ensemble which represents each stimulus is usually a subset of the whole vector or population of neurons so that interference between the stimuli or events is minimized.) These matrix operations thus provide a simple way of interfacing one population of neurons (perhaps an input population) to another population of neurons (perhaps an output population), with no need at any stage for a special "interpreter" or homunculus. In practice, in the brain, there are a series of matrix operations modified from this basic design, so that information processing proceeds through a series of specialized stages which categorize the stimulus before it is interfaced to motivational or motor systems (see below).

THE REPRESENTATION OF INFORMATION ACROSS ENSEMBLES OF NEURONS

One way in which the representation of information across ensembles of neurons in the brain is being investigated is by analyzing the responses of single neurons in the temporal lobe visual cortex which respond preferentially to faces. The question considered is whether information which could specify the face of one individual is represented by the firing of one neuron or whether the pattern of firing of an ensemble is needed to enable identification of the individual being seen.

Neurons which respond preferentially or selectively to faces are found in certain areas of the temporal lobe visual cortex which receive their inputs via a number of corticocortical stages from the primary visual cortex, the striate cortex, through prestriate visual areas ((14, 16, 83), see Fig. 7). The responses of these neurons to faces are selective in that they are 2-10 times as large to faces as to gratings, simple geometrical stimuli, or complex 3-D objects (4, 6, 52). They are probably a

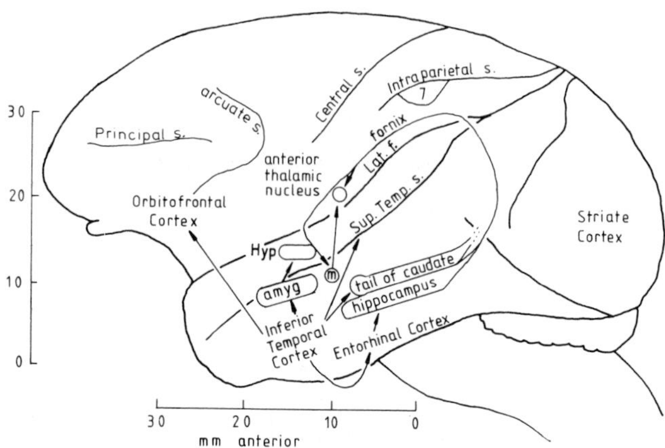

FIG. 7 - Some of the pathways described in the text are shown on this lateral view of the rhesus monkey brain. amyg = amygdala; central s = central sulcus; Hyp = hypothalamus / substantia innominata / basal forebrain; Lat f = lateral (or Sylvian) fissure; m = mammillary body; Sup Temp s = superior temporal sulcus; 7 = posterior parietal cortex, area 7.

specialized population for processing information from faces in that they are found primarily in architectonic areas TPO, TEa, and TEm and are not just the neurons with the most complex types of response found throughout the temporal lobe visual areas (6). The advantage of such a specialized system in the primate may lie in the importance of rapid and reliable recognition of other individuals using face recognition, so that appropriate social and emotional responses can be made (58).

In experiments to determine how information which could be used to specify an individual is represented by the firing of these neurons, it has been shown that in many cases (77% of one sample) these neurons are sensitive to differences between faces (4), but that each neuron does not respond to only one face. Instead, each neuron has a different pattern of responses to a set of faces, as illustrated in Fig. 8.

Such evidence shows that the responses of each of these neurons in the cortex of the superior temporal sulcus do not code uniquely for the face of a particular individual. Instead, across a population of such cells, information is conveyed which would be useful in making different behavioral responses to different faces. Thus information which specifies an individual face is present across an ensemble of such cells.

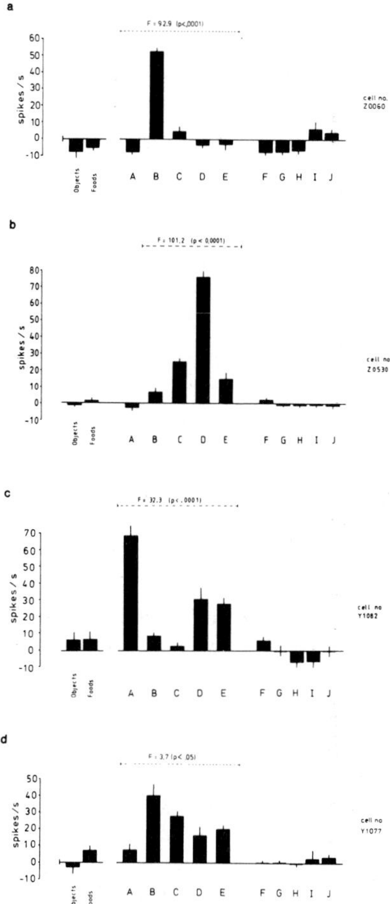

FIG. 8 – The responses of four cells (a-d) in the cortex of the superior temporal sulcus to a variety of face (A-E) and nonface (F-J) stimuli. The responses to nonface objects and to foods are shown on the left of the diagram. The bar represents the mean firing rate response above the spontaneous baseline firing rate with the standard error calculated over 4-10 presentations. The F ratio for the analysis of variance calculated over the face set indicates that the units shown range from very selective (Z0060) to relatively nonselective (Y1077) (from (4)).

In that each neuron does not respond to only one face, and in that a particular face can activate many neurons, these are not "grandmother" cells (2). However, because their responses are relatively specialized both for the class "faces" and within this class, they could contribute to relatively economic coding of information over relatively few cells (see Barlow, (2)). It should be noted that even if individual neurons in this population are not completely tuned to respond specifically to only face stimuli, it is nevertheless the case that the output of such an ensemble of neurons would be useful for distinguishing between different faces. The appropriateness of these neurons for such a function is enhanced by their relative constancy of response over some physical transforms, such as size, contrast, and color (52, 67). These findings lead to the hypotheses that such neurons are filters, the output of which could be used for recognition of different individuals and in emotional responses made to different individuals. Their different responses to different faces, and also their different responses to different parts of faces (52) and to different parts of the spatial frequency spectrum present in faces (5, 68), provide further evidence for understanding them as filters.

It is unlikely that there are further processing areas beyond those described where ensemble coding changes into grandmother cell encoding. Anatomically there does not appear to be a whole, further set of visual processing areas present in the brain beyond the temporal lobe visual areas such as those described, from which outputs are taken to limbic and related regions such as the amygdala and via the entorhinal cortex to the hippocampus. Indeed, tracing this pathway onwards, Leonard *et al.* (35) have found a population of neurons with face-selective responses in the amygdala, and in the majority of these neurons different responses occur to different faces with ensemble (not unique) coding still being present. After interfacing with limbic circuits in this way, there is evidence for further links which may be important in the behavioral output via the connections of the amygdala to the ventral striatum (which includes the nucleus accumbens), for in the ventral striatum a small number of neurons are found which also respond to faces (see Rolls, (64)).

INFORMATION CATEGORIZATION IN SENSORY SYSTEMS

The example of information representation described above shows that information needed to specify an individual face is represented across the population of neurons studied efficiently in terms of what is appropriate for a distributed information processing system illustrated by the properties of matrix memories. In particular, each neuron responds to only some faces and has graded responses to the faces to which it does respond. This would maintain interference at a reasonably low level in the matrix memory, yet would allow the beneficial properties such as completion, generalization, and graceful degradation to occur. The fundamental problem which the sensory systems of the brain have is how to reduce the redundancy present in the input signals and to extract a functionally useful information representation of the type just described. It may be noted, for example, that discrimination between faces based on gray level pixel images would be extremely difficult because of the great correlation or lack of orthogonality present between such images. The way in which information changes across successive processing stages in order to achieve efficient categorization is described with an example from the taste system.

The first central synapse of the gustatory system is in the rostral part of the nucleus of the solitary tract (NTS) (7, 8). In order to investigate the tuning of neurons in the nucleus of the solitary tract, the response of single NTS neurons to the prototypical stimuli (NaCl, glucose, HCl, and quinine), to water, and to a complex stimulus (blackcurrant juice) were measured in the macaque monkey. It was found that NTS neurons are relatively broadly tuned to the prototypical taste stimuli ((80, see Fig. 9). The breadth of tuning index used was that of Smith and Travers (84). This is a measure derived from information theory of entropy, calculated as

$$H = -k \sum_{i=1}^{n} P_i \log P_i$$

where H= breadth of responsiveness, k = scaling constant (set so that H = 1.0 when the neuron responds equally well to all stimuli in the set of size n), p_i = the response to stimulus i expressed as a proportion of the total response to all the stimuli in the set.

The NTS projects via the thalamic taste area to the frontal opercular taste cortex and insula (7). In these regions gustatory areas were found, and it was discovered that the breadth of tuning of the neurons in these areas was finer than in the NTS ((81, 95), see Fig. 9). The frontal opercular taste cortex projects into a fourth order gustatory area in the caudolateral orbitofrontal cortex (77), and here it was found that the tuning of gustatory neurons was even finer ((93), see Fig. 9). This analysis shows that one change which takes place in the representation of information in the gustatory system is that entropy (in terms of breadth of tuning described above) is reduced; that is, neurons become better able to differentiate between different stimuli or, equivalently, the correlation between the responses of a given neuron to different

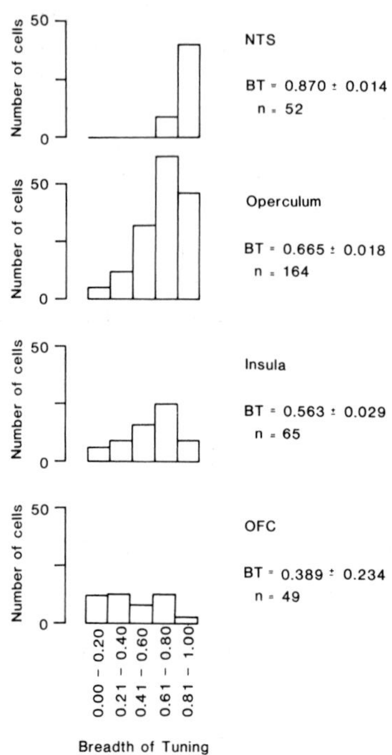

FIG. 9 – The breadths of tuning of neurons in different stages of the taste system. A value of 1 represents equal responses to all stimuli (i.e., very broad tuning) and a value of 0 represents a response to only one of the stimuli (see text). The stimuli used were 1 M glucose, 1 M NaCl, 0.01 M HCl, 0.001 M quinine HCl, water, and 20% blackcurrant juice.

stimuli becomes less. This is ideal for a distributed information processing system because it reduces interference in memories and interfacing systems, as illustrated by the properties of matrix memories described above.

Another important principle of nervous system function may be illustrated by information processing in the taste system. It is only after several or many stages of sensory information processing (which produce efficient categorization of the stimulus) that there is an interface to motivational systems, to other modalities, or to systems involved in association memory. Thus in the taste system of the primate neuronal responses to gustatory stimuli in the NTS, opercular taste cortex, and insular taste cortex are not affected by hunger (96, 97). It is only in the orbitofrontal taste area that neuronal responses are modulated by hunger, ceasing to occur, for example, to glucose if glucose has just been eaten to satiety (75). The reason for this is probably as follows. If satiety were to operate at an early level of sensory analysis, then because of the broadness of tuning of neurons, responses to non-foods would become attentuated as well as responses to foods (and this could be dangerous if poisonous non-foods became undetectable). This argument becomes even more compelling when it is realized that satiety typically shows some specificity for the particular food eaten, with other foods not eaten in the meal remaining relatively pleasant (59). Unless tuning were relatively fine this mechanism could not operate, for reduction in neuronal firing after one food had been eaten would inevitably reduce behavioral responsiveness to other foods. Indeed, it is of interest to note that such a sensory-specific satiety mechanism can be built by arranging for tuning to particular foods to become relatively specific at one level of the nervous system (as a result of categorization processing in earlier stages), and then at this stage (but not at prior stages) to allow habituation to be a property of the synapses. This would result in a decreased response to the taste of a food which had just been eaten but not to another taste unless they were very similar. It appears that precisely this mechanism is found in the gustatory system (75).

The point about interfacing to other modalities and to association memory can also be made with the taste system. In the rostral NTS, the frontal opercular taste cortex and the insular taste cortex, the neurons found are mainly gustatory, and other modalities are not represented. On the other hand, after these stages (that is when tuning has become fine) taste processing is interfaced to other modalities. For example, in and near to the orbitofrontal taste area, neurons with visual and somatosensory responses are found (87). Also, in the amygdala, which receives from the insular taste cortex (40), different modalities are brought together. Indeed, the visual projections to the amygdala follow the same rule in that visual projections are not found to the amygdala from early stages of sensory analysis but only from temporal lobe visual areas, that is after much earlier processing (9, 88, 89). The probable reason for this is again that it is only possible to allow modalities to interact in order to form associations (for example, after much processing in each modality), so that interference due to lack of orthogonalization of the representations of the stimuli can be minimized (see above). That is, it is only possible to form associations in distributed memory processing systems of the matrix memory type after the neuronal representations of the stimuli have been at least partly orthogonalized in order to minimize interference.

NEURONAL MECHANISMS OF CATEGORIZATION

The neuronal mechanisms which perform the categorization or orthogonalization evident in, for example, the taste and visual systems as described above are not yet well understood, but the following ideas may be useful.

One simple neuronal mechanism of orthogonalization is lateral inhibition. It orthogonalizes in that it tends to decorrelate two signals by high-pass spatial frequency filtering them. Consider two different square wave signals represented in a sensory system. To the extent that they overlap, there will be neuronal elements which will respond to both, and this overlap will produce interference in, and reduce the capacity of, matrix memories. If, however, both signals are high-pass filtered by lateral inhibition then the signals have neural elements in common only at the edges of the square waves and most of the overlap will have been reduced. This is so important for any matrix memory or interface operation that it is probably the most important function of lateral inhibition.

A much more sophisticated computation which results in categorization appears to be performed by the neocortex (cf. Marr, (36)). Some theoretical insight into this may come from considering the neocortex as a variant of the matrix memory as described above.

Consider a matrix memory in which the probability that a horizontal axon makes a synapse with every (vertical) neuron it passes is not near 1 (as in Fig. 1) but is much lower, perhaps in the range 0.1 - 0.001. If these contacts are made randomly then different input patterns on the horizontal axons will tend to activate different neurons. (An alternative design is to form the matrix with random numbers of synapses at each intersection or with random strengths of synapses initially at each intersection.) The tendency for each pattern to select or activate different neurons can then be enhanced by a) increasing the synaptic weights at those synapses where there is both pre- and postsynaptic activity and b) providing inhibition throughout (or alternatively locally within) the matrix from neurons which are already responding to a stimulus to prevent too many neurons becoming allocated to that stimulus. An example of the operation of such a matrix with low contact probability to produce classification is shown in Fig. 10. Such a categorization process effectively selects different neurons to respond to

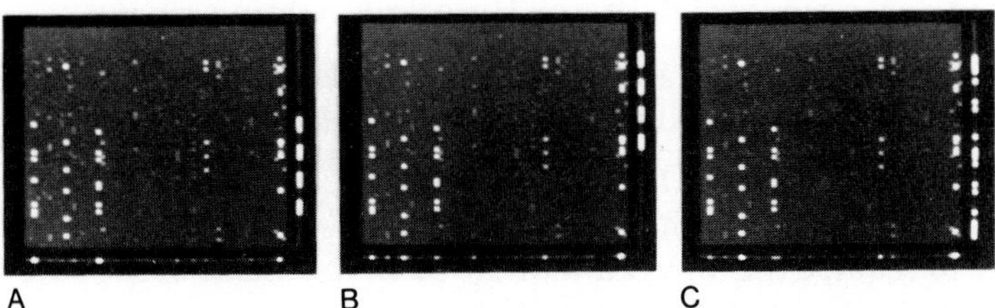

FIG. 10 – Categorization in a matrix memory with a low contact probability between a horizontal axon and a vertical dendrite (cf. Fig. 1). The contact probability was 0.13 in the 64 by 64 neuron matrix. Each panel shows the application of a stimulus (at the right of each panel) to the matrix. The resulting firing of the (vertical) neurons is shown by the output vector across the bottom of each panel. The brightness of the input and output vectors is proportional to the firing rate. The brightness of each position in the 64 by 64 connectivity matrix (with only 13% contact probability) is proportional to the strength of that synapse. Several iterations of learning with lateral inhibition to enhance the hill climbing (see text) preceded the stage shown. It is shown that after learning each complex input stimulus resulted in a different pattern of firing coded primarily across four output (vertical) neurons, the synapses of which had primarily been modified during the learning.

different combinations of active input horizontal lines. Major inputs which unconditionally activate the vertical neurons are not necessary for the operation of this system (although they may guide the mountain climbing (36, 37)). It should be noted that this categorization finds natural clusters in the input events, orthogonalizes the input events (overlap in input events can become coded onto output neurons with less overlap and many active input lines may be coded onto few active output lines), and does not allocate neurons to events which never occur (cf. Marr (36, 37)).

One way in which this theory of operation of the neocortex is being tested is by investigating whether, when completely novel faces are shown to a monkey, the neurons in the cortex of the superior temporal sulcus, which appear to be involved in the classification of different faces (4, 58), alter their responses as predicted by the theory. The theory predicts that a single neuron in such a classification system might show changes in its response to a novel stimulus within its potential classification repertoire (in this case faces) over a number of presentations of the new face and/or to familiar faces as a result of inhibition produced if other neurons in the matrix were activated by the novel face. Some evidence for the latter form of modification is being found in experiments of Rolls and Hasselmo, now in progress.

Other theoretical approaches to categorization in neuronal networks have been described by Kohonen (32) and by Cooper *et al.* (13).

ASSOCIATION MEMORY

Pathways for the cross-model association of complex, patterned stimuli appear to require the amygdala in the primate. Some of the evidence for this is that lesions of the amygdala impair the learning of a one-trial, object-reward association (85) and of a tactual-to-visual, cross-modal association (46, 47). Also, many of the symptoms of the Kluver-Bucy syndrome (in which monkeys with amygdala damage, for example, select non-food as well as food objects) can be interpreted as a failure to make normal associations between stimuli such as the sight of food and reinforcement provided, for example, by its taste (28, 31, 53-63). Moreover, the amygdala is well placed anatomically for this function. It receives highly processed inputs from higher (but not lower) stages of the visual, auditory, and gustatory systems in the primate, as well as olfactory and visceral inputs. It has outputs to the autonomic centers of the brainstem, hypothalamus, and other limbic (as well as cortical) structures, through which autonomic (as well as behavioral) responses learned to stimuli, which have been paired with other stimuli including reinforcers, can be produced (9, 24, 29, 58, 60-62).

It was therefore of interest to investigate the decoding of visual information through the inferior temporal visual cortex-amygdala-hypothalamic pathway, in order to determine at which stage visual information reflected the association of visual stimuli with reinforcement such as the taste of food. It was found that in the inferior temporal visual cortex the significance of a stimulus in terms of its association with reward or dependence on motivational state (hunger) was not a factor in determining the responses of the neurons (71). In the amygdala, neurons were found which responded to reinforcing stimuli such as food, but these neurons typically responded also to one or several neutral or even aversive stimuli, so that they did not completely code specifically for the reinforcement value of visual stimuli (79). Also, these neurons did not appear to reflect the changing reinforcement associations of stimuli during visual discrimination reversals (79). There is also a population of neurons in the basal accessory nucleus of the amygdala which responds to faces, and these neurons may be involved in emotional responses (35, 58, 60-62). This evidence thus suggests that the amygdala may be important in motivational and emotional responses to reinforcing stimuli, but that another system (perhaps the orbitofrontal cortex, see below) may be important in the rapid and readily reversible association of visual stimuli with reinforcement in visual discrimination tasks. At a further stage of information processing, the lateral hypothalamus and substantia innominata, which receive projections from the amygdala and orbitofrontal cortex (61) (approximately 13.4% in one sample of 764 neurons), had responses to the sight and/or taste of food (53, 54, 59, 63, 79). These neurons came through learning to respond to the sight of food as opposed to non-food visual stimuli. Their responses became associated with the sight of a previously neutral stimulus which signified food in a visual discrimination task, showed extinction if a stimulus no longer signified food, and showed reversal in the reversal of a visual discrimination task (45, 74). For example, when a monkey had to choose whether to initiate feeding in the visual discrimination task, it was found that the responses of these neurons occurred to the visual stimulus which signified that a lick response could be initiated to obtain food but not to the visual stimulus which indicated that the monkey should not lick or he would obtain aversive hypertonic saline. The latency of the discriminative responses of these neurons was 140-200 ms, compared to 250-350 ms for the EMG responses associated with licks made at 350-450 ms (74). Therefore the responses of these neurons preceded and predicted the initiation of feeding responses by the monkey (74). This evidence is consistent with the hypothesis that neuronal responses, which represent the reward value of the stimulus and thus reflect an output of an association memory, are elaborated along this pathway but are not fully evident until the stage of the ventral forebrain neurons (for further discussion see (53-63, 70)). Consistent also with this hypothesis are the latencies of neuronal firings which are approximately 100 ms in the inferior temporal visual cortex, 110 ms in the amygdala, and 140 ms in the basal forebrain (53-63, 71, 74, 79). It is of interest to note that relatively simple reward-related coding is evident at the hypothalamic level. This may be because from here the interface is to autonomic and endocrine systems so that neuronal firing has to be at a level at which the outputs of a reinforcement related system (which might include, for example, salivation to the sight of food) can be realized.

It should be noted that this cortico-amygdaloid system (and the cortico-orbitofrontal cortex system, see below) is particularly appropriate for the association of complex stimuli, given the cortical areas from which the amygdala receives its inputs. Although there are changes in neuronal responses to a tone-conditioned stimulus in the rabbit amygdala during the acquisition of an aversive Pavlovian conditioning procedure (1, 30), associations involving simple stimuli which do not require cortical processing, such as pure tones, can probably in some cases be made at an earlier stage of information processing in the brain, (e.g., in the magnocellular medial geniculate nuclei; see (92)). However, this relatively peripheral type of altered neuronal responsiveness may not be the normal mode of association formation, as this probably involves complex patterned stimuli in the natural environment. Similarly, although Berger *et al.* (10) have found neurons in the hippocampus which come to respond to the conditioned stimulus during tone-eye blink conditioning in the rabbit, these neurons must have some function other than the formation of the association because hippocampal damage does not impair the learning of this task. It is now thought that the association of a simple stimulus, such as a tone, with a simple motor response of this type involves the cerebellum because damage to this impairs the learning, and neuronal responses become modified here during the learning (86). The types of memory for which the hippocampus is crucial and the modification of neuronal activity in it during these types of learning in the primate are considered below.

Another area thought to be important in association memory in the primate is the orbitofrontal cortex. Damage to it impairs the flexible association of environmental stimuli with reinforcement. Examples of the situations in which a behavioral deficit is produced by orbitofrontal lesions include a) extinction, in that behavioral responses continue to be made to the previously reinforced stimulus; b) reversals of visual discriminations, in that the monkeys make responses to the previously reinforced stimulus or object; c) Go/Nogo tasks, in that responses are made to the stimulus which is not associated with food reward; and d) passive avoidance, in that feeding responses are made even when they are punished (11, 19, 27, 61, 78).

To investigate how the orbitofrontal cortex may be involved in the flexible association of visual stimuli with reinforcement and the reversal of such associations, recordings were made of the activity of 494 orbitofrontal cortex neurons during the performance of a Go/Nogo visual discrimination task, reversals of the visual discrimination task, extinction, and passive avoidance (87). First, neurons were found which responded a) in relation to the preparatory auditory or visual signal used before each trial (15.1%) or b) nondiscriminatively during the period in which the discriminative visual stimuli were shown (37.8%).

Thus, visual information reaches the orbitofrontal cortex, which anatomically receives connections from the inferior temporal visual cortex and the amygdala (61). Second, 8.6% of neurons had responses which occurred discriminatively during the period in which the visual stimuli were shown. It was shown using reversals of the visual discrimination that the majority of these neurons responded to whichever visual stimulus was associated with reward; the stimulus to which they responded changed during reversal. However, 6 of these neurons required a combination of a particular visual stimulus in the discrimination and reward in order to respond. Further, none of this second group of neurons responded to all the reward-related stimuli including different foods which were shown so that in general this group of neurons coded for a combination of one or several visual stimuli and reward. Thus information that particular visual stimuli were currently associated with reinforcement was represented in the responses of orbitofrontal neurons. Third, 9.7% of neurons had responses which occurred after the lick response was made in the task to obtain reward. Some of these responded independently of whether fruit juice reward was obtained. Aversive hypertonic saline was obtained on trials on which the monkey licked in error or was given saline in the first trials of a reversal. Through these neurons information that a lick had been made was represented in the orbitofrontal cortex. Other neurons in this third group responded only when fruit juice was obtained, and thus through these neurons information that reward had been given on that trial was represented in the orbitofrontal cortex. Other neurons in this group (3.6% of the total sample) responded when saline was obtained when a response was made in error, when saline was obtained on the first few trials of a reversal (but not in either case when saline was simply placed in the mouth), when reward was not given in extinction, or when food was taken away instead of being given to the monkey, but did not respond in all these situations in which reinforcement was omitted or punishment was given. Thus through these neurons task-selective information that reward had been omitted or punishment given was represented in the responses of these neurons.

These three groups of neurons found in the orbitofrontal cortex could together provide for computation of whether the reinforcement previously associated with a particular stimulus was still being obtained and generation of a signal if a match was not obtained. This signal could be partly reflected in the responses of the last subset of neurons with task-selective responses to nonreward or unexpected punishment. This signal could be used to alter the monkey's behavior leading, for example, to reversal to one particular stimulus but not to other stimuli, to extinction to one stimulus but not to others, etc. It could also lead to the altered responses of the orbitofrontal differential neurons found as a result of learning in reversal so that their responses indicate appropriately whether a particular stimulus is now associated with reinforcement.

In another part of the primate brain, the head of the caudate nucleus, neurons are found with activity related to another form of association. These neurons come by learning to respond to significant environmental events which signal, for example, that a trial of a task is about to begin (76). It is likely that the actual site of learning is the dorsolateral prefrontal cortex, which projects into this part of the striatum, for in this part of the cortex similar neurons are found (Rolls and Baylis, unpublished observations). This is probably part of a system for ensuring that the animal switches his behavior to significant environmental events (64).

FUNCTIONS OF THE PRIMATE HIPPOCAMPUS IN MEMORY

It is known that damage to certain regions of the temporal lobe in man produces anterograde amnesia evident as a major deficit following the damage in learning to recognize new stimuli (42, 82). The anterograde amnesia has been attributed to damage to the hippocampus, which is within the temporal lobe, and to its associated pathways such as the fornix (20, 21, 42, 50, 82). This has, however, been questioned. Alternatively, it has been suggested that damage to both the hippocampus and amygdala is crucial in producing anterograde amnesia, in that combined but not separate damage to the hippocampus and amygdala produced severe difficulty with visual and tactual recognition tasks in the monkey (43, 44, 46, 47). In investigations of the particular aspects of memory for which the hippocampus may be essential, it has been shown that monkeys with damage to the hippocampo-fornical system have a learning deficit on memory tasks which require them to make associations between a stimulus (e.g., a picture) and a motor response, such as touching one part of a screen (22). Impairment is also seen on memory tasks which require complex combinations of stimulus attributes to be processed together, such as memory not only for which object was shown but where it was shown (23).

In order to analyze the functions being performed by the hippocampus in these tasks requiring complex conjuctions of stimulus attributes or of stimuli with motor responses, the activity of 1510 single hippocampal neurons was recorded in rhesus monkeys learning and performing these memory tasks, which are known to be impaired by damage to the hippocampus or fornix (72).

In an object-place memory task in which the monkey had to remember not only which object had been seen in the previous 7-15 trials but also the position where it had appeared on a video monitor, neurons were found which responded differentially depending on which place on the screen the objects were shown. These neurons comprised 5.7% of the population recorded. It is notable that these neurons responded to particular positions in space (whereas "place" cells in the rat respond when the rat is in a particular place, (49)). In addition, 1.0% of neurons responded to a combination of place and novelty; they responded more to a stimulus the first time it was shown in a particular position than the second time. Most of these neurons had response latencies in the range 100-200 ms compared to typical behavioral response latencies of 300 ms.

In tasks in which the monkeys had to acquire associations between visual stimuli and spatial motor responses, 10.6% of neurons responded to particular combinations of stimuli and responses. For example, in a task in which the monkey had to perform an approach response (touching a screen 3 times) when one visual stimulus was shown to obtain reward, but had to perform a withholding response for 3 s to obtain reward when a different stimulus was shown (22), 9.2% of neurons responded to one of the stimuli if it was linked to one of the responses in this task. The same neurons typically did not respond if the same stimuli or the same responses were used in different tasks or if other stimuli were associated with the same responses in this task.

It was possible to study the activity of 41 hippocampal neurons while the monkeys learned new associations between visual stimuli and motor responses. In some cases it was possible to show that the activity of these neurons became modified during this learning. This is consistent with the hypothesis that the new learned associations are represented by the changed responses of an ensemble of hippocampal neurons.

In recognition memory tasks, a small proportion of neurons (0.7%) responded differently to novel, as compared to familiar, stimuli. In addition, some further neurons responded to novel stimuli in other memory tasks such as a delayed match to sample.

These results show that hippocampal neurons in the primate have responses related to certain types of memory. One type of memory involves complex conjunctions of environmental information, for example when information about position in space (perhaps reflecting information from the parietal cortex) must be memorized in conjunction with what that objects is (perhaps reflecting information from the temporal lobe visual areas), so that where a particular object was seen in space can be remembered. The hippocampus is ideally placed anatomically for detecting such conjunctions in that it receives highly processed information from association areas such as the parietal cortex (conveying information about position in space), the inferior temporal visual cortex (conveying a visual specification of an object), and the superior temporal cortex (conveying an auditory specification of a stimulus) (90). The positions of stimuli in space may be represented by the firing of hippocampal neurons as described above so that conjunctions of, for example, objects and their position can be formed. It may also be that conjunctions between sets of stimuli in different parts of space can be formed onto hippocampal neurons to provide a map of space (cf. O'Keefe (49)).

A second type of memory to which the activity of hippocampal neurons appears to be related is the learning of which spatial responses should be made to particular stimuli. It is important to note that these tasks involve symmetrical reinforcement (e.g., response A to stimulus 1 to obtain reward, and response B to stimulus 2 to obtain reward); if a task can be solved by stimulus-reinforcement associations it can then be learned without the hippocampus (22). The activity of hippocampal neurons often reflects a combination or conjunction of a particular stimulus and motor response in these tasks so that in this case also conjunction or combination learning appears to be an important aspect of hippocampal function. It is suggested that if the hippocampus is involved in determining which locomotor response must be made to which stimulus, then this provides a way of implementing a spatial map of the environment in which the readout might involve appropriate locomotor responses to conjunctions of stimuli in the environment. In this context it is of interest that the "place" cells in the rat hippocampus fire much more when a rat is actively moving in space that when it is passive in one position (O'Keefe, personal communication), that is when stimulus to bodily response conjunctions are being processed.

A possible theoretical basis for these results, and in particular how the hippocampus may perform the conjunction or combination learning just described, is now considered (cf. Marr (37)). The proposal is that the hippocampus is another modification of the basic design of a matrix memory as described below. A diagram to show some of the features of the connections of the hippocampus is shown in Fig. 11. It consists of a cascade of stages in each of which axons run orthogonally across dendrites, and the probability of contact of each axon with a dendrite is low – perhaps in the range 0.1-0.001. These synapses are modifiable. The modification rule is that when many inputs to a particular dendrite (or neuron) are active (which may produce postsynaptic effects important in the modification), those synapses increase in strength. As in the neocortex, with suitable inhibition from the neurons most active to a given stimulus, this tends to produce classification of clusters of information onto single neurons, when then tend to respond in the future only to such complex conjunctions or combinations of stimuli. An example of this is illustrated in Fig. 12. An additional feature of the hippocampus (particularly of the CA3 pyramidal cells) is the presence of strong recurrent collaterals which return from the output of the matrix to cross over the neurons of the matrix, as shown in Fig. 11. These synapses are also modifiable by the same learning rule. The effect of such recurrent collaterals is to make that part of the matrix into an autocorrelation matrix. The autocorrelation arises because the output of the matrix, expressed as the firing rate of the CA3 pyramidal cells, is fed back along the horizontally running axons so that the pattern of activity in this part of the matrix (the CA3 pyramidal cells) is autocorrelated with itself (see Kohonen *et al.* (34)). The importance of the autocorrelation performed by this part of the matrix is that it forms a recognition memory with all the advantageous properties of a matrix memory. The property which is particularly relevant here is completion in that if part of a stimulus (or event) occurs then the autocorrelation part of the matrix completes that event. It should be noted that the results of long-term potentiation experiments are consistent with the proposed operation of the hippocampus (39).

Taken together, these properties of each stage of hippocampal circuitry result in complex conjunctions or combinations of events being coded onto (i.e., resulting in the firing of) hippocampal neurons, with completion being possible with only a fraction of the original pattern. That is, recall of the whole of a complex event is achieved when only a part of it occurs later. One reason for the several cascades of hippocampal circuitry may be that early stages (such as the dentate granule cells) must be broken up into a number of separate parallel substages, each of which receives from only a part of the total afferent barrage received by the hippocampus. This may be necessary in order to keep the proportion of neurons firing at any one time in the matrix low,

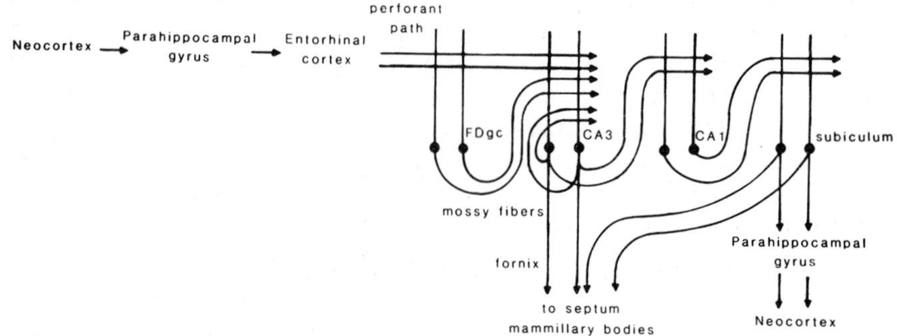

FIG. 11 – Schematic diagram of hippocampal connections. FDgc - dentate granule cells; CA3 and CA1 - pyramidal cells.

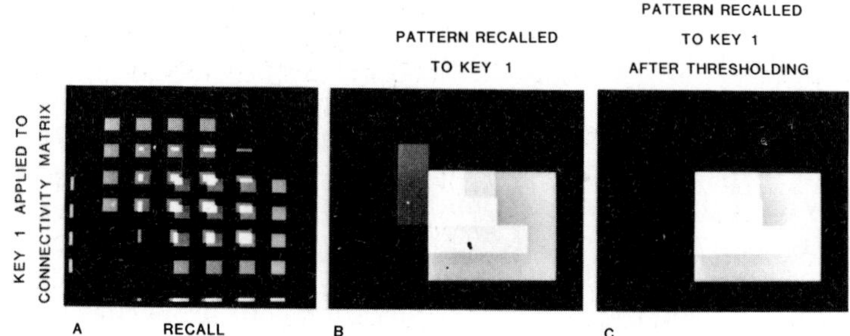

FIG. 12 – The recall of information from a recognition memory. The three stimuli shown in Fig. 2a were first stored in the matrix by applying each of the stimuli simultaneously to the vertical neurons and the horizontal axons to form an autocorrelation matrix. (Collaterals would perform this in a neuronal network.) Then, as shown in Fig. 12A, stimulus 1 was applied to the matrix. Stimulus 1 was recalled from the matrix, as shown before and after thresholding in B and C.

so as to keep interference down. After some classification has been performed by early stages, and the number of active neurons necessary to represent the input information has been reduced, all information may be brought together in the final stage of this hippocampal circuitry in the CA1 pyramids. This final bringing together of inputs received originally by the whole of the hippocampus, and thus representing highly processed neocortical information received from every sensory modality, may thus be a feature of what the hippocampus can achieve.

For example, it can detect, and classify onto a few specifically responding neurons, complex conjunctions of complex (cortically processed) events, such as that a particular object (presumably reflecting temporal lobe visual processing) has appeared in a particular position in space (probably reflecting parietal input). Another example might be that a particular stimulus should be associated with a particular body response. One should remember that this is the type of specific information which comes to activate different hippocampal neurons, as described above.

It should be noted that this computation involves recoding of the original input event into an information rich pattern of firing of a few hippocampal neurons. The exact ways in which this information is used by the rest of the brain are not quite understood. The recoding may take place over several trials, as shown by the neurophysiological experiments described above. The information represented may thus indicate what information should be stored in the neocortex. A path back from the hippocampal formation (through the subiculum and parahippocampal gyrus) to the neocortex (90) might perform this function. The evidence that the hippocampus may be involved in the storage process, but is not itself the location where the information is stored, is that hippocampal damage may impair the learning but not necessarily the retention of memory tasks of the type described above. Another important output of the hippocampus is via the fornix to the anterior thalamic nuclei and thus via the cingulate cortex to the supplementary motor area.

SHORT-TERM MEMORIES

The simplest way to build a short-term memory is to use an ordinary matrix memory (of the autocorrelation type if recognition is required), but to make it a property of the synapses that their strength decays with the required time constant. One example of such a memory is provided by some neurons in the inferior temporal visual cortex. This population has the property that after a stimulus is shown, that stimulus produces a smaller response (or for other neurons a larger response) the next time it is shown (41). To test whether these neurons could take part in a longer term form of recency memory, Baylis and Rolls (3) measured their responses when monkeys had to remember lists of visual stimuli with up to 17 stimuli intervening between the first and second presentations of a given stimulus. It was found that the majority of the neurons would remember the stimulus only providing that there were no intervening stimuli, with just a few neurons remembering over 1 or 2 intervening stimuli. Thus these neuron in the inferior temporal visual cortex do provide a short-term sensory memory but this particular memory has little resistance to disruption by intervening stimuli.

In a region which receives inputs from the inferior temporal visual cortex, the tail of the caudate nucleus, visual responses are found to the types of visual stimuli effective in exciting inferior temporal cortex neurons, but the majority of neurons in the tail of the caudate nucleus show rapid pattern-specific habituation which can be dishabituated by presentation of another visual stimulus. This thus provides a short-term visual memory system suitable for detecting changes in patterned visual stimuli (12).

In longer term recency memory, for whether a stimulus has been seen in the preceding 10-100 trials, a system with inputs to neurons at the rostral border of the thalamus is implicated (73). The inputs which drive these neurons may come from the amygdala and the hippocampus, in both of which there is a small proportion of neurons with responses which occur differently to novel and familiar stimuli in a serial recognition task (Wilson and Rolls, unpublished observations; (72)).

There is another way in which some parts of the brain provide a short-term memory suitable for bridging a delay with no intervening stimuli. This is by holding a particular pattern of firing in the delay period. For example, neurons in the dorsolateral prefrontal cortex fire in a 2-5 s delay in which a monkey must remember a position to which he must respond (i.e., in a delayed response task) (19, 48). Some of these neurons code in the delay for the position in which the stimulus has been seen and others for the response which the monkey has to make at the end of the interval (48). In the hippocampus, neurons with responses in the delay period of a delayed response task have also been found (91). It has been shown that some of these neurons reflect holding information in memory about the response required in that the same neurons do not fire when the monkey has to remember the same stimulus in a delayed matching-to-sample task (72).

NEURONAL ACTIVITY IN THE BASAL NUCLEUS OF MEYNERT DURING MOTIVATIONAL BEHAVIOR AND LEARNING

It is known that the neural changes in Alzheimer's disease include degeneration of neurons in the basal nucleus of Meynert (15, 38). In order to investigate the functions of these neurons their activity has been analyzed during a recognition memory task (in which the monkey must remember which stimuli he has seen in the previous 17 presentations) as well as in a visual discrimination task which requires association memory. It is shown in Table 1 that some neurons in these memory tasks responded only to novel stimuli and were thus influenced by recognition memory, and that others were activated by rewarding visual stimuli in the visual discrimination task. Another large proportion of these neurons responded to the tone cue signal which preceded each trial in these tasks to enable the monkey to pay attention to the video screen (94).

TABLE 1 – Neuronal populations in the basal forebrain during memory tasks.

	No. of cells	%
Responses to novel visual stimuli (recognition memory)	39	2.0
Responses to rewarding visual stimuli (association memory)	104	5.2
Nondiscriminating visual responses	623	31.1
Responses during tone signal	257	12.8
Responses during licking or reaching	37	1.8
Unresponsive neurons	944	47.1
Total number of neurons recorded	2004	100

These results show that the basal nucleus projects to the neocortex signals which depend on whether a new visual stimulus is shown, whether a rewarding visual stimulus is shown, or whether a stimulus which informs the monkey that he should pay attention has occurred. These signals are tightly time-locked to the onset of these stimuli with latencies for the visual responses of 140-180 ms. It is suggested that a function of this signal, and of these neurons, is to enhance activation or consolidation in the neocortex at an appropriate time (that is when new, rewarding, or significant environmental stimuli occur) and that failure of this function could contribute to some of the symptoms of Alzheimer's disease.

Acknowledgements. The author has worked on some of the experiments described here with G.C. Baylis, M.J. Burton, P. Cahusac, M. Hasselmo, L. Hughes, C.M. Leonard, F. Mora, D.I. Perrett, M.K. Sanghera, T.R. Scott, S.J. Thorpe, F.A.W. Wilson, and S. Yaxley. Their collaboration is sincerely acknowledged. This research was supported by the Medical Research Council and the Wellcome Trust.

REFERENCES

(1) Applegate, C.D.; Frysinger, R.C.; Kapp, B.S.; and Gallagher, M. 1982. Multiple unit activity recorded from amygdala central nucleus during heart rate conditioning. *Brain Res.* 238: 457-462.

(2) Barlow, H.B. 1972. Single units and sensation: a neuron doctrine for perceptual psychology? *Perception* 1: 371-394.

(3) Baylis, G.C., and Rolls, E.T. 1983. Responses of neurons in the inferior temporal visual cortex in long and short term memory tasks. *Exp. Brain Res.*, in press..

(4) Baylis, G.C.; Rolls, E.T.; and Leonard, C.M. 1985. Selectivity between faces in the responses of a population of neurons in the cortex in the superior temporal sulcus of the monkey. *Brain Res.* 342: 91-102.

(5) Baylis, G.C.; Rolls, E.T.; and Hasselmo, M. 1986. Responses of neurons in the cortex in the superior temporal sulcus of the monkey to spatial frequency band-limited face stimuli. *Vision Res.*, in press.

(6) Baylis, G.C.; Rolls, E.T.; and Leonard, C.M. 1986. Functional subdivisions of temporal lobe neocortex. *J. Neurosci.*, in press.

(7) Beckstead, R.M.; Morse, J.R.; and Norgen, R. 1980. The nucleus of the solitary tract in the monkey: projections to the thalamus and brainstem nuclei. *J. Comp. Neur.* 190: 259-282.

(8) Beckstead, R.M., and Norgren, R. 1979. An autoradiographic examination of the central distribution of the trigeminal, facial, glossopharyngeal, and vagal nerves in the monkey. *J. Comp. Neur.* 184: 455-472.

(9) Ben-Ari, Y., ed. 1981. The Amygdaloid Complex. Amsterdam: Elsevier.

(10) Berger, T.W. 1984. Neural representation of associative learning in the hippocampus. In *The Neuropsychology of Memory*, eds. L.W. Squire and N. Butters, pp. 443-461. New York: Guilford Press.

(11) Butter, C.M. 1969. Perseveration in extinction and in discrimination reversal tasks following selective prefrontal ablations in *Macaca mulatta*. *Physl. Behav.* 4: 163-171.

(12) Caan, W.; Perrett, D.I.; and Rolls, E.T. 1984. Responses of striatal neurons in the behaving monkey. 2. Visual processing in the caudal neostriatum. *Brain Res.* 290: 53-65.

(13) Cooper, L.N.; Liberman, F.; and Oja, F. 1979. A theory for the acquisition and loss of neuron specificity in visual cortex. *Biol. Cybern.* 33: 9-28.

(14) Cowey, A. 1979. Cortical maps and visual perception. *Q. J. Exp. Psych.* 31: 1-17.

(15) Davies, P. 1979 Neurotransmitter-related enzymes in senile dementia of the Alzheimer type. *Brain Res.* 171: 319-327.

(16) Desimone, R., and Gross, C.G. 1979. Visual areas in the temporal lobe of the macaque. *Brain Res.* 178: 363-380.

(17) Erickson, R.P. 1963. Stimulus encoding in topographic and nontopographic modalities: on the significance of the activity of individual sensory neurons. *Psychol. Rev.* 75: 447-465.

(18) Erickson, R.P. 1982. The across-fiber pattern theory: an organizing principle for molar neural function. *Contr. Sen. Physiol.* 6: 79-110.

(19) Fuster, J. 1980. The Prefrontal Cortex. New York: Raven Press.

(20) Gaffan, D. 1974. Recognition impaired and association intact in the memory of monkeys after transection of the fornix. *J. Comp. Phys. Psych.* 86: 1100-1109.

(21) Gaffan, D. 1977. Monkey's recognition memory for complex pictures and the effects of fornix transection. *Q. J. Exp. Psych.* 29: 505-514.

(22) Gaffan, D. 1985. Hippocampus: memory, habit and voluntary movement. *Phil. T. Roy. Soc. B* 308: 87-99.

(23) Gaffan, D., and Saunders, R.C. 1985. Running recognition of configural stimuli by fornix transected monkeys. *Q. J. Exp. Psych.* 37B: 61-71.

(24) Herzog, A.G., and Van Hoesen, G.W. 1976. Temporal neocortical afferent connections to amygdala in the rhesus monkey. *Brain Res.* 115: 57-69.

(25) Hinton, G.E., and Anderson, J.A. 1981. Parallel Models of Associative Memory. New Jersey: Erlbaum.

(26) Ito, M. 1984. The Cerebellum and Neural Control. New York: Raven Press.

(27) Iversen, S.D., and Mishkin, M. 1970. Perseverative interference in monkey following selective lesions of the inferior prefrontal convexity. *Exp. Brain Res.* 11: 376-386.

(28) Jones, B., and Mishkin, M. 1972. Limbic lesions and the problem of stimulus-reinforcement associations. *Exp. Neurol.* 36: 362-377.

(29) Jones, E.G., and Powell, T.P.S. 1970. An anatomical study of converging sensory pathways within the cerebral cortex of the monkey. *Brain* 93: 793-820.

(30) Kapp, B.S.; Pascoe, J.P.; and Bixler, M.A. 1984. The amgydala: a neuroanatomical systems approach to its contribution to aversive conditioning. In *The Neuropsychology of Memory*, eds. L.W. Squire and N. Butters, pp. 473-488. New York: Guilford Press.

(31) Kluver, H., and Bucy, P.C. 1939. Preliminary analysis of functions of the temporal lobes in monkeys. *Arch. Neurol. Psychiatr.* 42: 979-1000.

(32) Kohonen, T. 1984. Self-Organization and Associative Memory. Berlin: Springer-Verlag.

(33) Kohonen, T.; Lehtio, P.; Rovamo, J.; Hyvarinen, J.; Bry, K.; and Vainio, L. 1977. A principle of neural associative memory. *Neuroscience* 2: 1065-1076.

(34) Kohonen, T.; Oja, E.; and Lehtio, P. 1981. Storage and processing of information in distributed associative memory systems. In *Parallel Models of Associative Memory*, eds. G.E. Hinton and J.A. Anderson, pp. 105-143. New Jersey: Erlbaum.

(35) Leonard, C.M.; Rolls, E.T.; Wilson, F.A.W.; and Baylis, G.C. 1985. Neurons in the amygdala of the monkey with responses selective for faces. *Beh. Brain Res.* 15: 159-176.

(36) Marr, D. 1970. A theory for cerebral cortex. *P. Roy. Soc. B* 176: 161-234.

(37) Marr, D. 1971. Simple memory: a theory for archicortex. *Phil. T. Roy. Soc. B* 262: 23-81.

(38) McGeer, E.G., and McGeer, P.L. 1981. Cholinergic mechanisms in central disorders. In *Neuropharmacology of Central Nervous System and Behavioral Disorders*, ed. G.C. Palmer, pp. 479-505. New York: Academic Press.

(39) McNaughton, B.L. 1984. Activity dependent modulation of hippocampal synaptic efficacy: some implications for memory processes. In *Neurobiology of the Hippocampus*, ed. W. Seifert, pp. 231-252. London: Academic Press.

(40) Mesulam, M.-M., and Mufson, E.J. 1982. Insula of the old world monkey. III: Efferent cortical output and comments on function. *J. Comp. Neurol.* 212: 38-52.

(41) Mikami, A., and Kubota, K. 1980. Inferotemporal neuron activities and color discrimination with delay. *Brain Res.* 182: 65-78.

(42) Milner, B. 1972. Disorders of learning and memory after temporal lobe lesions in man. *Clin. Neurosur.* 19: 421-446.

(43) Mishkin, M. 1978. Memory severely impaired by combined but not separate removal of amygdala and hippocampus. *Nature* 273: 297-298.

(44) Mishkin, M. 1982. A memory system in the monkey. *Phil. T. Roy. Soc. B* 298: 85-95.

(45) Mora, F.; Rolls, E.T.; and Burton, M.J. 1976. Modulation during learning of the responses of neurons in the lateral hypothalamus to the sight of food. *Exp. Neurol.* 53: 508-519.

(46) Murray, E.A., and Mishkin, M. 1984. Severe tactual as well as visual memory deficits follow combined removal of the amgydala and hippocampus in monkeys. *J. Neurosci.* 4: 2565-2580.

(47) Murray, E.A., and Mishkin, M. 1985. Amygdalectomy impairs crossmodal association in monkeys. *Science* 228: 604-606.

(48) Niki, H., and Watanabe, M. 1976. Prefrontal unit activity and delayed response: relation to cue location versus direction of response. *Brain Res.* 105: 79-88.

(49) O'Keefe, J. 1984. Spatial memory within and without the hippocampal system. In *Neurobiology of the Hippocampus*, ed. W. Seifert, pp. 375-403. London: Academic Press.

(50) Olton, D.S. 1984. Memory functions and the hippocampus. In *Neurobiology of the Hippocampus*, ed. W. Seifert, pp. 335-373. London: Academic Press.

(51) Palm, G. 1982. Neural Assemblies. Berlin: Springer-Verlag.

(52) Perrett, D.I.; Rolls, E.T.; and Caan, W. 1982. Visual neurons responsive to faces in the monkey temporal cortex. *Exp. Brain Res.* 47: 329-342.

(53) Rolls, E.T. 1981. Processing beyond the inferior temporal visual cortex related to feeding, learning, and striatal function. In *Brain Mechanisms of Sensation*, eds. Y. Katsuki, R. Norgren, and M. Sato, pp. 241-269. New York: Wiley.

(54) Rolls, E.T. 1981. Responses of amygdaloid neurons in the primate. In *The Amygdaloid Complex*, ed. Y. Ben-Ari, pp. 383-393. Amsterdam: Elsevier.

(55) Rolls, E.T. 1982. Feeding and reward. In *The Neural Basis of Feeding and Reward*, eds. D. Novin and G.B. Hoebel. Brunswick, Maine: Haer Institute for Electrophysiological Research.

(56) Rolls, E.T. 1982. Neuronal mechanisms underlying the formation and disconnection of associations between visual stimuli and reinforcement in primates. In *Conditioning*, ed. C.D. Woody. New York: Plenum Press.

(57) Rolls, E.T. 1984. Activity of neurons in different regions of the striatum of the monkey. In *The Basal Ganglia: Structure and Function*, eds. J.S. McKenzie, R.E. Kemm, and L.N. Wilcox, pp. 467-493. New York: Plenum.

(58) Rolls, E.T. 1984. Neurons in the cortex of the temporal lobe and in the amygdala of the monkey with responses selective for faces. *Human Neurobiol.* 3: 209-222.

(59) Rolls, E.T. 1984. The neurophysiology of feeding. *Int. J. Obes., Supp.* 1 8: 139-150.

(60) Rolls, E.T. 1985. A theory of emotion, and its application to understanding the neural basis of emotion. In *Neuronal and Endogenous Chemical Control Mechanisms in Emotional Behavior*, ed. Y. Oomura. Berlin: Japan Scientific Societies Press and Springer-Verlag.

(61) Rolls, E.T. 1985. Connections, functions and dysfunctions of limbic structures, the prefrontal cortex, and hypothalamus. In *The Scientific Basis of Clinical Neurology*, eds. M. Swash and C. Kennard, pp. 201-213. London: Churchill Livingstone.

(62) Rolls, E.T. 1985. Neural systems involved in emotion in primates. In *Biological Foundations of Emotion*, eds. R. Plutchik and H. Kellerman, pp. 125-143. New York: Academic Press.

(63) Rolls, E.T. 1986. Neuronal activity related to the control of feeding. In *Neural and Humoral Controls of Food Intake*, eds. R. Ritter and S. Ritter. New York: Academic Press.

(64) Rolls, E.T. 1986. Investigations of the functions of different regions of the basal ganglia. In *Parkinson's Disease*, ed. G. Stern. London: Chapman and Hall.

(65) Rolls, E.T. 1986. Sensory to motor information processing in the primate brain. In *Textbook of Clinical Neurophysiology*, eds. A.M. Halliday, R. Paul, and S.R. Butler. London: Wiley.

(66) Rolls, E.T. 1986. The Brain and Memory, in press.

(67) Rolls, E.T., and Baylis, G.C. 1986. Size and contrast have only small effects on the responses to faces of neurons in the cortex in the superior temporal sulcus of the monkey. *Exp. Brain Res.*, in press.

(68) Rolls, E.T.; Baylis, G.C.; and Leonard, C.M. 1985. Role of low and high spatial frequencies in the face-selective responses of neurons

in the cortex in the superior temporal sulcus. *Vision Res.* 25: 1021-1035.

(69) Rolls, E.T.; Burton, M.J.; and Mora, F. 1976. Hypothalamic neuronal responses associated with the sight of food. *Brain Res.* 111: 53-66.

(70) Rolls, E.T.; Burton, M.J.; and Mora, F. 1980. Neurophysiological analysis of brain-stimulation reward in the monkey. *Brain Res.* 194: 339-357.

(71) Rolls, E.T.; Judge, S.J.; and Sanghera, M. 1977. Activity of neurons in the inferotemporal cortex of the alert monkey. *Brain Res.* 130: 229-238.

(72) Rolls, E.T.; Miyashita, Y.; Cahusac, P.; and Kesner, R.P. 1985. The responses of single neurons in the primate hippocampus related to the performance of memory tasks. *Soc. Neurosci. Abstr.* 11: 525.

(73) Rolls, E.T.; Perrett, D.I.; Caan, A.W.; and Wilson, F.A.W. 1982. Neuronal responses related to visual recognition. *Brain* 105: 611-646.

(74) Rolls, E.T.; Sanghera, M.K.; and Roper Hall, A. 1979. The latency of activation of neurons in the lateral hypothalamus and substantia innominata during feeding in the monkey. *Brain Res.* 164: 121-135.

(75) Rolls, E.T.; Sienkiewicz, Z.J.; and Yaxley, S. 1986. Hunger modulates the responses to gustatory stimuli of single neurons in the orbitofrontal cortex, submitted.

(76) Rolls, E.T.; Thorpe, S.J.; and Maddison, S.P. 1983. Responses of striatal neurons in the behaving monkey. 1. Head of the caudate nucleus. *Beh. Brain Res.* 7: 179-210.

(77) Rolls, E.T.; Yaxley, S.; and Sienkiewicz, Z.J. 1986. Gustatory responses of single neurons in the orbitofrontal cortex of the macaque monkey, submitted.

(78) Rosenkilde, C.E. 1979. Functional heterogeneity of the prefrontal cortex in the monkey: a review. *Behav. Neur. Biol.* 25: 301-345.

(79) Sanghera, M.K.; Rolls, E.T.; and Roper-Hall, A. 1979. Visual responses of neurons in the dorsolateral amygdala of the alert monkey. *Exp. Neurol.* 63: 610-626.

(80) Scott, T.R.; Yaxley, S.; Sienkiewicz, Z.J.; and Rolls, E.T. 1986. Taste responses in the nucleus tractus solitarius of the behaving monkey. *J. Neurophysl.*, in press.

(81) Scott, R.T.; Yaxley, S.; Sienkiewicz, Z.J.; and Rolls, E.T. 1986. Taste responses in the gustatory cortex of the behaving monkey. *J. Neurophysl.*, in press.

(82) Scoville, W.B., and Milner, B. 1957. Loss of recent memory after bilateral hippocampal lesions. *J. Neurol. Neurosurg. Psychiat.* 20: 11-21.

(83) Seltzer, B., and Pandya, D.N. 1978. Afferent cortical connections and architectonics of the superior temporal sulcus and surrounding cortex in the rhesus monkey. *Brain Res.* 149: 1-24.

(84) Smith, D.V., and Travers, J.B. 1979. A metric for the breadth of tuning of gustatory neurons. *Chem. Senses and Flavour* 4: 215-229.

(85) Spiegler, B.J., and Mishkin, M. 1981. Evidence for the sequential participation of inferior temporal visual cortex and amygdala in the formation of stimulus-reward associations. *Beh. Brain Res.* 3: 303-417.

(86) Thompson, R.F.; Clark, G.A.; Donegan, N.H.; Lavond, D.G.; Madden, J.; Mamounas, L.A.; Mauk, M.D.; and McCormick, D.A. 1984. Neuronal substrates of basic associative learning. In *The Neuropsychology of Memory*, eds. L.W. Squire and N. Butters, pp. 424-442. New York: Guilford Press.

(87) Thorpe, S.J.; Rolls, E.T.; and Maddison, S. 1983. Neuronal activity in the orbitofrontal cortex of the behaving monkey. *Exp. Brain Res.* 49: 93-115.

(88) Turner, B.H.; Mishkin, M.; and Knapp, M. 1980. Organization of the amygdalopetal modality-specific cortical association areas in the monkey. *J. Comp. Neurol.* 191: 515-543.

(89) Van Hoesen, G.W. 1981. The differential distribution, diversity and sprouting of cortical projections to the amygdala in the rhesus monkey. In *The Amygdaloid Complex*, ed. Y. Ben-Ari, pp. 79-90. Amsterdam: Elsevier.

(90) Van Hoesen, G.W. 1982. The parahippocampal gyrus. New observations regarding its cortical connections in the monkey. *Trends Neur.* 5: 345-350.

(91) Watanabe, T., and Niki, H. 1985. Hippocampal unit activity and delayed response in the monkey. *Brain Res.* 325: 241-254.

(92) Weinberger, N. 1984. The neurophysiology of memory. A view from the sensory side. In *The Neuropsychology of Memory*, eds. L.W. Squire and N. Butters, pp. 489-503. New York: Guilford Press.

(93) Wiggins, L.L.; Baylis, G.C.; Rolls, E.T.; and Yaxley, S. 1986. Afferent connections of the orbitofrontal cortex taste area of the primate, submitted.

(94) Wilson, F.A.W.; Rolls, E.T.; Yaxley, S.; Thorpe, S.J.; Williams, G.V.; and Simpson, S.J. 1984. Responses of neurons in the basal forebrain of the behaving monkey. *Soc. Neurosci. Abstr.* 10: 128

(95) Yaxley, S.; Rolls, E.T.; and Sienkiewicz, Z.J. 1986. Gustatory responses of single neurons in the insula of the macaque monkey, submitted.

(96) Yaxley, S.; Rolls, E.T.; and Sienkiewicz, Z.J. 1986. Hunger does not modulate the responses of neurons in the insular taste cortex of the macaque monkey, submitted.

(97) Yaxley, S.; Scott, T.R.; Rolls, E.T.; and Sienkiewicz, Z.J. 1985. Satiety does not affect gustatory activity in the nucleus of the solitary tract of the alert monkey. *Brain Res.* 347: 85-93.

List of Participants with Fields of Research

ALKON, D.L.
Section on Neural Systems
Laboratory of Biophysics, NINCDS
Marine Biological Laboratory
Woods Hole, MA 02543
USA

Biophysics and biochemistry of learning

AMARI, S.-I.
Faculty of Engineering
University of Tokyo
Hongo 7-3-1, Bunkyo-ku
Tokyo 113
Japan

Mathematical theory on self-organization of neural systems

ANDERSEN, P.
Institute of Neurophysiology
Karl Johans Gate 47
0162 Oslo 1
Norway

Mechanisms of neuronal integration, in cortical cells particularly, mechanisms of synaptic plasticity (long-term potentiation)

BAUDRY, M.
Center for the Neurobiology of Learning and Memory
University of California
Irvine, CA 92717
USA

Biochemistry of learning and memory

BEAR, M.F.
Center for Neural Science
Box G
Brown University
Providence, RI 02912
USA

Experience-dependent synaptic modification in the visual cortex

BICKER, G.
Institut für Tierphysiologie-Neurobiologie der
Freien Universität Berlin
Königin-Luise-Strasse 28-30
1000 Berlin (West) 33

Neurobiology of invertebrate behavior

BIENENSTOCK, E.
Laboratoire de Neurobiologie du Développement, bâtiment 440
Université de Paris-Sud
91405 Orsay Cédex
France

Mathematical modeling of dynamical processes in neuronal networks; special emphasis on learning and perception

BLISS, T.V.P.
National Institute for Medical Research
Mill Hill
London NW7 1AA
England

Mechanisms of synaptic plasticity in the hippocampus, particularly long-term potentiation

BYRNE, J.H.
Dept. of Physiology and Cell Biology
University of Texas Medical School
P.O. Box 20708
Houston, TX 77225
USA

Neural and molecular mechanisms underlying information storage

CAREW, T.J.
Dept. of Psychology
Yale University
P.O. Box 11A Yale Station
New Haven, CT 06520
USA

Cellular mechanisms of learning and memory

CHANGEUX, J.-P.
Neurobiologie Moléculaire
Institut Pasteur
28, rue du Dr. Roux
75724 Paris Cédex 15
France

Acetylcholine receptor

COTMAN, C.W.
Dept. of Psychobiology
University of California
Irvine, CA 92717
USA

Synapse turnover in the central nervous system

DEHAENE, S.
Ecole normale supérieure,
Chambre 331
45, rue d'Ulm
75005 Paris
France

Learning by selection in neural networks: dynamic aspects

DUDAI, Y.
Dept. of Neurobiology
Weizmann Institute of Science
Rehovot 76100
Israel

Molecular mechanisms of learning and memory

EBENDAL, T.L.
Dept. of Zoology
Uppsala University
Box 561
751 22 Uppsala
Sweden

Regulation of nerve growth factor (NGF) expression in the brain and PNS (development, denervation)

FUSTER, J.M.
Dept. of Psychiatry
UCLA Neuropsychiatric Institute
760 Westwood Plaza
Los Angeles, CA 90024
USA

Behavioral neurophysiology: neuronal representation of behaviorally relevant stimuli in association cortex and limbic structures

GERSCHENFELD, H.M.
Laboratoire de Neurobiologie
École normale supérieure
46, rue d'Ulm
75230 Paris Cédex 05
France

Neurobiology (mechanisms of neuronal modulation by synaptic transmitters)

GODDARD, G.V.
Dept. of Psychology
University of Otago
P.O. Box 56
Dunedin
New Zealand

Modulation of long-term potentiation in fascia dentata by inputs from other areas of the brain

HEISENBERG, M.
Institut für Genetik und Mikrobiologie der Universität Würzburg
Röntgenring 11
8700 Würzburg
F.R. Germany

Neurogenetics (Drosophila)

HENDERSON, C.E.
Neurobiologie Moléculaire
Institut Pasteur
25, rue du Dr. Roux
75724 Paris Cédex 15
France

Growth factors for spinal motoneurons

HUTTNER, W.B.
European Molecular Biology Laboratory
Postfach 10.2209
6900 Heidelberg
F.R. Germany

Posttranslational modifications of proteins in neuronal and nonneuronal cells

INNOCENTI, G.M.
Institut d'Anatomie
9, rue du Bugnon
1011 Lausanne
Switzerland

Development and plasticity of corticocortical connections

ITO, M.
Dept. of Physiology
Faculty of Medicine
University of Tokyo
7-3-1 Hongo, Bunkyo-ku
Tokyo 113
Japan

Neurophysiology, synaptic plasticity, vestibular function, cerebellum

KANDEL, E.R.
Center for Neurobiology and Behavior
Howard Hughes Medical Institute
College of Physicians and Surgeons
Columbia University
722 West 168th St.
New York, NY 10032
USA

Neurobiology of behavior

KENNEDY, M.B.
Division of Biology 216-76
California Institute of Technology
Pasadena, CA 91125
USA

Synaptic Ca^{2+}/calmodulin-dependent protein kinase

KONISHI, M.
Division of Biology 216-76
California Institute of Technology
Pasadena, CA 91125
USA

Neuroethology

LØMO, T.
Institute of Neurophysiology
Karl Johans Gate 47
Oslo 1
Norway

Neuromuscular system

MALLET, J.B.
Centre National de la Recherche Scientifique
Laboratoire de Neurobiologie Céllulaire et Moléculaire
1, avenue de la Terrasse
91190 Gif-sur-Yvette
France

Molecular genetics; neurotransmission

MENZEL, R.
Institut für Tierphysiologie-Neurobiologie der Freien Universität Berlin
Königin-Luise-Strasse 28-30
1000 Berlin (West) 33

Neurobiology of invertebrates, neural basis of learning and memory

MERZENICH, M.M.
Coleman Laboratory, 871 HSE
University of California Medical School
3rd and Parnassus Avenues
San Francisco, CA 94143
USA

CNS, neurophysiology

MEYER, R.L.
Developmental Biology Center
University of California
Irvine, CA 92717
USA

Formation of selective axonal connections: effect of activity

MISHKIN, M.
Laboratory of Neuropsychology
Bldg. 9, Rm. 1N107, NIH
Bethesda, MD 20205
USA

Neurobiology of cognitive functions in primates

MÜLLER, C.M.
Institut für Zoologie
Technische Hochschule Darmstadt
Schnittspahnstr. 3
6100 Darmstadt
F.R. Germany

Mechanisms of the reticular control of sensory systems; physiology and pharmacology of auditory information processing

MULLE, C.
Laboratoire de Neurobiologie Moléculaire
Institut Pasteur
28, rue du Dr. Roux
75724 Paris Cédex 15
France

Cellular and molecular basis of long-term potentiation in the neocortex

NICOLL, R.
Dept. of Pharmacology
University of California
San Francisco, CA 94143
USA

Neurotransmitter action in the CNS, with particular emphasis on slow modulatory actions in the hippocampus

RAKIC, P.
Section of Neuroanatomy
Yale University School of Medicine
333 Cedar Street
New Haven, CT 06510
USA

Developmental neurobiology; organization of primate brain

ROLLS, E.T.
Dept. of Experimental Psychology
University of Oxford
South Parks Road
Oxford OX1 3UD
England

Neurophysiology of information processing and memory in primates; computational models of memory

SCHMIDT, R.
AK Neurochemie
Zoologisches Institut
Universität Frankfurt
Siesmayerstr. 70
6000 Frankfurt
F.R. Germany

Biochemistry of memory and learning

SCHWEGLER, H.H.
Institut für Anthropologie und Humangenetik
Universität Heidelberg
Im Neuenheimer Feld 328
6900 Heidelberg
F.R. Germany

Genetic variability of the brain morphology accounting for behavioral differences

SEIFERT, W.
Max-Planck-Institut für Biophysikalische Chemie
Abt. Neurobiologie
Postfach 2841
3400 Göttingen
F.R. Germany

Neurobiology of the hippocampus, role of gangliosides in neuronal plasticity

SINGER, W.
Max-Planck-Institut für Hirnforschung
Deutschordenstr. 46
6000 Frankfurt 71
F.R. Germany

Development and plasticity of the cerebral cortex

SOTELO, C.
INSERM U-106
42, rue Desbassayns de Richemont
92150 Suresnes
France

Development of the cerebellum; synaptic plasticity; cerebellar transplantations

STENT, G.S.
Dept. of Molecular Biology
University of California
Berkeley, CA 94720
USA

Developmental neurobiology

STÜRMER, C.A.O.
Max-Planck-Institut für Entwicklungsbiologie
Abt. Physikalische Biologie
Spemannstr. 35
7400 Tübingen 1
F.R. Germany

Developmental neurobiology; growth and regeneration; fiber organizations and specificity of termination; retinotectal system; lower vertebrates

THOENEN, H.
Max-Planck-Institut für Psychiatrie
Abt. Neurochemie
8033 Planegg-Martinsried
F.R. Germany

Molecular neurobiology with focus on development

THOMPSON, R.F.
Dept. of Psychology
Stanford University
Jordan Hall, Bldg. 420
Stanford, CA 94305
USA

Neural mechanisms of learning and memory in the mammalian brain

THOMPSON, W.J.
Dept. of Zoology
University of Texas
Austin, TX 78712
USA

Development of neuromuscular junctions

VON DER MALSBURG, C.
Max-Planck-Institut für Biophysikalische Chemie
Postfach 2841
3400 Göttingen
F.R. Germany

Theoretical neurobiology

WILLMUND, R.
Institut für Biologie III
Universität Freiburg
Schänzlestr. 1
7800 Freiburg
F.R. Germany

Molecular mechanisms of behavioral plasticity in Drosophila

YANIV, M.
Dépt. de Biologie Moléculaire
Institut Pasteur
25, rue du Dr. Roux
75724 Paris Cédex 15
France

Molecular biology

Subject Index

Author Index

Dahlem Workshop Reports

Life Sciences Research Reports (LS)

LS 35 Biotechnology: Potentials and Limitations
Editor: S. Silver (1986)

LS 34 The Molecular Mechanism of Photoreception
Editor: H. Stieve (1986)

LS 33 The Importance of Chemical Speciation in Environmental Processes
Editors: M. Bernhard, F. E. Brinckman, P. J. Sadler (1986, in press)

LS 32 Exploitation of Marine Communities
Editor: R. M. May (1984)

LS 31 Microbial Adhesion and Aggregation
Editor: K. C. Marshall (1984)

LS 30 Leukemia
Editor: I. L. Weissman (1985)

LS 29 The Biology of Learning
Editors: P. Marler, H. S. Terrace (1984)

LS 28 Changing Metal Cycles and Human Health
Editor: J. O. Nriagu (1984)

LS 27 Minorities: Community and Identity
Editor: C. Fried (1983)

LS 26 The Origins of Depression: Current Concepts and Approaches
Editor: J. Angst (1983)

LS 25 Population Biology of Infectious Diseases
Editors: R. M. Anderson, R. M. May (1982)

LS 24 Repair and Regeneration of the Nervous System
Editor: J. G. Nicholls (1982)

LS 23 Biological Mineralization and Demineralization
Editor: G. H. Nancollas (1982)

LS 22 Evolution and Development
Editor: J. T. Bonner (1982)

LS 21 Animal Mind - Human Mind
Editor: D. R. Griffin (1982)

LS 20 Neuronal-glial Cell Interrelationships.
Editor: T. A. Sears (1982)

Physical, Chemical and Earth Sciences Research Reports (PC)

PC 5 Patterns of Change in Earth Evolution
Editors: H. D. Holland, A. F. Trendall (1984)

PC 4 Atmospheric Chemistry
Editor: E. D. Goldberg (1982)

PC 3 Mineral Deposits and the Evolution of the Biosphere
Editors: H. D. Holland, M. Schidlowski (1982)

Springer-Verlag
Berlin Heidelberg New York Tokyo

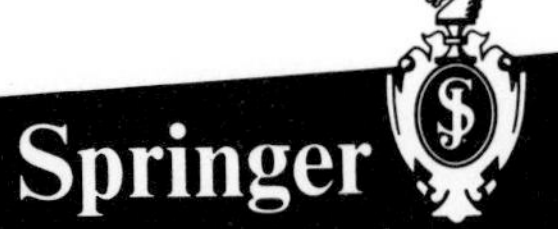